Primary Preventive Dentistry

SEVENTH EDITION

Norman O. Harris, DDS, MSD, FACD

Professor (Retired), Department of Community Dentistry
University of Texas Health Science Center at San Antonio

Franklin García-Godoy, DDS, MS, FICD

Professor and Associate Dean for Research, College of Dental Medicine
Nova Southeastern University

Christine Nielsen Nathe, RDH, MS

Professor and Graduate Program Director
University of New Mexico
Division of Dental Hygiene

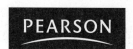
PEARSON

Upper Saddle River, New Jersey 07458

Library of Congress Cataloging-in-Publication Data

Primary preventive dentistry / [edited by] Norman O. Harris,
Franklin Garcia-Godoy, Christine Nielsen Nathe. — 7th ed.
    p. ; cm.
    Includes bibliographical references and index.
    ISBN-13: 978-0-13-241223-0
    ISBN-10: 0-13-241223-3
    1. Preventive dentistry.   2. Preventive dentistry—
Examinations, questions, etc.   I. Harris, Norman O.
II. García-Godoy, Franklin.   III. Nathe, Christine Nielsen.
    [DNLM: 1. Preventive Dentistry—methods.   2. Dental
Plaque—prevention & control.   3. Primary Prevention—
methods.   WU 113 P9522 2009]
    RK60.7.H37 2009
    617.6'01—dc22
                                        2008031941

Publisher: Julie Levin Alexander
Assistant to Publisher: Regina Bruno
Executive Editor: Mark Cohen
Development Editor: Melissa Kerian
Editorial Assistant: Nicole Ragonese
Managing Production Editor: Patrick Walsh
Production Liaison: Christina Zingone
Production Editor: Bruce Hobart, Pine Tree Composition
Manufacturing Manager: Ilene Sanford
Manufacturing Buyer: Pat Brown
Creative Design Director: Christy Mahon
Design Coordinator: Christopher Weigand
Cover Designer: Rob Aleman
Director of Marketing: Karen Allman

Executive Marketing Manager: Katrin Beacom
Marketing Assistant: Lauren Castellano
Marketing Specialist: Michael Sirinides
Director, Image Resource Center: Melinda Patelli
Manager, Rights and Permissions: Zina Arabia
Manager, Visual Research: Beth Brenzel
Manager, Cover Visual Research & Permissions:
    Karen Sanatar
Image Permission Coordinator: Vicki Menanteaux
Composition: Pine Tree Composition, Inc.
Printer/Binder: Edwards Brothers
Cover Printer: Phoenix Color Corporation
Cover Image: Stanley Flegler/Visuals Unlimited/
    Getty Images, Inc.

Pearson Education Ltd., *London*
Pearson Education Australia PTY. Limited
Pearson Education Singapore, Pte. Ltd.
Pearson Education North Asia Ltd., *Hong Kong*
Pearson Education Canada, Inc.

Pearson Educación de Mexico, S. A. de C. V.
Pearson Education—Japan
Pearson Education Malaysia, Pte. Ltd.
Pearson Education, Upper Saddle River, New Jersey

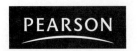

10 9 8 7 6 5 4
ISBN-13: 978-0-13-241223-0
ISBN-10:   0-13-241223-3

CONTENTS

Preface   xix
Contributors   xx
Reviewers   xxii

UNIT 1   **Primary Preventive Dental Concepts**

1   Introduction to Primary Preventive Dentistry   1
Christine N. Nathe

Objectives   1
Introduction   2
Historical Aspect of Preventive Dental Care   2
Dental Diseases and Systemic Health   5
Health Defined and Primary Preventive Care   6
Primary Prevention   7
Secondary and Tertiary Prevention   8
Preventive Care   8
Categories of Oral Diseases   9
Plaque Prevention   9
Summary   11

UNIT 2   **Etiology of Dental Diseases and Conditions**

2   Dental Plaque   13
Melissa McDougal-Plese

Objectives   13
Introduction   14
Dental Plaque: A Microbial Biofilm   14
Bacterial Colonization of the Mouth   15
The Acquired Pellicle   17
Dental Plaque Formation   17
Molecular Mechanisms of Bacterial Adhesion   18
Bacteria in the Dental Plaque   19
Dental Plaque Matrix   20

Dental Plaque Metabolism 20
Dental Calculus 22
   Attachment of Calculus to the Teeth 24
   Inhibition of Calculus Formation 24
Summary 25

3 Carious Lesions 29
Patricia Regener Campbell

Objectives 29
Introduction 30
Multifactorial Disease Process 30
Dental Caries Description 31
Physical and Microscopic Features of Incipient Caries 31
   Pore Spaces of the Different Zones 34
   Direct Connection of the Bacterial Biofilm to the Body
   of the Lesion 34
Cariogenic Bacteria 35
   Mutans Streptococci and Caries 36
   Lactobacilli and Caries 37
Adherence of Bacteria to Tooth 37
Ecology of Caries Development 37
   Caries Transmission 37
   Coronal Dentin Caries 38
   Root Caries 38
   Secondary, or Recurrent, Caries 39
   Measuring Plaque pH, the Stephan's Curve 40
   The Relationship of Saturation to pH 40
Demineralization and Remineralization Principles 41
   The Relationship between HAP, FHA, and CaF_2 41
   Depth of Remineralization 41
Summary 42

4 Periodontal Diseases 46
Kathleen O. Hodges

Objectives 46
Introduction 47
The Periodontium 49
The Gingival Sulcus 53
Periodontal Microflora 53
The Developing Gingival Lesion 54
The Deepening Pocket 56
Cellular Defense in the Periodontal Disease Process 57
Classifications of Periodontal Diseases 58

Risk Factors   60
Primary Prevention of Periodontal Diseases   62
Summary   63

5   Oral Cancer   67
Sandra J. Maurizio

Objectives   67
Introduction   68
Epidemiology of Oral Cancer   71
Risk Factors   72
  Tobacco   72
  Alcohol   72
  Age   73
  Race and Ethnicity   73
  Actinic Radiation (Ultraviolet Light) Exposure   73
  Potentially Malignant Oral Epithelial Lesions   74
Signs and Symptoms of Oral Cavity or Oropharyngeal
Cancer   76
Detection and Diagnosis of Oral Cancer   76
Health History   76
Oral Cancer Screening/Examination   78
  Biopsy Types   82
  Imaging   85
Prognosis of Oral Cancer: Staging System   86
Treatment Options for Oral Cancer   86
  Considerations Regarding Treatment Options   86
  Surgery   88
  Radiation Therapy   88
  Reconstruction   90
Management of Side Effects from Treatment of Oral
Cancer   91
Role of the Dental Team   93
  Education   93
  Public Health Screening for Oral and Pharyngeal Cancers   94
  Cultural Sensitivity   94
Summary   94

6   Dental Trauma   99
Gary Cuttrell

Objectives   99
Introduction   100
Etiology   101
Initial Examination   102

Soft Tissue Injuries   103
Categories of Traumatic Dental Injuries   103
Primary Teeth   104
  Intruded Primary Teeth   104
  Avulsed Primary Teeth   104
Permanent Teeth   104
  Avulsed Secondary Teeth   104
  Fractured Secondary Teeth   105
  Intruded Secondary Teeth   106
Public Education on Dental Truama   106
Research   106
  On Dental Truama
Summary   107

7   Host Defense Mechanisms in the Oral Cavity   109
     Beth E. McKinney

Objectives   109
Introduction   110
Anatomic Barriers: The Great Wall of Mesenchyme   110
Normal Oral Flora   113
The Immune System in the Oral Cavity   113
Saliva and Its Role in Promoting Oral Homeostasis   115
  Salivary Glands   115
  Organic Components of Saliva   118
Summary   119

UNIT 3   **Preventive Strategies**

8   Toothbrushes and Toothbrushing Methods   121
     Elaine Sanchez Dils

Objectives   121
Introduction   122
The History of the Toothbrush   123
Manual Toothbrush Designs   129
Toothbrush Profiles   129
Nylon versus Natural Bristles   129
Bristle Shape and Texture   129
Handle Designs   129
Manual Toothbrushing Methods   130
  Bass Method   131
  Rolling Method   132
  Stillman Method   132

Charters Method   132
Fones Method   132
Leonard Method   132
Horizontal Method   133
Smith Method   133
Scrub Toothbrushing Method   133
Modified Brushing Methods   133
Powered Toothbrushes   133
Design   133
Powered Toothbrush Methods and Uses   135
Toothbrush Efficiency and Safety Evaluations   138
Clinical Assessments of Toothbrushing   138
Toothbrush Replacement   139
Dentures and Removable Orthodontic Appliances   139
Tongue Brushing   139
The American Dental Association Acceptance Program   139
Summary   140

9   Dentifrices, Mouthrinses, and Chewing Gums   141
Meg Horst Zayan

Objectives   141
Introduction   142
Safety and Efficacy   143
Dentifrices   144
Packaging   145
Dentifrice Ingredients   145
Abrasives   146
Humectants   147
Soaps and Detergents   147
Flavoring and Sweetening Agents   148
Sweetening Agents   148
Baking-Soda Dentifrices   148
Methods of Controlling Plaque and Gingivitis   148
Therapeutic Dentifrices   148
Anti-calculus Dentifrices   150
Antihypersensitivity Products   150
Whiteners   151
Mouthrinses   151
Cosmetic Mouthrinses: Halitosis   152
Xerostomia Mouthrinses   152
Therapeutic Mouthrinse Agents   153
Chewing Gum   154
Summary   156

10   Self-Care Measures to Supplement Toothbrushing   161
     Christine French Beatty
     Nahid S. Nikpour

     Objectives   161
     Introduction   162
     Oral Health Self-Care   166
     Frequency of Self-Care   166
     Dental Floss   167
       Dental Flossing Methods   169
       Dental Floss Holder   173
       Dental Floss Threader   174
     Other Interdental Aids   175
       Automated Flosser   176
       Interproximal Brush   177
       Uni-Tuft Brush   179
       Toothpick   180
       Rubber or Plastic Tip   183
       Knitting Yarn   184
       Pipe Cleaner   184
       Gauze Strip   184
       Rinsing   185
       Irrigation   187
     Oral Malodor and the Tongue   189
       Tongue Cleaners   190
     Peri-Implant Self-Care   192
     Self-Care of Dentures   193
       Patient Education   195
       Cleaning the Denture   195
       Disinfection of the Denture   199
       Denture Liners   200
       Denture Adhesives   200
       Xerostomia and the Denture Patient   200
     Summary   201

11   Community Water Fluoridation   212
     William D. Bailey

     Objectives   212
     Introduction   213
     Definition and Background   213
     History of Community Water Fluoridation   215
     Mechanisms of Action of Fluoride   220
     Benefits and Effectiveness of Fluoridation   223
     Effects of Discontinuation of Water Fluoridation   226

Enamel Fluorosis   227
Reducing the Risk for Enamel Fluorosis   230
Optimal Fluoride Levels   231
Engineering Aspects: Chemicals and Technical Systems Used   232
Monitoring and Surveillance of Fluoridation   233
Cost of Community Water Fluoridation   234
Other Fluoride Vehicles   235
Risk Communication   236
Myths and Actions Related to Risk Communication   237
Principles of Risk Communication   238
Summary   238

12 Topical Fluoride Therapy   245
Patricia Regener Campbell

Objectives   245
Introduction   246
Mechanism of Action of Topical Fluoride Treatments   246
Effects of Fluoride on Plaque and Bacterial Metabolism   250
Topical Fluoride Applications   250
Available Forms   250
Application Procedures   251
Application Frequency   253
Efficacy of Topical Fluoride Therapy   254
Root-Surface Caries   255
Recommendations: Topical Fluoride Treatments   257
Fluoride Varnishes   257
Initiation of Therapy   257
Disadvantages of Fluoride Treatments   258
Multiple Fluoride Therapy   259
Fluoride Rinses   260
Fluoride Gels for Oral Self-Care   261
Fluoride-Releasing Dental Materials   262
Toxicology of Fluoride   262
Fluoride Toxicity   262
Emergency Treatment   263
Chronic Fluoride Exposure   264
Home Security of Fluoride Products   264
Summary   265

13 Dental Sealants   272
Denise Muesch Helm

Objectives   272
Introduction   273

Historical Perspective   273
Sealant Use in Dental Care   273
Polymerization of Sealants   274
  Light-Cured Sealants   275
  Self-Cured Sealants   275
Types of Sealants   276
  Glass Ionomer Cement Sealants   276
  Sealants with Bonding Agents   276
  Self-Etching Light-Cured Sealants   276
  Fluoride-Releasing Sealants   276
  Colored versus Clear Sealants   276
Sealant Retention   277
Criteria for Selecting Teeth for Sealant Placement   277
Sealant Placement   279
  Increasing the Surface Area   279
  Pit-and-Fissure Depth   279
  Surface Cleanliness   279
  Preparing the Tooth for Sealant Application   280
  Drying the Tooth Surface   280
  Sealant Application   281
  Occlusal and Interproximal Discrepancies   282
  Evaluating Retention of Sealants   282
Placement of Sealants over Carious Lesions   282
Dental Providers   282
Economics   283
Disparities in Dental Sealant Use   283
Summary   283

14 Nutrition, Diet, and Associated Oral Conditions   287
Carole A. Palmer

Linda D. Boyd

Objectives   287
Introduction   288
Diet Assessment and Counseling in Dental Care   289
  Primary Prevention   289
  Secondary Prevention   289
  Tertiary Prevention   289
The Basis for a Healthy Diet   289
  Dietary Reference Intakes   289
  Dietary Guidelines for Americans   290
  MyPyramid   293
  Food Labels   294
Nutritional Factors Affecting the Oral Cavity   295
  Protein/Calorie Malnutrition   296

Minerals   298
Vitamins   298
Diet and Enamel Demineralization   299
Diet and Dental Caries   300
Role of Carbohydrates   300
Effects of Eating Patterns and Physical Form of Foods   301
Caries-Protective Foods and Nutrients   301
Measuring the Cariogenic Potential of Foods   302
Nutrition and Periodontal Diseases   303
Lifestyle Diet and Oral Health Issues   305
Early Childhood Caries   305
Eating Disorders   305
Aging Issues   307
Dental and Nutritional Implications of Common Chronic
Conditions   308
Diabetes Mellitus   308
Immunocompromising Conditions   308
Oral Surgery and Intermaxillary Fixation   309
Summary   311

15   Sugar and Other Sweeteners   316
Michelle L. Sensat

Jill L. Stoltenberg

Objectives   316
Introduction   317
Taste Perception and Sensation   317
History of Sweeteners   318
Sucrose and Constituents   320
Uses of Sucrose   320
Evaluation of the Health Aspects of Sucrose   321
Sugars and Dental Caries Formation   321
The Polyols as Sweeteners   324
Sorbitol   324
Mannitol   324
Xylitol   324
Intense Sweeteners   326
Saccharin   327
Aspartame   327
Acesulfame-K   327
Sucralose   327
Neotame   328
Non-nutritive Sweeteners Not Approved
in the United States   328
Alitame   328

Cyclamate   328
Neohesperidine   328
Stevia (Steveoside)   328
Thaumatin   328
Health Considerations   328
Obesity   328
Diabetes and Glycemic Response   328
Hyperlipidemias   329
Behavioral Disorders   329
Summary   329

16   Professional Dental Hygiene Care   332
Kathleen O'Neill-Smith

Carolyn Horton Ray

Objectives   332
Introduction   333
Assessment   333
Medical/Dental History   334
Vital Signs   334
Extraoral/Intraoral Examination   334
Dental/Periodontal Examination   334
Self-Care Evaluation   338
Diagnostic Radiographs   338
Diagnosis   338
Planning   340
Implementation   340
Evaluation   343
Summary   345

17   Health Education and Promotion Theories   347
Mary Catherine Hollister

Objectives   347
Introduction   348
History of Health Education   348
Health Belief Model   349
Oral Health Applications   350
Transtheoretical Model and Stages of Change   350
Oral Health Application   351
Theory of Reasoned Action   352
Oral Health Applications   353
Social Learning Theory   354
Locus of Control   354
Oral Health Applications   356

Sense of Coherence   356
  Oral Health Applications   357
Implementing Health Education Models   359
Adult Health Education   359
Motivating Patients   360
Motivational Interviewing   360
Oral Health Application   361
Summary   361

18   Tobacco Cessation   364
Joan M. Davis

Objectives   364
Introduction   365
Tobacco Use: Morbidity, Mortality, and U.S. Population
Trends   365
Tobacco-Related Oral Diseases and Lesions   366
  Oral Cancer/Precancerous Lesions   367
  Periodontal Diseases   368
  Smokeless Tobacco and Periodontal Disease   369
Tobacco Types, Toxins, and Carcinogens   369
Nicotine Use: A Biochemical Dependence   372
Tobacco Use: A Behavioral and Social Addiction   373
  Pharmacotherapy for Treatment of Nicotine Dependence   374
  First-Line Medications   374
  Proper Dosing of Nicotine Replacement   375
  Non-NRT Cessation Medications   376
  Second-Line Therapies   376
Alternative Cessation Methods   377
Components of an Effective Tobacco-Cessation
Intervention   377
  The PHS Guidelines' 5 A's   377
  PHS's 5 R's   379
Levels of a TCI   379
  Brief Intervention (1+ minute)   379
  Moderate Intervention (5 to 10 minutes)   380
  Intensive Intervention (20+ minutes)   380
Establishing a TCI Program   380
  Step One   380
  Step Two   381
  Step Three   381
Tobacco-Prevention Strategies—In-Office
and Community   381
Summary   382

19 Athletic Mouthguards   387
Christine N. Nathe

    Objectives   387
    Introduction   388
    Historical Perspective   388
    Mouthguard Use   388
    Contact Sport Injuries   389
    Mouthguard Protection and Prevention   390
    Types of Mouthguards   391
    Fabrication of the Custom-Made, Vacuum-Formed
    Mouthguard   392
    Dental Provider's Role in Mouthguard Use   394
    Summary   394

20 Technological Advances in Primary Dental Care   397
Vicki Gianopoulos

    Objectives   397
    Introduction   398
    Immunizations in Oral Health   398
      Dental Caries   399
      Periodontal Diseases   400
    Genetics   401
      Dental Caries   402
      Periodontal Diseases   402
    Gene Therapy   403
    Stem Cells in Oral Health   403
    Summary   404

UNIT 4 **Public Health and Target Populations**

21 Public Health Programs   406
Scott L. Tomar

    Objectives   406
    Introduction   407
    Public Health Defined   407
    Dental Public Health Science and Practice   408
    Public Health Approaches   408
      Population versus Individual Approach   409
      Reach versus Intensity   409
      Balancing Individual Rights and Societal Protection   410
    Dental Public Health Organization and Infrastructure   410
      International Agencies   410
      U.S. Federal Agencies   411

State and Local Dental Public Health Programs   412
Professional Organizations in Dental Public Health   413
Dental Public Health Activities   413
Assessment   413
Policy Development   415
Assurance in Dental Public Health   416
Summary   419

22   Pregnancy and Infancy   422
Sharon G. Peterson

Objectives   422
Introduction   423
Target Populations and Preventive Strategies   423
Population Characteristics   423
Pregnant Women   423
Infants   424
Common Oral Manifestations   424
Pregnant Women   424
Infants   425
Preventive Strategies   427
Pregnant Women   427
Infants   428
Summary   434

23   Pediatrics   437
Tamara L. Donald

Objectives   437
Introduction   438
Population Characteristics   438
Child Development   439
Early Childhood Development: 2 to 5 Years of Age   440
School-Aged Development: 6 to 11 Years of Age   443
Adolescent Development: 12 to 19 Years of Age   444
Children's Development and Behavior   444
Common Oral Manifestations   445
Early Childhood Caries   445
Preventive Strategies   445
Communication   446
Tell-Show-Do   448
Voice Control   448
Positive Reinforcement   448
Distraction   448
Summary   448

24   Adult Dental Care   451
      Maria Perno Goldie

         Objectives   451
         Introduction   452
         Population Characteristics   452
            Adolescence to Young Adulthood: 13–20 Years of Age   452
            Early Adulthood: 21–39 Years of Age   452
            Mature Adulthood: 40–60 Years of Age   452
         Common Oral Manifestations   453
            Dental Caries   453
            Periodontal Diseases   455
            Oral and Pharyngeal Cancer   455
            Women's Oral Health   456
         Preventive Strategies   457
            Adolescence to Young Adulthood: 13–20 Years of Age   457
            Early Adulthood: 21–39 Years of Age   457
            Mature Adulthood: 40–60 Years of Age   458
         Summary   460

25   Geriatrics   462
      Charles D. Tatlock

         Objectives   462
         Introduction   463
         Population Characteristics   463
            Frail Elderly   465
            Health   466
            Physiologic Changes   467
            Functional Status   467
            Cognitive Changes   468
         Common Oral Manifestations   469
            Long-Term Care   470
            Surgeon General's Report   470
         Preventive Strategies   471
            Senior-Friendly Dental Practice   471
            Health Promotion   471
            Public Policy   472
            Dental Providers   473
         Summary   473

26   Medically Compromised Populations   476
      Elaine Sanchez Dils

         Objectives   476
         Introduction   477

Arthritis   477
  Population Characteristics and Common Oral Manifestations   477
  Strategies to Prevent Oral Manifestations   477
Bulimia   478
  Population Characteristics and Common Oral Manifestations   478
  Strategies to Prevent Oral Manifestations   478
Cancer   478
  Population Characteristics and Common Oral Manifestations   478
  Strategies to Prevent Oral Manifestations   478
Cardiac Arrhythmias   479
  Population Characteristics and Common Oral Manifestations   479
  Strategies to Prevent Oral Manifestations   479
Congestive Heart Failure   479
  Population Characteristics and Common Oral Manifestations   479
  Strategies to Prevent Oral Manifestations   479
Depression   479
  Population Characteristics and Common Oral Manifestations   479
  Strategies to Prevent Oral Manifestations   480
Diabetes   480
  Population Characteristics and Common Oral Manifestations   480
  Strategies to Prevent Oral Manifestations   480
Epilepsy   480
  Population Characteristics and Common Oral Manifestations   480
  Strategies to Prevent Oral Manifestations   481
Hemophilia   481
  Population Characteristics and Common Oral Manifestations   481
  Strategies to Prevent Oral Manifestations   481
HIV and AIDS   481
  Population Characteristics and Common Oral Manifestations   481
  Strategies to Prevent Oral Manifestations   483
Hypertension   483
  Population Characteristics and Common Oral Manifestations   483
  Strategies to Prevent Oral Manifestations   484
Organ Transplants   484
  Population Characteristics and Common Oral Manifestations   484
  Strategies to Prevent Oral Manifestations   484
Pulmonary Disease   484
  Population Characteristics and Common Oral Manifestations   484
  Strategies to Prevent Oral Manifestations   484
Renal Disease/Failure   485
  Population Characteristics and Common Oral Manifestations   485
  Strategies to Prevent Oral Manifestations   485

Substance Abuse Disorders   485
  Population Characteristics of Alcohol Abuse and Common Oral
  Manifestations   485
  Population Characteristics of Tobacco Use and Common Oral
  Manifestations   485
  Population Characteristics of Marijuana Use and Common Oral
  Manifestations   486
  Population Characteristics of Cocaine Abuse and Common Oral
  Manifestations   486
  Population Characteristics of Methamphetamine Abuse and Common
  Oral Manifestations   487
  Strategies to Prevent Oral Manifestations   487
Thyroid Dysfunction   487
  Population Characteristics and Common Oral Manifestations   487
  Strategies to Prevent Oral Manifestations   488
Summary   488

27 Populations with Developmental Disabilities   495
    Elaine Sanchez Dils

Objectives   495
Introduction   496
Mental Retardation   496
  Population Characteristics and Common Oral Manifestations   496
  Preventive Strategies   497
Autism   497
  Population Characteristics and Common Oral Manifestations   497
  Preventive Strategies   497
Cerebral Palsy   497
  Population Characteristics and Common Oral Manifestations   497
  Preventive Strategies   498
Down Syndrome   499
  Population Characteristics and Common Oral Manifestations   499
  Preventive Strategies   499
Summary   499

Glossary   502

Index   517

PREFACE

The guiding principles that have sustained *Primary Preventive Dentistry* throughout the last several decades remain consistent. *Primary Preventive Dentistry* comprehensively presents the science and practice of assessment and treatment modalities of preventive dental care. This seventh edition strives to enhance the readability of this book for dental hygiene and dental students. Moreover, the web site has been enhanced to provide further opportunities for student study.

The book is sequenced in units to further organize the material for reader understanding and comprehension. The beginning unit focuses on a comprehensive discussion on preventive dental concepts with an emphasis on the historical perspective and creation of prevention in health care today. The relationship between prevention, and urgent and restorative care is presented to help dental providers understand *all* facets of dental care delivery. A thorough discussion of assessment, diagnostic, and therapeutic sciences of dental care is addressed.

The second unit focuses on oral disease etiology and contributing risk factors. This unit includes chapters on plaque, dental caries, periodontal disease, oral cancer, dental trauma, and host mechanisms. The etiology of all diseases is comprehensively discussed so that students completely understand the disease before prevention is discussed. The third unit addresses strategies to prevent these diseases/conditions and to maintain health. These chapters include toothbrushing, dentifrices, toothpastes and mouthrinses, oral hygiene aids, fluorides, dental sealants, nutrition, mouthguards, tobacco cessation, and health education and promotion theories.

The final unit includes chapters on target populations and public health approaches to preventing disease and maintaining health in these populations. These populations include infants, children, individuals with medical conditions and/or diseases, older adults, and hospitalized individuals.

Christine Nielsen Nathe

CONTRIBUTORS

William D. Bailey, DDS, MPH
Dental Officer
National Center for Disease Prevention
  and Health Promotion
Centers for Disease Control and Prevention
Atlanta, Georgia

Christine French Beatty, RDH, PhD
Professor, Dental Hygiene
Texas Woman's University
Denton, Texas

Linda D. Boyd, RDH, RD, EdD
Associate Professor and Director, Dental Hygiene
Division of Graduate Studies
Idaho State University
Pocatello, Idaho

Patricia Regener Campbell, RDH, MS
Associate Professor and Graduate Program Director
Caruth School of Dental Hygiene
Baylor College of Dentistry
Dallas, Texas

Gary Cuttrell, DDS, JD
Associate Professor, Dental Services
University of New Mexico
Albuquerque, New Mexico

Joan M. Davis, RDH, MS
Associate Professor, Dental Hygiene
Southern Illinois University
Carbondale, Illinois

Tamara L. Donald, RDH, MS
Private Practice
Santa Fe, New Mexico

Vicky Gianopoulos, RDH, MS
Assistant Professor, Dental Hygiene
University of New Mexico
Albuquerque, New Mexico

Maria Perno Goldie, RDH, BA, MS
President Elect, International Federation
  of Dental Hygienists
San Carlos, California

Denise Muesch Helm, RDH, MS
Associate Professor and Chair, Dental Hygiene
Northern Arizona University
Flagstaff, Arizona

Kathleen O. Hodges, RDH, MS
Professor and Chair, Dental Hygiene
Idaho State University
Pocatello, Idaho

Mary Catherine Hollister, RDH, MS, PhD
US Public Health Service
United South and Eastern Tribes, Inc.
Nashville, Tennessee

Sandra J. Maurizio, RDH, PhD
Associate Professor, Dental Hygiene
Southern Illinois University
Carbondale, Illinois

Melissa McDougal-Plese, RDH, MS
Assistant Professor, Dental Hygiene
University of New Mexico
Albuquerque, New Mexico

Beth E. McKinney, RDH, MS
Public Health Dental Hygienist
Montgomery County Government
Rockville, Maryland

Nahid S. Nikpour, RDH, PhD
Assistant Clinical Professor, Dental Hygiene
Texas Woman's University
Denton, Texas

Kathleen O'Neill-Smith, RDH, MS
Director
Hu-Friedy Manufacturing Company
Dallas, Texas

Carole A. Palmer, RD, Ed.D
Professor and Head, Nutrition and Oral
  Health Promotion
Department of Public Health and Community Service
Tufts University School of Dental Medicine
Boston, Massachusetts

Sharon G. Peterson, RDH, MEd
Professor, Dental Hygiene
College of Southern Nevada
Las Vegas, Nevada

Carolyn Horton Ray, RDH, MS
Clinical Associate Professor, Dental Hygiene
Oklahoma University College of Dentistry
Oklahoma City, Oklahoma

Elaine Sanchez Dils, RDH, MA
Assistant Professor, Dental Hygiene
University of New Mexico
Albuquerque, New Mexico

Michelle L. Sensat, BSDH, MS
Adjunct Assistant Professor, Dental Hygiene
School of Dentistry
University of Minnesota
Minneapolis, Minnesota

Jill L. Stoltenberg, RDH, MA, RF
Associate Professor, Dental Hygiene
School of Dentistry
University of Minnesota
Minneapolis, Minnesota

Charles D. Tatlock, DDS, MPH
Associate Professor, Dental Services
University of New Mexico
Albuquerque, New Mexico

Scott L. Tomar, DMD, MPH, DrPH
Professor and Chair, Community Dentistry
  and Behavioral Science
University of Florida College of Dentistry
Gainesville, Florida

Meg Horst Zayan, RDH, MPH, EdD
Associate Professor and Dean
Fones School of Dental Hygiene
University of Bridgeport
Bridgeport, Connecticut

REVIEWERS

Barbara Adams, RDH, MA
Program Director, Dental Assisting/Dental Hygiene
Wallace State Community College
Hanceville, Alabama

June Biss, RDH, MS
Instructor, Dental Hygiene
Sheridan College
Sheridan, Wyoming

Lydia Duffy, RDH, BHS
Assistant Professor, Dental Hygiene
Palm Beach Community College
Lake Worth, Florida

Michelle Oristian Fellona, RDH, MS
Professor, Dental Programs
Florida Community College at Jacksonville
Jacksonville, Florida

Jacqueline Freudenthal, RDH, MHE
Assistant Professor, Dental Hygiene
Idaho State University
Pocatello, Idaho

Barbara M. Gonzalez, RDH, MHS
Assistant Professor, Dental Hygiene
Wichita State University
Wichita, Kansas

Connie Henry, RDH, BA
Instructor, Dental Hygiene
Laramie County Community College
Cheyenne, Wyoming

Annette M. Russell, RDH, MS
Program/Clinical Director, Dental Hygiene
Baltimore City Community College
Baltimore, Maryland

Nicole Scoles, BSDH, RDH, MA
Instructor, Dental Hygiene
Chabot College
Hayward, California

Kathi R. Shepherd, RDH, BS, MS
Director, Dental Hygiene
University of Detroit Mercy
Detroit, Michigan

Adele Spencer, RDH, MS
Assistant Professor, Dental Hygiene
Farmingdale State University
Farmingdale, New York

Chapter 1

Introduction to Primary Preventive Dentistry

Christine N. Nathe

OBJECTIVES

After studying this chapter, the student should be able to:

1. Define and apply the following key terms: primary, secondary, and tertiary prevention.
2. Describe the historical aspect of preventive dental care.
3. Describe the state of dental health in the United States.
4. Describe categories that aid in classifying diseases.

KEY TERMS

Periodontal diseases
Caries
Restorations
Extractions
Dentures
Constitutional
Systemic diseases
Dental sealants
Health disparities
Health
Preventive dentistry
Primary preventive care
Therapeutic modality
Diagnostic modality
Primary prevention
Secondary prevention
Restorative care
Tertiary prevention
Reconstructive care
Plaque
Self-care
Periodontal debridement
Water fluoridation

(continued)

KEY TERMS (CONTINUED)

Remineralization
Sugar discipline
Radiographic oral examination
Incipient lesions
Gingivitis
Prevalence
Dentate
Opportunistic infections
Craniofacial disorders
Sequelae
Plaque diseases
Incidence
Etiology
Overt cavitation
Periodontitis
Cementum
Contiguous gingiva

Histologically
Clinical pathology
In situ
Demineralization
Sulcular epithelium
Gingival sulcus
Noninvasive caries
Interproximally
Apical
Cervical
Occlusal fissures
Buccal
Lingual
Overt
Periodontium
Apical migration
Apex

INTRODUCTION

The mission of dental care focuses on the ability to help individuals achieve and maintain maximum oral health throughout their lives. Success in attaining this mission is highlighted by the dramatic reduction in tooth loss among adults in the United States. This progress has been attributed mainly to the prevention of dental disease by the use of fluoride, the initiation of the practice of dental hygiene, and the subsequent acceptance and practice of primary preventive care.

This textbook will discuss effective strategies that markedly can reduce the number of carious (decayed) teeth, better control **periodontal diseases,** prevent the devastating effects of trauma caused by accidents, increase the early detection of oral cancer, decrease the lifestyle choices that increase disease susceptibility, and increase healthy behaviors. The U.S. Surgeon General stated that mouth and throat diseases, which range from dental **caries** to cancer, cause pain and disability for millions of Americans, even though most oral diseases can be prevented.[1] In dental health, lack of preventive dental care results in the further progression of disease and in the increased number of **restorations, extractions,** surgeries, and **dentures.**

HISTORICAL ASPECT OF PREVENTIVE DENTAL CARE

Dr. Alfred C. Fones (Figure 1–1 ■), the founder of dental hygiene and preventive dentistry, eloquently stated, in 1916, that hundreds of millions of dollars in public and private funds are expended to restore the sick to health, but only a relatively small portion of this amount is spent to maintain the health of well people, even though it is definitely known that the most common physical defects and illnesses are preventable.[2] He envisioned the tremendous effect of prevention before it was routinely practiced and promoted in health care.

The first college textbook on preventive dentistry, written by Fones, states that the mouth is the show window in which the body displays its physical wares.[2] This statement is reminiscent of the 2000 report of oral health in America, in which the Surgeon General states that, indeed, the phrase "the mouth is the mirror," has been

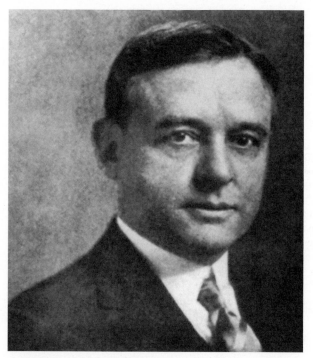

■ **FIGURE 1-1**   Alfred C. Fones, DDS, founder of dental hygiene. (American Dental Hygienists Association)

TEXTBOOK TABLE OF CONTENTS

Fones, AC. *Preventive Dentistry for Dental Students.*

Philadelphia: Lea & Febiger. 1925.

The Normal Histology of Dental Tissues

The Alveolar Process

The Enamel and the Saliva

Normal Occlusion

Brief Pathology of the Dental Tissues

Dental Caries: Immunity and Susceptibility

Dietetics: Elements of the Human Body

The Unnatural Dietary Habits of Civilized Nations

Modern Methods of Preparing and Cooking Food

Principles of Dental Prophylaxis

The Prophylactic Treatment

Prevention Through Public Education

■ **FIGURE 1-2**   Topics covered in the first book on preventive dentistry.

used to illustrate the wealth of information that can be derived from examining oral tissues.[1]

Fones continued to discuss the need for preventive dentistry departments in dental schools and the need to further enhance the dental hygienist movement.[2] Figure 1-2 ■ lists the topics covered in this first college textbook on preventive dentistry. Moreover, Fones stated that the research field in preventive dental care was broadening into a study of **constitutional** causes, that is, causes related to **systemic diseases,** which affect one or more organs, or the whole body; these diseases are believed to have an influence on the general health and, consequently, on dental health.[2–6] In addition, this statement is similar to the Surgeon General's recommendation that dental providers need to help change perceptions regarding oral health and ideas so that oral health becomes an accepted component of general health.[1]

Preventive dentistry is flourishing as a science and practice. In fact, most dental insurance companies routinely cover preventive care because of the long-term benefit and cost effectiveness of prevention in dental health. Moreover, many communities voluntarily add fluoride to their water supplies as a method of preventing dental disease. And most recently, to aid in the prevention of dental disease, many school systems offer their students **dental sealants** through dental health providers.

Although many individuals studied and practiced preventive dental measures, it was Fones who actually initiated the practice of dental hygiene, which began the prevention movement in dental care witnessed today. Some may propose that the creation of dental hygiene, a preventive-based science and practice, truly was the primary component of the prevention movement in health care. A decade after dental hygiene began, Fones stated that it was no longer a theory that the service of the dental hygienist improved dental and overall health in the community, and that those who were initially skeptical are finding it difficult indeed to suggest any other means by which similar good results can be accomplished for the community.[4] Interestingly, skeptics at the time could not dispute the effectiveness of primary preventive dentistry delivered by dental hygienists.

Many interesting issues were addressed in the 2000 Surgeon General's oral health report and are included in Table 1–1 ■. This report provided more details on the meaning of oral health and explained why oral health is essential to general health and well-being. The major themes included:

- Oral health means much more than healthy teeth.
- Oral health is essential to general health.

- Safe and effective disease prevention measures exist so that everyone can voluntarily decide to improve oral health and prevent disease.

Major findings and a framework for action from the report are listed in Tables 1–2 ■ and 1–3 ■.[1] The Surgeon General published a subsequent document titled *A National*

■ **Table 1–1** The Burden of Oral Diseases and Disorders

Oral diseases are progressive and cumulative, and become more complex over time. They can affect our ability to eat, the foods we choose, how we look, and the way we communicate. These diseases can affect economic productivity and compromise our ability to work at home, at school, or on the job. Health disparities exist across population groups at all ages. Over one third of the U.S. population (100 million people) has no access to community water fluoridation. Over 108 million children and adults lack dental insurance, which is over 2.5 times the number who lack [*sic*] medical insurance. The following are highlights of oral health data for children, adults, and the elderly. (Refer to the full report for details of these data and their sources.)

Children
- Cleft lip/palate, one of the most common birth defects, is estimated to affect 1 out of 600 live births for whites and 1 out of 1,850 live births for African Americans.
- Other birth defects, such as hereditary ectodermal dysplasias[a] where all or most teeth are missing or misshapen, cause lifetime problems that can be devastating to children and adults.
- Dental caries (tooth decay) is the single most common chronic childhood disease—5 times more common than asthma and 7 times more common than hay fever.
- Over 50 percent of 5- to 9-year-old children have at least one cavity or filling, and that proportion increases to 78 percent among 17-year-olds. Nevertheless, these figures represent improvements in the oral health of children compared to a generation ago.
- There are striking disparities in dental disease by income. Poor children suffer twice as much dental caries as their more affluent peers, and their disease is more likely to be untreated. These poor–nonpoor differences continue into adolescence. One out of four children in America is born into poverty, and children living below the poverty line (annual income of $17,000 for a family of four) have more severe and untreated decay.
- Unintentional injuries, many of which include head, mouth, and neck injuries, are common in children.
- Intentional injuries commonly affect the craniofacial tissues.
- Tobacco-related oral lesions are prevalent in adolescents who currently use smokeless (chewing) tobacco.
- Professional care is necessary for maintaining oral health, yet 25% of poor children have not seen a dentist before entering kindergarten.
- Medical insurance is a strong predictor of access to dental care. Uninsured children are 2.5 times less likely than insured children to receive dental care. Children from families without dental insurance are 3 times more likely to have dental needs than children with either public or private insurance. For each child without medical insurance, there are at least 2.6 children without dental insurance.
- Medicaid has not been able to fill the gap in providing dental care to poor children. Fewer than one in five Medicaid-covered children received a single dental visit in a recent yearlong study period. Although new programs such as the State Children's Health Insurance Program (SCHIP) may increase the number of insured children, many will still be left without effective dental coverage.
- The social impact of oral diseases in children is substantial. More than 51 million school hours are lost each year to dental-related illness. Poor children suffer nearly 12 times more restricted-activity days than children from higher-income families. Pain and suffering due to untreated diseases can lead to problems in eating, speaking, and attending to learning.

[a] Ectodermal dysplasia is the abnormal development of the outer layer of cells in an embryo.
Source: U.S. Department of Health and Human Services. (2000). *Oral health in America: A report of the Surgeon General—Executive summary.* Rockville, MD: U.S. Department of Health and Human Services, National Institute of Dental and Craniofacial Research, National Institutes of Health, 2–3.

■ **Table 1–2**   Major Findings from the Surgeon General's Report

- Oral diseases and disorders in and of themselves affect health and well-being throughout life.
- Safe and effective measures exist to prevent the most common dental diseases: dental caries and periodontal diseases.
- Lifestyle behaviors that affect general health, such as tobacco use, excessive alcohol use, and poor dietary choices, affect oral and craniofacial health as well.
- There are profound and consequential oral health disparities within the U.S. population.
- More information is needed to improve America's oral health and eliminate health disparities.
- The mouth reflects general health and well-being.
- Oral diseases and conditions are associated with other health problems.
- Scientific research is the key to further reduction in the burden of diseases and disorders that affect the face, mouth, and teeth.

Source: U.S. Department of Health and Human Services. (2000). *Oral health in America: A report of the Surgeon General—Executive summary.* Rockville, MD: U.S. Department of Health and Human Services, National Institute of Dental and Craniofacial Research, National Institutes of Health.

■ **Table 1–3**   Framework for Action

- Change perceptions regarding oral health and disease, so that oral health becomes an accepted component of general health.
- Accelerate the building of the science and evidence base, and apply science effectively to improve oral health.
- Build an effective health infrastructure that meets the oral health needs of all Americans and integrates oral health effectively into overall health.
- Remove known barriers between people and oral health services.
- Use public-private partnerships to improve the oral health of those who still suffer disproportionately from oral diseases.

Source: U.S. Department of Health and Human Services. (2000). *Oral health in America: A report of the Surgeon General—Executive summary.* Rockville, MD: U.S. Department of Health and Human Services, National Institute of Dental and Craniofacial Research, National Institutes of Health.

Call to Action to Promote Oral Health: A Public-Private Partnership under the leadership of the Surgeon General. This publication was an invitation to expand plans, activities, and programs designed to promote oral health and prevent disease, especially to reduce the **health disparities,** that is, the marked difference in quality of health status among populations. These disparities usually affect members of racial and ethnic groups, lower-income populations, many who are geographically isolated, and others who are vulnerable because of oral health care needs.[7] Prevention is a common thread within these documents.

DENTAL DISEASES AND SYSTEMIC HEALTH

Although dental diseases are preventable, dental health in the United States remains an issue. In fact, frequently it is claimed that oral health is a major unmet need in this country. And although more than 80% of 17-year-old children have experienced dental decay, the burden of this disease is not evenly distributed.[8,9] Children who experience the majority of the decay are from lower-income households or ethnic minorities, and many times they have special needs.

The consequences of this widespread problem are alarming. More than half of parents report unmet dental needs for their children, which is nearly 5 times the number reporting the need for eyeglasses.[10] Untreated dental disease results in children who have constant pain, difficulty eating and speaking, chronic infections, increased use of pain medicine, and embarrassment over the appearance of their teeth. Unfortunately, emergency room and operating room staffs regularly see large numbers of children presenting with unrelenting toothaches and caries that cannot be managed in the dental office.[11,12] Emergency visits usually consist of antibiotic therapies and can require hospitalization if not treated in an effective manner.

Moreover, oral health and its relationship to total health underscore the need for preventive dental care. Research has linked periodontal diseases to systemic diseases, such as cardiovascular and respiratory diseases, diabetes, cancer, premature and low-birth-weight babies, and a number of other systemic diseases.[1] Oral health is not a minor health concern; it affects overall health and well-being throughout life.

HEALTH DEFINED AND PRIMARY PREVENTIVE CARE

Although health can be defined as the period of time that an individual is not ill, it truly is much more expansive. The wellness scale defines a continuum from a state of health to a state of illness and death, with areas in between for quality-of-life indicators (Figure 1–3 ■).[13] Quality-of-life indicators define those areas between total health and death, when illness, injury, conditions, and diseases can affect the quality of life. For instance, an individual who sprained an ankle while playing basketball would not be experiencing total health, even though the individual may not be close to fatal illness or death. Prevention focuses on maintaining quality of life by actively focusing on healthy behaviors that prevent diseases and maintain health.

Furthermore, it has been accepted that the individual is a multidimensional being who consists of five dimensions (Figure 1–4 ■). This updated model shows the physical, mental, and social aspects of the first model, and adds the spiritual and emotional aspects.[14] By accepting the concept of multidimensional health, health care providers believe that, to experience total health, an individual must attain each dimension of health. This theory focuses on the need to address more than the physical dimension of health that previously defined health. Preventive strategies need to be focused on all multidisciplinary dimensions of health, realizing that all facets affect overall health.

The World Health Organization (WHO) defines **health** as the state of complete physical, mental, and social well-being and not merely the absence of disease or infirmity.[15] The WHO definition and other definitions are not without criticism, as some argue that health cannot be defined as a state at all, but must be seen as a process of continuous adjustment to the changing demands of living and of the changing meanings individuals give to life. If health is not described as merely the absence of disease, prevention then becomes an essential component of health and the definition of health. For instance, some individuals

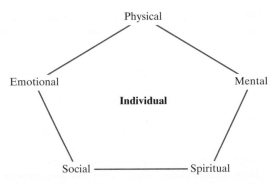

■ **FIGURE 1–4** Five-dimensional health model. (From R. Eberst (1984). Defining health: A multidimensional model. *Journal of School Health*, 54:99–104. Blackwell Publishing.)

may actually be in excellent health but believe, for some reason logical to them, that they have oral cancer. These individuals do not have optimum mental well-being and will continue to worry until they are somehow convinced otherwise that they are indeed healthy. Another person may be functionally healthy but physically disfigured and consequently shunned socially throughout life. Thus, health can at times be what the patient thinks and not the actual condition of the body.

Even the terminology **preventive dentistry** has different meanings to different people. **Primary preventive care** focuses on the preventive aspects of the dental hygiene sciences and emphasizes the use of diagnostic and therapeutic modalities to prevent disease. A **therapeutic modality** is a *method* of applying or using any therapeutic agent, whereas a **diagnostic modality** is a method used to diagnose a condition. Preventive care can be defined and classified into three different levels.

1. **Primary prevention** uses strategies and agents to prevent the onset of disease, reverse the progress of disease, or arrest the disease process before secondary preventive treatment becomes necessary. This level is sometimes thought of as dental hygiene.
2. **Secondary prevention** uses routine treatment methods to terminate a disease process and/or restore tissues to as near normal as possible. This level can be termed **restorative care.**
3. **Tertiary prevention** uses measures necessary to replace lost tissues and rehabilitate patients to as near normal as possible. This level can be termed **reconstructive care.**

Some examples of each stage of prevention in dental care are described in Table 1–4 ■.

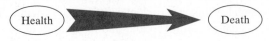

■ **FIGURE 1–3** Health wellness scale.

■ **Table 1–4** Levels of Dental Preventive Care

Levels of Prevention	Therapies and Services
Primary prevention	Oral evaluation
	Dental prophylaxis
	Fluoride as a preventive agent
	Dental sealants
	Health education
	Health promotion
Secondary prevention	Dental restorations
	Periodontal debridement
	Fluoride use on incipient caries
	Dental sealants on incipient caries (ART)
	ART, alternative restorative treatment
	Endodontics
Tertiary prevention	Prosthodontics
	Implants
	Oromaxillofacial surgery

Primary Prevention

The general approaches to the primary prevention of dental caries and periodontal diseases involve the following measures:

- Professional oral assessments.
- Patient involvement in the control of **plaque,** a naturally acquired bacterial biofilm that develops on the teeth. This process is called **self-care** and is accomplished by brushing and flossing teeth, and using other preventive products.
- Professional **periodontal debridement** (removal of hard deposits from the teeth using manual or ultrasonic dental instruments).
- **Water fluoridation** (addition of fluoride to a water supply).
- Use of fluoride products for self-care and for professionally initiated **remineralization** procedures (i.e., replacement of lost minerals in teeth).[16]
- Use of antimicrobial agents to reduce plaque biofilm.
- Use of dental sealants.

- Practice of nutritionally healthy habits including **sugar discipline** (limitation of amount of sugar in the diet to prevent a nutrient source for oral bacteria).

Tables 1–5 ■ lists the responsibilities of the dental practitioner and the patient in implementing these preventive strategies. In addition, patients have access to the dental provider, who performs diagnoses, risk assessments, comprehensive care, and planned maintenance programs. The comprehensiveness with which these preventive measures should be prescribed and used is indicated by the information obtained from the clinical and **radiographic oral examination,** dietary analysis, patient history, and laboratory tests.

At the time of the clinical and radiographic examinations, the first step should be to look for **incipient lesions**—the initial stage of tooth decay— and **gingivitis** (inflammation of the gingiva). Then preventive strategies could be applied that would result in a reversal or control of either or both of these diseases caused by plaque. It is essential for the profession and the public to realize that biologic repair of incipient lesions and cure of gingivitis are preferred alternatives to restorations or periodontal treatment.

■ **Table 1–5** Preventive Strategies for the Reduction of Dental Caries and Periodontal Diseases (Associated with Plaque Biofilm)

Preventive Strategy	*Dental Provider*	*Patient*
Mechanical reduction of plaque biofilm	Periodontal debridement	Toothbrush, dental floss, supplemental aids
Chemical reduction of plaque biofilm	Antibiotic therapies	Antimicrobial mouthrinses
Demineralization and remineralization of dental caries	Professionally applied fluoride, prescription fluoride, fluoride custom trays	Toothpaste with fluoride, mouthrinse with fluoride, fluoridated water, products with ACP[a]
Prevention of a host surface	Dental sealants	Chewing gums and lozenges with xylitol
Diet	Nutritional counseling	Sugar discipline
Knowledge	Dental health education and promotion	Seeking information and care

[a]ACP, amorphous calcium phosphate.

Even if these primary preventive dental modalities fail, tooth loss can still be avoided. In practice, the early identification and expeditious treatment of caries and periodontal diseases greatly minimizes the loss of teeth. When such routine diagnostic and treatment services are linked with an effective dental hygiene program that includes an annual dental examination and appropriate recall appointments that are based on risk assessment, tooth loss can realistically be expected to be reduced to zero or near-zero.

Secondary and Tertiary Prevention

When prevention is not practiced, disease and infection frequently cause the undesirable effects of pain and discomfort. Furthermore, the shift from primary to tertiary prevention results in an extremely rapid increase in the cost of health care, with a proportional decrease in patient satisfaction.

An excellent example of the comparative cost of secondary and tertiary prevention is the treatment of an individual with poliomyelitis. Recently the cost of the polio vaccine was only a few dollars. The use of the polio vaccine to prevent the onset of the disease was highly effective. But, for someone who was not adequately immunized, the cost of treatment for poliomyelitis and subsequent rehabilitation was close to $50,000 or more for the first 7 weeks of hospitalization and outpatient care (Easter Seal Foundation, San Antonio, Texas, personal communication, 1997). Yet, the individual receiving the

$50,000 worth of tertiary preventive treatment, who became disabled as a result, certainly was not as happy as the one who benefited from only a few dollars' worth of primary preventive care.

A dentally related example is the fluoridation of drinking water. This process costs approximately $0.50 per year per individual, yet it reduces the incidence of dental caries in the community by 20% to 40%. If this primary preventive measure is not available, the necessary restorative dentistry (secondary prevention) can cost approximately 100 times more or at least $50 per restoration.[16] Finally, if secondary prevention fails, as it often does, dentures can be constructed at even greater costs.

Preventive Care

Possibly the most important benefit of preventive dental care is the fulfillment of the moral commitment to the Hippocratic oath, which is taken by health providers upon graduation: "To render help to those in need, and to do no harm." Dental providers should derive a deep sense of satisfaction by helping individuals maintain their oral structures in a state of maximum function, comfort, and esthetics. Comprehensive dental care actively seeks to prevent disease and care for those individuals for whom prevention has failed. Further, comprehensive preventive care involves the collaboration of dental hygienists providing assessment, primary preventive services, and referral to other health care providers and dentists who provide secondary and tertiary services and referrals. Comprehensive preventive care should become a vital component in the health care delivery system, to enhance the overall health and well-being of the population.

Moreover, for the individual who thinks in terms of economic benefits and enjoyment of life, prevention is tremendously effective. Many studies document **prevalence** of dental diseases, which is the number of people in a population affected with a dental disease at the time of an epidemiology survey. But behind these numbers there is little mention of the adverse affects on humans caused by dental neglect. One study suggests that 51% of **dentate** patients (those who have teeth) have been affected in some way by their oral health, and for 8% of them, the impact was sufficient to have reduced their quality of life.[17] If preventive programs are started early by an individual (or the parents/guardians), long-range freedom from diseases caused by plaque is possible. It is a sound cost–benefit investment. Teeth are essential for many dimensions of total health. In contrast, as stated earlier in this chapter, the absence of teeth or presence of broken-down teeth often results in pain, infection, disfigured appearance, and subsequent loss of self-esteem. These effects minimize employment opportunities and often reduce social interaction.

Another example of prevention is of the ordinary seat belt in a car. This strategy illustrates how a simple preventive measure can greatly reduce facial injuries suffered in car accidents. Looming in the not-too-distant future is the very real possibility that many acquired health problems will be corrected or improved for total populations by the use of vaccines, genetic engineering, or specifically targeted drugs ("magic bullets"), which will be discussed in Chapter 20.

CATEGORIES OF ORAL DISEASES

Oral diseases and abnormalities can be conveniently grouped into three categories:

1. Dental caries and periodontal disease, both of which are acquired conditions.
2. Acquired oral conditions other than dental caries and periodontal diseases such as oral cancer, HIV/AIDS, and **opportunistic infections,** which are infections caused by a usually harmless microorganism that can become capable of causing disease when the host's resistance is impaired.

3. **Craniofacial disorders,** or disorders that involve both the cranium (portion of the skull that encases the brain) and the face, which would include a wide variety of conditions ranging from heredity to accidents.[18,19]

The treatment of caries and periodontal diseases, and their **sequelae** (after effects of the diseases) account for most of the estimated $60 billion U.S. dental bill for the year 2000.[20] Both caries and periodontal diseases are caused by the presence of pathogenic dental plaque on the surfaces of the teeth and therefore are known as the **plaque diseases.** Any major reduction in the **incidence** of caries and periodontal disease will release resources for the investigation and treatment of conditions included in the acquired and craniofacial category. *Incidence* is defined as the number of new cases that occurs *between* two epidemiology surveys conducted over an agreed-upon time period. In contrast, *prevalence* is a measurement of the number of existing cases *at the time* of a survey.

Plaque Prevention

The ideal or long-range planning objectives for coping with both dental caries and periodontal diseases should be the development of a preventive delivery system and methods to eventually attain a zero or near-zero disease incidence for the target population. However, a more realistic and feasible shorter-term goal is the attainment of a zero or near-zero rate of tooth loss from these diseases by integrated preventive and treatment procedures. Because of the varied **etiology** (cause) of acquired conditions other than caries and periodontal diseases, and of craniofacial malformations and diseases, the planning for the control of each of these problem areas must be individually addressed and placed within the priorities of any overall health plan.

In the quest for a zero or near-zero incidence of the plaque diseases, it is critical that dental professionals identify the signs and symptoms of disease that is about to occur at a time when progression to more-advanced stages can be prevented, arrested, or reversed. Examples are progression of an incipient caries lesion to **overt cavitation** (i.e., when undermined tooth enamel has demineralized into a carious lesion) and the progression of gingivitis to **periodontitis** and subsequent bone loss. Three notable factors make this preventive objective feasible:

1. Both dental caries and periodontitis are the result of a prolonged presence of pathogenic plaques affecting the enamel, **cementum** (a specialized

bony layer of connective tissue that covers the root), and/or **contiguous gingiva** (gingiva in contact with the tooth).

2. In most cases, both diseases can be controlled by mechanical and chemical plaque control regimens.
3. Both of the plaque diseases must go through a continuum of two reversible interim stages from histological normalcy to clinical pathology.

Both of the plaque diseases must go through a continuum of two reversible interim stages from a **histologically** normal state (i.e., having normal tissue structure or organization) to a state of **clinical pathology,** defined as structural and functional deviations from the normal that constitute disease or characterize a particular disease.

The earliest stage of the plaque diseases is **in situ** involvement, or involvement that does not extend beyond the site of origin. For caries, this stage is marked by the microscopic **demineralization** (loss of minerals) of the components that make up the tooth enamel.[21] For periodontal disease, it is the early infiltration of inflammatory cells beneath the **sulcular epithelium,** the tissue that lines the shallow space between the gingiva and the root of the tooth; this space is called the **gingival sulcus.**[22] Neither the early demineralization of caries nor the early cellular infiltration of gingivitis can be directly seen. Although these microscopic beginnings of plaque disease are not visible to the eye, they can be *suspected* on the basis of **noninvasive caries** (decay that has not penetrated tooth enamel), and periodontal risk assessment tests and indices that are *now* available to dental providers.

An in situ involvement, unless arrested or reversed, merges into the next stage of progression of the caries process, the incipient lesion. In caries, the lesion's clinical appearance is that of a "white spot" on the enamel, which is due to a more extensive subsurface demineralization of enamel.[23] Incipient lesions can occur on any surface as a precaries lesion. They may occur on the following areas of the tooth:

- **Interproximally** (on the contact areas of adjacent teeth; i.e., between teeth).
- **Apical** to the contact point (i.e., toward the area near the end of the root).
- On the **cervical** part of the tooth (i.e., near the junction of the crown and root).
- On the walls of the deep **occlusal fissures,** which are grooves on chewing surfaces of posterior teeth; the grooves developed during formation of the teeth.
- On **buccal** surfaces (surfaces located adjacent to the inside of the cheek).
- On **lingual** surfaces (surfaces located adjacent to the tongue).

Incipient lesions are found basically wherever there is plaque stagnation. These precaries lesions can be easily seen on dry, well-lighted buccal, lingual, and gingival enamel surfaces.[24] They are more difficult to detect on the occlusal surface where "sticky" pits and fissures should always be highly suspect as having incipient carious lesions or even early undetected carious lesions.[25] The presence of white spots on the smooth interproximal surfaces are usually identified first in radiographs.[26,27] In periodontal disease, the incipient lesion is gingivitis, with gingival bleeding being one of the first noticeable manifestations.[28] The incipient lesions of *both* caries and gingivitis can be reversed to histological normality, which by definition represents a cure.

The third and final stage of the plaque diseases is the **overt,** or clinically evident, lesion. In caries development, the overt lesion is characterized by cavitation with bacterial infiltration. For periodontal disease, an overt lesion is characterized by *irreversible* changes in the **periodontium** (tissue that surrounds the tooth) such as an **apical migration** of the epithelial attachment, which involves movement of the zone of soft tissue normally attached to the tooth toward the **apex** of the tooth root (i.e., area near the end of the root). If still untreated, the disease will usually progress to bone loss. At the overt lesion stage of the plaque diseases, treatment is usually indicated. However, two noninvasive preventive regimens may reverse overt caries: the use of antibacterial agents and/or remineralization therapy to arrest root decay, and the use of sealants to arrest early pit-and-fissure caries.[29,30]

Not all in situ lesions progress to the incipient stage, nor do all the incipient lesions progress to the overt stage of caries and/or periodontitis.[31] However, it is extremely important to note that no overt plaque disease lesion occurs at any site without first beginning as an in situ manifestation, and then progressing to an incipient lesion before becoming overt. Thus, any prevention program must focus on identifying and reversing the in situ and incipient stages of the plaque diseases with the same, or greater, diligence that is now given to searching for and treating overt disease. Achievement of primary prevention will allow the profession to move from a traditional emphasis on secondary and tertiary preventive dentistry to a primary preventive focus and commitment.

SUMMARY

This text emphasizes primary prevention and specifically focuses on primary prevention as it applies to oral health. Each year more than $60 billion is spent in the United States for dental care, mainly for the treatment of dental caries, periodontal disease, or their sequelae. Yet, strategies now exist that, with patient knowledge and cooperation, could greatly aid in preventing, arresting, or reversing the onset of caries or periodontal disease.

This introductory chapter has briefly pointed out some of the problems of dental care and the means by which the dental and dental hygiene professions can make primary preventive dental care its hallmark. The remaining chapters provide the detailed background that can make this challenge become a reality.

REFERENCES

1. U.S. Department of Health and Human Services. (2000). *Oral health in America: A report of the Surgeon General.* Rockville, MD: U.S. Department of Health and Human Services, National Institute of Dental and Craniofacial Research, National Institutes of Health.
2. Fones, A. C. (1916). *Mouth hygiene.* Philadelphia: Lea & Febiger.
3. Fones, A. C. (1921). *Mouth hygiene* (2nd ed.). Philadelphia: Lea & Febiger.
4. Fones, A. C. (1927). *Mouth hygiene* (3rd ed.). Philadelphia: Lea & Febiger.
5. Fones, A. C. (1934). *Mouth hygiene* (4th ed.). Philadelphia: Lea & Febiger.
6. Fones, A. C. (1925). *Preventive dentistry.* Philadelphia: Lea & Febiger.
7. U.S. Department of Health and Human Services. (May 2003). *A national call to action to promote oral health* (NIH Publication No. 03-5303). Rockville, MD: U.S. Department of Health and Human Services, Public Health Service, Centers for Disease Control and Prevention and the National Institutes of Health, National Institute of Dental and Craniofacial Research.
8. Collins, R. J. (1994). Celebrating the year of oral health: Changing public expectation and challenges for the profession. *J Amer Coll Dent,* 61:6–12.
9. Kaste, L. M., Selwitz, R. J., Oldakowski, R. J., Brunelle, J. A., Winn, D. M., Brown, L. J. (1996). Coronal caries in the primary and permanent dentition of children and adolescents 1–17 years of age. *J Dent Res,* 75:631–41.
10. U.S. Department of Health and Human Services. (1997). *Healthy people 2000: Review 1997.* Hyattsville, MD: U.S. Department of Health and Human Services, National Center for Health Statistics.
11. Wilson, S., Smith, G. A., Preish, J., & Casamassimo, P. S. (1997). Nontraumatic dental emergencies in a pediatric emergency department. *Clin Ped,* 36:333–37.
12. Sheller, B., Williams, B. J., & Lombardi, S. M. (1997). Diagnosis and treatment of dental caries-related emergencies in children's hospital. *Ped Dent,* 19:470–75.
13. Nathe, C. (2005). *Dental public health* (3rd ed.). Upper Saddle River, NJ: Prentice Hall.
14. Eberst, R. (1984). Defining health: A multidimensional model. *J School Health,* 54:99–104.
15. Health Definition. World Health Organization. (1948). World Health Organization: Geneva, Switzerland.
16. Blair, K. P. (1992). Fluoridation in the 1990s. *J Am Coll Dent,* 59:3.
17. Nuttal, N. M., Steele, J. G., Pine, C. M., White, D., & Pitts, N. B. (2001). The impact of oral health on people in the UK in 1998. *Brit Dent J,* 190:121–26.
18. Mouradian, W. E. (1995). Who decides? Patients, parents or gatekeeper: Pediatric decisions in the craniofacial setting. *Cleft Palate Craniofac J,* 32:510–14.
19. Haug, R. H., & Foss J. (2000). Maxillofacial injuries in the pediatric patient. *Oral Surg Oral Med Oral Path and Oral Radiol Endod,* 90:126–34.
20. Health Care Financing Administration (HCFA), National Health Expenditures Projections: 1998–2000. Office of the Actuary. http//www.hefa.gov/stats/NHE-Proj, April 25.
21. Barakow, F., Imfeld, T., & Lutz, F. (1991). Enamel re-mineralization: How to explain it to the patients. *Quint Int,* 22:141–47.
22. Brecx, M. C., Schlegel, K., Gehr, P., & Lang, N. P. (1987). Comparison between histological and clinic parameters during human experimental gingivitis. *J Periodontol Res.,* 22:52–57.
23. Von der Fehr, F. R., Löe, H., & Theilade, E. (1970). Experimental caries in man. *Caries Res.,* 4:131–48.
24. Nelson, A., & Pitts, N. B. (1991). The clinical behavior of free smooth surface carious lesions monitored over 2 years in a group of Scottish children. *Br Dent J.,* 171:313–18.
25. Konig, K. G. (1963). Dental morphology in relation to caries resistance with special reference to fissures in susceptible areas. *J Dent Res.,* 42:461–76.
26. Wenzel, A., Pitts, N., Verdonschot, E. H., & Kalsbeck, H. (1993). Developments in radiographic diagnosis. *J Dent Res.,* 21:131–40.
27. Espolid, I., & Tveit, A. B. (1984). Radiographic diagnosis of mineral loss in approximal enamel. *Car Res.,* 18:141–48.

28. Lang, N. P., Adler, A., Joss, A., & Nyman, S. (1990). Absence of bleeding on probing: An indicator of periodontal stability. *J Clin Periodontol,* 7:714–21.

29. Markitziu, A., Rajstein, J., Deutsch, D., Rahdmim, E., & Gedalia, I. (1988). Arrest of incipient cervical caries by topical chemotherapy. *Gerodontics,* 4:293–98.

30. Mertz-Fairhurst, E. J. (1992). Editorial: Pit-and-fissure sealants: A global lack of science transfer? *J Dent Res,* 71:1543–44.

31. Silverstone, L. M. (1984). The significance of demineralization in caries prevention. *J Canad Dent Assoc,* 50:157–67.

Chapter **2**

Dental Plaque

Melissa McDougal-Plese

OBJECTIVES

After studying this chapter, the student should be able to:

1. Differentiate between organic coatings of endogenous and exogenous (acquired) origin.
2. Describe why dental plaque is not unique among naturally occurring microbial layers.
3. Describe the mechanisms proposed to explain bacterial adhesion to the acquired pellicle.
4. Distinguish between primary and secondary bacterial colonizers in dental plaque, and cite examples of each.
5. Identify the primary sites of calculus formation, explain how calculus forms, and detail the differences between supragingival and subgingival calculus.
6. Describe the basis for the involvement of the acquired pellicle, bacterial dental plaque, and dental calculus in caries and the inflammatory periodontal diseases.

KEY TERMS
Dental caries
Periodontal diseases
Pathogenic
Dental plaque
Bacterial biofilm
Facial
Maxilla
Interproximally
Incis
Mineralized
Calculus
Extracellular
Exogenous antimicrobial agents
Gingiva
Alimentary tract
Gingival recession
Mucosal
Enamel-forming organ
Subsurface pellicle
Endogenous origin
Pellicle
Exogenous
Adsorption
Absorption
Ameloblasts

(continued)

KEY TERMS (CONTINUED)

Microbiota
Acquired pellicle
Prophylaxis
Dental restorations
Dental prosthetics
Gingival sulcus
Stagnation
Mastication
Occlusal fissures
Apical
Hemidesmosomes
Desquamated
Materia alba
Hydrophobicity
Glucosyltransferase
Glucans
Adhesins
Fimbriae
Pilin
Calcium bridging
Chelating
Supragingival
Subgingival

Primary colonizers
Secondary colonizers
Cocci
Proximal surfaces
Approximal plaque
Palisades
Ecologic niche
Symbiosis
Acidogenesis
Demineralize
Cavitation
Systemic conditions
Distal
Hydroxyapatite
Brushite
Whitlockite
Coronal
Lingual
Mandibular
Lingual
Inflammatory exudate
Perikymata
Sharpey's fibers
Dentifrices

INTRODUCTION

The dental professional comes into contact with two of the most widespread of all human maladies, **dental caries** and **periodontal diseases** (Figure 2–1 ■). Unlike typical infectious diseases, dental caries and periodontal diseases are not caused by a single **pathogenic** microorganism. Rather, these oral diseases result from the accumulation of many different species of bacteria that form **dental plaque,** a naturally acquired **bacterial biofilm** that develops on the teeth (Figure 2–2 ■).[1,2] Given that dental plaque is a multi-species biofilm, it should be taken into account that some bacterial species may be of greater relevance in the development of caries and periodontal diseases. Bacterial species are found in the plaque in a healthy mouth,

in the plaque associated with caries, and in the plaque of an individual with inflammatory periodontal disease.[3,4]

To understand the role of dental plaque in caries and inflammatory periodontal diseases, one must first know how dental plaque forms, and how changes in the proportions of different plaque bacteria can contribute to the development of oral diseases.[5,6]

DENTAL PLAQUE: A MICROBIAL BIOFILM

Most natural surfaces have their own coating of microorganisms, or biofilm, adapted to their individual habitats. The features of dental plaque formation are by no means unique; they merely reflect a single instance of a widespread and ancient natural phenomenon. One of the first

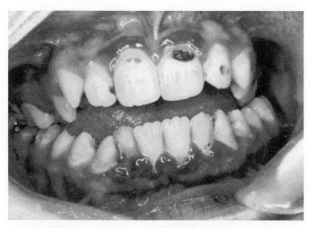

■ **FIGURE 2–1**   A 13-year-old female with dental caries on the **facial** surface of the incisors in the **maxilla** and swollen, discolored gingival tissues around the mandibular incisors, which is characteristic of chronic gingivitis.
(Courtesy of Dr. W. K. Grigsby, University of Iowa College of Dentistry, Iowa City.)

known examples of life is **mineralized** bacteria, or algae, attached to rocks from the Precambrian era.[7,8] These organic organisms were converted into a mineral (i.e., inorganic) format. Bacterial adhesion to surfaces, as seen with these mineralized organisms, primarily involves two types of reactions: physicochemical and biochemical.

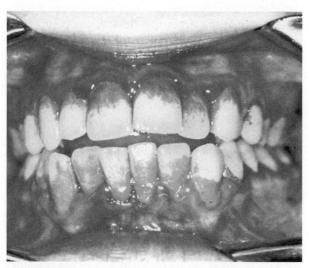

■ **FIGURE 2–2**   The dental plaque on these teeth has been stained with a discoloring solution and rinsed. Note the presence of plaque **interproximally** and adjacent to the gingiva, but relatively absent closer to the **incis**.
(Courtesy of Dr. W. K. Grigsby, University of Iowa College of Dentistry, Iowa City.)

These same interactions occur in the formation of plaque and calculus on oral structures.[9–11] **Calculus** is a hard calcified deposit of plaque that has become mineralized. For example, all living cells in nature, including bacterial plaque cells, have a net-negative surface charge. The cells can, therefore, be attracted to oppositely charged surfaces on such items as rocks in a stream, skin, or, as in the case of bacterial plaque, the surfaces of cells, teeth, and soft tissues of the oral cavity. In an attempt to prolong the existence of biofilms, the microorganisms within bacterial plaque and in other environments can produce (**extracellular** coatings) such as slime layers; they can also produce a variety of surface fibrils, or appendages, that extend from their cell walls. These mechanisms mediate (indirectly cause) attachment of bacteria to a substrate by providing additional attachment structures between the tooth surface and the plaque, thus allowing the formation of adherent matrices.[9,12]

Because biofilm is composed of various species of organisms, interactions with other members of the multispecies community in the oral cavity can influence the behavior of dental bacterial plaque. The mixed-species bacteria engulfed within the biofilm population behave differently from planktonic, liquid-phase, mono-species cells. This difference in behavior has significant clinical implications. Current research indicates that bacteria growing in biofilms are more resistant to the effects of **exogenous antimicrobial agents** (agents applied to the surface of the organism), than when these same cells are placed in a liquid suspension of antimicrobial agents.[13–15] This resistance could be attributed to the fact that biofilm communities house an assortment of microorganisms that have individual fluctuations in cellular structures. As a result, not all microorganisms within the biofilm population react uniformly to antimicrobial treatment at a given time. Thus, it is very important to include mechanical oral hygiene practices to disturb the attached biofilm, in addition to using antimicrobial therapy.

BACTERIAL COLONIZATION OF THE MOUTH

Microorganisms found in the oral cavity are naturally acquired from the environment. Bacteria are acquired from the atmosphere, food, human contact, and even from contact with animals, such as pets. The bacteria subsequently form colonies between saliva and oral soft tissues such as the **gingiva,** tongue, cheeks, and **alimentary tract.** Bacteria also form colonies between saliva and hard tissues such as erupted teeth, and exposed root cementum and dentin. Cementum and dentin become exposed during a process called **gingival recession.** The tongue and tonsils are covered by a **mucosal** surface (a surface covered by a membrane that secretes mucus). Mucosal surfaces may serve as reservoirs for organisms that form dental plaque, including those related to disease.[16]

Prior to eruption, the external surface of tooth enamel is lined by remnants of the **enamel-forming organ.** These tissue remnants are the reduced enamel epithelium and the basal lamina. The basal lamina connects the epithelium to the enamel surface. The basal lamina is also continuous with organic material that fills the microscopic voids in the superficial enamel. This subsurface organic material appears as a fringe-like struc-

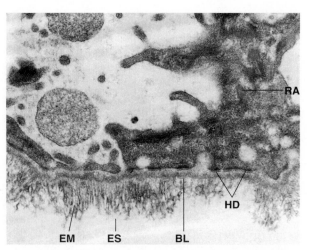

■ FIGURE 2–4 Junction of reduced enamel epithelium and enamel. The reduced **ameloblasts** (RA) are attached to the enamel by hemidesmosomes (HD) and a basal lamina (BL). EM, enamel matrix remnants form a subsurface pellicle; ES, enamel space. Original magnification × 45,000. (Courtesy of Dr. M. A Listgarten, University of Pennsylvania School of Dental Medicine, Philadelphia.)

ture attached to the basal lamina and is composed of residual enamel matrix proteins (Figures 2–3 ■ and 2–4 ■). This material is referred to as a **subsurface pellicle.** The pellicle originates from local cells during tooth formation; therefore, it is considered to be of **endogenous origin.** When the tooth emerges into the oral cavity, the remnants of the reduced enamel epithelium are worn off or digested by salivary and bacterial enzymes.[17]

An erupted tooth immediately becomes covered by a thin, microscopic coating of saliva materials. The salivary components become adsorbed[a] to the surface of the enamel within seconds. This coating is also referred to as a **pellicle.** Because it is acquired after eruption of teeth, it is said to have an **exogenous** origin—that is, the pellicle was formed by a substance from outside the tooth, rather than during the development of teeth. Tooth surfaces are also exposed to the oral **microbiota** (microscopic organisms found in a specific area). The oral bacteria can form colonies in the pellicle.[17]

Thus, the tooth surface, during development or after eruption, is almost always coated by a variety of structures

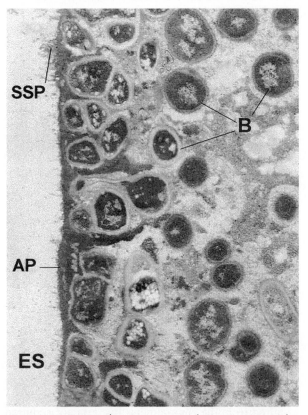

■ FIGURE 2–3 This transmission electron micrograph demonstrates remnants of the subsurface pellicle (SSP) and the acquired pellicle (AP) between the enamel (ES) surface and the bacterial cells (B) of the dental plaque. (Courtesy of Dr. M. A. Listgarten, University of Pennsylvania School of Dental Medicine, Philadelphia.)

[a]In a dental context, **adsorption** is the process in which a solid substance, such as tooth enamel, attracts and holds a liquid suspension, such as the salivary components, to its surface. In contrast, **absorption** involves the incorporation of a substance into the tooth.

that are either of endogenous origin (derived from cells of the dental organ) or of exogenous origin (acquired following eruption of the teeth into the oral cavity).[17]

THE ACQUIRED PELLICLE

The coating of salivary origin that forms on exposed tooth surfaces is called the **acquired pellicle**.[18,19] It is acellular and consists primarily of glycoproteins[b] derived from saliva (Figure 2–3). The pellicle also occupies the millions of microscopic voids in the erupted tooth caused by chemical and mechanical interactions of the tooth surface with the oral environment. Collectively, these organic fringe-like projections form a subsurface pellicle, which is of exogenous, or acquired, origin. Oral fluids and small molecules can slowly diffuse through the acquired pellicle into the superficial enamel. If the pellicle is displaced, for example by a **prophylaxis,** the pellicle begins to reform immediately.[20,21] It takes about a week for the pellicle to develop its condensed, mature structure, which may also incorporate bacterial products.[22–24]

An acquired pellicle also forms on artificial surfaces, such as **dental restorations** and **dental prosthetics** (i.e., dentures and partials). These organic coatings are similar to the pellicles on natural teeth and may be colonized by bacteria.[25–27] Colonization of the acquired pellicle can be beneficial for the bacteria, because the pellicle components can serve as nutrients.[28] For example, proline-rich salivary proteins may be degraded by bacterial collagenases. This action releases peptides, free amino acids, and salivary mucins that may enhance the growth of dental plaque organisms, such as actinomycetes and spirochetes.[29,30]

The carbohydrate components of certain pellicle glycoproteins may serve as receptors for proteins that bind bacteria to surfaces (e.g., adhesins), thereby contributing to bacterial adhesion to the tooth.[31–33] There is competition for the binding sites on the pellicle, not only by receptors on bacteria, but also from host proteins, including immunoglobulins (i.e., antibodies), the enzyme lysozyme, and proteins of the complement system, which are found in the blood and help to support the body's immune defenses. These host proteins originate from saliva and **gingival sulcus** fluid.[34,35] Once a pellicle site is occupied by one of the competing entities, occupancy by another is inhibited.[36] Not only does

competition arise for occupancy of binding sites, but an antagonistic relationship often exists between different types of bacteria competing for the binding sites. For example, it has been shown that some streptococci synthesize and release proteins called bacteriocins, which can inhibit some strains of *Actinomyces* and *Actinobacillus* species.[37,38]

DENTAL PLAQUE FORMATION

All bacteria that initiate plaque formation come in contact with the organically coated tooth surface by chance. Forces exist that tend either to allow bacteria to accumulate on teeth or to remove them. Shifts in these forces determine whether more or less plaque accumulates at a given site on a tooth. Many factors, ranging from simple to complex, influence the buildup of plaque. The simple factors include mechanical displacement, **stagnation** (colonization in a sheltered or undisturbed environment), and availability of nutrients. The complex factors include interactions between the microbes and the host's inflammatory–immune systems.[39] (Chapter 7 discusses these host defense mechanisms.) Bacteria tend to be removed from the teeth during **mastication** of foods, by the tongue, and by toothbrushing and other oral hygiene activities. For this reason, bacteria tend to accumulate on teeth in sheltered, undisturbed environments, which basically are sites at risk. These sites include the **occlusal fissures,** the surfaces **apical** to the contact between adjacent teeth, and in the gingival sulcus.

Therefore, it is no coincidence that the major plaque-based diseases—caries and inflammatory periodontal diseases—arise at these sites where plaque is most abundant and stagnant. Initial plaque formation may take as long as 2 hours.[40] Binding sites and the affinity of individual bacterial strains for a given surface vary considerably.[41,42] Colonization begins as a series of isolated colonies, often confined to microscopic tooth surface irregularities.[23] With the aid of nutrients from saliva and host food, the colonizing bacteria begin to multiply. About 2 days are required for the plaque to double in mass, during which time the bacterial colonies have been growing together.[43] The most dramatic change in bacterial numbers occurs during the first 4 or 5 days of plaque formation.[44,45] After approximately 21 days, bacterial replication slows, and plaque accumulation becomes relatively stable.[46] The increasing thickness of the plaque limits the diffusion of oxygen to the entrapped

---

[b]A glycoprotein is a protein molecule that includes an attached carbohydrate component.

original, oxygen-tolerant populations of bacteria. As a result, the organisms that survive in the deeper aspects of the developing plaque are either facultative or obligate anaerobes.[c]

The forming bacterial colonies are rapidly covered by saliva.[47] When seen with the scanning electron microscope, growing colonies protrude from the surface of the plaque as domes (**hemidesmosomes**), giving the appearance of a cluster of igloos beneath newly fallen snow (Figure 2–5 ■). In individuals with poor oral hygiene, superficial dental plaque may incorporate food debris and human cells such as epithelial cells shed by oral tissues (**desquamated** cells) and leukocytes. This debris is called **materia alba,** which literally means "white matter." Unlike plaque, it is usually removed easily by rinsing with water.[18] At times, the plaque demonstrates staining, which is caused by sources including tea, heavy metal salts, drugs, and chromogenic bacteria, which produce a brown pigment.

MOLECULAR MECHANISMS OF BACTERIAL ADHESION

The initial bacterial attachment to the acquired pellicle (Figure 2–6A ■) is thought to involve physicochemical interactions (e.g., electrostatic forces and hydrophobic bonding) between molecules or portions of molecules, such as the side chains of the amino acids phenylalanine and leucine.[48–51] It has been suggested that the **hydrophobicity** of some streptococci, a major plaque group, is caused by cell wall–associated molecules including **glucosyltransferase,** an enzyme that converts the glucose portion of the sugar, sucrose, into extracellular polysaccharide. Some glucosyltransferases have been designated as hydrophobins.[52] These polysaccharides include "sticky" **glucans** that, through hydrogen bonding, are thought to contribute to the mediation of bacterial adhesion (Figure 2–6C).[53] Once the bacteria adhere, they are often "entombed" as additional glucan is produced.[54]

Bacteria also have external cell-surface proteins termed **adhesins,** which have lectin-like[d] activity, because they can bind to carbohydrate components of glycoproteins.[32,33,55,56] These molecules are believed to aid colonization of the acquired pellicle.[57,58] Some

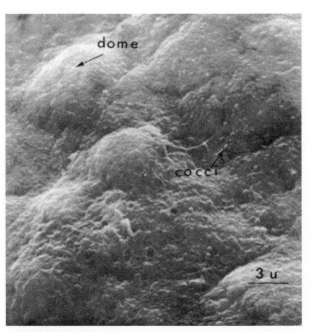

■ **FIGURE 2–5** Scanning electron micrograph of dome formation in the plaque.
(From Brady, J. M. (1973). *J Periodontol,* 44:416–28.)

researchers have suggested the adhesins may be located on bacterial surface appendages, such as **fimbriae** (Figure 2–6D ■). Fimbria-associated adhesins probably mediate bacterial adhesion via ionic or hydrogen-bonding interactions. Adhesins and fimbria may function together to promote bacterial attachment to pellicle-coated surfaces.[59] For example, **pilin,** a structural protein that constitutes the bulk of some fimbria, is hydrophobic because of its amino-acid content.[60] These fibrillar surface appendages extend from the bacterial surface and may reduce or mask the repelling effect of the net-negative surface charges. Carbohydrate-binding adhesins have been shown to link actinomycetes to streptococci in early dental-plaque formation.[61,62]

Another molecular mechanism of bacterial adhesion is **calcium bridging.** In this process *positively* charged, divalent calcium ions in the saliva help to link the *negatively* charged cell surfaces of bacteria to the *negatively* charged acquired pellicle (Figure 2–6B ■).[63,64,65] Calcium bridging may be important in only early plaque formation, because recently formed plaque is readily disrupted by exposure to a calcium-complexing (**chelating**) agent, such as ethylenediaminetetraacetic acid (EDTA).[66]

---

[c]Facultative anaerobes can exist in an environment with or without oxygen; obligate anaerobes cannot exist in an environment with oxygen.
[d]Lectins are plant proteins with receptor sites that bind specific sugars.

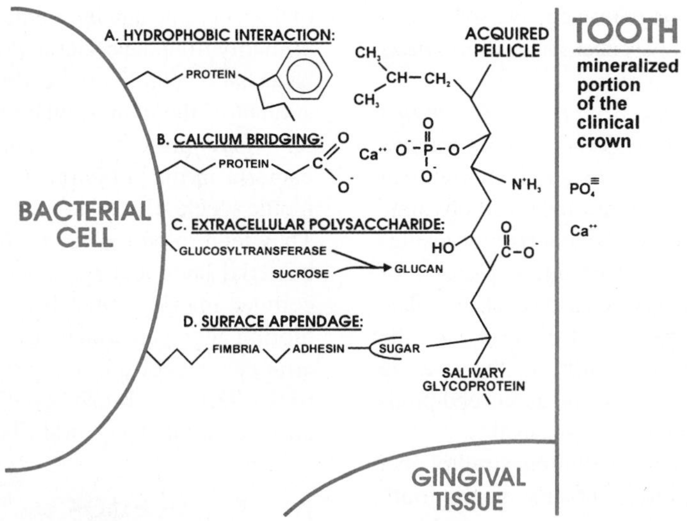

■ **FIGURE 2–6**   This diagram illustrates some of the possible molecular mechanisms that mediate attachment of bacteria to teeth during dental plaque formation. **A.** A side chain of a phenylalanine component of a bacterial protein interacts via hydrophobic bonding with a side chain of a leucine component of a salivary glycoprotein in the acquired pellicle. **B.** The negatively charged carboxyl group of a bacterial protein is attracted to a positively charged calcium ion (i.e., electrostatic attraction), which in turn is attracted to a negatively charged phosphate group of a salivary phosphoprotein in the acquired pellicle. **C.** The host's dietary sucrose is converted by the bacterial enzyme, glucosyltransferase, to the extracellular polysaccharide, glucan, which has many hydrophobic groups and can interact with amino acid side-chain groups, such as serine, tyrosine, and threonine. **D.** The fimbrial surface appendage extends from the bacterial cell to permit the terminal adhesin portion to bind to a sugar component of a salivary glycoprotein in the acquired pellicle.

While some or all of the above-described mechanisms may play a role in the attachment of bacteria to one another and to the tooth surface, the nature of the actual linking molecules in plaque, or between plaque and tooth surface coatings, is not known.

BACTERIA IN THE DENTAL PLAQUE

Within the mouth of any one individual, plaque bacteria vary in number and proportions from time to time and site to site. The diversity is even greater between individuals, between races, and between **supragingival** and **subgingival** plaques.[67–69] The only abundant bacteria found almost universally in the mouths of humans and animals are streptococci and actinomycetes.

The bacteria colonize the teeth in a reasonably predictable sequence. The first to adhere are **primary colonizers,** sometimes referred to as "pioneer species." These are microorganisms that are able to stick directly to the acquired pellicle. Those that arrive later are **secondary colonizers.** They may be able to colonize an existing bacterial layer, but they are unable to act as primary colonizers. Generally speaking, the primary colonizers are not pathogenic. If the plaque is allowed to remain undisturbed, it eventually becomes populated with secondary colonizers that are the likely etiologic agents of dental caries and periodontal diseases.

The earliest colonizers are overwhelmingly **cocci** (spherical bacteria), especially streptococci, which constitute 47% to 85% of the cultivable cells found during the first 4 hours after professional tooth cleaning.[1,69–71] These organisms tend to be followed by short rods and filamentous bacteria. Because of stagnation, the most abundant colonization is on the **proximal surfaces,** in the fissures of teeth, and in the gingival sulcus region.[72]

Cocci are probably the first to adhere because they are small and round and, therefore, have a smaller energy barrier to overcome than other bacterial forms.[73] The first or primary colonizers tend to be aerobic (oxygen-tolerant) bacteria including *Neisseria* and *Rothia*. The streptococci, the gram-positive facultative rods, and the actinomycetes are the main organisms in plaque found in early fissures and **approximal plaque**).[73–75] As plaque oxygen levels fall, the proportions of gram-negative rods (e.g., fusobacteria) and gram-negative cocci such as *Veillonella* tend to increase.

Of the early colonizers, *Streptococcus sanguis* often appears first, followed by *Streptococcus mutans* (*S. mutans*).[76] Both depend on a sheltered environment for growth and the presence of extracellular carbohydrate (e.g., sucrose). Sucrose is used to synthesize intracellular polysaccharides that serve as an internal source of energy, as well as external polysaccharide coats.[77,78] The polysaccharide coating helps protect the cell from the osmotic effects of sucrose. In addition, the coating reduces the inhibitory effect of toxic metabolic end products, such as lactic acid, on bacterial survival.

Whereas non-motile cells, including streptococci and actinomycetes, come into contact with the tooth randomly, motile cells such as the spirochetes are likely to be attracted by chemotactic factors (e.g., nutrients). Surface receptors probably provide a means of attachment for secondary colonizers onto the initial bacterial layer.[79] Bacteria that cannot adhere easily to the tooth initially via organic coatings can probably attach by strong lectin-like, cell-to-cell interactions with similar or dissimilar bacteria that are already attached (i.e., the primary colonizers).[33,80,81]

Gram-negative, anaerobic species such as *Treponema*, *Porphyromonas*, *Prevotella*, and *Fusobacterium* species predominate in the subgingival plaque during the later phases of plaque development, but they may also be present in early plaque.[82] There is evidence that oxygen does not penetrate more than 0.1 mm into the dental plaque, a fact that may explain the presence of anaerobic bacteria in early plaque.[83-84]

DENTAL PLAQUE MATRIX

A great variety of factors affect the colonization of bacteria on teeth. Dental plaque consists of different species of bacteria that are not uniformly distributed, because different species colonize the tooth surface at different times and under different circumstances. The newly formed supragingival biofilm frequently exhibits **"palisades"** (columnar microcolonies of cells) made up of firmly attached cocci, rods, or filaments. The organisms are positioned perpendicular to the tooth surface as a result of competitive colonization. The bacterial cells in the biofilm are surrounded by an intercellular plaque matrix (Figure 2–7 ■).[1,56,69,85] The matrix is composed of both organic and inorganic components that originate primarily from the bacteria. Polysaccharides derived from bacterial metabolism of carbohydrates are a major constituent of the matrix, whereas salivary and serum proteins/glycoproteins represent minor components. The bacteria in the subgingival biofilm consist of several motile species that do not form distinctive microcolonies. They tend to be located on the surface of the adherent bacterial layer and are separated by an abundant intercellular matrix. Some bacteria on the surface of the biofilm aggregate into distinctive structures that include arrangements of cocci ("corn-cob" configurations) and rods ("test-tube brush" configurations)[1,2,69,86] radially arranged around a central filament (Figure 2–8 ■).

DENTAL PLAQUE METABOLISM

For metabolism to occur, a source of energy is required. For the caries-related *S. mutans* and many other acid-forming organisms, this energy source can be sucrose.[87]

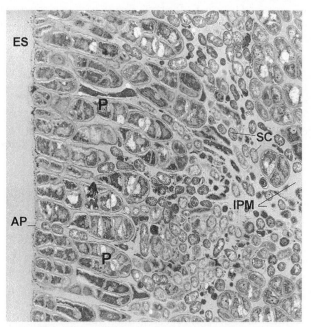

■ **FIGURE 2–7** An electron micrograph showing palisades (P) of bacteria perpendicular to the enamel surface (ES), bacterial cells that are probably secondary colonizers (SC), the intercellular plaque matrix (IPM), and the acquired pellicle (AP).

(Courtesy of Dr. M. A Listgarten, University of Pennsylvania School of Dental Medicine, Philadelphia.)

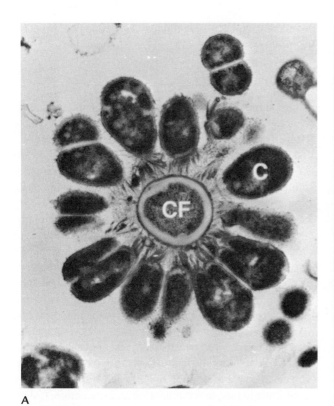
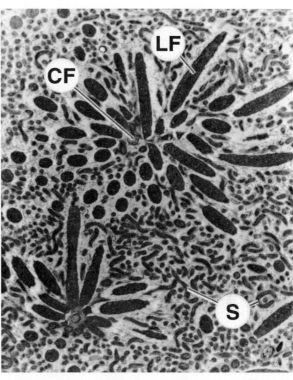

A   B

■ **FIGURE 2–8**   **A.** Cross section of "corn cob" from 2-month-old plaque. A coarse fibrillar material attaches the cocci (C) to the central filament (CF). Original magnification × 22,500.
(From Listgarten, M. A., Mayo, H. E., & Tremblay, R. (1975). *J Periodontol,* 46:10–26.)
B. Coarse "test-tube brush" formations consisting of central filament (CF) surrounded by large, filamentous bacteria with flagella uniformly distributed over its body (LF). Background consists of a spirochete-rich microbiota (S). Original magnification × 4,300.
(From Listgarten, M. A. (1976). *J Periodontol,* 47: 1–18.)

Almost immediately following exposure of these microorganisms to sucrose, they produce (1) acid, (2) intracellular polysaccharides, which provide a reserve source of energy for each bacterium, much like glycogen does for human cells,[88] and (3) extracellular polysaccharides including glucans (dextran)[89] and fructans (levan).[90] As mentioned previously, glucans can be viscid substances that help anchor the bacteria to the pellicle, as well as stabilize the plaque mass. Fructans can act as an energy source for any bacteria having the enzyme levanase.[91,92] Quantitatively, the glucans constitute up to approximately 20% of plaque dry weight, levans about 10%, and bacteria the remaining 70% to 80%. As stated earlier, the glucans and fructans are major contributors to the intercellular plaque matrix.[92]

Plaque organisms grow under adverse environmental conditions, which include varying pH, temperature, ionic strength, oxygen tension, nutrient levels, and antagonistic elements, such as competing organisms and the host inflammatory–immune response. The numerous fluctuations in the oral environment can influence many aspects of the initial colonization, maturation, and survival of microorganisms within oral plaque. Variations of the aforementioned conditions can affect the primary and extended adherence of microorganisms to the surface, as well the diffusion of essential elements (i.e., oxygen and nutrients), all of which are required for the prolonged existence of bacterial biofilm. To cope with this hostile environment, the plaque organisms must find a safe haven in relation to their neighbors and the oral environment. Such a favorable location is termed an **ecologic niche.**[5] Normally, once the niches are established, the bacteria of the resident microbiota coexist with the host and the surrounding microcosm. This relationship is referred to as **symbiosis,** and it results in a resistance to colonization by subsequent nonindigenous organisms. In this manner, the resident microbiota can protect the host against infection by major primary pathogens (e.g., *Corynebacterium diphtheriae* and *Streptococcus pyogenes*).

With dietary sugars entering the plaque, anaerobic glycolysis results in **acidogenesis** (acid production) and accumulation of acid in the plaque.[5] If no acid-consuming organisms (e.g., *Veillonella*) are available to use the acids, the plaque pH drops rapidly from 7.0 to below 4.5. This drop is important because enamel begins to **demineralize** between pH 5.0 and 5.5. One possible outcome of the drop in pH may be the dissolution of the mineralized tooth surface adjacent to the plaque, resulting in carious **cavitation** of the tooth.[77] This process provides the bacteria access to the inorganic elements (e.g., calcium and phosphate) needed for their nutritional requirements. By adhering to the tooth surface via an organic layer of salivary origin, dental plaque bacteria can also gain access to a supply of organic nutrients, a widespread phenomenon.[47] The same search for nutrients may explain the extension of bacteria from the supragingival plaque into the gingival sulcus.[93,94] To prevent or reduce subgingival colonization, the host tissues defend against the bacterial challenge with antibacterial strategies, such as the passage of antibodies and the emigration of polymorphonuclear neutrophils from the adjacent connective tissue into the gingival sulcus. The continued metabolic activity of plaque in the subgingival environment initiates the inflammatory response of the gingival tissues (gingivitis) and also may eventually lead to progressive destruction of the periodontium (periodontitis).[95,96]

Until supragingival plaque mineralizes as dental calculus, it can be removed by mechanical debridement (e.g., toothbrushing, flossing, or use of interdental aids).[97] Dental plaque cannot be removed by rinsing alone. As the plaque matures, it becomes more resistant to removal with a toothbrush. In one study, at 24, 48, and 72 hours after formation, 5.5, 7.8, and 14.0 g/cm² of pressure, respectively, were required to dislodge the plaque—almost 3 times as much pressure to remove it on the third day as on the first.[98] Once dental calculus is formed, use of professional instruments is necessary for its removal.

DENTAL CALCULUS

A last stage in the maturation of some dental plaques is characterized by the appearance of mineralization in the deeper portions of the plaque to form dental calculus.[99] The term *calculus* is derived from the Latin word meaning pebble or stone. The lay term *tartar* refers to an accumulated sediment or crust on the sides of a wine cask. Some people do not form calculus, others form only moderate amounts, and still others form heavy amounts.

Calculus itself is not harmful. However, a layer of unmineralized, viable, metabolically active bacteria that are closely associated with the external calculus surface is potentially pathogenic. Calculus cannot be removed by brushing or flossing. It is often difficult to remove all the calculus, even professionally, without damaging the tooth, especially the softer root cementum. However, calculus needs to be removed because its presence makes routine oral hygiene more difficult or even impossible by forming calculus spurs (Figure 2–9 ■). These structures may contribute to plaque accumulation and stagnation. Calculus removal is also a prerequisite to regenerating lost or damaged periodontal tissues after treatment.

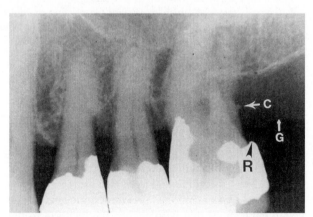

■ FIGURE 2–9 Radiograph demonstrating a "spur"-shaped deposit of calculus (C) on the **distal** side of the left first molar in the maxilla. The calculus is apical to the overhanging metallic restoration (R). The arrow (G) marks the coronal level of the gingival tissues, which indicates that this is a subgingival deposit of calculus.
(Courtesy of Dr. W. K. Grigsby, University of Iowa College of Dentistry, Iowa City.)

In addition to local factors, calculus formation may be affected by behavioral factors, and **systemic conditions.** For example, smoking causes an accelerated formation of calculus.[100] Children afflicted with asthma or cystic fibrosis form calculus at approximately twice the rate of other children.[101] Similarly, non-ambulatory, mentally handicapped individuals, tube-fed over long periods, may develop heavy calculus within 30 days, despite the fact that no food passes through the mouth.[102] Conversely, medications such as beta-blockers, diuretics, and anticholinergics can result in significantly reduced levels of calculus. The authors of the study that made this determination concluded that either the medications were excreted directly into the saliva, affecting the rate of crystallization, or altered the composition of the saliva and thus indirectly affected calculus formation.[103]

Calculus formation is related to the fact that saliva is saturated with respect to calcium and phosphate ions.[104] Precipitation of these elements leads to mineralization of dental plaque, which gives rise to calculus. The crystals in calculus include **hydroxyapatite, brushite,** and **whitlockite,** all of which have different proportions of calcium and phosphate in combination with other ions, such as magnesium, zinc, fluoride, and carbonate. Supragingival calculus forming on the tooth **coronal** to the gingival margin frequently develops opposite the duct orifices of the major salivary glands. It is often found where saliva pools on the **lingual** surfaces of the **mandibular** incisors (Figure 2–10 ■). Supragingival calculus can also form in the fissures of teeth. Subgingival calculus forms from calcium phosphate and organic materials derived from blood serum, which contribute to mineralization of subgingival plaque.

One of the means by which formation and growth of calculus may be studied is by ligating thin plastic strips around the teeth and then removing the strips at various intervals.[105] Within 12 hours after placement, x-ray diffraction studies demonstrate mineral elements in the forming plaque. By 3 to 4 days, the concentration of calcium and phosphate is significantly higher in the plaque of those with heavy calculus formation than in the plaque of those with no calculus formation.

Subgingival calculus is about 60% mineralized, whereas supragingival calculus is only about 30% mineralized.[106] Because subgingival calculus is harder, thinner, and more closely adapted to tooth surface

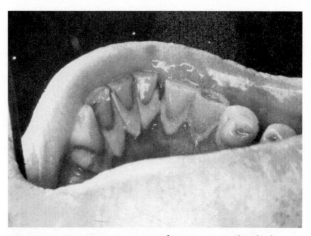

■ **FIGURE 2–10**   Deposits of supragingival calculus on the **lingual** surface of incisors and canines that could not be removed by brushing.
(Courtesy of Dr. W. K. Grigsby, University of Iowa College of Dentistry, Iowa City.)

imperfections, it can be more difficult to remove than supragingival calculus. The two types of calculus may differ in color. Supragingival calculus, which derives its mineral content from saliva, usually appears as a yellow to white mass with a chalky consistency. Subgingival calculus derives its minerals from the **inflammatory exudate** in the sulcus and periodontal pocket. Subgingival calculus appears gray to black in color and has a flint-like consistency. The dark coloration may be caused by bacterial degradation of components of the hemorrhagic exudate that accompanies gingival inflammation.

Alkaline conditions in dental plaque may be an important predisposing factor for calculus formation.[107] Calculus formation is not restricted to one bacterial species, or even to those growing at neutral or slightly acidic pHs. This is evidenced by the fact that caries-related streptococci may mineralize.[108] Not all plaques mineralize, but a plaque that is destined to mineralize begins to do so within a few days of its initial formation, even though this early change is not detectable at a clinical level. Mineralization usually begins in the intercellular plaque matrix but eventually occurs within the bacterial cells (Figure 2–11 ■). Bacterial phospholipids and other cell-wall constituents may act as initiators of mineralization, in which case mineralization may begin in the cell wall and subsequently extend to

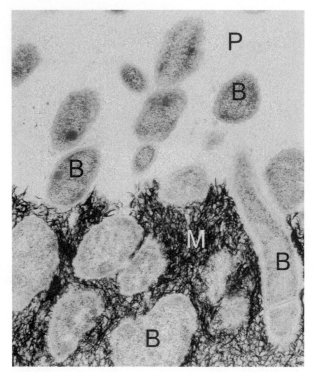

■ FIGURE 2–11 Typical pattern of dental plaque mineralization in which the initial mineralization occurs in the inter-bacterial plaque matrix (M), with bacterial cells (B) becoming mineralized secondarily. Original magnification × 40,000.
(Courtesy of Dr. M. A. Listgarten, University of Pennsylvania School of Dental Medicine, Philadelphia.)

the rest of the cell and into the surrounding matrix (Figure 2–12 ■).[109] Calculus may also form on the tooth surfaces of germ-free animals.[110] This type of calculus consists of an organic matrix of non-microbial origin, which becomes mineralized.

Attachment of Calculus to the Teeth

At the tooth interface with calculus, neither the enamel nor the root cementum is perfectly smooth, and invariably they contain a variety of surface imperfections. These normal irregularities, such as the **perikymata**[e] and the

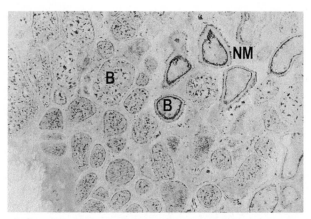

■ FIGURE 2–12 Atypical pattern of dental plaque mineralization in which bacterial cells (B) act as foci of initial mineralization, with the matrix (NM), becoming mineralized secondarily. Original magnification × 25,000.
(Courtesy of Dr. M. A. Listgarten, University of Pennsylvania School of Dental Medicine, Philadelphia.)

point of origin of **Sharpey's fibers**[f] on the cementum, appear to aid calculus attachment. Other defects in the enamel and cementum, including areas of demineralization and cemental tears, may also contribute to a stronger attachment of calculus to the tooth.[111] Electron micrographs indicate a very close relationship between the matrix of the tooth surface and the matrix of calculus; the crystalline structures of both are also very similar.[112]

Inhibition of Calculus Formation

Several agents are currently available to reduce calculus formation, including **dentifrices** that contain pyrophosphate or metal ions such as zinc.[113,114] One dentifrice contains two soluble phosphates, tetrasodium pyrophosphate and disodium dihydrogen pyrophosphate, in addition to fluoride.[114,115] The pyrophosphate ion is an analog of the orthophosphate ion, which means it differs structurally from the parent compound (orthophosphate) by a single element, but has many of the same functions. In the case of dental calculus, the pyrophosphate ion disrupts the formation of calcium phosphate crystals. This analog also inhibits some bacterial growth at concentrations significantly lower than the levels found in dentifrices without pyrophosphate.

---

[e]Perikymata are the numerous, small, transverse ridges on the exposed surface of the enamel of the permanent teeth.

---

[f]The tooth is anchored by connective tissue fibers that extend between the cementum and the bone; the ends embedded in the cementum and bone are known as Sharpey's fibers.

SUMMARY

Bacteria in dental plaque are the direct cause of the most widespread of all human diseases: dental caries and inflammatory periodontal diseases. These diseases, however, are not classic infections. They arise because of complex changes in plaque ecology and are affected by many factors in the host's protective responses. To understand the role of dental plaque in disease and how to prevent or control the plaque-associated diseases, it is essential to understand the nature of dental plaque. Plaque forms initially on the organic layer that coats the erupted tooth. This organic layer originates from salivary products that are deposited on the teeth, forming an acquired pellicle to which bacteria adhere. Adhesion is mediated by a variety of bonding mechanisms, including physicochemical and electrostatic interactions, as well as stereochemical interactions between bacterial adhesins and receptors in the acquired pellicle and bacterial surfaces.

The earliest of the primary bacterial colonizers are mainly gram-positive facultative cocci. They are followed by a variety of gram-positive and gram-negative species— the secondary colonizers. Caries-related bacterial species have a greater ability than others to adapt to excess sugars and their metabolites.

Supragingival plaque is associated with caries and gingivitis, whereas subgingival plaque is associated with gingivitis and periodontitis. With higher pH (i.e., less acidity), some plaques mineralize to form supragingival and subgingival dental calculus. In calculus formation, mineralization of dental plaque generally begins in the extracellular matrix and eventually spreads to include the bacteria. Rarely, mineralization may begin within the walls of bacterial cells and spread to the extracellular matrix. Calculus is generally covered by actively metabolizing bacteria, which can cause caries, gingivitis, and periodontitis. Regular toothbrushing and flossing can remove dental plaque and control its formation. Once dental plaque mineralizes to form calculus, use of professional instruments is necessary for its removal. Although calculus does contribute to inflammatory periodontal diseases, it is stagnation of pathogenic bacteria at critical sites that leads to both dental caries and periodontal diseases.

Later chapters deal with the wide range of methods, mechanical and chemical, increasingly used to control plaque and calculus formation. All of these methods have the aim of preventing, arresting, or reversing the progression of dental caries and periodontal tissue inflammation.

REFERENCES

1. Listgarten, M. A. (1976). Structure of the microbial flora associated with periodontal health and disease in man. A light and electron microscopic study. *J Periodontol*, 47:1–17.
2. Listgarten, M. A. (1999). Formation of dental plaque and other oral biofilms. In Newman, H. N., & Wilson, M., Eds. *Dental plaque revisited—Oral biofilms in health and disease.* Cardiff, U.K.: BioLine, 187–210.
3. Wolinsky, L. E. (1994). Caries and cariology. In Nisengard, R. J., & Newman, M. G., Eds. *Oral microbiology and immunology* (2nd ed.). Philadelphia: W. B. Saunders, 341–59.
4. Nisengard, R. J., Newman, M. G., & Zambon, J. J. (1994). Periodontal disease. In Nisengard, R. J., & Newman, M. G., Eds. *Oral microbiology and immunology* (2nd ed.). Philadelphia: W. B. Saunders, 360–84.
5. Marsh, P. D. (1999). Microbiologic aspects of dental plaque and dental caries. *Dent Clin North Am*, 43:599–614.
6. Chen, C. (2001). Periodontitis as a biofilm infection. *J Calif Dent Assoc*, 29:362–67.
7. Schopf, J. W. (1974). The development and diversification of Precambrian life. *Orig Life*, 5:119–35.
8. Schopf, J. W. (1975). The age of microscopic life. *Endeavor*, 34:51–58.
9. Costerton, J. W., Cheng, K. J., Geesey, G. G., Ladd, T. I., Nickel, J. C., Dasgupta, M., & Marrie, T. J. (1987). Bacterial biofilms in nature and disease. *Ann Rev Microbiol*, 41:435–64.
10. Costerton, J. W., Lewandowski, Z., Caldwell, D. E., Korber, D. R., & Lappin-Scott, H. M. (1995). Microbial biofilms. *Ann Rev Microbiol*, 49:711–45.
11. Costerton, J. W., Cook, G., & Lamont, R. (1999). The community architecture of biofilms: Dynamic structures and mechanisms. In Newman, H. N., & Wilson, M., Eds. *Dental plaque revisited—Oral biofilms in health and disease.* Cardiff, U.K.: BioLine, 5–14.
12. Newman, H. N. (1974). Microbial films in nature. *Microbios*, 9:247–57.
13. Gilbert, P., Das, J., & Foley, I. (1997). Biofilm susceptibility to antimicrobials. *Adv Dent Res*, 11:160–67.
14. Bowden, G. H. W., & Hamilton, I. R. (1998). Survival of oral bacteria. *Crit Rev Oral Biol Med*, 9:54–85.
15. Socransky, S. S., & Haffajee, A. D. (2002). Dental biofilms: Difficult therapeutic targets. *Periodontol*, 2000, 28:12–55.
16. Van der Velden, U., Van Winkelhoff, A. J., & Abbas de Graf, J. (1986). The habitat of periodontopathic microorganisms. *J Clin Periodontol*, 13:243–48.
17. Listgarten, M. A. (1976). Structure of surface coatings of teeth. A review. *J Periodontol*, 47:139–47.
18. Ericson, T. (1967). Adsorption to hydroxyapatite of proteins and conjugated proteins from human saliva. *Caries Res*, 1:52–58.

19. Meckel, A. R. (1965). The formation of biological films. *Swed Dent J,* 10:585–99.

20. Leach, S. A., Critchley, P., Kolendo, A. B., & Saxton, C. A. (1967). Salivary glycoproteins as components of the enamel integuments. *Caries Res,* 1:104–11.

21. Mayhall, C. W. (1970). Concerning the composition and source of the acquired enamel pellicle on human teeth. *Arch Oral Biol,* 15:1327–41.

22. Hardie, J. M., & Bowden, G. H. (1976). The microbial flora of dental plaque: Bacterial succession and isolation considerations. In Stiles, H. M., Loesche, W. J., & O'Brien, T. C., Eds. Proceedings Microbial Aspects of Dental Caries. *Microbiol Abstr,* 1 (Spec Suppl):63–87.

23. Lie, T., & Gusberti, F. (1979). Replica study of plaque formation on human tooth surfaces. *Acta Odontol Scand,* 79:65–72.

24. Baier, R. E. (1977). On the formation of biological films. *Swed Dent J,* 1:261–71.

25. Tullberg, A. (1986). An experimental study of the adhesion of bacterial layers to some restorative dental materials. *Scand J Dent Res,* 94:164–73.

26. Kawai, K., & Urano. M. (2001). Adherence of plaque components to different restorative materials. *Oper Dent,* 26:396–400.

27. Quirynen, M., De Soete, M. & van Steenberghe, D. (2002). Infectious risks for oral implants: A review of the literature. *Clin Oral Implant Res,* 13:1–19.

28. Leach, S. A., & Critchley, P. (1966). Bacterial degradation of glycoprotein sugars in human saliva. *Nature,* 209:506.

29. Hay, D. I., & Oppenheim, I. G. (1974). The isolation from human parotid saliva of a further group of proline-rich proteins. *Arch Oral Biol,* 19:627–32.

30. Glenister, D. A., Salamon, K. E., Smith, K., Beighton, D., & Keevil, C. W. Enhanced growth of complex communities of dental plaque bacteria in mucin-limited continuous culture. *Microbiol Ecol Health Dis,* 1:31–38.

31. Gibbons, R. J., & van Houte, J. (1975). Bacterial adherence in oral microbial ecology. *Ann Rev Microbiol,* 29:19–44.

32. Weerkamp, A. H., van der Mei, H. C., & Engelen, D. P., et al. (1984). Adhesion receptors (adhesins) of oral streptococci. In ten Cate, J. M., Leach, S. A., & Arends, J., Eds. *Bacterial adhesion and preventive dentistry.* Oxford: IRL Press, 85–97.

33. Rosan, B. R., & Lamont, R. J. (2000). Dental plaque formation. *Microbes Infect,* 2:1599–1607.

34. Kraus, F. W., Orstavik, D., Hurst, D. C., & Cook, C. H. (1973). The acquired pellicle: Variability and subject dependence of specific proteins. *J Oral Pathol Med,* 2:165–73.

35. Orstavik, D., & Kraus, F. W. (1973). The acquired pellicle: Immunofluorescent demonstration of specific proteins. *J Oral Pathol Med,* 2:68–76.

36. Williams, R. C., & Gibbons, R. J. (1975). Inhibition of streptococcal attachment to receptors or human buccal epithelial cells by antigenically similar salivary glycoproteins. *Infect Immun,* 11:711–18.

37. Rogers, A. H., van der Hoeven, J. S., & Mikx, F. (1978). Inhibition of *Actinomyces viscosus* by bacteriocin producing strains of *Streptococcus mutans* in the dental plaque of gnotobiotic rats. *Arch Oral Biol,* 23:477–83.

38. Hammond, B. F., Lillard, S. E., & Stevens, R. H. (1987). A bacteriocin of *Actinobacillus actinomycetemcomitans. Infect Immun,* 55:686–91.

39. Christersson, L. A., Grossi, S. G., Dunford, R. G., Nachtei, E. E., & Genco, R. J. (1992). Dental plaque and calculus: Risk indicators for their formation. *J Dent Res,* 71:1425–30.

40. Baier, R. E., & Glantz, P. O. (1979). Characterization of oral *in vivo* film formed on different types of solid surfaces. *Acta Odontol Scand,* 36:289–301.

41. Liljemark, W. F., & Schauer, S. V. (1977). Competitive binding among oral streptococci to hydroxyapatite. *J Dent Res,* 56:156–65.

42. Kuramitsu, H., & Ingersoll, L. (1977). Molecular basis for the different sucrose-dependent adherence properties of *Streptococcus mutans* and *Streptococcus sanguis. Infect Immun,* 17:330–37.

43. Tanzer, J. M., & Johnson, M. C. (1976). Gradients for growth within intact *Streptococcus mutans* plaque *in vitro* demonstrated by autoradiography. *Arch Oral Biol,* 21:555–59.

44. Bjorn, H., & Carlsson, J. (1964). Observations on a dental plaque morphogenesis. *Odontol Rev,* 15:23–28.

45. Furuichi, Y., Lindhe, J., Ramberg, P., & Volpe, A. R. (1992). Patterns of de novo plaque formation in the human dentition. *J Clin Periodontol,* 19:423–33.

46. Howell, A., Jr., Risso, A., & Paul, F. (1965). Cultivable bacteria in developing and mature human dental calculus. *Arch Oral Biol,* 10:307–13.

47. Rudney, J. D. (2000). Saliva and dental plaque. *Adv Dent Res,* 14:29–39.

48. Newman, H. N. (1974). Diet, attrition, plaque and dental disease. *Br Dent J,* 136:491–97.

49. Leach, S. A. (1979). On the nature of interactions associated with aggregation phenomena in the mouth. *J Dent,* 7:149–60.

50. Rosenberg, M., Judes, H., & Weiss, E. (1983). Cell surface hydrophobicity of dental plaque microorganisms. *Infect Immun,* 42:831–34.

51. Busscher, H. J., & van der Mei, H. C. (1997). Physicochemical interactions in initial microbial adhesion and relevance for biofilm formation. *Adv Dent Res,* 11:24–32.

52. Doyle, R. J., Rosenberg, M., & Drake, D. (1990). Hydrophobicity of oral bacteria. In Doyle, R. J., Rosenberg, M., Eds. *Microbial cell surface hydrophobicity.* Washington, DC: American Society for Microbiology, 387–419.

53. Edgar, W. M. (1979). Studies of the role of calcium in plaque formation and cohesion. *J Dent,* 7:174–79.

54. Matsukubo, T., Katow, T., & Takazoe, I. (1978). Significance of Ca-binding activity of early plaque bacteria. *Bull Tokyo Dent Coll,* 19:53–57.

55. Rose, R. K., Dibdin, G. H., & Shellis, R. P. (1993). A quantitative study of calcium binding and aggregation in selected oral bacteria. *J Dent Res,* 72:78–84.

56. Newman, M. N., & Britton, A. B. (1974). Dental plaque ultrastructure as revealed by freeze-etching. *J Periodontol,* 45:478–88.

57. Germaine, G. R., Harlander, S. K., Leung, W.-L. S., & Schachtele, C. F. (1977). *Streptococcus mutans* dextransucrase: Functioning of primer dextran and endogenous dextransucrase in water-soluble and water-insoluble glucan synthesis. *Infect Immun,* 16:637–48.

58. Gibbons, R. J., & van Houte, J. (1980). Bacterial adherence and the formation of dental plaque. Receptors and recognition. In Beachey, E. H., Ed. *Bacterial adherence.* London. Chapman and Hall, Ltd., 6:63–104.

59. Ofek, I., & Perry, A. (1985). Molecular basis of bacterial adherence to tissues. In Mergenhagen, S. E., & Rosan, B., Eds. *Molecular basis of oral microbial adhesion.* Washington, DC: American Society for Microbiology, 7–13.

60. Gibbons, R. J. (1984). Adherent interactions which may affect microbial ecology in the mouth. *J Dent Res,* 63:378–85.

61. Clark, W. B., Wheeler, T. T., Lane, M. D., & Cisar, J. O. (1986). Actinomyces adsorption mediated by type-I fimbriae. *J Dent Res,* 65:1166–68.

62. Kolenbrander, P. E., & London, J. (1992). Ecological significance of coaggregation among oral bacteria. *Adv Microb Ecol,* 12:183–217.

63. Handley, P. S., McNab, R., & Jenkinson, H. F. (1999). Adhesive surface structures on oral bacteria. In Newman, H. N., & Wilson, M., Eds. *Dental plaque revisited—Oral biofilms in health and disease.* Cardiff: BioLine, 145–70.

64. Irwin, R. T. (1990). Hydrophobicity of proteins and bacterial fimbriae. In Doyle, R. J., & Rosenberg, M., Eds. *Microbial cell surface hydrophobicity.* Washington, DC: American Society of Microbiology, 137–77.

65. Cisar, J. O., Brennan, M. J., & Sandberg, A. L. (1985). Lectin-specific interaction of *Actinomyces* fimbriae with oral streptococci. In Mergenhagen, S. E., & Rosan, B., Eds. *Molecular basis of oral microbial adhesion.* Washington, DC: American Society for Microbiology, 159–63.

66. Kolenbrander, P. E., & Andersen, R. N. (1985). Use of co-aggregation-defective mutants to study the relationship of cell-to-cell interactions and oral microbial ecology. In Mergenhagen, S. E., & Rosan, B., Eds. *Molecular basis of oral microbial adhesion.* Washington, DC: American Society for Microbiology, 164–66.

67. Rosenberg, E. S., Evian, C. I., & Listgarten, M. A. (1981). The composition of the subgingival microbiota after periodontal therapy. *J Periodontol,* 52:435–41.

68. Cao, C. F., Aeppli, D. M., Liljemark, W. F., Bloomquist, C. G., Brandt, C. L., & Wolff, L. F. (1990). Comparison of plaque microflora between Chinese and Caucasian population groups. *J Clin Periodontol,* 17:115–18.

69. Listgarten, M. A., Mayo, H. E., & Tremblay, R. (1975). Development of dental plaque on epoxy resin crowns in man. A light and electron microscopic study. *J Periodontol,* 46:10–26.

70. Lie, T. (1978). Ultrastructural study of early plaque formation. *J Periodont Res,* 13:391–409.

71. Kolenbrander, P. E., & London, J. (1993). Adhere today, here tomorrow: Oral bacterial adherence. *J Bacteriol,* 175:3247–52.

72. Theilade, J., Fejerskov, O., & Hørsted, M. (1976). A transmission electron microscopic study of 7-day-old bacterial plaque in human tooth fissures. *Arch Oral Biol,* 21:587–98.

73. Newman, H. N. (1980). Retention of bacteria on oral surfaces. In Bitton, G., & Marshall, K. C., Eds. *Adsorption of microorganisms to surfaces.* New York: Wiley-Intersciences, 207–51.

74. Hardie, J. M., & Bowden, G. H. (1974). The normal microbial flora of the mouth. In Skinner, F. A., & Carr, J. G., Eds. *The normal microbial flora of man.* London: Academic Press, 47–83.

75. Socransky, S. S. (1977). Microbiology of periodontal disease—Present status and future considerations. *J Periodontol,* 48:497–504.

76. van Houte, J., Gibbons, R. J., & Banghart, S. B. (1970). Adherence as a determinant of the presence of *Streptococcus salivarius* and *Streptococcus sanguis* on the human tooth surface. *Arch Oral Biol,* 15:1025–34.

77. Donoghue, H. D., & Newman, H. N. (1976). Effect of glucose and sucrose on survival in batch culture of *Streptococcus mutans* C67-1 and a non-cariogenic mutant, C67-25. *Infect Immun,* 13:16–21.

78. Kilian, M., & Rölla, G. (1976). Initial colonization of teeth in monkeys as related to diet. *Infect Immun,* 14:1022–27.

79. Weerkamp, A. H. (1985). Coaggregation of *Streptococcus salivarius* with Gram-negative oral bacteria: Mechanism and ecological significance. In Mergenhagen, S. E., & Rosan, B., Eds. *Molecular basis of oral microbial adhesion.* Washington, DC: American Society for Microbiology, 177–83.

80. Ciardi, J. E., McCray, G. F. A., Kolenbrander, P. E., & Lau, A. (1987). Cell-to-cell interaction of *Streptococcus sanguis* and *Propionibacterium acnes* on saliva-coated hydroxyapatite. *Infect Immun,* 55:1441–46.

81. Lamont, R. J., & Rosan, B. (1990). Adherence of mutans streptococci to other oral bacteria. *Infect Immun,* 58:1738–43.

82. Shah, H. N., & Gharbia, S. E. (1991). Microbial factors in the aetiology of chronic inflammatory periodontal disease. In Newman, H. N., & Williams, D. N., Eds. *Inflammation and immunology in chronic inflammatory periodontal disease.* Northwood, England: Science Reviews Limited, 1–32.

83. Van der Hoeven, J. S., de Jong, M. H., & Kolenbrander, P. D. (1985). *In vivo* studies of microbial adherence in

dental plaque. In Mergenhagen, S. E., & Rosan, B., Eds. *Molecular basis of oral microbial adhesion.* Washington, DC: American Society for Microbiology, 220–27.

84. Globerman, D. Y., & Kleinberg, I. (1979). Intra-oral pO_2 and its relation to bacterial accumulation on the oral tissues. In Kleinberg, I., Ellison, S. A., Mandel, I. D., Eds. *Proceedings: Saliva and dental caries.* (A special supplement for *Microbiol Abst*). New York: Information Retrieval, 275–92.

85. Newman, H. N. (1973). The organic films on enamel surfaces. 2. The dental plaque. *Br Dent J,* 135:106–11.

86. Kolenbrander, P. E. (1991). Coaggregation: Adherence in the human oral microbial ecosystem. In Dworkin, M., Ed. *Microbial cell-cell interactions.* Washington, DC: American Society for Microbiology, 316.

87. Simmonds, R. S., Tompkins, G. R., & Goerge, R. J. (2000). Dental caries and the microbial ecology of dental plaque: a review of recent advances. *N Z Dent J,* 96:44–49.

88. Mattingly, S. J., Daneo-Moor, L., & Shockman, G. D. (1977). Factors regulating cell wall thickening and intracellular iodophilic polysaccharide storage in *Streptococcus mutans. Infect Immun,* 16:967–73.

89. Critchley, P., Wood, J. M., Saxton, C. A., & Leach, S. A. (1967). The polymerization of dietary sugars by dental plaque. *Caries Res,* 112–29.

90. McDougall, W. F. (1964). Studies on the dental plaque. IV. Levans and the dental plaque. *Aust Dent J,* 9:1–5.

91. Da Costa, T., & Gibbons, R. J. Hydrolysis of levan by human plaque streptococci. *Arch Oral Biol,* 13:609–17.

92. Manly, R. S., & Richardson, D. T. (1968). Metabolism of levan by oral samples. *J Dent Res,* 47:1080–86.

93. Newman, H. N. (1972). Structure of approximal human dental plaque as observed by scanning electron microscopy. *Arch Oral Biol,* 17:1445–53.

94. Soames, J. V., & Davies, R. M. (1975). The structure of subgingival plaque in a beagle dog. *J Periodont Res,* 9:333–41.

95. Löe, H., Theilade, E., & Jensen, S. B. (1965). Experimental gingivitis in man. *J Periodontol,* 36:177–87.

96. Kinane, D. F. (2001). Causation and pathogenesis of periodontal disease. *Periodontol 2000,* 25:8–20.

97. Petersilka, G. J., Ehmke, B., & Flemmig, T. F. (2002). Antimicrobial effects of mechanical debridement. *Periodontol 2000,* 28:56–71.

98. Mehrotra, K. K., Kapoor, K. K., Pradhan, B. P., & Bhushan, A. (1983). Assessment of plaque tenacity on enamel surface. *J Periodont Res,* 18:386–92.

99. White, D. J. (1997). Dental calculus: Recent insights into occurrence, formation, prevention, removal and oral health effects of supragingival and subgingival deposits. *Eur J Oral Sci,* 105:508–22.

100. Feldman, R. S., Bravacos, J. S., & Rose, C. L. (1983). Association between smoking different tobacco products and periodontal disease indexes. *J Periodontol,* 54:481–88.

101. Wotman, S., Mercadante, J., Mandel, I. D., Goldman, R. S., & Denning, C. (1973). The occurrence of calculus in normal children, children with cystic fibrosis, and children with asthma. *J Periodontol,* 44:278–80.

102. Klein, F. K., & Dicks, J. L. (1984). Evaluation of accumulation of calculus in tube-fed mentally handicapped patients. *J Am Dent Assoc,* 108:352–54.

103. Turesky, S., Breur, M., & Coffman, G. (1992). The effect of certain systemic medications on oral calculus formation. *J Periodontol,* 63:871–75.

104. ten Cate, J. M. (1988). *Recent advances in the study of dental calculus.* Oxford: IRL Press, 143–259.

105. McDougall, W. A. (1985). Analytical transmission electron microscopy of the distribution of elements in human supragingival dental calculus. *Arch Oral Biol,* 30:603–608.

106. Galil, K. A., & Gwinnett, A. J. (1975). Human tooth-fissure contents and their progressive mineralization. *Arch Oral Biol,* 2:559–62.

107. Turesky, S., Renstrup, G., & Glickman, I. (1961). Histologic and histochemical observations regarding early calculus formation in children and adults. *J Periodontol,* 32:7–14, 69–100.

108. Sundberg, M., & Friskopp, J. (1985). Crystallograph of supragingival human dental calculus. *Scand J Dent Res,* 93:30–38.

109. Schroeder, H. E. (1969). *Formation and inhibition of dental calculus.* Bern, Switzerland: Hans Huber Publishers, 559–62.

110. Listgarten, M. A., & Heneghan, J. B. (1973). Observations on the periodontium and acquired pellicle of adult germfree dogs. *J Periodontol,* 44:85–91.

111. Moskow, B. S. (1969). Calculus attachment in cemental separations. *J Periodontol,* 4:1125–30.

112. Selvig, K. A. (1970). Attachment of plaque and calculus to tooth surfaces. *J Periodontol Res,* 5:8–18.

113. Zacherl, W. A., Pfeiffer, H. J., & Swancar, J. R. (1985). The effect of soluble pyrophosphates on dental calculus in adults. *J Am Dent Assoc,* 110:737–38.

114. Ciancio, S. G. (1995). Chemical agents: Plaque control, calculus reduction and treatment of dentinal hypersensitivity. *Periodontol 2000,* 8:75–86.

115. Drake, D. R., Chung, J., Grigsby, W., & Wu-Yuan, C. (1992). Synergistic effect of pyrophosphate and sodium dodecyl sulfate on periodontal pathogens. *J Periodontol,* 63:696–700.

Chapter 3

Carious Lesions

Patricia R. Campbell

OBJECTIVES

After studying this chapter, the student should be able to:

1. Describe the four general types of carious lesions that are found on the different surfaces of the teeth.
2. Describe the histologic characteristics of enamel and dentin that facilitate fluid flow throughout a tooth.
3. Describe the four zones of an incipient caries lesion.
4. Describe the conduits (pores) that directly conduct acid from the bacterial plaque to the body of the lesion.
5. List the two bacteria most often implicated in the caries process, and indicate when each is present in the greatest numbers during the caries process.
6. Describe the series of events in a cariogenic plaque and subsurface lesion from the time of bacterial exposure to sugar until the pH returns to a resting state.
7. Describe the characteristics of root caries, and explain the differences and similarities to coronal caries.
8. Describe why so much time is taken by the profession in treating secondary caries.
9. Describe the relationship between pH and the saturation of calcium and phosphorus ions in caries development.
10. Describe the protective relationship of calcium fluoride to hydroxyapatite and fluorhydroxyapatite during an acidogenic attack.

KEY TERMS
Dental caries
Edentulism
Acidogenesis
Dental plaque
Plaque
Cariogenic
Incipient lesion
Xerostomia
Carious
Pit-and-fissure caries
Smooth-surface caries
Root-surface caries
Secondary/recurrent caries
Dentinoenamel junction
Overt lesion
Frank lesion
Rampant dental caries
Etiologic
Histologic
Periapical radiograph
Bitewing radiograph
Coronally
Pore space

(continued)

KEY TERMS (CONTINUED)

Remineralization
Enamel rods
Striae of Retzius
Inter-rod space
Dentinal tubules
Pulp chamber
Cariogenic
Caries-inactive
Caries-free
Glucans
Aciduric
Colonization
Primary colonizers
Ameloblasts
Odontoblasts
Dental pulp
Odontoblastic process
Predentin

Peritubular dentin
Enamel spindles
Intertubular dentin
Mantle dentin
Canaliculi
Inter-rod areas
Sclerotic dentin
Reparative dentin
Dentition
Root caries
Cementum–dentin complex
Cemento–enamel junction
Arrested root caries
Secondary caries
Composites
Glass ionomers
Amalgams
Stephan curve

INTRODUCTION

Dental caries is one of the most common diseases in humans; caries causes pain and disability and can lead to infection, tooth loss, and **edentulism** (loss of all teeth).[1,2] Researchers have also discovered connections between chronic oral infections and other chronic diseases such as diabetes, cardiovascular diseases, osteoporosis, and obesity.[3]

One of the oldest theories of caries and toothache was that of the tooth worm, which allegedly lived in the center of the tooth.[4] Various therapies were used to eradicate the tooth worm such as fumigations with henbane seeds, magical formulas, and oaths.[5] In the early 1700s Pierre Fauchard, the father of modern dentistry, rejected the tooth worm theory, described caries as an erosion of the enamel, and recommended those areas be smoothed with the use of files. In 1881, two speakers at the International Medical Congress, Miles and Underwood, proposed that dental caries was caused by the presence and proliferation of organisms.[2]

In 1890 W. D. Miller, an American dentist teaching in Germany, published his chemicoparasitic theory of caries, which is still accepted, in concept, today.[6,7] As a result of his experimentation, Miller believed that extraction of the lime salts from the teeth was a result of bacterial **acidogenesis,** and was the first step in dental decay. However, Miller's work failed to identify **dental plaque** as the source of the bacteria and the bacterial acids. The chemicoparasitic theory became more convincing when combined with the findings of other contemporary dental researchers, including G. V. Black, who described the gelatinous microbic **plaque** as the source of the acids.[8]

MULTIFACTORIAL DISEASE PROCESS

Dental caries is a multifactorial disease process, often represented by the interlocking circles and an arrow depicting the passage of time (Figure 3–1 ■). For caries to develop, four conditions must occur simultaneously: (1) There must be a susceptible tooth and host; (2) **cariogenic** microorganisms must be present in a sufficient quantity; (3) there

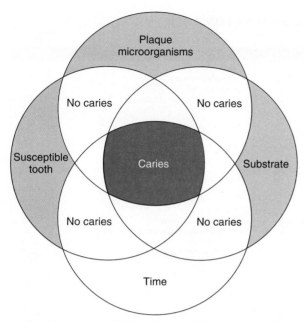

■ **FIGURE 3–1**   Dental caries: multifactorial disease process.

must be frequent excessive consumption of refined carbohydrates; and (4) this process must occur over a sufficiently long period of time. When a tooth covered with cariogenic bacteria is exposed to a suitable substrate, such as a refined carbohydrate, the bacteria produce acid. If these conditions persist over a sufficiently long period of time, an incipient lesion develops. An **incipient lesion** is the initial stage of tooth decay that has not penetrated the outer surface of the tooth. The lesion looks like a white spot on the enamel.

Each of these main factors includes a number of secondary factors, which can be introduced to either protect or further damage the tooth. For example, in the susceptible tooth/host condition, fluoride incorporated into dental enamel increases tooth resistance. Conversely, **xerostomia** greatly increases the caries risk of a susceptible tooth/host.

A risk assessment form for dental caries is shown in Figure 3–2 ■. This form includes existing conditions and risk factors that may contribute to the development of dental carious lesions, and preventive strategies to reduce the occurrence of dental caries.

DENTAL CARIES DESCRIPTION

Carious lesions occur in four general areas of the tooth:

1. **Pit-and-fissure caries** are found mainly on the occlusal surfaces of posterior teeth; in lingual pits

of the maxillary incisors; and in buccal pits located on the surfaces of lower molars;
2. **Smooth-surface caries** arise on intact smooth enamel surfaces other than at the location of the pits and fissures.
3. **Root-surface caries** might involve any surface of the root.
4. **Secondary/recurrent caries** occur on the tooth surface adjacent to an existing restoration.

Smooth-surface caries can be further divided into (1) caries that affect the buccal and lingual tooth surfaces, and (2) interproximal caries, which affect the contact area of adjoining tooth surfaces (i.e., mesial or distal surfaces).

PHYSICAL AND MICROSCOPIC FEATURES OF INCIPIENT CARIES

The development of a carious lesion occurs in three distinct stages (Figure 3–3 ■). The earliest stage is the incipient lesion, which is accompanied by histologic changes of the enamel. The changes include demineralization, which, simply put, is loss of calcium and phosphorus and other ions from the enamel. The second stage includes the progress of demineralization toward the **dentinoenamel junction** (DEJ), the point at which the dentin of the tooth and the enamel meet. Demineralization then continues into the dentin. The final phase of caries development is the development of the **overt,** or **frank, lesion,** which is characterized by actual cavitation. If the time between the onset of the incipient lesion in one or more teeth and the development of cavitation is rapid and extensive, the condition is referred to as **rampant dental caries.** Usually rampant caries occurs after either the excessive and frequent intake of sucrose, or the presence of severe xerostomia, or both. The early identification of the incipient lesion is extremely important, because it is during this stage that the carious process can be arrested or reversed. The overt lesion can be treated *only* by operative intervention.

Clinically, it is often difficult to recognize and diagnose the early lesion; for this reason it is important to be familiar with its features from **etiologic** and **histologic** standpoints.[9] The incipient lesion is macroscopically evidenced on the tooth surface by the appearance of an area of opacity, the white spot lesion. At this earliest clinically visible stage, the subsurface demineralization at the microscopic level is well established, with a number of recognizable zones. Interestingly, the surface of the enamel appears relatively intact, although the electron

ORAL DISEASE RISK ASSESSMENT FOR ADULTS

RISK CATEGORY	EXISTING CONDITIONS		TREATMENT CONSIDERATIONS	CODE
Caries Risk	*Please use a check mark to indicate caries risk*	☑		

Low	No carious lesions in previous 3 years
	Adequately restored dentition
	Adequate oral hygiene
	Regular dental visits
	Diet History:
	    Consumes food/beverages<five times daily
	    Chews sugar-free gum
	    Avoids sweetened beverages between meals
	    Avoids refined sugars and/or fermentable
	        carbohydrates between meals
	    Drinks milk or eats cheese every day
			Review oral hygiene practices
			Review dietary factors
			Recommend fluoride dentifrice
			One year recall (repeat ODRA)
				1330
				1310
				
				0170

Moderate	One carious lesion in previous 3 years
	Exposed roots
	Fair oral hygiene
	Presence of white spots lesions (not fluorosis)
	Presence of interproximal radiolucencies (not into dentin)
	Irregular dental visits
	Orthodontic treatment (planned or in progress)
	Diet History:
	    Eats food or drinks beverages five or more times daily
	    Chews regular (non-sugar-free) gum
	    Drinks sweetened beverages between meals
	    Eats refined sugars and/or fermentable carbohydrates
	        between meals
	    Does not drink milk or eat cheese every day
			Pit and Fissure Caries:
			    Oral hygiene instructions
			    Nutritional counseling
			    Sealants
			    Preventive resins
			Smooth Surface, Recurrent and root Caries:
			    Oral hygiene instructions
			    Nutritional counseling
			Professionally applies topical fluoride
			Recommend fluoride dentifrice
			Rx for self-applied fluoride
			Six month recall (repeat ODRA)
				
				1330
				1310
				1351
				2391
				
				1330
				1310
				1360
				
				1340
				0170

High	Two carious lesions in previous three years
	Previous root caries or numerous exposed roots
	Deep pits and fissures
	Poor oral hygiene
	Frequent sugar intake
	Inadequate use of topical fluoride
	Irregular dental visits
	Inadequate saliva flow
	Orthodontic treatment (planned or in progress)
	Diet History: (As described in moderate caries risk above)
			Pit and Fissure Caries:
			    Oral hygiene instructions
			    Nutritional counseling
			    Sealants
			    Preventive resins
			Smooth Surface, Recurrent and root Caries:
			    Oral hygiene instructions
			    Nutritional counseling
			Professionally applies topical fluoride
			Recommend fluoride dentifrice
			Rx for self-applied fluoride
			3-6 month recall (repeat ODRA)
			Antimicrobial agents
				
				1330
				1310
				1351
				2391
				
				1330
				1310
				1360
				
				1340
				0170
				4381

Other Risks	*Please use Y (yes) or N (no) to indicate risk.*	*Y/N*		

Xerostomia	Patient's mouth dry when eating a meal
	Difficulty in swallowing food
	Liquid needed to aid swallowing
	"Too little" saliva in mouth most of the time
	Medications with potential to cause Xerostomia
	Head & neck radiation therapy
			Evaluate for stimulated and un-stimulated
			    flow reduction
			Evaluate contributing factors
			Fluoride therapy (see above)
			Oral hygiene instructions (special products)
			Select appropriate restorative materials
			Nutritional and hydration counseling
			Referral for salivary dysfunction evaluation
			    (unless medication - induced)
				
				0415

Regressive Alterations or Injury	Evidence of tooth erosion/abrasion Evidence of tooth attrition/bruxism Evidence of maladaptive oral habits Risk of oral injury (contact sport, no seatbelt use, physical abuse)		Oral hygiene instructions Occlusal guard Athletic mouth guard	1330 9940
Periodontal Risks	History of periodontitis Soft tissue disease Diabetes Genetics Tobacco or marijuana use		Follow periodontal treatment protocol Advise patient of potential risks	
Cancer Risks	HX of oral cancer Tobacco user past or present Heavy alcohol use Sunlight exposure/fair-skinned patient		Schedule intraoral/extraoral examination annually Teach patient oral self-examination Tobacco counseling to control/prevent oral disease: 5A program, RX nicotine cessation, refer as appropriate)	0120 1301 1320

Date: ___/___/___   Student: [_____]   Faculty: [_____]
        MO   DAY   YR   SIGNATURE STAMP   SIGNATURE STAMP

■ **FIGURE 3-2**   Oral disease risk assessment worksheet.

(Baylor School of Dentistry, Texas A&M Health Science Center, Dallas. Used with permission.)

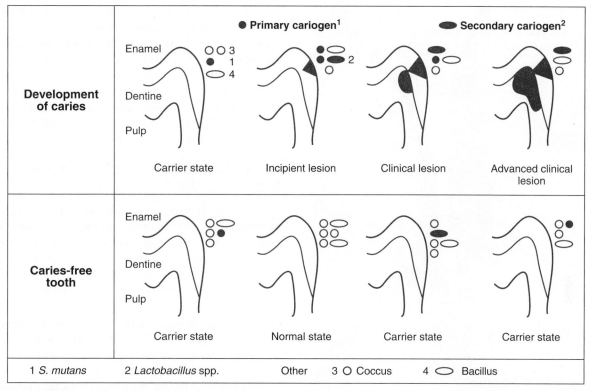

Primary cariogen[1] ● **Secondary cariogen[2]** ◗

Enamel
Dentine
Pulp

Development of caries

Carrier state / Incipient lesion / Clinical lesion / Advanced clinical lesion

Caries-free tooth

Carrier state / Normal state / Carrier state / Carrier state

| 1 *S. mutans* | 2 *Lactobacillus* spp. | Other | 3 ○ Coccus | 4 ◯ Bacillus |

■ **FIGURE 3–3** Development of a carious lesion.
(Retrieved June 27, 2007, from http://www.gsbs.utmb.edu/microbook/ch099.htm. Used with permission.)

microscope shows a surface that is more porous than sound enamel. On the buccal and lingual surface of a tooth, the white spot may be localized, or it can extend along the entire gingival area of the tooth, or along multiple teeth at places where food tends to lodge between the teeth. Interproximally, the incipient lesion is usually first detected on a **periapical** or **bitewing radiograph.** The lesion usually starts as a small radiolucency located immediately on the gingival side of the contact point, and then gradually expands to a small kidney shape, with the indentation of the kidney contour directed **coronally.**[10] In fissure caries, the initial lesion, comparable to the "white spot," usually occurs bilaterally on the two surfaces of the fissure at its orifice. The lesion eventually coalesces at the base of the fissure (Figures 3–4 ■ and 3–5 ■).[11] Occasionally, lesion formation begins below the tooth surface along the wall of the fissure or at its base, either unilaterally or bilaterally.[11]

During the early stages, the incipient lesion is not a surface lesion in which loss of outer enamel can be detected. Instead, the mature surface layer remains intact. If an explorer is used, the surface enamel feels hard and provides no indication of demineralization. However, microscopic pores extend through the mature surface layer to the point where subsurface demineralization occurs; the main body of the lesion is located and enlarges from this point.

The incipient lesion has been extensively studied and is best described by Silverstone.[10] Many of the observations of the incipient lesion have been based on the use of a polarizing microscope. This microscope permits precise measurements of the amount of space, called **pore space,** which exists in normal enamel and to a greater extent in enamel defects. Thus, as demineralization progresses, more pore space occurs; in contrast, during **remineralization,** less pore space is present.

In the incipient lesion as described by Silverstone, four zones are usually present. Starting from the tooth surface, the four zones are the (1) surface zone, (2) body of the lesion, (3) dark zone, and (4) the translucent zone.

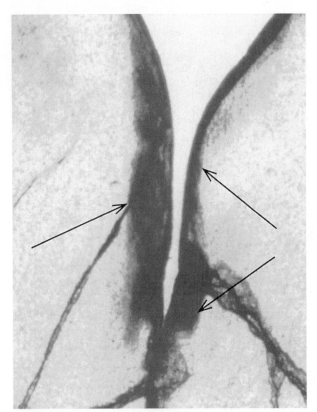

■ FIGURE 3–4 Incipient caries in an occlusal fissure. The bilaterality of the lesion is evident in the microradiograph.
(Courtesy of J. S. Wefel, University of Iowa College of Dentistry, Iowa City.)

Pore Spaces of the Different Zones

The translucent zone, the deepest zone, is seen in approximately 50% of the carious lesions examined.[10] In this zone, which is the advancing front of the lesion, slight demineralization occurs, resulting in a 1% pore space, compared with 0.1% for intact enamel. In contrast, the dark zone occurs in approximately 95% of carious lesions and has a pore volume of 2% to 4%. When teeth showing no dark zone are placed in a remineralizing solution, the dark zone becomes visible in its expected position between the translucent zone and the body of the lesion.[12] On the basis of this phenomenon, it is suggested that this dark zone is the site where remineralization can occur, and that a wider dark zone requires a greater amount, or a longer period, of remineralization.

Peripheral to the dark zone lies the main body of the lesion. In this zone, pore volume ranges from approximately 5% on the fringes of the lesion to about 25% in the center.[10] Despite this considerable amount of demineralization, the remaining crystals still maintain their basic orientation on the protein matrix. Finally, the surface zone has a near-normal pore space of approximately 1%. The surface zone and the dark zone are the remineralization zones of the incipient lesion.

Direct Connection of the Bacterial Biofilm to the Body of the Lesion

Tooth enamel is made up of interlocking structures called **enamel rods,** which contain billions of crystals. The pores present between the crystals and the rods form a network of channels that allow fluid diffusion of ions and small molecules found in the enamel cap. Other structures such as the **striae of Retzius** extend this network into deeper layers of the enamel. This diffusion network allows remineralization of the tooth throughout its life; however, the channels also allow plaque acids to enter the interior enamel, causing demineralization.

Demineralization of the surface enamel produces a ragged profile; in fact, the initial attack may be on the ends of the enamel rods, between the rods, or both.[13] There is a subsequent widening of the areas between adjacent rods (**inter-rod space**).[14] When conditions are optimum, this ragged interface between surface and subsurface can be remineralized, either by the body defenses, such as calcium and phosphate and other ions from the saliva, or by man-made strategies, such as fluoride therapy and reduction of fermentable carbohydrates in the diet.

En route to the DEJ, the striae of Retzius allow access out of the inter-rod space into the center of the intact or damaged rods and crystals. Once at the DEJ, any fluid flow, whether it causes demineralization or remineralization, can trichotomize (go in three directions), either along the hypomineralized DEJ in either direction, or into the **dentinal tubules** to the **pulp chamber** (Figure 3–6 ■). The speed of progression of the caries front depends on such factors as ion concentration, pH, saliva flow, and buffering actions—all of which are continually changing. In summary, there is a trail of interconnecting channels for diffusion of fluids moving from the bacterial plaque to the pulp chamber. Any chemical changes in the plaque can soon be reflected throughout the enamel and dentin as part of the incipient lesion.

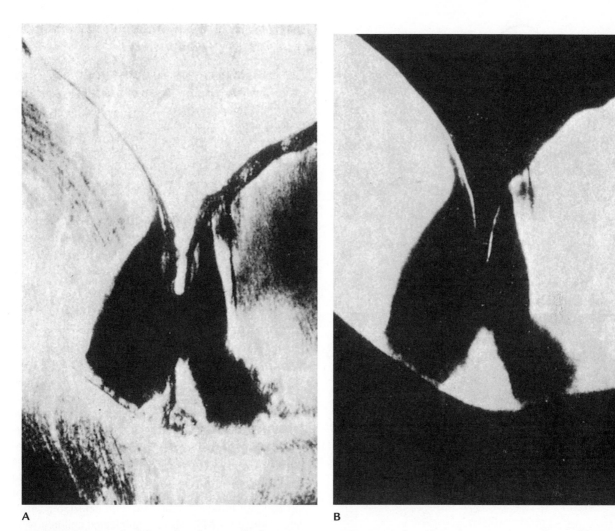

A

B

■ **FIGURE 3–5**   The bilaterality of caries development. Note coalescence of two lateral carious areas at base of fissure. (From Konig, K. G. (1963). Dental morphology in relation to carious resistance with special reference to fissures as susceptible areas. *J Dent Res,* 42:461–76.)

The pores allow plaque acids to exit directly to the subsurface region. The initial acid attack preferentially dissolves the magnesium and carbonate ions, followed by removal of the less-soluble calcium, phosphate, and other ions that are part of the crystal.

Eventually the undermined surface zone collapses. At the same time, the more soluble proteins are lost from the subsurface matrix. Once cavitation occurs, the zones of the incipient lesion become less clearly defined because of mineral loss and the presence of bacteria, bacterial end products, biofilm, and residual substrate, which may support further lesion development with cavitation.

The lesion is no longer an incipient lesion—but an overt caries lesion requiring operative intervention.

CARIOGENIC BACTERIA

Following Miller's works in the 1890s, it was not until 1954 that fundamental experimental evidence proved bacteria were the agents of acid production. Orland and colleagues demonstrated that gnotobiotic rats (rats grown in a germ-free environment) did not develop caries when fed a **cariogenic** diet that promotes tooth decay. However, they did develop caries when acidogenic bacteria,

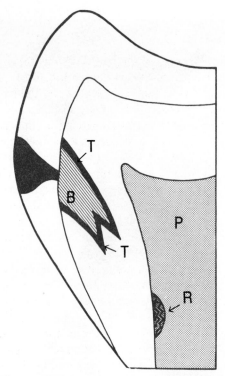

■ FIGURE 3–6 Diagram of a trichotomized lesion attributable to diffusion of acids in both directions under the enamel and directly into the body of the lesion in the dentin. T, translucent zone; B, body of the lesion; R, reactionary dentin; P, pulp.

(From Silverstone L. M., & Hicks, M. J. (1985). The structure and ultrastructure of the carious lesion in human dentin. *Gerodontics,* 1:185–93.)

plus a cariogenic diet, were introduced into the previous germ-free environment.[15] The transmissible nature of caries in animals was later demonstrated by the experiments of Keyes, who showed that previously gnotobiotic hamsters who were **caries-inactive** (i.e., had incipient lesions but no cavitation) developed caries after contact with animals.[16]

Mutans Streptococci and Caries

For caries to develop, acidogenic bacteria must be present, and a means must exist to prevent the acid from being washed away from the point where the carious lesion is to develop. Dental plaque fulfills both of these functions. It helps protect the bacterial colonies from being flushed, neutralized, or affected by antimicrobials in the saliva by enveloping the colonies in a cocoon of gel-like glucan, an insoluble extracellular polysaccharide.

Of the 300-or-more species of microorganisms inhabiting the plaque, the great majority are not directly involved in the caries process. Two bacterial genera are of special interest in cariogenesis: (1) the mutans streptococci and (2) the lactobacilli.[17,18] Mutans streptococci (MS) are a group of bacterial species characterized by their ability to produce extracellular glucans from sucrose and by their acid production in animal and human studies. One species in this group, *Streptococcus mutans,* received its name in 1924 when J. K. Clarke, in England, isolated organisms from human carious lesions. He noted that they were more oval than round and assumed them to be a mutant form of a streptococcus.[19]

Mutans streptococci are now considered to be the major pathogenic bacterial species involved in the caries process.[20–29] Mutans streptococci are usually found in relatively large numbers in the plaque that occurs immediately over developing smooth-surface lesions. In one study, specific sites were periodically sampled for the presence of MS, and the teeth were later examined for caries. Teeth destined to become carious exhibited a significant increase in the proportions of MS from 6 to 24 months before the eventual diagnosis of caries.[30] Similarly, dental plaques isolated from sites overlying white spot lesions have a significantly higher proportion of MS than plaques sampled from sound enamel sites.[31] Increased numbers of MS in the saliva also parallel the development of the smooth-surface lesion. In another study, MS counts from the saliva of 200 children indicated that 93% with detectable caries were positive for MS, whereas uninfected children were almost always **caries-free.**[32]

Certain physiologic characteristics of the MS favor their reputation as a prime agent in caries. These traits include the ability to adhere to tooth surfaces, production of abundant **glucans** from sucrose, rapid production of lactic acid from a number of sugar substrates, acid tolerance, and the production of intracellular polysaccharide (energy) stores. These features help the MS survive in an unfriendly environment related to periods of very low availability of substrate (i.e., between meals and snacks). As a general rule, the cariogenic bacteria metabolize sugars to produce the energy required for their growth and reproduction. The byproducts of this metabolism are acids, which are released into the plaque fluid. The damage caused by MS is mainly caused by lactic acid, although other acids, such as butyric and propionic, are present within the plaque.[33]

Lactobacilli and Caries

Lactobacilli (LB) are cariogenic, acidogenic, and **aciduric.** From the early 1920s until the 1950s, LB was considered the essential bacteria that caused caries. It was not until 1954 when the studies of Orland demonstrated that if rodents living in a germ-free environment were infected with lactic acid–producing enterococci, but no LB, they still developed caries.[15] This was the first knowledge that LB were not required for caries development. Often, the number of LB isolated from either saliva or plaque was too low in number to be considered capable of producing the range of pH values required for initiation of caries.[34] However, once a caries lesion develops, the stability of the immediate plaque population changes rapidly. The low pH environment of LB often eliminates, or at least suppresses, the continuity of **colonization** of MS (i.e., its formation of compact groups of bacteria).[35,36]

This phenomenon, of a lowering pH causing MS to be displaced by LB, is seen after irradiation therapy for head and neck cancer. During the treatment, multiple caries lesions develop rapidly because of the destruction of the salivary glands.[37] During the initial phases of the developing carious lesions, large numbers of MS are involved, only to decrease in number later as the LB population increases. This decrease is believed to be caused by LB creating a sufficiently low pH to establish a monopoly of the environment.

ADHERENCE OF BACTERIA TO TEETH

Continuous adherence to the solid tooth surface by MS is necessary both before and after initial colonization. The first bacteria must establish a foothold on the acquired pellicle on the tooth surface, and then maintain their positions while other bacteria continue to colonize in other protected areas offered by the interproximal spaces, along the gingiva, or in the pits and fissures. Otherwise the bacteria would be swept away by the saliva.

Children who consume little or no sucrose because of sucrase or fructase enzyme deficiencies have a less-cariogenic plaque. Similarly, patients receiving long-term nourishment via a stomach tube have less plaque and fewer MS.[38] Individuals restricting their sucrose intake have a decreased proportion of MS in their plaque, but the MS increases when sucrose is reintroduced into the diet.[39] Dietary restriction of sugar has also been shown to reduce the acidogenicity of dental plaque.[40,41]

ECOLOGY OF CARIES DEVELOPMENT
Caries Transmission

Several studies support the possibility that the first bacteria to adhere to teeth (**primary colonizers**) can help determine the eventual pathogenicity of the plaque.[30] Once a species of bacteria has established a haven safe from competing bacteria and saliva (i.e., its ecologic niche), other bacteria introduced at a later date appear to have a more difficult task in colonizing. Once established, a niche can last a long time. For instance, children with the highest number of MS for primary teeth usually experience a higher attack rate for the later permanent teeth.[42]

Mutans streptococci require a solid surface, the tooth surface, for successful colonization. During the first year of life before eruption of the primary teeth, very few MS are found in the mouth.[43] When teething begins at approximately 8 months, MS often rapidly colonize the plaque of newly erupting teeth.[44] It has been shown that an important source of infection of infants by MS is from the caregivers, usually the mother, by mouth-to-mouth transmission via kissing, or by sharing a spoon during feeding.[45] Mothers with the highest MS counts often have infants with similarly high counts of caries lesions.[46] Because early infection by MS is associated with high decay rates, it has been strongly suggested that an effective means of preventing caries in young children would be to reduce the number of MS in the parents' and siblings' mouths before a child's birth.[47] There is growing evidence that mothers using xylitol gums or lozenges have decreased levels of MS and do not transmit these cariogenic bacteria as readily to their children.[48] Xylitol is a sugar alcohol that has a sweet taste, but is less cariogenic than sucrose.

At the time of eruption, no populations of bacteria are entrenched on the tooth's surface; therefore, primary colonizers probably have little difficulty in establishing their ecologic niches on the acquired pellicle and in the saliva. After tooth eruption, many bacteria already present in the mouth participate in the formation of plaque. Each firmly established niche can act as a "seeding" area for other areas of the mouth. Mutans streptococci decrease in number as teeth are lost throughout life and practically disappear after full-mouth extraction.[49] After dentures are inserted, MS reappear, only to disappear again when the dentures are removed for an extended period.

Coronal Dentin Caries

During the embryonic stage of the tooth, the ameloblasts and the odontoblasts are lined up at the location of the future DEJ.[50] **Ameloblasts** are responsible for the formation of enamel, which becomes the future surface of the tooth, whereas **odontoblasts** are responsible for the formation of the dentin, which becomes the border of the dental pulp. The primary function of enamel is to protect the underlying dentin. In turn, the dentin forms a protective layer around the dental pulp. Dentin also contains a network of tubules that allows the transport of fluids to and from the dental pulp. The **dental pulp** is located at the center of the tooth and contains nerves and blood vessels, which provide nutrients to the tooth through the dentinal tubules. A detailed description of these processes follows.

During the period of tooth formation, each day each odontoblast lays down a trailing **odontoblastic process,** which is an extension of the odontoblast into the dentinal tubules. The substance secreted by an odontoblast (i.e., **predentin**) travels through the odontoblastic process and is deposited at the edge of the dental pulp. The participation of numerous odontoblasts in this process results in the formation of a concentric, incremental layer of predentin. Each succeeding day the predentin becomes a calcified layer of dentin and forms a tubule around the odontoblastic process. The lining of the tubule is a hypercalcified layer called the **peritubular dentin.** Most of these tubules extend from the DEJ to the dental pulp, and a few extend into the enamel as **enamel spindles.**

Between the tubules there is **intertubular dentin,** also called **mantle dentin.**[51] The tubules contain fluid that originates from the pulp chamber. There is intertubular communication and fluid transport, via secondary tubules and smaller-sized **canaliculi.** All tubules act as channels for the convection flow of fluids that flow outward from the pulp.[52] Dentinal fluid is constantly pumped into tubules by the forces of mastication, with a return of the fluid to the pulp upon release of the pressure.[53] When infection products, such as caries, arrive in the tubules, more fluid is forced into the tubule.[54,55] The pulp fluid also contains important calcium, phosphate, and secretory immunoglobulin A.[55,56]

When enamel caries reach the DEJ, many of the odontoblastic processes underlying the carious **inter-rod areas** of the enamel will lose their vitality. These tubules become dead tracts and may begin to partially or wholly calcify. The complete calcification results in a hard calcified group of tubules, called **sclerotic dentin,** which acts as a protective barrier to the advancing caries. At the same time, the odontoblasts located on the periphery of the pulp are triggered to begin laying down increments of amorphous **reparative dentin** to further protect the pulp.

In summary, the millions of diffusion and convection channels in the enamel and dentin, respectively, permit movement of fluid from the tooth surface to the pulp.[57,58] The intertubular secondary canals and the canaliculi provide permeability within the dentin, whereas the DEJ allows acid to move laterally in these channels, which can undermine the enamel and aid in its collapse to form an overt caries lesion. According to in vitro studies, if an x-ray shows a radiolucency that extends even into deep dentin, the entire precaries lesion can theoretically and slowly be remineralized *if* the surface zone where the caries began has not broken down into an overt cavity.[59]

Root Caries

A general demographic shift is continually occurring in the United States, with each successive generation living longer and retaining more of their natural **dentition.** This increase can be attributed to the success of dental hygiene in preventing and controlling infectious diseases during the last century.[60,61] Older adults are retaining much of their natural dentition, which provides a longer time for gingival recession and root caries to take place. In addition, this population is consuming an increasing number of medications that are known to reduce saliva production and cause **root caries.**[62] Katz and colleagues estimated that individuals entering their thirties have about 1 in 100 surfaces with recession and root caries. When they enter their sixties, about 1 of 5 exposed surfaces is involved. The roots of the molars in the mandible are at greatest risk, whereas the mandibular incisors are at the least risk.[63]

The Third National Health and Nutrition Examination Survey found that the percentage of persons with at least one decayed or filled root surface increased from 20.8% in those aged 35 to 44 years to 55.9% in those aged 75 years and older.[64] A Canadian study concluded that the increase in the prevalence of root decay with age may not be due to aging per se; instead, the increase may be the result of neglect of oral health during the years of growing older. Older adults with continual good oral health still had low rates of root decay.[65] A study of

5000 subjects in Finland found that men had 1.1 to 2.5 times more root caries than women. The greatest difference was in the group 60 to 69 years of age.[66]

A number of risk factors have been identified for root caries development, including age, gender, fluoride exposure, systemic illness, medications, oral hygiene, and diet.[67,68] In terms of the microbiology of root caries, despite early indications of a strong association between the *Actinomyces* species and progressive root lesions,[69,70] more recent studies indicate that plaque and salivary concentrations of MS are correlated positively with the presence of root-surface caries.[69–72]

Root caries differs from coronal caries in several aspects. A critical difference is that the tissues affected, enamel versus cementum, are fundamentally dissimilar. Enamel on the tooth surface is much more highly mineralized than the cementum, which covers the root surface, or the dentin. Because of the lower mineral content and higher organic content of the **cementum–dentin complex,** root caries may progress both by acid demineralization of the inorganic structure and by proteolysis of the organic component.[73] In proteolysis, the organic components (proteins) are broken down into simpler substances, usually through the action of enzymes. These tissue variations determine the differences in the rate of lesion formation, its histologic and visual appearance, and the potential for and rate of remineralization.[74] Clinically, the lesion is initially non-cavitated. The carious material is soft and has a yellowish-brown coloration. The lesion can eventually assume any outline and may involve multiple root surfaces (Figure 3–7 ■). When cavitation is evident, lesions tend to spread laterally, have a depth of approximately 0.5 to 1.0 mm, and have a dark-brown appearance.[75] The lesions appear immediately below the **cemento–enamel junction,** undermining but not involving the enamel.

Root caries differ from coronal caries in that bacterial invasion of cementum and dentin occurs quickly once the cariogenic process begins. At times in the invasion, columns of organisms appear between spikes of relatively intact cementum. At other times, a complete loss of cementum exposes the dentin. Similar to enamel caries, root caries are amenable to remineralization and/or arrest.[74] **Arrested root caries** demonstrate three physical characteristics: (1) an outer barrier of hypermineralized surface dentin; (2) a sclerotic inner barrier between carious and sound dentin; and (3) mineralization occurring within the dentinal tubules.[75] Clinically, such remineralized lesions may appear dark

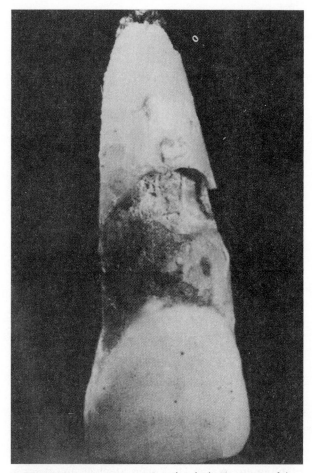

■ **FIGURE 3–7** Root caries. The darker staining of the coronal half of the root indicates considerable gingival recession, which is a prerequisite to lesion development.

and hard; tactile examination with a dental explorer easily distinguishes the smooth, hard, and glassy feel of arrested lesions from the leathery feel of active root caries.

Secondary, or Recurrent, Caries

Secondary caries start with small imperfections or restoration overhangs that exist between the tooth surface and the margins of a restoration.[76] Also, some tooth-colored fillings (**composites**) have a higher affinity for plaque.[77] Bacteria are able to colonize and multiply at these vulnerable sites, sheltered from the protective effects of saliva and patients' self-care efforts. Eventually, a lesion develops between the cavity margin and the restoration.

Diagnosis of these lesions is difficult.[78,79] In one study, extracted teeth were cut so that the section included both a clinically sound amalgam margin and one defined as "ditched." The prevalence of recurrent lesions in both sound and ditched restorations was close to 50%, although it is unknown whether these lesions were truly recurrent or due to residual caries left during a previous cavity preparation.[80] The magnitude of the problem of secondary decay is illustrated by studies indicating that the median survival time of restorations ranges from 5 to 10 years.[81] Prevention of the number of primary lesions will help and would be the best solution. Some future relief may be forthcoming from the use of materials that bond directly to the tooth tissue, thus eliminating the gap between tooth and filling, or from restorative materials that slowly release fluoride. Fluoride-releasing materials include **glass ionomers,** and the newer fluoride-releasing composites and **amalgams.**[82–84]

Measuring Plaque pH, the Stephan Curve

There is a continuous pH change in the plaque every time food is consumed. In many studies, pH microelectrodes have been inserted in bridges and telemonitored to determine these changes. There is an almost immediate drop in pH when sugar or sugary snacks are eaten, followed by a longer recovery period than when other foods are eaten. This drop-and-recovery curve has been termed the **Stephan curve** after Dr. Robert Stephan, an officer in the United States Public Health Service, who first reported the continuous changes in pH that followed eating and drinking of different foods and beverages.[85] Plaque pH responses to simple sugar rinses performed by caries-free and caries-active individuals exhibited different drops in pH and different lengths of time to return to normal. Thus, different individuals have different capabilities to buffer acid production (Figure 3–8 ■). Similar pH studies have identified foods that are not hazardous to the teeth, as well as those that are accompanied by a drop past the critical pH of 5.5 to 5.0, such as dried fruits, white bread, cereals, and starchy foods. These lists are of considerable value when counseling patients.[86]

The Relationship of Saturation to pH

The concentration of calcium and phosphate ions in the plaque fluid bathing the tooth at the plaque–tooth interface is extremely important, because these are the same elements that compose the hydroxyapatite crystal found

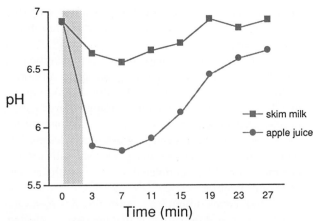

■ **FIGURE 3–8**   Stephan curves. These curves show the typical plaque pH response to an oral glucose rinse (indicated by the screened area). An immediate fall in the pH is followed by a gradual return to resting values after about 40 minutes. Each curve represents the mean of 12 subjects; the pH was measured by sampling method and therefore is an average value for the whole-mouth plaque pH. In individual sites away from the salivary buffers, the pH values may fall close to 4.0. The upper curve was obtained from reconstituted skim milk and the lower one from an apple-flavored drink, showing a large difference in the acidogenicity of these two drinks.
(Courtesy of M. W. J. Dodds, University of Texas Dental School, San Antonio.)

in the enamel. If the fluid adjacent to the tooth is supersaturated with calcium and phosphate ions at a given pH, the enamel cannot undergo demineralization.

The saliva in contact with the teeth is normally supersaturated with calcium and phosphate, compared with the levels of these minerals in enamel.[15] The bacterial plaque can concentrate these ions to an even greater extent. For instance, the number of calcium and phosphate ions in plaque is 3 times greater than the number in the saliva.[87] This increased concentration is of practical importance because calcium and phosphate levels tend to be inversely related to the caries score.[47] It is also of great importance because the plaque fluid determines the eventual caries status.

As the pH drops in an acid attack, the level of supersaturation also drops, and the risk of demineralization increases. There is no exact pH at which demineralization begins, only a general range of 5.5 to 5.0. The range is rather large because demineralization is a function of both a drop in pH and the length of time that the enamel surface is exposed to the acidic environment. Different plaques have different initial pHs, buffering potentials, and concentrations of calcium and phosphate in different parts of the mouth. A change in any of these variables results in a different level of supersaturation in the tooth environment.

DEMINERALIZATION AND REMINERALIZATION PRINCIPLES

Throughout this book, there will continue to be many references to demineralization and remineralization of teeth, both as a pathologic and a therapeutic process. Demineralization is caused by plaque acids, which dissolve the tooth minerals making up the basic calcium, phosphate, and hydroxyl crystals of the enamel, dentin, and cementum. Remineralization, on the other hand, requires the availability of the same ions, preferably with fluoride as a catalyst to reconstruct the missing or damaged rods, a process that ten Cate aptly calls *non-restorative repair*.[88] Recent studies have shown that products containing amorphous calcium phosphate (ACP) can stimulate remineralization of tooth enamel. Products containing ACP, or ingredients that form ACP, can be found in toothpastes, mouthrinses, artificial saliva, chewing gums, topically applied coatings, and other vehicles for topical use.[89–92]

There are many calcium and phosphate compounds in the body that vary in chemical composition and with changes in pH. The crystals and fluoride compound of most dental interest in the demineralization and remineralization process are hydroxyapatite (HAP), fluorhydroxyapatite (FHA), and calcium fluoride (CaF_2).

The long-term exposure of teeth to low concentrations of fluoride (as found in fluoridated water) results in the gradual incorporation of fluoride into the existing hydroxyapatite (HAP) crystals to form fluorhydroxyapatite (FHA), which is more resistant to acid damage. Conversely, a higher concentration of fluoride (as occurs with the use of topical fluoride applications, fluoride dentifrices, foams, and varnishes, etc.) results in the formation of surface globules of CaF_2 (as seen in electron microscope images). If phosphates and proteins of the saliva coat these globules, the globules become more insoluble.[93] When the fluoride is incorporated into HAP to form FHA, it is said to be firmly bound, whereas loosely bound fluoride is in the form of CaF_2, which is adsorbed onto the surface of HAP and FHA crystals.[94]

The Relationship between HAP, FHA, and CaF_2

After an attack by plaque acid(s), CaF_2 dissolves first, followed in sequence by HAP, and finally, FHA (with its fluoride substitutions). As the attack continues, the dissociated ions increase the saturation level of the immediate fluid sufficiently to slow crystal dissolution and eventually arrest further solution of the crystals. As the pH begins to return to normal, crystals begin to re-form from the complex pool of dissolved ions, some as HAP, some as FHA (with many of the fluoride ions coming from the previous CaF_2). Finally, newly adsorbed CaF_2 is precipitated. Any deficiencies are subsequently replaced, in time, by calcium, phosphate, and fluoride from sources such as the saliva, water, and toothpastes. In observing the above process, one must marvel at the body's defense system. Although components of the lymph system that provide cellular or humoral immunity are absent in the enamel, the body can use a chemical system to maintain a state of equilibrium (homeostasis)—one in which CaF_2 provides a reservoir for fluoride that is immediately available when and where it is needed.[95] The only time the system breaks down is when the attacks are too frequent and too prolonged. (See Chapter 7 for further discussion of the oral cavity's defense system.)

Depth of Remineralization

There is little controversy about the success of topical procedures in stimulating surface remineralization, and of the use of commercial fluoride products such a dentifrices, gels, and varnish to compensate for the daily wear and tear of demineralization. In the New Zealand School System, incipient lesions with x-ray lucencies that extend midway through the enamel are considered candidates for remineralization. An in vitro study performed by ten Cate showed that both the inner enamel and dentin could be remineralized, but very slowly. Only the outer part of the enamel appeared to be responsive to fluoride diffusion and remineralization.[88]

Some researchers believe that remineralization is a reasonable objective even for lesions reaching to the dentin. The test for remineralization in these cases is the lack of demonstrable caries progress for 2 to 3 years. However, the important fact is that no reported studies indicate whether deep remineralization is or is not successful.

SUMMARY

Dental caries is a multifactorial disease involving an interaction of bacteria, diet, host resistance, and time. Cavitation can occur only when demineralization outstrips the body's defensive capability for remineralizations over a period of time. The embryology and histology of the enamel are favorable for either the demineralization or the remineralization of the enamel. The residual matrix and spacial relationships of rod-to-rod and crystalite-to-crystalite, as well as the less-calcified structures such as the stria of Retzius, lamellae, and tufts, allow fluids to diffuse throughout the enamel. Like the wick of an oil lamp, this network is available for the in-and-out movement of tooth-mineral ions and plaque acids. Even when an incipient lesion penetrates the enamel cap, this precaries lesion can often be remineralized without the need for a restoration. Possibly months or years will elapse before cavitation occurs, or a natural remineralization that entirely reverses the caries progression may even occur. There are several acidogenic bacteria that cause caries production, with mutans streptococci and lactobacilli being the most studied.

Silverstone opened up the possibility of a new non-restorative repair era when he described the demineralizing and remineralizing zones of an incipient lesion. If those in the dental care profession and research can bring remineralization to fruition, millions of teeth can be saved from the dentist's drill. The polarizing and electron microscopes allow one to see the details of how the plaque acids can easily flow into the body of the lesion and beyond. To simultaneously increase tooth resistance and the probability of remineralizing any known or unknown incipient lesions, individuals must use mechanical strategies for plaque control (e.g., tooth brushing, flossing, and irrigation) to remove the plaque. Chemical plaque control stratagems involve the use of antimicrobials to kill or suppress the cariogenic bacteria. And use of fluoride in the forms of water fluoridation, in-office topical applications, or fluoride rinses or dentifrices improves tooth resistance. Means now exist to greatly reduce the toll of dental caries, yet patients need access to examination and treatment systems that are based on early identification and treatment of risk factors before these measures become treatment requirements. Throughout this book, emphasis will be placed on the various strategies now available for preventing or limiting demineralization, or of enhancing remineralization.

REFERENCES

1. Centers for Disease Control and Prevention. (2005). Surveillance for dental caries, dental sealants, retention, edentulism, and enamel fluorosis United States, 1988–1994 and 1999–2002. *MMWR Morb Mortal Wkly Rep,* 54(03):1–44.

2. Ismal, A. I., Hasson, H., & Sohn, W. (2001). Dental caries in the second millennium. *J Dent Ed,* 65:953–58.

3. The oral health and chronic disease connection. (2002). Retrieved from http://www.astho.org/docs/access/ohcd.htm on February 29, 2008.

4. Ring, M. E., Ed. (1985.) *Dentistry: An illustrated history.* New York: Harry N. Abrams, Inc.

5. Gerabek, W. E. (1999). The tooth-worm: Historical aspects of a popular medical belief. *Clin Oral Investig,* 3:1–6.

6. Ring, M. E., & W.E. Miller. (2002). The pioneer who laid the foundation for modern dental research. *N Y State Dent J,* 68:34–37.

7. Miller, W. D. (1973). *The microorganisms of the human mouth.* Philadelphia: SS White Dental Manufacturing Company; 1890. Reprinted Basel, Switzerland: Karger.

8. Black, G. V. (1898). Dr. Black's conclusions reviewed again. *Dental Cosmos,* 40:440–51.

9. Dodds, M. W. J. (1993). Dilemmas in caries diagnosis—Applications to current practice, and need for research. *J Dent Educ,* 57:433–38.

10. Silverstone, L. M. (1973). The structure of carious enamel, including the early lesion. *Oral Sci Rev,* 3:100–160.

11. Juhl, M. (1983). Localization of carious lesions in occlusal pits and fissures of human premolars. *Scand J Dent Res,* 91:251–55.

12. Silverstone, I. M. (1977). Remineralization phenomena. *Caries Res,* 11 (Suppl 1):59–84.

13. Johnson, N. W. (1967). Some aspects of the ultrastructure of early human enamel caries seen with the electron microscope. *Arch Oral Biol,* 12:1505–21.

14. Haikel, Y., Frank, R. M., & Voegel, J. C. (1983). Scanning electron microscopy of the human enamel surface layer of incipient enamel lesions. *Caries Res,* 17:1–13.

15. Orland, F. J., Blayney, J. R., Harrison, R. W., Reynzers, J. A., Trexler, P. C., Wagner, M., Gordon, H. A., & Luckey, T. D. (1954). Use of germ-free animal technic in the study of experimental dental caries. I. Basic observations on rats reared free of all microorganisms. *J Dent Res,* 33:147–74.

16. Keyes, P. H. (1960). The infections and transmissible nature of experimental dental caries—Findings and implications. *Arch Oral Biol,* 1:304–20.

17. Loesche, W. J. (1986). Role of Streptococcus mutans in human dental decay. *Microbiol Rev,* 50:353–80.

18. Tanzer, J. M. (1989). On changing the cariogenic chemistry of coronal plaque. *J Dent Res,* 68 (Spec Iss):1576–87.

19. Clarke, J. K. (1924). On the bacterial factor in the aetiology of dental caries. *Br J Exp Pathol,* 5:141–47.

20. Twetman, S., & Frostnec, N. (1991). Salivary mutans streptomutans and caries prevalence in 8-year-old Swedish schoolchildren. *Swed Dent J,* 15:145–51.

21. Keene, H. J., & Shklair, I. L. (1975). Relationship of Streptococcus mutans carrier status to the lesions in initially caries free recruits. *J Dent Res,* 53:1295.

22. Loesche, W. J., Rowan, J., Straffon, L. H., Loos, P. J. (1975). Association of Streptococcus mutans with human dental decay. *Infect Immun,* 11:1252–60.

23. Tenuta, L. M., Ricomini, F. A. P., Del Bel Cury, A. A., & Cury, J. A. (2006). Effect of sucrose on the selection of mutans streptococci and lactobacilli in dental biofilm formed in situ. *Caries Res,* 40:546–49.

24. Winston, A. E., & Bhaskar, S. N. (1998). Caries prevention in the 21st century. *J Am Dent Assoc,* 129:1579–87.

25. Thibodeau, E. A., & O'Sullivan, D. M. (1999). Salivary mutans streptococci and caries development in the primary and mixed dentitions of children. *Community Dent Oral Epidemiol,* 27:406–12.

26. Fure, S. (1998). Five-year incidence of caries, salivary and microbial conditions in 60-, 70-, and 80-year-old Swedish individuals. *Caries Res,* 32:166–74.

27. Kohler, B., Bjarnason, S., Care, R., Mackevica, I., & Pence, I. (1995). Mutans streptococci and dental caries prevalence in a group of Latvian preschool children. *Eur J Oral Sci,* 103:264–66.

28. Alaluusua, S., Kleemola-Jujala, E., Gronroos, L., & Evalahti, M. (1990). Salivary caries-related tests as predictors of future caries increment in teenagers. A three-year longitudinal study. *Oral Microbiol,* 5:77–81.

29. Shi, S., Liang, Q., Hayashi, Y., Yakushiji, M., & Achida, Y. (1998). The relationship between caries activity and the status of dental caries—Application of the Dentocult SM method. *Chin J Dent Res,* 1:52–55.

30. Loesche, W. J., Eklund, S., Earnest, R., & Burt, B. (1984). Longitudinal investigation of bacteriology of human fissure decay: Epidemiological studies in molars shortly after eruption. *Infect Immun,* 46:765–72.

31. Van Houte, J., Sansone, C., Joshipura, K., & Kent, R. (1991). *In vitro* acidogenic potential and mutans streptococci on human smooth-surface plaque associated with initial caries lesions and sound enamel. *J Dent Res,* 70:497–502.

32. Edelstein, B., & Tinanoff, N. (1989). Screening preschool children for dental caries using a microbial test. *Pediatr Dent,* 11:129–32.

33. Geddes, D. A. M. (1975). Acids produced by human dental plaque metabolism *in situ. Caries Res,* 9:98–109.

34. Gibbons, R. J. (1964). Bacteriology of dental caries. *J Dent Res,* 43:1021–28.

35. Burne, R. A. (1998). Oral streptococci . . . Products of their environment. *J Dent Res,* 77:445–52.

36. Quivey, R. G., Kuhnert, W. L., & Hahan, K. (2001). Genetics of acid adaption in oral streptococci. *Crit Rev Oral Biol Med,* 12:301–14.

37. Brown, L. R., Dreizen, S., & Handler, S. (1976). Effects of elected caries regimens on microbial changes following radiation-induced xerostomia in cancer patients. In Stiles, H. M., Loesche, W. J., & O'Brien, T. C., Eds. *Proceedings: Microbial aspects of dental caries.* Washington, DC: Information Retrieval, 275–90.

38. Littleton, N. W., McCabe, R. M., & Carter, C. H. (1967). Studies of oral health in persons nourished by stomach tube. II. Acidogenic properties and selected bacterial components of plaque material. *Arch Oral Biol,* 12:601–609.

39. De Stoppelar, S. D., van Houte, J. S., & Backer-Dirks, O. (1970). The effect of carbohydrate restriction on the presence of *Streptococcus mutans, Streptococcus sanguis* and iodophilic polysaccharide-producing bacteria in human dental plaque. *Caries Res,* 4:114–23.

40. Dodds, M. W. J., & Edgar, W. M. (1986). Effects of dietary sucrose levels on pH fall and acid–anion profile in human dental plaque after a starch mouthrinse. *Arch Oral Biol,* 31:509–12.

41. Sgan-Cohen, H. D., Newbrun, E., Huber, R., Tenebaum, G., & Sela, M. N. (1988). The effect of previous diet on plaque pH response to different foods. *J Dent Res,* 67:1434–37.

42. Zickert, I., Emilson, C.-G., & Krasse, B. (1982). Effect of caries preventive measures in children highly infected with the bacterium Streptococcus mutans. *Arch Oral Biol,* 27:861–68.

43. Carlsson, J., Grahnen, H., & Jonsson, G. (1975). Lactobacilli and streptococci in the mouth of children. *Caries Res,* 9:333–39.

44. Suhonen, J. (1992). Mutans streptococci and their specific oral target: New implications to prevent dental caries. *Schweiz Monafsschr Zahnmed,* 102:286–91.

45. Alalluusia, S. (1991). Transmission of mutans streptococci. *Proc Finn Dent Soc,* 87:443–47.

46. Köhler, B., & Bratthall, D. (1978). Intrafamilial levels of Streptococcus mutans and some aspects of the bacterial transmission. *Scand J Dent Res,* 86:35–42.

47. Zickert, I., Emilson, C.-G., & Krasse, B. (1983). Correlation of level and duration of Streptococcus mutans infection with incidence of dental caries. *Infect Immun,* 39:982–85.

48. Modesto, A. & Drake, D. R. (2006) Multiple exposures to chlorhexidine and Xylitol: adhesion and biofilm formation by streptococcus mutans. *Curr Microbiol.*

49. Carlsson, J., Soderholm, G., & Almfedt, I. (1969). Prevalence of Streptococcus sanguis and Streptococcus mutans in the mouth of persons wearing full-dentures. *Arch Oral Biol,* 14:243–49.

50. Avery, J. K. (2000). *Essentials of oral histology and embryology: A clinical approach* (2nd ed.). St Louis: C.V. Mosby, 94–106.

51. Silverstone, L. M., & Hicks, M. J. (1985). The structure and ultra structure of the carious lesion in human dentin. *Gerodontics,* 1:185–93.

52. Pashley, D. H., & Matthews, W. G. (1993). The affects of outward forced convective flow on inward diffusion in human dentine in vitro. *Arch Oral Biol,* 38:577–82.

53. Ciucchi, B., Bouillaguet, S., Holz, J., & Pashley, D. (1995). Dentinal fluid dynamics in human teeth, in vivo. *J Endod,* 21:191–94.

54. Heyeraas, K. J., & Berggreen, E. (1999). Interstitial fluid pressure in normal and inflamed puls. *Crit Rev Oral Biol Med,* 10:328–36.

55. Ahn, C. L., & Overton, B. (1997). The effects of immunoglobulins on the convective permeability of human dentine *in vitro. Arch Oral Biol Med,* 42:835–43.

56. Pashley, D. H. (1996). Dynamics of the pulpo-dentin complex. *Crit Rev Oral Biol Med,* 7:104–33.

57. Pashley, D. H. (1992). Dentin permeability and dentine sensitivity. *Proc Finn Dent Soc,* 88 (Suppl. 1):13–37.

58. Pashley, D. H. (1991). Clinical correlations of dentin structure and function. *J Prosthet Dent,* 66:777–81.

59. ten Cate, J. M. (2001). Remineralization of caries lesions extending into dentin. *J Dent Res,* 80:1407–11.

60. Shay, K. (2004). The evolving impact of aging America on dental practice. *J Contemp Dent Pract,* 15:101–10.

61. Saunders, R. H., Jr., & Meyerowitz, C. (2005). Dental caries in older adults. *Dent Clin North Am,* 49:293–308.

62. Tugnait, A., & Clerehugh, V. (2001). Gingival recession— Its significance and management. *J Dent,* 29:381–94.

63. Katz, R. V., Hazen, S. P., Chilton, N. W., & Mumm, R. D., Jr. (1982). Prevalence and intraoral distribution of root caries in an adult population. *Caries Res,* 16:265–71.

64. Winn, D. M., Brunelle, J. A., Selwitz, R. H., Oblakowski, R. J., Kingmon, A., & Brown, L. J. (1996). Coronal and root caries in the dentition of adults in the United States, 1988–1991 *J Dent Res,* 75:642–51.

65. Locker, D., Slade, G. D., & Leake, J. L. (1989). Prevalence of and factors associated with root decay in older adults in Canada. *J Dent Res,* 68:768–72.

66. Vehkalahti, M. M., & Paunlo, I. K. (1988). Occurrence of root caries in relation to dental health behavior. *J Dent Res,* 67:911–14.

67. Banting, D. W. (1986). Epidemiology of root caries. *Gerodontology,* 5:5–11.

68. Petersen, P. E. (2005). Sociobehavioural risk factors in dental caries—International perspectives. *Community Dent Oral Epidemiol,* 33:274–79.

69. Jordan, H. V., & Hammond, B. F. (1972). Filamentous bacteria isolated from human root surface caries. *Arch Oral Biol,* 17:1333–42.

70. Sumney, D., & Jordan, H. (1974). Characterization of bacteria isolated from human root surface carious lesions. *J Dent Res,* 63:343–51.

71. Van Houte, J., Jordan, H. V., Laraway, R., Kent, R., Sopark, P. M., & DePaula P. F. (1990). Association of the microbial flora of dental plaque and saliva with human root-surface caries. *J Dent Res,* 69:1463–68.

72. Bowden, G. H. W. (1990). Microbiology of root surface caries in humans. *J Dent Res,* 69:1205–10.

73. Dung, S. Z. (1999). Effects of mutans streptococci, Actinomyces species and Porphyromona gingivalis on collagen degenerations. *Chung Hua I, Hsueh Tsa Chihi* (Taipai), 62:764–74.

74. Mellberg, J. R. (1986). Demineralization and remineralization of root surface caries. *Gerodontology,* 5:25–31.

75. Nyvad, B., & Fejerskov, O. (1986). Active root surface caries converted into inactive caries as a response to oral hygiene. *Scand J Dent Res,* 94:281–84.

76. Wallman, C., & Krasse, B. (1992). Mutans streptococci on margins of fillings and crowns. *J Dent,* 20:163–66.

77. Lindquist, B., & Emlson, C. G. (1990). Distribution and prevalence of mutans streptococci in the human dentition. *J Dent Res,* 69:1160–66.

78. Kidd, E. A. M. (1990). Caries diagnosis within restored teeth. *Adv Dent Res,* 4:10–13.

79. Fontana, M., & Zero, D. (2006). Assessing patient's caries risk. *J Am Dent Assoc,* 137:1231–39.

80. Kidd, E. A. M., & O'Hara, J. W. (1990). The caries status of occlusal amalgam restorations with marginal defects. *J Dent Res,* 69:1275–77.

81. Elderton, R. J. (1983). Longitudinal study of dental treatment in the General Dental Service in Scotland. *Br Dent J,* 155:91–96.

82. Skartveit, L., Wefel, J. S., & Ekstrand, J. (1991). Effect of fluoride amalgams on artificial recurrent enamel and root caries. *Scand J Dent Res,* 99:287–94.

83. Dijkman, G. E. H. M., de Vries, J., Lodding, A., & Arenda, J. (1993). Long-term fluoride release of visible light-activated composites *in vitro:* A correlation with in situ demineralization data. *Caries Res,* 27:117–23.

84. Hudson, P. (2004). Conservative treatment of the Class I lesion: A new paradigm. *J Am Dent Assoc,* 135:1514, 1516.

85. Stephan, R. M. (1910). Changes in hydrogen–ion concentration on tooth surfaces and in carious lesions. *JADA,* 27:718–23.

86. Dodds, M. W. J., & Edgar, W. M. (1998). The relationship between plaque pH, plaque acid anion profiles and oral carbohydrate retention after ingestion of several 'reference foods' by human subjects. *J Dent Res,* 67:861–65.

87. ten Cate, J. M. (1992). Saliva a physiological medium. *Ned Tijdschr Tandheelkr,* 99:82–84.

88. ten Cate, J. M. (2001). Remineralization of caries lesions extending into dentin. *J Dent Res,* 80:1407–11.

89. Tung, M. S., & Eichmiller, F. C. (2004). Amorphous calcium phosphates for tooth mineralization. *Compend Contin Educ Dent,* 25 (9 Suppl 1): 9–13.

90. Tung, M. S. Malerman, R., Huang, S., & McHale, W.A. (2005) Reactivity of prophylaxis paste containing calcium, phosphate and fluoride salts. *J Dental Res,* 84:Special Issue A, IADR Abstracts.

91. Ramalingam, L., Messer, L. B., & Reynolds, E. C. (2005). Adding casaein phosphopeptide-amorphous calcium phosphate to sports drinks to eliminate in vitro erosion. *Pediatr Dent,* 27:61–67.

92. Giniger, M., Spaid, M., MacDonald, J., & Felix, H. (2005) A 180-day clinical investigation of the tooth whitening efficacy of a bleaching gel with added amorphous calcium phosphate. *J Clin Dent,* 16:11–16.

93. Ogaard, B. (1999). The cariostatic mechanism of fluoride. *Comp Contin Educ Dent,* 20 (1 Suppl):10–17.

94. ten Cate, J. M., & Loveren, van C. (1999). Fluoride mechanisms. *Dent Clinics North Am,* 43:713–42.

95. Rosin-Grget, K., & Lincir, J. (2001). Current concept on the anticaries fluoride mechanism of the action. *Coll Antropol,* 25:703–12.

Chapter 4

Periodontal Diseases

Kathleen O. Hodges

OBJECTIVES

After studying this chapter, the student will be able to:

1. Name and describe the functions of the four components of the periodontium.
2. Describe the normal gingival sulcus.
3. Differentiate between gingivitis and periodontitis.
4. Describe the role of clinical attachment loss in making the correct diagnosis between gingivitis and periodontitis.
5. Describe characteristic microflora associated with periodontal health, gingivitis, and periodontitis.
6. Describe how periodontal disease progresses, starting with a healthy periodontium and ending with advanced periodontitis.
7. Describe the relationship of supragingival plaque and subgingival plaque biofilm to periodontal diseases.
8. Describe the role of the host defenses involved in periodontal disease.
9. Discuss the purposes of a classification system for periodontal diseases.
10. Describe the classification system categories for gingivitis and periodontitis.
11. Define a "risk factor" for periodontal diseases.
12. List the risk factors associated with periodontal diseases.

KEY TERMS

Loss of attachment
Junctional epithelium
Bidirectional synergism
Periodontal pockets
Prognosis
Alveolar process
Marginal gingiva
Free marginal groove
Gingival fibers
Circular fibers
Circumferential fibers
Gingivodental fibers
Dentogingival fibers
Crest
Periosteum
Dentoperiosteal fibers
Alveologingival fibers
Transseptal fibers
Interdental gingiva
Papillae
Interdental papillae
Col
Mucogingival junction

(continued)

KEY TERMS (CONTINUED)

Alveolar mucosa
Gingival crevice
Sulcular epithelium
Periodontal ligament
Alveolar crest fibers
Horizontal fibers
Oblique fibers
Apical fibers
Occlusal forces
Interradicular fibers
Furcation
Dentogingival unit
Dentogingival junction
Oral vestibule
Palate
Gingival crevicular fluid
Nonspecific plaque hypothesis
Specific plaque hypothesis
Manifestations

Oral prophylaxis
Immunopathologic
Instrumentation
Chemotactic
Vasculitis
Edema
Necrotizing disease
Endodontic
Chronic periodontitis
Aggressive periodontitis
Necrotizing ulcerative gingivitis
Necrotizing ulcerative periodontitis
Periodontal abscess
Pericoronal
Developmental deformities and conditions
Acquired deformities and conditions
Risk factor
Genomics
Refractory periodontal disease
Adjunct

INTRODUCTION

Periodontal diseases are diseases induced by biofilm (dental plaque).[1] The mildest form of periodontal disease is characterized by slight inflammatory changes of the gingiva surrounding the teeth. The severest form is a massive loss of tooth-supporting structures, including alveolar bone, and subsequent tooth loss[2] (Figure 4–1 ■). Early periodontal disease that is limited to the gingiva is referred to as *gingivitis*. Gingivitis is a common clinical finding that affects nearly everyone at some time during the life cycle. It usually can be reversed by the use of primary preventive measures.

Periodontal disease that affects the tooth-supporting structures and alveolar bone is referred to as periodontitis. Damage caused by periodontitis usually is not reversible with primary preventive measures; however, these procedures aid in the control of periodontitis. Loss of attachment is the primary clinical and diagnostic difference between gingivitis and periodontitis. Specifically, **loss of attachment** is the detachment of collagen fibers from the cementum and subsequent movement of the zone of soft tissue attached to the teeth (i.e., the **junctional epithelium**) toward the apex of the root. The presence of gingival inflammation without loss of attachment is gingivitis. Gingival inflammation accompanied by a pathological loss of attachment is classified as periodontitis.[3]

Periodontal disease is a broad term that encompasses multiple types of plaque-induced periodontal diseases. These diseases are infections associated with specific groups of bacteria. An individual's susceptibility to periodontal diseases depends on the person's host response to the oral bacteria. This host susceptibility explains why individuals present with varying clinical findings, types, and extents of the disease. The progression of periodontal disease also depends on risk factors that modify the host's susceptibility to the bacterial infection. Risk factors include medical or systemic conditions, environmental factors, and genetic diseases.[4–12] Examples of risk factors that affect the progress of periodontal disease are (1) the close relationship between the severity of periodontal disease and the severity of type 2 diabetes mellitus; (2) the strong relationship between periodontal disease and exposure to tobacco and tobacco products such as cigarettes and spit (chewing) tobacco, as well as the environmental exposure of nonsmokers to cigarette smoke; and (3) the less-strong relationship between genetically influenced inflammatory mediators and periodontitis.[13–17]

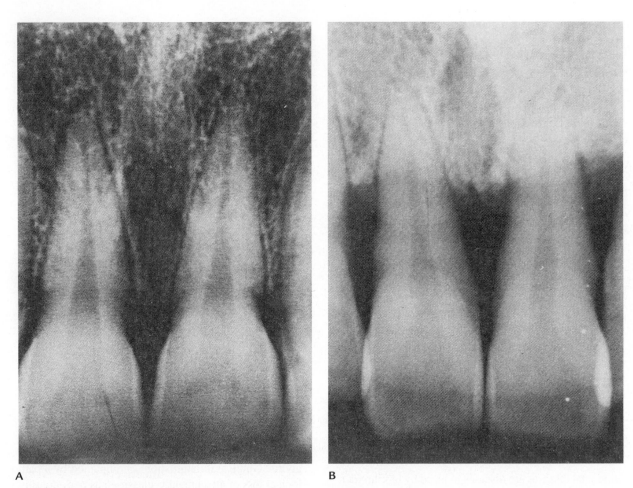

A   B

■ **FIGURE 4–1**   Maxillary central incisors. Bone loss on radiographs. **A.** Slight interproximal bone loss. **B.** Greater bone loss is seen in advanced periodontal disease.
(Courtesy of Dr. O. Langland, University of Texas Dental School at San Antonio.)

Periodontal diseases are widespread and world-wide. Gingivitis is found in children, adolescents, and young adults, but seems to decline in the older adult. In fact, gingivitis is almost universal in children and adolescents, and the prevalence of destructive forms of periodontal disease is lower in young adults than in adults.[18] Loss of attachment and bone loss are both rather uncommon in young individuals; however, incidence does increase in adolescents who are 12 to 17 years of age in comparison with children who are 5 to 11 years old.[18] The prevalence of severe attachment loss among children and young adults seems to be minimal; however, children, adolescents, and young adult patients should receive periodontal evaluation and relevant self-care education when seeking oral health care.[18,19]

Some form of periodontitis has been estimated to affect the majority of adults in the United States, with severe generalized periodontitis affecting 5% to 15% of the overall population.[20] Periodontitis is age related; however, this statement can be misleading, because it implies that periodontal disease is directly related to the aging process. Instead, studies have shown that the periodontal health of older adults is closely related to self-care and the cumulative effects of the disease process, rather than to age.

At one time, it was believed that the systemic disease and periodontal disease relationship was unidirectional, meaning that periodontitis could adversely affect a systemic disease, but not vice versa. It is clear today, however, that the presence of certain systemic diseases affects the periodontal health and treatment outcomes of some patients. There are three ways that systemic disease and periodontal diseases are related. First, systemic relationships might be suspected in individual situations in which periodontal disease appears to be disproportional to the local irritants.[21] The systemic disease itself affects the response to local irritants. Second, genetic (e.g., Down syndrome, Papillon-Lefevre syndrome, Cohen syndrome) or hematologic diseases (e.g., acute leukemia or acquired neutropenia) can cause periodontitis. Third, a complex relationship also exists between periodontitis and systemic diseases such as cardiovascular diseases, diabetes mellitus, pregnancy outcomes, and osteoporosis. This relationship has been referred to as **bidirectional synergism,** meaning that periodontal disease is a risk factor for adverse systemic diseases or conditions.[22–25] Periodontal medicine is an emerging discipline that strives to define the relationship between systemic disease and periodontal diseases through scientific inquiry.[23] Periodontal medicine focuses on periodontal disease as a risk factor for adverse systemic diseases or conditions.[26]

The prevalence of periodontal diseases in the United States may increase in the future, because longer life spans are increasing the time that teeth are at risk. Also, people are taking better care of their teeth and maintaining their teeth longer, which, in turn increases the number of teeth at risk. Also, improved diagnosis and detection of periodontal diseases by oral health professionals could, perhaps, increase the prevalence of periodontal diseases. On the other hand, the prevalence of periodontal disease in the United States might decrease, because access to information about periodontal disease has exploded, making more people aware of preventive measures. Improvements in the early diagnosis and treatment of periodontal disease are still needed, because some people will not have access to the manpower-intensive periodontal care needed for the repeated monitoring and treatment of this lifelong disease. [27]

Although there are many scientific advances in the diagnosis and treatment of periodontal diseases, oral health care professionals still face challenges. It is not possible to predict periodontal disease risk accurately.[28,29] The presence of **periodontal pockets** or clinical attachment loss is not an indicator of the actual activity of disease at the time of examination. Thus, from 3% to 5% of periodontal patients have frequent episodes of rapid disease progression that cannot be identified until an examination months or years later confirms that periodontal destruction has already occurred.[30,31] Genetic research, however, is being conducted to find a marker that will help predict periods of disease activity, which might, in turn, lead to more efficacious treatment.[32] The successful completion of the Human Genome Project to decode the DNA molecule offers the possibility of developing genetic approaches to prevention, diagnosis, nonsurgical treatment, **prognosis,** and vaccination.

THE PERIODONTIUM

Four anatomical structures support the teeth: (1) gingiva, (2) periodontal ligament, (3) cementum, and (4) alveolar bone (Figure 4–2 ■). Collectively these structures

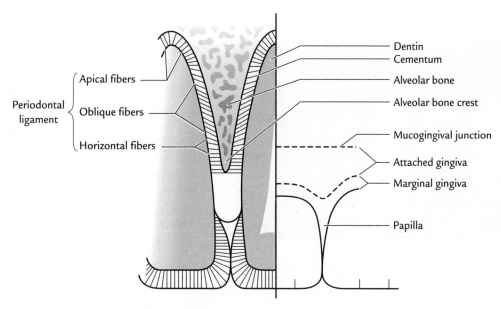

■ **FIGURE 4–2**   Parts of the periodontium.

comprise the periodontium. The tissues of the periodontium attach the tooth to the **alveolar process.**

The gingiva covers the cervical and root portions of the teeth, and the maxillary and mandibular alveolar processes. The gingiva consists of the free (or marginal) gingiva, interdental papillae, and attached gingiva (Figure 4–3 ■). The **marginal gingiva** surrounds each tooth in a "cuff-like" fashion and is not attached to the tooth. The most coronal portion of the marginal gingiva is the edge of the gingiva that touches the tooth. Its most apical portion is the **free marginal groove,** which defines the boundary between the attached and marginal gingiva. In health, the gingival margin should be flat against the bone with scalloped coronal edges that follow the tooth contour. The marginal gingiva is about 1 mm wide on the facial and lingual surfaces.

The marginal gingiva is held firmly against the tooth by a complex arrangement of collagen fiber groups: circumferential, gingivodental, and transseptal. The **gingival fibers** aid the tissue in withstanding the forces of mastication, and connect the marginal gingiva with the cementum and the attached gingiva. These fibers, which are arranged in bundles, are divided into groups according to their orientation and insertion into the periodontal tissues. Fibers that encircle the tooth within the marginal gingiva are called **circular** or **circumferential fibers**. These fibers are attached to other collagen fibers much like those in Figure 4–4 ■. A second group of fibers, known as the **gingivodental** (or **dentogingival**) **fibers,** are inserted into the cementum,

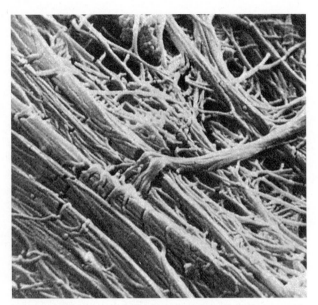

■ **FIGURE 4–4** Electron scanning microscopic view of collagen bundles in the periodontal ligament space. Note narrow bundle crossing thick bundle at right angle.
(From Svejda J., & Skach M. (1973). The periodontium of the human teeth in the scanning electron microscope (stereoscan). *J Periodont,* 44:478–84.)

and extend into the **crest** (upper ridge) and the **periosteum** (connective tissue surrounding the alveolar bone) of the alveolar bone just beneath the epithelium at the base of the gingival sulcus (Figure 4–3). These fibers are located in the facial, lingual, and interproximal

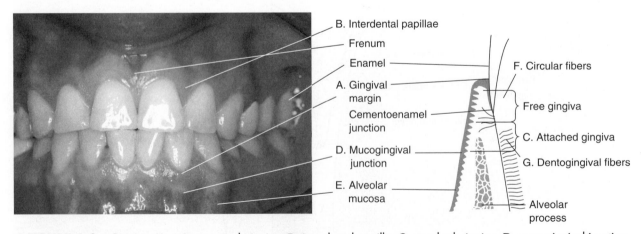

■ **FIGURE 4–3** Gingiva. Key: **A.** marginal gingiva, **B.** interdental papilla, **C.** attached gingiva, **D.** mucogingival junction, **E.** alveolar mucosa, **F.** circular fibers, **G.** dentogingival fibers.
(Adapted from J. Lindhe and T. Karring. Wiley Publishers. Anatomy of the periodontium, in *Clinical Periodontology and Implant Dentistry,* ed. J. Lindhe. Copenhagen: Munksgaard, © 2003.)

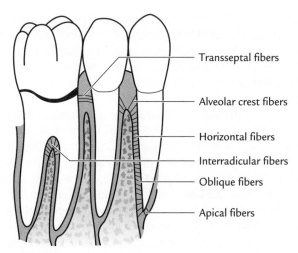

■ **FIGURE 4–5**   Principal fibers of the periodontal ligament.

Transseptal fibers

Alveolar crest fibers

Horizontal fibers

Interradicular fibers

Oblique fibers

Apical fibers

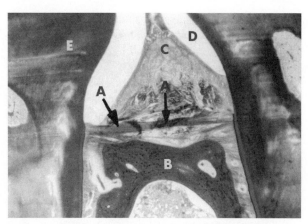

■ **FIGURE 4–6**   Cross-sectional view of interdental papillae showing **A.** transseptal fibers, **B.** alveolar crest, **C.** dental papilla, **D.** enamel space, and **E.** dentin. (Courtesy of Dr. Don Willman, University of Texas Dental School at San Antonio.)

surfaces. Also, two other fiber groups are present: the dentoperiosteal and the alveologingival groups; the **dentoperiosteal fibers** anchor the tooth to the bone, whereas the **alveologingival fibers** extend from the alveolar crest to the marginal and attached gingiva (Figure 4–5 ■). **Transseptal fibers** are located interproximally and extend from the cementum of one tooth, over the alveolar crest of interproximal bone, and into the cementum of the adjacent teeth (Figures 4–5 and 4–6 ■). Together, these fibers serve to maintain the close, tight contact of the free marginal gingiva against the tooth.

The **interdental gingiva** is composed of two **papillae,** which fill the interproximal space between adjacent teeth and are also called **interdental papillae:** One papilla is located on the facial side of the teeth; the other is on the lingual side. The two papillae are connected beneath the tooth contact by a concave-shaped nonkeratinized tissue termed the **col** (Figure 4–7 ■). The attached gingiva is apical to the marginal gingiva and extends from the free marginal groove to the **mucogingival junction,** where it meets the loose and moveable **alveolar mucosa** (Figure 4–3). The alveolar mucosa is a thin, nonkeratinized mucosal layer that is loosely attached to the

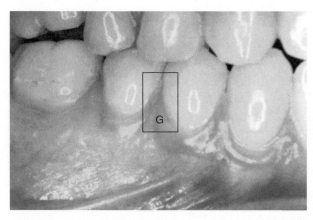

A

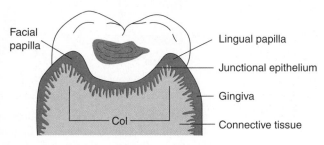

Facial papilla

Lingual papilla

Junctional epithelium

Gingiva

Connective tissue

Col

B

■ **FIGURE 4–7**   Col area. Proximal view of tooth and gingiva. G, Interdental gingiva fills the gingival embrasure. (From P. F. Fedi, Jr., and A. R. Vernino. The Periodontic Syllabus. Copyright © 2000 by Lippincott Williams & Wilkins.)

alveolar process; the alveolar mucosa extends into the cheek, lips, tongue, and palate. In contrast, the attached gingiva is firm, keratinized, and tightly attached to the periosteum of the alveolar bone.

The marginal gingiva attaches to the tooth at the base of the gingival sulcus (also called the **gingival crevice**), which is the shallow space around each tooth (Figure 4–8B ■ and 4–8C ■). The boundaries of the gingival sulcus are the cementum on one side, the **sulcular epithelium** of the marginal gingiva on the other side, and the epithelial attachment at the base or apical portion of the sulcus. The orifice of this sulcus opens into the oral cavity. The depth of the gingival sulcus is an important characteristic of health or disease; its depth is measured with a periodontal probe. The gingival sulcus measures 1 to 2 mm facially and lingually, and 1 to 3 mm proximally in health. In disease, edema or enlargement and/or erythema may create inflammation, increasing the depth of the sulcus more than 2 to 3 mm, or the gingival mar-

gin may recede below the cementoenamel junction. With disease, gingival bleeding might occur spontaneously or because of provocation (periodontal probing or patient self-care). Inflammation affects the interdental gingiva first, the marginal facial and lingual gingiva second, and the attached gingiva last.

The **periodontal ligament** is a network of collagen fibers. This structure surrounds the tooth root and connects it with the alveolar bone (Figure 4–8B). Its collagen fibers embed into the cementum of the root on one side and into the alveolar bone on the other side. The five principal fibers of the periodontal ligament have different orientations and functions at various levels on the tooth root. They are arranged in bundles called alveolar crest, horizontal, oblique, apical, and interradicular fiber groups (Figure 4–5). The **alveolar crest fibers** extend obliquely from the cementum to the alveolar crest. They prevent lateral movement and extrusion of the tooth. The **horizontal fibers** are located at the cer-

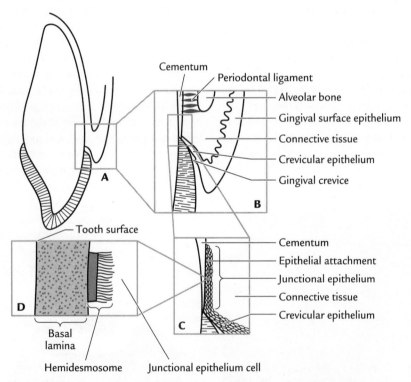

■ **FIGURE 4–8** Dentogingival junction: **A.** and **B.** The junction between the tooth and gingival soft tissues. **C.** This junction occurs where there are a few layers of junctional epithelial cells. **D.** The attachment mechanism for these cells consists of hemidesmosomes in each cell, and a basal lamina between the cell body and tooth.

vical area and also resist lateral forces. The **oblique fibers** extend in an oblique fashion from the alveolar bone to the cementum and bear the stress of chewing. The **apical fibers** form at the tooth apex and are generally parallel to the long axis of the tooth to help cushion the tooth from **occlusal forces.** The **interradicular fibers** are found in the **furcation** area of a multi-rooted tooth and connect the cementum and tooth. In addition, a network of blood vessels within the periodontal ligament protects the bone and periodontal fibers from excessive occlusal forces.

The junctional epithelium is found at the apical termination of the gingival sulcular/crevicular epithelium, which lines the gingival sulcus (Figure 4–8C ■). The junctional epithelium is attached to the tooth by gingival fibers that hold the marginal gingiva against the tooth as previously described. The junctional epithelium and the gingival fibers are considered a functional unit called the **dentogingival unit** or **dentogingival junction.** The junctional epithelium is several layers thick when it initially forms, and the number of layers increases with age. The length of the junctional epithelium ranges from 0.25 to 1.35 mm. This very special epithelium is actually attached to the enamel, forming a seal between the soft tissue and the tooth surface. This biologic seal functions to anchor the sulcular epithelium to the tooth surface and to protect the underlying periodontal fibers from the hostile oral environment (Figure 4–8 ■). The junctional epithelium is one of the most important structures in the practice of periodontics. The junctional epithelial cells are joined to the tooth surface by hemidesmosomes, which consist of a few layers of epithelial cells that initially extend a short distance along the enamel surface at the cementoenamel junction[33] (Figure 4–8D ■). Inflammation, especially chronic inflammation such as in periodontitis, can result in apical migration of the cells, first over the cementoenamel junction, and then apically onto the cementum.

For each millimeter of apical migration of the attachment, there is also an accompanying loss of 1 mm of periodontal fibers attached between the cementum and bone. As the junctional epithelium migrates apically in more advanced disease, there is loss of alveolar bone and exposure of the cementum to which the fibers were originally attached. The migration also causes a deepening of the sulcus to form a periodontal pocket. This apical migration of the junctional epithelium and consequent loss of attachment (clinical attachment loss) is the hallmark sign for diagnosing periodontitis.

THE GINGIVAL SULCUS

In a longitudinal section of the free gingiva (Figure 4–8A ■), the tissues encountered from the sulcus to the **oral vestibule** or **palate** are (1) sulcular/crevicular epithelium, (2) connective tissue, and (3) attached gingiva surface epithelium. The sulcular and attached gingiva merge at the crest of the free gingival margin (Figure 4–3). The connective tissue between the sulcular and attached gingiva contain blood vessels, lymphatics, and nerves that supply both surfaces. The connective tissues immediately beneath the sulcular epithelium contain the oral cavity's (i.e., host) cellular and humoral defense system, which helps minimize the detrimental effects of bacteria in the plaque biofilm. (See Chapter 7 for discussion of host defense mechanisms.)

In an inflamed disease state, fluid flows from the depths of the gingival sulcus. This **gingival crevicular fluid** (GCF) is a transudate, which contains a few cells and proteins as opposed to exudates which is inflammatory in nature. Gingival crevicular fluid is derived from blood vessels in the connective tissue adjacent to the sulcus. An increase in GCF flow is one of the first detectable signs of impending gingivitis. Increased GCF flow is present prior to development of overt signs of inflammation, and the flow rate depends primarily on the severity of inflammation.[34] After patients stop dental self-care, an increase of GCF can be observed as early as the ninth day.[35]

Gingival crevicular fluid serves several protective functions. It helps clear bacteria from the gingival sulcus, and it is the vehicle for leukocytes, complement, antibodies, and assorted enzymes that help protect the enamel and the periodontium from bacterial attack. Gingival crevicular fluid serves as one of the first lines of host defense against the bacteria that cause periodontal disease and the bacteria that cause caries. The presence of an increasing flow of GCF has been related to the presence and increasing severity of gingivitis, but not to the severity of periodontitis.

PERIODONTAL MICROFLORA

Historically, two hypotheses have guided thinking about periodontal microflora: the nonspecific plaque hypothesis and the specific plaque hypothesis. The **nonspecific plaque hypothesis** simply relates periodontal disease to the overall amount of plaque present. As the amount of plaque increases, inflammation and disease increase. In the 1960s, Loe and others recognized a causal relationship between bacterial plaque and gingivitis.[36] Gingivitis would result when plaque was not removed by self-care, and gingivitis would reverse when self-care was resumed. This landmark study seems to be the basis for the nonspecific plaque hypothesis. At that time, a single-disease concept was advocated, which said periodontal disease was caused by the transition from health to gingivitis to periodontitis in relation to the presence of bacterial plaque over time. All individuals were equally susceptible, gingivitis always progressed to periodontitis, and treatment was standard for each patient. This theory came into question, however, because clinical findings did not reflect this hypothesis. For example, some patients who had a vast accumulation of bacterial plaque had minimal disease.

When plaque bacteria could be cultured, researchers were able to differentiate between various bacterial species, and the specific plaque hypothesis became prevalent and accepted. The **specific plaque hypothesis** attributes the various demonstrations of signs or symptoms (**manifestations**) of the periodontal plaque-related diseases to "specific," although not necessarily known, bacteria. Quality of bacterial plaque biofilm is more important than the quantity. In other words, specific types and complexes of bacteria and their pathogenic potential are more important than the amount of plaque biofilm present. Also, not all plaque biofilm is associated with disease. Therefore, all individuals are not equally susceptible, gingivitis does not always progress to periodontitis, and treatment interventions vary depending on the type of disease.

Experimental gingivitis in children, versus adults, reveals increased subgingival levels of *Actinomyces* species, *Capnocytophaga* species, *Leptotrichia* species, and *Selenomonas* species. These species, therefore, might be important in the etiology and pathogenesis of gingivitis.[37,38] Periodontitis appears to conform to the specific plaque hypothesis, because certain bacterial species have been associated with the most destructive periodontal diseases.[10] Substantial evidence identifies certain microorganisms or combinations of organisms as etiologic factors.[11] For example, the microbial species that appear to be associated with chronic periodontitis—the most common variety of periodontitis—are *Actinobacillus actinomycetemcomitans* (AA), *Porphyromonas gingivalis*, *Prevotella intermedia*, *Bacteroides forsythus*, *Fusobacterium* species, *Campylobacter rectus,* and *Treponema denticola.* This list may seem long, but 300 to 500 different species of bacteria are estimated to inhabit the oral cavity.[39,40] Despite this presumptive evidence of etiology, none of the suspected organisms has yet been successfully implanted into a test animal to duplicate the original disease.

As the status of the marginal gingiva deteriorates from health to gingivitis, a proportional shift begins to take place in the plaque biofilm bacteria, going first from aerobic, nonmotile, gram-positive cocci and rods[36,41,42] to facultative anaerobic bacteria, and then to anaerobic, gram-negative, motile species. This major shift in the plaque biofilm bacteria indicates the onset of gingivitis. Microscopic examination reveals an increase in numbers of both motile rods and spirochetes, with the two comprising approximately 20% of the microorganisms.[36,41,43]

THE DEVELOPING GINGIVAL LESION

There are four stages of inflammation in the periodontal lesion[44] (Table 4–1 ■). A sample of sulcular/crevicular fluid from healthy, tightly adapted marginal gingiva reveals only a few forms of bacteria in the sulcus. They include nonmotile coccal forms and motile vibrio. In a diseased gingival sulcus, the flora is markedly different and includes many motile bacteria, as seen in Figure 4–9 ■.

The free margin of the gingiva constitutes the first line of defense for the periodontium, and it is usually the initial site of gingival disease. If plaque biofilm is allowed to accumulate on a tooth surface adjacent to the gingiva, inflammation of the free margin results. If self-care of a healthy mouth is stopped, gingivitis is observed clinically (i.e., changes in color, size, and/or texture) in only 9 to 21 days. Presumably, inflammation might manifest itself sooner in some cases.

With gingivitis, the extent of the gingival inflammation parallels the extent of plaque biofilm accumulation. Early gingival clinical changes include alterations in color, contour changes from knife-edge-to-rolled, and a consistency change from firm-to-spongy. The free margin often bleeds on gentle manipulation such as from toothbrushing or probing. In the early stages, the developing inflammatory process can be completely reversed by professional oral health care interventions and patient self-care strategies as shown in Figures 4–10 ■ and 4–11 ■.

Not all gingival pathology is caused solely by bacterial plaque biofilm. Systemic conditions such as pregnancy or other hormonal changes cause the tissues to react more readily to the bacterial insult. There can also be gingival changes caused by inherited diseases such as hereditary fibromatosis and by drug therapy such as

■ **Table 4–1** Inflammation in the Periodontal Lesion

Stages	Time Interval	Histologic Changes	Clinical Changes
I. Initial lesion • Initial response of tissues to bacterial plaque • Subclinical gingivitis	2–4 days	Brief vasoconstriction followed by vasodilation, margination, emigration, and migration of PMN Slight alteration of junctional epithelium Increase in gingival crevicular fluid	None
II. Early lesion • Acute gingivitis	4–7 days	Continuation of initial lesion Macrophages and lymphocytes appear (chronic inflammatory cells) Junctional epithelium invaginates (folds in) with rete pegs Sulcular epithelium ulcerations Connective tissue fiber destruction	Redness Bleeding upon probing Loss of tissue tone
III. Established lesion • Chronic gingivitis	14 or more days	Continuation of changes in early lesion Plasma cells predominate Chronic inflammation; blood vessels congested; blood flow impaired; increase in collagenase and other enzymes Elongated rete pegs in junctional epithelium extending deep into connective tissue; breakdown of connective fibers	Moderate-to-severe inflammation An underlying bluish hue might be present In addition to color, changes in consistency will be evident
IV. Advanced lesion • Transition from gingivitis to periodontitis	Dependent on host response	Continuation of changes in established lesion Inflammation extending into connective tissue attachment and alveolar bone Repair manifests as fibrotic tissue Bone resorption by osteoclasts and mononuclear cells; bone formation might occur	True periodontal pockets Attachment loss Bone loss

PMN, polymorphonuclear leukocyte.

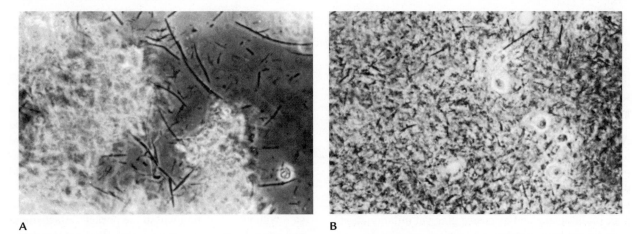

A   B

■ **FIGURE 4–9** **A.** A few plaque organisms (dark figures) from a relatively healthy sulcus as seen with a phase microscope. **B.** Great increase in number of organisms seen in moderate-to-severe marginal gingivitis.

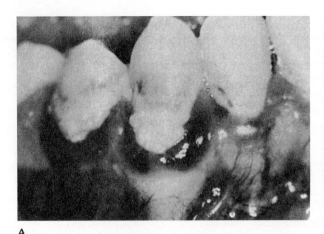

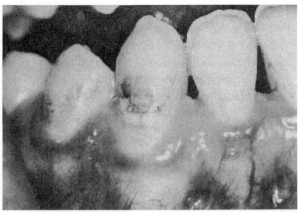

A   B

■ **FIGURE 4–10** **A.** A severe gingivitis with calculus, food debris, and poor self-care. Note the rolled and edematous gingiva. **B.** After a few days of diligent use of a brush, floss, and irrigation.
(Courtesy of Dr. Donald Willmann, University of Texas Dental School at San Antonio.)

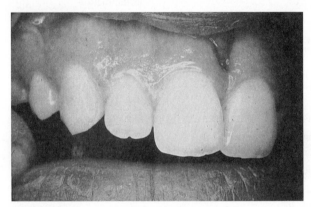

■ **FIGURE 4–11**   Healthy periodontium.
(Courtesy of Dr. Donald Willmann, University of Texas Dental School at San Antonio.)

phenytoin used to control seizure disorders.[45,46] Control of these latter conditions can be shared medical–dental responsibilities for the patient.

THE DEEPENING POCKET

All periodontitis is preceded by gingivitis, but not all untreated gingivitis progresses to periodontitis. For example, Ronderos completed a study of the indigenous people of the Amazon rain forest and found that most individuals had a loss of epithelial attachment. Despite poor oral hygiene and extensive gingival inflammation, they did not have severe periodontal destruction.[47]

A diagnosis of gingivitis implies that the actual level of the junctional epithelial attachment has migrated apically, but is still on the enamel or on the cementoenamel junction. A diagnosis of periodontitis implies that the junctional epithelium has migrated apically 2, 3, or more millimeters from its original level at the cementoenamel junction. This migration creates a deeper gingival sulcus, which is a periodontal pocket. The formation of the periodontal pocket with its inaccessible subgingival plaque biofilm creates the need for periodontal treatment.

As the pocket deepens, subgingival plaque acquires new characteristics that differentiate it from the supragingival plaque. In the supragingival plaque, the bacteria and the interbacterial matrix are well confined to the enamel. This biofilm can easily be removed by **oral prophylaxis,** which is defined as the removal of plaque (biofilm), calculus, and stains by supragingival and subgingival instrumentation combined with selective coronal polishing.[48] (See Chapter 16 for discussion of dental hygiene procedures.) Oral prophylaxis maintains health or converts gingivitis to health. In the subgingival plaque, a two-compartment subgingival plaque system begins to evolve, and that system is made up of (1) tooth-associated subgingival plaque, a biofilm on the cementum, and (2) a more fluid environment referred to as epithelium-associated plaque that bathes the cementum. This fluid consists of purulent fluids (pus), food debris, body defense cells, and saliva confined under low-oxygen tension without circulation within the pocket.[49] Bacteroides and spirochetes are present in this fluid environment.

The gram-negative organisms that extend deep into the pocket are believed to be the plaque biofilm responsible for the continued damage and migration of the epithelial attachment.

The tooth-associated subgingival plaque is initially an apical extension of the supragingival plaque into the deepening crevicular area. The bacterial population may still include some mutans streptococci, although their numbers decrease as the distance increases below the gingiva.[50] Subgingival calculus complicates disease control by sheltering plaque bacteria from routine plaque control measures.

In the late 1970s, researchers also differentiated between adherent (attached) plaque and loosely adherent, unattached plaque as causative factors in periodontal disease.[51,52] It was suggested that the pathogenic potential of loosely adherent plaque was greater than that of adherent or attached plaque. The relationship of the specific periodontal pathogens and the host response was then explored. In the 1980s, the specific plaque hypothesis, as previously discussed, was studied and periodontal diseases were reclassified to reflect bacteriologically and immunologically distinct forms of periodontal diseases. The result was the premise that the presence of pathogens is not enough to initiate disease; the host must also be susceptible to disease.

At this same time, researchers clarified similarities and differences between supragingival and subgingival plaque. It was clear that inflammation caused by supragingival plaque resulted in an altered relationship between the gingival margin and the tooth. This change in the environment permits subgingival bacteria to colonize into bacterial plaque on the root, or in the sulcus. Next, aerobic bacteria become organized subgingivally in attached and unattached plaque. Toxins, enzymes, and metabolic byproducts then injure the periodontium, and cause an immune response that results in indirect toxicity. As the host responds to the irritant, periodontal destruction occurs by **immunopathologic** reaction, that is, periodontal tissues are altered as a result of immune or allergic reactions to the irritant.

In conclusion, elimination of supragingival plaque is critical in preventing periodontal diseases. In addition, control of supragingival and subgingival plaque biofilm is critical to successful periodontal therapy. Patients are continually challenged to remove plaque biofilm. It is difficult for a patient to be 100% effective in controlling plaque, especially when it is located subgingivally; therefore, self-care without professional mechanical removal,

such as periodontal instrumentation, results in less healing.[53–55] Obviously, professional subgingival mechanical **instrumentation** is mandatory to complement patient self-care to achieve and maintain periodontal health.[56] Nonsurgical periodontal therapy is the professional treatment rendered and is defined as "plaque (biofilm) removal, plaque (biofilm) control, supragingival and subgingival scaling, root planing, and the adjunctive use of chemical agents."[57] Presently, the relationship between bacterial plaque and forms of periodontal diseases is complex; however, approaches to clinical care and self-care therapies for patients are improving rapidly.

CELLULAR DEFENSE IN THE PERIODONTAL DISEASE PROCESS

The body has three key functions of immunologic defense: (1) to protect it from outside invaders (antigens); (2) to destroy or neutralize the antigens that do penetrate the epithelial defenses; and (3) to repair any damage caused by the antigen–antibody reactions. To accomplish this task, the body uses cellular immunity and humoral immunity. The cells responsible for the cellular defense are the granular cells, which consist of granulocytes (basophils, eosinophils, and polymorphonuclear neutrophils [PMN, polys]), monocytes (macrophages), and those cells of lymphoid origin, and T and B lymphocytes.

During the cellular response to a periodontal infection, there is first a **chemotactic** (movement of a cell along a chemical concentration gradient away from the chemical stimulus) signal from an inflamed gingival site, which initiates the cellular immune response.[58,59] This signal could possibly arise from the epithelial cells under bacterial attack. For example, in laboratory studies, it was demonstrated that the gingival epithelial cells can cause an increase in the secretion of potent neutrophil chemotactic interleukin-8 following *Actinobacillus actinomycetemcomitans* challenge.[60] The defense cells then arrive at the inflamed site in a definite sequence. Initially, during the acute phase of inflammation, large numbers of PMN enter the connective tissue underlying the sulcus. The acute phase may last from a few days to a few weeks. However, if the inflammation continues, the number of PMN decreases and they are replaced by lymphocytes. This stage lasts a few weeks to a few months. Finally, if healing does not occur, the lymphocytes are replaced largely by plasma cells, macrophages, and mast cells. The inflammation is now in the chronic stage.

The above immune response can be linked to predictable histopathologic events. Within 2 to 4 days of plaque biofilm accumulation, the microscopic picture of the connective tissue is one of early inflammation. **Vasculitis** (inflammation of blood vessels) is present and extravascular PMN begin to appear in large numbers in the connective tissue. **Edema** (excessive fluid in local body tissues) is present because of fluid permeation through the capillary walls. After 4 to 7 days, the vasculitis becomes clinically apparent with the four primary signs of inflammation (i.e., heat, redness, swelling, and pain). Cellular infiltrate is predominated by lymphocytes.

The heat and the change of color of the marginal gingiva from pink to red are caused by the increased blood flow to the area. The gingival swelling is caused by the edema that is caused by leakage from the dilated (enlarged) capillaries. The fluid pressure of edema on nerve endings can cause an acute soreness. When the pain and swelling of the gingiva are sufficiently painful, altered eating habits can result. At this point, if the gingivitis is treated by professional care and self-care, the gingiva can make a complete return to normal. The shallow sulcus is soon cleared of destroyed bacteria and dead cells by the GCF, while the saliva flushes and neutralizes residual oral debris.

The development of a chronic stage of gingivitis, especially with pocket formation, is accompanied by a different series of reactions. The bacteria possess enzymes that can be lethal to the defense cells,[61] and the defense cells contain enzymes to destroy the bacteria. Thus, there are cellular or humoral reactions, such as dying cells and dying bacteria in the inflamed area, while destruction of epithelial cells, fibroblasts, and bone occurs. Also, the macrophage kills agents such as oxygen and nitrogen, as well as hypochlorite.[62] Other products of an activated macrophage include numerous proteins that affect coagulation and multiplication of cells that generate new tissue and repair damaged tissue.[63] This bacteria–epithelial–defense cell exchange is continuously taking place in the small pocket area. The low oxygen tension and low circulation within the pocket aid in perpetuating the pathogenicity of the inflamed periodontal site. Table 4–1 provides an overview of the stages of inflammation in the periodontal lesion.

Because of its complexity, a detailed discussion of the humoral defense of the periodontal site is beyond the scope of this book. (See Chapter 7 for discussion of host defense mechanisms.) Growing evidence points to the immune system playing an important role in the pathogenesis of periodontitis. One genetic factor, interleukin-1 should be mentioned, because it has received attention as a marker that can help predict the risk for periodontal disease.[64] Interleukin-1 is a proinflammatory cytokine that is a key regulator of host responses to microbial infection, and it is a major modulator of the catabolism (breakdown) of extracellular matrix and bone resorption.[65] There are other cytokines involved in tissue destruction such as interleukin-8, interleukin-10, and interleukin-11.[66]

Because interleukin-1 is a genetic factor, it may serve as a marker for a lifetime risk factor. A great advantage of such a marker is that it would help identify higher-risk individuals early in the periodontal disease process.[67] A positive genetic marker would serve to focus immediate attention on the daily requirement for meticulous mechanical and chemical biofilm control to negate the effect of the plaque bacteria. For a clinical practice, the genetic marker would aid in developing the periodontal care plan, an appropriately planned and individualized reevaluation, and follow-up visit intervals.[68] There is a test for interleukin-1 on the market; thus, this genetic marker is currently being used to help predict the future course of the disease.

In conclusion, as the chronic inflammation continues, the epithelial attachment slowly migrates apically on the cementum. Alveolar bone and soft tissue continue to be lost, and the periodontal pocket becomes deeper, making the control of disease difficult. Eventually, this continuing loss of tooth support results in a loosening of the tooth or teeth. The destruction of hard and soft tissues can continue until little or no support remains for the tooth or teeth if professional nonsurgical and/or surgical care is not sought. Extraction might become necessary, at which time all components of the periodontium are lost. Infrequently, even with professional care, tooth loss is inevitable.

CLASSIFICATIONS OF PERIODONTAL DISEASES

The most current classification system for periodontal diseases was developed in 1998. Classification systems aid in studying the etiology, pathogenesis, and treatment of diseases, and provide a way to organize the health care needs of patients.[69] Classification systems also enhance communication about periodontal diseases among oral health professionals and other health care providers, and serve to classify periodontal diseases for insurance-reporting purposes. The previous classification system from 1989 was changed because it had overlapping disease categories, no gingival disease category, an inappropriate emphasis on age of onset of disease and its progression rate, and inadequate or unclear classification criteria.[69]

There are two major categories of gingival diseases: plaque-induced and non–plaque-induced. Gingivitis that is initiated by plaque biofilm (i.e., plaque-induced) can be modified by systemic factors, medications, and malnutrition. Non–plaque-induced gingival lesions include diseases of bacterial, viral, or fungal origin, genetic manifestations of systemic conditions, traumatic lesions, or foreign body reactions.

There are seven categories of periodontitis: chronic, aggressive, and systemic periodontitis; **necrotizing disease;** abscesses; **endodontic** lesions; and developmental or acquired deformities and conditions.[69] **Chronic periodontitis** is the most commonly diagnosed disease category. Chronic periodontitis implies disease that occurs over a period of time, disease that is usually treatable and can be controlled, and disease that is usually responsive to appropriate treatment. Generally, this disease state progresses slowly; however, some patients experience short periods of rapid progression. There are three stages of chronic periodontitis: slight (early), moderate, and advanced (severe). Each stage has specific therapeutic goals, clinical features, treatment options, and prognoses or outcomes.[70,71]

Aggressive periodontitis is a highly destructive form of periodontal disease that can be localized or generalized. It occurs in otherwise healthy individuals and has a familial aggregation (i.e., tends to occur in most members of a family). Characteristics of aggressive periodontitis include (1) microbial deposit accumulation that is inconsistent with the severity of the disease (i.e., not much deposit but significant destruction) and (2) advancement of loss of attachment and bone loss that can be self-arresting (stopped on its own without recent treatment). Features of the localized form include onset around puberty, destruction to permanent first molars and incisors, association with the periodontal pathogen *Actinobacillus actinomycetemcomitans,* and abnormalities in neutrophil function.[72]

Although there are exceptions, generalized aggressive periodontitis usually affects people under the age of 30 years. Generalized attachment loss is present, and affects at least three permanent teeth in addition to the first molars and incisors. The loss of attachment occurs in major episodic periods of destruction, and it is also associated with *Actinobacillus actinomycetemcomitans,* and *Porphyromonas gingivalis,* as well as abnormalities in neutrophil function.[72]

Periodontitis as a manifestation of systemic disease includes diseases associated with hematologic disorders (e.g., leukemias), and genetic disorders, such as cyclic neutropenia, Down syndrome, Papillon-Lefevre syndrome, Cohen syndrome, and hypophosphatasia, to name a few.[69] These diseases actually cause periodontal destruction and loss of attachment.

Necrotizing periodontal diseases encompass necrotizing ulcerative gingivitis (NUG) and necrotizing ulcerative periodontitis (NUP). **Necrotizing ulcerative gingivitis** is a condition of sudden onset, and the patient might have a history of stress, change in living habits, inadequate rest, debilitating disease, and/or respiratory tract infection. In NUG, the lesions appear punched out and crater-like; the necrotic tissue separates from the healthy gingiva, forming a gray pseudomembrane (false membrane); and the gingiva shows pronounced linear erythema (redness). Spontaneous bleeding is another characteristic accompanied by a fetid odor and increased salivation. If left untreated, NUG might advance to the supporting structures. When bone loss occurs the condition has become **necrotizing ulcerative periodontitis.**

The **periodontal abscess** category relates to gingival, periodontal, or **pericoronal** lesions (gingival lesions close to the crown), which require special diagnostic and treatment approaches. Also, the periodontic–endodontic lesion classification recognizes the possible connection between periodontitis and endodontic lesions.

The last category of periodontal diseases, **developmental** or **acquired deformities and conditions,** refers to modifiers of the susceptibility to periodontal diseases and not to separate diseases. These modifiers such as recession, lack of keratinized gingiva, or decreased depth of the vestibule directly influence the outcomes of nonsurgical or surgical treatment.[69]

Future classifications are inevitable as more is learned about the etiology and pathogenesis of periodontal diseases. The reader is referred to the American Academy of Periodontology Web site (www.perio.org) for scientific and position papers related to the specific categories of periodontal diseases.

RISK FACTORS

A **risk factor** is a behavior, inherent characteristic, or environmental exposure associated with a disease.[73] Risk factors are associated with incidence, extent, and progression of periodontal diseases, and are usually identified through longitudinal studies (research studies in which the subjects are followed for a long period of time to study the natural course of a disease). Risk assessment can help dental professionals assess a patient's risk of developing periodontal disease and also helps to improve clinical decision making related to oral health care and prognosis. Risk assessment has the potential to reduce the need for complex periodontal therapy, and to improve patient outcomes that will lead to reduced cost for oral health care.[74,75] Specific examples of risk factors for periodontal diseases are age, gender, socioeconomic status, genetics, plaque biofilm, self-care, tobacco, stress, and diabetes.[76] Some risk factors cannot be changed or modified (non-modifiable or determinant), such as age and gender, whereas others are modifiable, such as smoking and plaque biofilm. The difference between these two types of risk factors is important in educating patients about risk factors that can be changed in the future. Through education and risk assessment in the dental practice, patients will understand the significance of their individual risk factors and be motivated to strive to change and/or control those factors that are modifiable. This model represents the medical or wellness model of patient care versus the "repair" or treatment model that was used formerly for dental care.[74]

Periodontal disease is not a disease of aging; however, greater periodontal destruction is found in the elderly population as a result of lifetime disease accumulation rather than an age-specific condition.[76] By the time 90% of persons are 55 years of age, they have at least one site of 2 mm or more clinical attachment loss, and 53.6% have 4 mm or greater loss of attachment at one or more sites.[77] Clinical attachment loss does increase with age; however, extensive loss of tooth function in the affected teeth is not prevalent. Pocket depth also relates somewhat to age.[76] Periodontitis seen in youth and early adulthood could be diagnosed as aggressive periodontitis, as previously discussed, depending on clinical conditions and other findings. The most rapid disease progression with periodontitis is seen in the small number of patients who manifest disease at an early age. Genetic predisposition probably contributes to this aggressive periodontitis.[72,78,79]

In reference to gender, clinical attachment loss is more prevalent in males than females.[77] This finding has been consistent in national surveys conducted over the years.[76] Genetic factors are not thought to be responsible for this gender difference in clinical attachment loss. Rather, it is thought that males are less compliant with self-care and routine oral health care visits, and have a less positive attitude toward oral health.

Socioeconomic status is another risk factor for periodontal diseases that is complex and multifactorial, and includes a variety of cultural factors.[76] It is accepted that patients who are well educated, relatively wealthy, and live in advantageous circumstances have better health status than those who are less educated and not wealthy, and live in poorer conditions. Gingivitis and poor oral hygiene are clearly related to socioeconomic status; however, the relationship of periodontitis to socioeconomic status is less established.[76] Even though racial and ethnic differences are evident in periodontal status, these differences are not due to true genetic differences. Instead, they are due to enhanced self-care among the better educated, positive health attitudes, and a greater frequency of health care visits for those who are aware of the need and who have insurance.[76] This risk factor points to the need for culturally relevant education related to self-care practices and biofilm bacteria.[80]

Genomics is the study of structure and function of organisms in terms of their DNA sequences.[81] Genomics provides the means to discovering hereditary factors in disease. Genes, by themselves, do not determine disease; however, genetic factors alter how patients interrelate with environmental agents such as smoking. The key to a patient's development of periodontitis appears to be controlled by the response to microflora.[81] The first reported genetic components in periodontitis were discovered in 1997.[65] A specific genotype of a polymorphic interleukin-1 gene cluster, which is a key regulator of the host response to microbial infection, is associated with only severe periodontitis in nonsmokers. This finding means that the genetic factor was not as strong a risk factor as smoking.

There is little doubt that the genetic component is a factor in periodontitis; however, the strength of the component is currently being studied. Most research is based on clinical and laboratory procedures versus epidemiologic surveys (i.e., incidence, distribution, and control of disease in a population); therefore, future studies of patients with and without disease are necessary to determine the genetic contribution to the initiation and progression of periodontitis.[76] Genetic studies have been conducted in relation to aggressive and chronic forms of periodontitis. Aggressive periodontitis appears to have several forms, and it currently is not clear how many genes may be responsible for this disease.[82] The difficulty of studying the gene identification for this disease is its rarity.[81] The genetic component for chronic periodontitis comes from studying twins in whom 50% of the susceptibility may be due to genetic factors.[83] Hopefully, the future will reveal how genetic information will help in identifying, managing, and treating those with periodontitis.

Plaque biofilm and self-care (oral hygiene) are two very significant risk factors for periodontal disease; dental professionals routinely educate patients about these factors. Plaque biofilm or, more specifically, the microbiota was previously discussed in this chapter. It is thought that the current culprits of disease are the gram-negative anaerobes found at many disease sites including *Actinomyces actinomycetemcomitans, Bacteroides forsythus* now known as *Tannerella forsythensis, Porphyromonas gingivalis, Prevotella intermedia, Fusobacterium nucleatum, Campylobacter rectus,* and *Treponema denticola.* It is not known if all gram-negative anaerobes are pathogenic; however, they are found most often in the broad gram-negative groupings of bacteria from disease sites.[76] It is important for patients to realize that not all types of bacteria are equally detrimental to their periodontal health, and that this variation is why the amount of plaque biofilm deposit is not as important to health as the quality or type of bacteria. Unfortunately, without efficient and cost-effective chairside tests, practitioners usually teach patients that the less plaque biofilm one has, the less chance there will be of developing periodontal disease or perpetuating an existing disease. This information is somewhat of a problem, because patients often leave the education session believing quantity or amount is more important than quality of plaque biofilm.

It is clear there is a relationship between poor oral hygiene and manifestation of gingivitis.[76] In fact, the better the self-care, the less gingivitis one seems to develop. On the other hand, oral hygiene positively affects the subgingival microflora in shallow and moderate pocket depths; however, self-care has little effect on the microflora in deep pockets.[84] Some of the detrimental gram-negative pathogens identified above can be established in young children; these pathogens are found in supragingival plaque. Supragingival plaque microflora

can migrate subgingivally when the host response is overwhelmed in the individual. Therefore, frequent supragingival prophylaxis and good self-care together can have a beneficial effect on subgingival microflora in shallow to moderately deep pockets.[84] In conclusion, it is important to educate the patient about the importance of removing supragingival plaque to prevent and arrest progression of periodontitis.

Tobacco use is a health behavior that causes or contributes, as a major environmental factor, to various oral diseases and adverse conditions including periodontal disease. There is no doubt that tobacco users are at more risk for periodontal diseases than nonusers. Increased risk for periodontal disease is 2.5 to 6.0 times greater if one smokes.[85] Smokers make up 90% of individuals with **refractory periodontal disease** (periodontal disease that continues to progress or recur despite professional care and self-care).[86] In fact, smoking is one of the most significant risk factors for periodontal disease.[87] Smoking produces heat that may enhance attachment loss, that reduces collagen synthesis and protein secretion, and that inhibits bone formation. It also inhibits immunologic function and negatively affects immunoglobulin levels, which may increase susceptibility to microbial pathogens.[80] Also, most research concludes that healing is slower in smokers, possibly because of the suppressed growth and attachment of fibroblasts in the periodontal ligament of smokers, and the slower reduction of white blood cells and neutrophils after therapy.[76] It is thought that smokers display a favorable environment for the detrimental periodontal pathogens to grow; therefore, they may have a higher prevalence of subgingival pathogenic species.[76] Some studies show more calculus and plaque accumulates in smokers, and other studies show the opposite.

It seems that further study on how smoking affects gingival bleeding is needed. Some studies show that smoking masks the signs of inflammation; therefore, smokers have less bleeding than nonsmokers. In contrast, other studies show that bleeding is increased in smokers because of increased vascularity. Still other studies show that bleeding is equal among smokers and nonsmokers.[76] Smoking also seems to inhibit granulocyte function, and interactions between smoking and the interleukin-1 gene cluster have also been identified, as mentioned previously. Dentists and dental hygienists are responsible for educating patients about tobacco use as a risk factor for periodontitis, and about prevention strategies and cessation programs. Jones[88] points out that *Healthy People 2000* [89] called for an "increase to at least 75 percent the proportion of primary care and oral health care providers who routinely advise cessation and provide assistance and follow-up for all their tobacco using patients." The dental office is a credible source of information about smoking and tobacco use intervention.

It is also known that stress is a risk factor for many different diseases. Likewise, stress seems to be associated with the progression of periodontitis, lending credibility to the theory that periodontitis is related to systemic diseases.[76]

There is strong evidence suggesting that diabetes, an abnormal elevation in blood glucose levels, is a risk factor for both gingivitis and periodontitis, and that the level of glycemic control appears to be important in this relationship.[90] Diabetes is a very prevalent disease, affecting 21 million Americans, 6 million of whom are unaware they have the disease, because it is undiagnosed.[90] Older individuals, Hispanics, Native Americans, and non-Hispanic blacks are groups who have more diabetes compared with younger people and non-Hispanic whites.[90] Multiple studies indicate that the presence of diabetes is usually associated with increased gingival inflammation and that the level of glycemic control may be a factor in how the gingiva responds to plaque biofilm. Not only does diabetes increase the risk of periodontitis, it does so at any age. Also, poorly controlled diabetes increases the extent and severity of periodontitis as well as the progression of periodontal destruction. The dental professional should always be mindful of this relationship when reviewing health histories, educating patients, and assessing and treating periodontal diseases.

A risk calculator is available to assess a patient's risk of periodontal disease. It is a computer-based risk assessment tool called the Periodontal Risk Calculator (Dental Medicine International, Inc., Philadelphia, Pennsylvania). Page and others report that one study showed valid and accurate prediction of risk of periodontal deterioration, as measured by change in alveolar bone status and tooth loss with the use of the calculator.[74] The findings show a strong association between the assigned risk score and the actual periodontal deterioration observed during a 15-year period.[74,75] Risk assessment factors, tools, and models of the future will aid clinicians in the ability to help patients prevent and control disease, as well as aid practitioners in selecting and delivering appropriate individualized periodontal therapy.

PRIMARY PREVENTION OF PERIODONTAL DISEASES

The most important strategy for preventing periodontal disease is to exercise prevention from the earliest age. Prevention requires daily mechanical plaque control (toothbrushing and interdental cleaning) often supplemented with chemical control measures for plaque biofilm (e.g., chlorhexidine, triclosan, or essential-oil mouthrinses) as an additional component (**adjunct**) of the primary treatment. Fluoride mouthrinses can be used to aid in preventing root and coronal caries.

Bleeding gingiva is a first sign of periodontal disease; patients who report "bleeding gums" should be treated by a dentist and dental hygienist. A thorough prophylaxis, including removal of plaque-retention factors (e.g., calculus and overhanging restorations) plus more diligent self-care are indicated for gingivitis. For patients with early-to-moderate periodontitis, nonsurgical periodontal therapy is indicated, with treatment focused on removal of plaque biofilm and calcified deposits from the cementum and disruption of subgingival microbial flora. Thorough debridement (scaling and root planing) of tooth surfaces is performed by manual (hand) or ultrasonic instrumentation. Flushing out toxins from the epithelial-related plaque biofilm can be achieved with some irrigation units with special tips that permit patients to irrigate shallow pockets (4 to 5 mm).[91]

Some patients have advanced periodontitis with vast tissue destruction, deep pockets (greater than 5 mm), and furcation involvement, which indicate a need for periodontal surgery. Even if complex surgical procedures or intensive therapy is used to treat patients, primary preventive measures play a critical role in helping to maintain disease control after periodontal health has been reestablished.

A major challenge in primary preventive dentistry is to increase public awareness that patient self-care can maintain excellent oral health. Effective removal of supragingival plaque biofilm coupled with regular professional examination and appropriate oral health care established early in life will minimize periodontal disease. It was long believed that, once the subgingival plaque biofilm was permanently organized, supragingival plaque control (self-care) activities had no effect on the subgingival plaque. However, more recent evidence has demonstrated that meticulous supragingival plaque control measures can delay the initiation and organization of the subgingival plaque.[92–94]

SUMMARY

Periodontitis is a disease involving pathology of one or more of the four components of the periodontium: the epithelial attachment, alveolar bone, cementum, and periodontal ligament. The term *periodontal disease* is an umbrella term for several clinically similar types of diseases attributable to different bacteria and different modifying factors. Gingivitis, by definition, becomes periodontitis when the epithelial attachment migrates apically, causing a loss of the level of clinical attachment and alveolar bone. Periodontitis is caused by a combination of bacterial species. Estimation of these variables can be made by studying clinical signs of inflammation and past disease behavior. The bacteria associated with healthy gingiva are usually composed of aerobic, nonmotile, gram-positive cocci. In contrast, the microorganisms for the subgingival plaque that are associated with disease usually are anaerobic, gram-negative motile rods and treponema. The most common form of gingivitis is plaque-induced, and the most common form of periodontitis is chronic periodontitis.

The supragingival plaque biofilm is on the enamel, and the tooth-associated subgingival plaque biofilm is on the cementum. In the area separating the supragingival from the subgingival plaque, there is a melding of bacteria of the two biofilms. To combat the bacterial challenge, when there is a site of inflammation, the body recognizes chemotactic signals that bring both cellular and humoral immune responses to the inflamed areas.

Predicting risk of periodontitis is a complex issue. It is difficult to study the effects of one risk factor in a population for many reasons. Multiple risk factors enhance the ability of an individual to acquire periodontal disease and for it to progress. It is evident, however, that tobacco use is clearly a single indicator that affects one's risk of disease development and progression.

In patients with periodontal disease, it currently is not possible to predict speed of development and severity of the disease with complete accuracy. Research is being conducted in genetics to identify etiologic bacteria, aid in diagnosis, and enhance treatment. The Human Genome Project, a worldwide effort that decoded the DNA molecule, is expected to enhance these efforts in the future. Studies of interleukin-1, a cytokine, have indicated that laboratory evaluation of this cytokine can help identify those individuals at higher risk for developing severe periodontal diseases. Interleukin-1 is also related to bleeding on dental probing. Because interleukin-1 is a lifetime genetic factor, one test for this factor may suffice to assign risk for a lifetime. This test may also be used in developing treatment plans for individual patients.[95] Because bacteria are essential for periodontitis, a positive (high blood level) of interleukin-1 should alert the dental professional and the patient to the importance of complying with daily mechanical and chemical plaque control therapies.

REFERENCES

1. Socransky, S. S., & Haffajee, A. D. (1992). The bacterial etiology of destructive periodontal disease. *J Periodontol, 63*:322–31.
2. The American Academy of Periodontology. (1999). The pathogenesis of periodontal diseases. (Position paper). *J Periodontol, 70*:457–70.
3. The American Academy of Periodontology. (2003). Diagnosis of periodontal diseases. (Position paper). *J Periodontol, 74*:1237–47.
4. Kiane, D. F., & Marshall, G. J. (2001). Periodontal manifestations of systemic disease. *Aust Dent J, 46*:2–12.
5. Cichon, P., Crawford, L., & Grimm, W. D. (1998). Early onset periodontitis associated with Down's syndrome—Clinical intervention study. *Ann Periodontol, 3*:370–80.
6. Nuabe, Y., Ogawa, T., Kamoi, H., Kiyonobu, K., Sato, S., Kamoi, K., & Deguchi, S. (1998). Phagocytic function of salivary PMN after smoking or secondary smoking. *Ann Periodontol, 3*:370–80.
7. Janson, L., Lavstedt, S., Frithiof, L., & Theobold, H. (2000). Relation between oral health and mortality in cardiovascular diseases. *J Clin Periodont, 28*:762–68.
8. Hashim, R., Thomson, W. M., & Pack, A. R. (2001). Smoking in adolescence as a predictor of early loss of periodontal attachment. *Comm Dent Oral Epidemiol, 29*:130–35.
9. Wilson, T. G., Jr. (1998). Effects of smoking on the periodontium. *Quintessence Int, 29*:265–66.
10. Michalowicz, B. S., Diehl, S. R., Gunsolley, J. C., Sparks, B. S., Brooks, B. S., Koetge, T. E., Califano, J. V., Burmeister, J. A., & Schenkein, H. A. (2000). Evidence of a substantial genetic basis of risk of adult periodontitis. *J Periodontol, 71*:1699–1707.
11. Kornman, K. S., Knobelman, C., & Wang, N.-Y. (2000). Is periodontitis genetic The answer may be yes! *Mass Dent Soc, 49*:2–6.
12. Salvi, G. E., Lawrence, H. P., Offenbacher, S., & Beck, J. D. (1997). Influence of risk factors on the pathogenesis of periodontitis. *Periodontol 2000, 14*:173–201.
13. Taylor, G. W., Loesche, W. J., & Terpenning, M. S. (2000). Impact of oral diseases on systemic health in the elderly: diabetes mellitus and aspiration pneumonia. *J Public Health Dent, 60*:313–20.

14. Stewart, J. E., Wager, K. H., Friedlander, A. H., & Zadek, N. H. (2001). The effect of periodontal treatment on glycemic control in patients with type 2 diabetes mellitus. *J Clin Periodontol,* 28:306–10.

15. Tonetti, M. S. (1998). Cigarette smoking and periodontal diseases; etiology and management of disease. *Ann Periodontol,* 25:88–101.

16. Arbes, S. J., Jr, Agerstsdottier, H., & Slade, G. D. (2001). Environmental tobacco smoke and periodontal disease in the United States. *Am J Public Health,* 91:253–57.

17. Lerner, U. H., Modeer, T., Krekmanova, L., Claesson, R., & Rasmussen, L. (1998). Gingival crevicular fluid from patients with periodontitis contains bone resorbing activity. *Eur J Oral Sci,* 106:778–87.

18. The American Academy of Periodontology. (2003). Periodontal diseases of children and adolescents. (Position paper). *J Periodontol,* 74:1696–1704.

19. Loe, H., & Brown, L. J. (1991). Early onset periodontitis in the United States of America. *J Periodontol,* 62:608–16.

20. The American Academy of Periodontology. (2005). Epidemiology of periodontal diseases. (Position paper). *J Periodontol,* 76:1406–19.

21. The American Academy of Periodontology. (2000). Parameter on periodontitis associated with systemic conditions. *J Periodontol,* 71 (Suppl):876–79.

22. Kim, J., & Amar, S. (2006). Periodontal disease and systemic conditions: a bidirectional relationship. *Odontology,* 94:10–21.

23. Paquette, D. W., Madianos, P., Offenbacher, S., Beck, J. D., & Williams, R.C. (1999). The concept of "risk" and the emerging discipline of periodontal medicine. *J Contemp Dent Pract,* 15:1–8.

24. Fowler, E. B., Brealt, L. G., & Cuenin, M. F. (2001). Periodontal disease and its association with systemic disease. *Mil Med,* 166:85–89.

25. Brandtzaeg, P. (2001). Inflammatory bowel disease: Clinics and pathology. Do inflammatory bowel disease and periodontal disease have similar immunopathogeneses? *Acta Odontol Scand,* 59:235–43.

26. Klokkevold, P. R. (1999). Periodontal medicine: assessment of risk factors for disease. *J Calif Dent Assoc,* 27:135–42.

27. U.S. Department of Health and Human Services. (2000). *Oral health in America: A report of the Surgeon General—Executive summary.* Rockville, MD: U.S. Department of Health and Human Services, National Institute of Dental and Craniofacial Research, National Institutes of Health.

28. Pearlman, B. (2000). Prognosis: The dilemma of modern periodontics. *Ann R Australas Coll Dent Surg,* 15:141–43.

29. Socransky, S. S., & Haffajee, A. D. (1997). The nature of periodontal diseases. *Ann Periodontol,* 2:3–10.

30. Page, R. C. (1998). A new paradigm. *J Dent Edu,* 62:812–20.

31. Hart, T. C., & Kornman, K. S. (1997). Genetic factors in the pathogenesis of periodontitis. *J Periodontol,* 14:141–43.

32. Cattabriga, M., Rotundo, R., Muzzi, L., Nieri, M., Verrocchi, G., Cairo, F., & Pine Prato, G. (2001). Retrospective evaluation of the influence of the interleukin-1 genotype on radiographic bone levels in treated periodontal patients over 10 years. *J Periodontol,* 72:767–73.

33. Hormia, M., Owaribe, K., & Virt, I. (2001). The dento-epithelial junction cell adhesion by Type I hemidesmosomes in the absence of true basal lamina. *J Periodontol,* 72:788–97.

34. Griffiths, G. S., Sterne, J. A., Wilton, J. M., Eaton, K. A, & Johnson, N. W. (1992). Associations between volume and flow rate of gingival crevicular fluid and clinical assessments of gingival inflammation in a population of British male adolescents. *J Clin Periodontol,* 19:464–70.

35. Weidlich, P., Lopez de Souza, M. A., & Opperman, R. V. (2001). Evaluation of the dentogingival area during early plaque formation. *J Periodontol,* 72:901–10.

36. Löe, H., Theilade, E., & Jensen, S. B. (1965). Experimental gingivitis in man. *J Periodontol,* 36:177–83.

37. Moore, W., Holdeman L., Smibert, R., Cato, E. P., Burmeister, J. A., Palcanis, K. G., Ranney, R. R. (1984). Bacteriology of experimental gingivitis in children. *Infect Immun,* 46:1–6.

38. Slots, J., Möenbo, D., Langebaek, J., & Frandsen, A. (1978). Microbiota of gingivitis in man. *Scand J Dent,* 86:174–81.

39. Socransky, S. S., & Haffajee, A. D. (1991). Microbial mechanisms in the pathogenesis of destructive periodontal diseases: A critical assessment. *J Periodontol Res,* 26:195–212.

40. Paster, B. J., Boches, S. K., Galvin, J. L., Ericson, R. E., Lau, C. N., Levanios, V. A., Sahasrabudhe, A., & Dewhirst, F. E. (2001). Bacterial diversity in human subgingival plaque. *J Bacteriol,* 183:3770–83.

41. Friedman, M. T., Barber, P. M., Mardan, N. J., & Newman, H. N. (1992). The "plaque-free zone" in health and disease: A scanning electron microscope study. *J Periodontol,* 63:890–96.

42. *Periodontal literature review.* (1996). Chicago: The American Academy of Periodontology, 68–72.

43. Moore, W. E. C., & Moore, L. V. H. (1994). The bacteria of periodontal diseases. *Periodontol 2000,* 5:66–77.

44. Page, R. C., & Schroeder, H. E. (1977). Pathogenic mechanisms. In Schluger, S., Ysudelis, R., & Page, R. C., Eds. *Periodontal disease: Basic phenomena clinical management and restorative interrelationships.* Philadelphia: Lea & Febiger.

45. Bhowmick, S. K., Giduani, V. K., & Retting, K. R. (2001). Hereditary gingival fibromatosis and growth retardation. *Endocr Prac,* 7:383–87.

46. Majola, M. P., McFadyen, M. L., Connolly, C., Nair, Y. P., Govender, M., Laher, M. H. E. (2000). Factors influencing phenytoin-induced gingival enlargement. *J Clin Periodontol,* 27:506–12.

47. Ronderas, M., Pihlstrom, B. L., & Hodges, J. S. (2001). Periodontal disease among indigenous people in the Amazon rain forest. *J Clin Periodontol,* 28:995–1003.

48. Bowen, D. M. (1998). Introduction to nonsurgical periodontal therapy. In Hodges, K. O., Ed. *Concepts in nonsurgical periodontal therapy.* Albany: Delmar Publishers.

49. Sanz, M., & Newman, M. G. (1988). Dental plaque and calculus. In Newman, M. G., & Nisengard, R., Eds. *Oral microbiology and immunology.* Philadelphia: W.B. Saunders, 367–80.

50. Berghton, D., Lynch, E., & Heath, M. R. (1993). A microbiological study of primary root caries lesions with different treatment needs. *J Dent Res,* 72:623–29.

51. Fine, D. H., Tabak, L., Oshrain, H., Salkind, A., & Siegel, K. (1978). Studies in plaque pathogenicity. Plaque collection limulus lysate screening of adherent and loosely adherent plaque. *J Periodontol Res,* 13:17–22.

52. Fine, D. H., Tabak, L., Oshrain, H., Salkind, A., & Siegel, K. (1978). Studies in plaque pathogenicity. II. A technique for the specific detection of endotoxin in plaque samples using the limulus lysate assay. *J Periodontol Res,* 13:127–133.

53. Caton, J., Bouwsma, O., Polson, A., & Epseland, M. (1989). Effect of personal oral hygiene and subgingival scaling on bleeding interdental gingiva. *J Periodontol,* 60: 84–90.

54. Cercek, J. F., Kiger, R. D., Garrett, S., & Egelberg, J. (1983). Relative effects of plaque control and instrumentation on the clinical parameters of human periodontal disease. *J Periodontol,* 10:46–56.

55. Kho, P., Smales, F., & Hardie, J. (1985). The effect of supragingival plaque control on subgingival microflora. *J Clin Periodontol,* 12:676–86.

56. Greenstein, G. (1992). Periodontal response to mechanical non-surgical therapy: A review. *J Periodontol,* 63:118–30.

57. Ciancio, S. G. (1989). Non-surgical periodontal treatment. In *Proceedings of the world workshop in clinical periodontics* (Section II). Chicago: American Academy of Periodontology.

58. Boch, J. A., Wara-aswapati, N., & Auron, P. E. (2000). Interleukin 1. Signal transduction—Current concepts and relavence to periodontitis. *J Dent Res,* 80:400–407.

59. Flood, P. M., Washington, O., Stevens, D. P., & Ptak, W. (1992). Immunological signals which control T cell responses. *J Endod,* 18:435–39.

60. Huang, G. T., Haake, S. K., & Park, N. H. (1998). Gingival epithelial cells increase interleukin-8 secretion in response to Actinobacillus actinomycetemcomitans challenge. *J Periodontol,* 69:1105–10.

61. Guthmiller, J. M., Lally, E. T., & Korostoff, J. (2001). Beyond the specific plaque hypothesis: Are highly leukotoxic strains of Actinobacillus actinomycetemcomitans a paradigm of periodontal pathogenesis? *Crit Rev Oral Biol Med,*12:116–24.

62. Widmann, F. K., & Itatani, C. A., Eds. (1998). *An introduction to clinical immunology and serology.* Philadelphia: F.A. Davis Company, 473.

63. Gustafasson, A., Asman, B., & Bergstrom, K. (2001). Increased release of IL-B from monocytes for patients with chronic periodontitis. *J Dent Res,* 80:Special Issue, Abstract No. 007.

64. McGuire, M. K., & Nunn, M. E. (1999). Prognosis versus actual outcome. IV. The effectiveness of clinical parameters and IL-1 genotype in accurately predicting prognoses and tooth survival. *J Periodontol,* 70:49–56.

65. Kornman, K. S., Crane, A., Wang, H-Y., diGiovine, F. S., Newman, M. G., Pink, F. W., Wilson, T. G., Jr., Higginbottom, F. L. & Duff, G. W. (1997). The interleukin-1 genotype as a severity factor in adult periodontal disease. *J Clin Periodontol,* 24:72–77.

66. Seymour, G. J., & Gemmell, E. (2001). Cytokines in periodontal disease: where to from here. *Acta Odonto Scan,* 59:167–73.

67. Schenkein, H. A. (1998). Inheritance as a determinant of susceptibility for periodontitis. *J Dent Edu,* 62:840–51.

68. McDevitt, M. J., & Wang, H-Y. (2000). Interleukin-1 genetic association with periodontitis in clinical practice. *J Periodontol,* 71:156–62.

69. Armitage, G. C. (1999). Development of a classification system for periodontal diseases and conditions. *Ann Periodontol,* 4:1.

70. American Academy of Periodontology. (2000). Parameter on chronic periodontitis with slight to moderate loss of periodontal support. *J Periodontol,* 71 (Suppl):853–55.

71. American Academy of Periodontology. (2000). Parameter on chronic periodontitis with advanced loss of periodontal support. *J Periodontol,* 71 (Suppl):856–58.

72. American Academy of Periodontology. (2000). Parameter on aggressive periodontitis. *J Periodontol,* 71 (Suppl):867–69.

73. Last, J. M., Ed. (2001). *A dictionary of epidemiology* (4th ed.). New York: Oxford University Press, 91, 140, 160.

74. Page, R. C., Krall, E. A., Martin J., Mancl, L., & Garcia, R. I. (2002). Validity and accuracy of a risk calculator in predicting periodontal disease. *J Am Dent Assoc,* 133:569–76.

75. Persson, G. R., Mancl, L. A., Martin, J., & Page, R. C. (2003). Assessing periodontal disease risk. *J Am Dent Assoc,* 134:575–82.

76. American Academy of Periodontology. (2005). Epidemiology of periodontal diseases. (Position Paper). *J Periodontol,* 76:1406–19.

77. U.S. Public Health Service, National Institute of Dental Research. (1987). *Oral health of United States adults: National findings* (NIH Publication Number 87-2868). Bethesda, MD: National Institute of Dental Research.

78. Thompson, W. M., Edwards, S. J., Dobson-Le, D. P., Tompkins, G. R., Poulton, R., Knight, D. A., Braithwaite, A. W. IL-1 genotypes and adult periodontitis among young New Zealanders. *J Dent Res,* 80:1700–703.

79. Parkhill, J. M., Hennig, B. J., Chapple, I. L, Heasman, P. A., & Taylor, J. J. Association of interleukin-1 gene polymorphisms with early-onset peridontitis. *J Clin Periodontol,* 27:682–89.

80. Douglass, C. W. Risk assessment and management of periodontal disease. *J Am Dent Assoc,* 137 (Suppl 3):27–32.

81. American Academy of Periodontology. (2005). Informational paper: Implications of genetic technology for the management of periodontal diseases. *J Periodontol,* 76:850–57.

82. Li, Y., Xu, L., Hasturk, H., Kantarci, A., DePalma, S. R., & van Dyke, T. E. (2004). Localized aggressive periodontitis is linked to human chromosome 1q25. *Hum Genet,* 114:291–97.

83. Michalowicz, B. S., Diehl, S. R., Gunsolley, J. C., Sparks, B. S., Brooks, C. N., Koertge, T. E., Califano, J. V., Burmeister, J. A., Schenkein, H. A. (2000). Evidence of a substantial genetic basis for risk of adult periodontitis. *J Periodontol,* 71:1699–1701.

84. Westfelt, E. (1996). Rationale of mechanical plaque control. *J Clin Periodontol,* 23:263–67.

85. Bergstrom, J., & Preber, H. (1994). Tobacco use as a risk factor. *J Periodontol,* 65:545–50.

86. Johnson, G. K., Slach, N. A. (2001). Impact of tobacco use on periodontal status. *J Dent Educ,* 65:313–21.

87. American Academy of Periodontology. (1999). Tobacco use and the periodontal patient. (Position Paper). *J Peridontol,* 70:1419–27.

88. Jones, R. B. (2000). Tobacco or oral health: Past progress, impending challenge. *J Am Dent Assoc,* 131:1130–36.

89. U.S. Department of Health and Human Services. (1990). *Healthy people 2000* (DHHS Publication 91-50212). Washington, DC: U.S. Department of Health and Human Services, Public Health Service.

90. American Academy of Periodontology. (2006). Diabetes mellitus and periodontal diseases. *J Periodontol,* 77:1289–303.

91. Cutler, C. W., Stanford, T. W., Abraham, C., Cederberg, R. A., Boardman, T. J., & Ross, C. (2000). Clinical benefits of oral irrigation for periodontitis are related to reduction of proinflammatory cytokine levels and plaque. *J Clin Periodontol,* 27:134–43.

92. Dahlen, G., Lindhe, J., Sato, K., Hanamura, H., & Okamoto, H. (1992). The effect of supragingival plaque control on the subgingival microbiota in subjects with periodontal disease. *J Clin Periodontol,* 19:802–809.

93. Katsanoulas, T., Renee, I., & Attstrom, R. The effect of supragingival plaque control on the composition of the subgingival flora in periodontal pockets. *J Clin Periodontol,* 19:760–65.

94. Corbet, E. F., & Davies, W. I. (1993). The role of supragingival plaque in the control of progressive periodontal disease: A review. *J Clin Periodontol,* 20:307–13.

95. Bowers, J. E. (1999). Genetic testing. One part of periodontal risk assessment. *Pract Hygiene,* 27:627–39.

Chapter 5

Oral Cancer

Sandra J. Maurizio

OBJECTIVES

After studying this chapter, the student should be able to:

1. Describe the epidemiology of oral cancer.
2. Identify risk factors that contribute to oral cancer.
3. Identify signs and symptoms of oral cancer.
4. Identify factors to prevent oral cancer.
5. Identify clinical manifestations of oral cancer and conditions that mimic it.
6. Describe the common locations for oropharyngeal cancers.
7. Describe the various screening and diagnostic tools used to detect oral cancer.
8. Describe the steps in a complete oral cancer examination.
9. Identify the staging system used for oral cancer.
10. Identify appropriate referral sites.
11. Describe treatment options.
12. Identify resources available to health care providers and patients.

KEY TERMS

Neoplasm
Proliferation
Apoptosis
Carcinomas
Oral cancers
Oropharynx
Pharynx
Oral cavity
Vermilion (red) border
Pharyngeal arches
Soft palate
Palatoglossus
Palatopharyngeal
Palate
Tonsillar fossae
Epithelial dysplasia
Growth regulation
Differentiation
Replicative senescence
Angiogenesis
DNA repair
Tissue remodeling and migration
Immune evasion
Incidence rates

(continued)

KEY TERMS (CONTINUED)

Stage
Mortality rate
Human papillomavirus infection
Carcinogenesis
Actinic cheilitis
Leukoplakia
Erythroplakia
Erythroleukoplakia
Chemopreventive agents
Lichen planus
Human papillomavirus
Symptom
Sign
Palpation
Tolonium chloride
Carcinoma in situ
Exfoliative cytology
Oral brush test
Adjunct
Fine-needle aspiration biopsy
Punch biopsy
Incisional biopsy
Excisional biopsy
Otolaryngologist
Maxillofacial surgeon

Prognosis
Grading
Staging
Wide local excision
Resection
Marginal resections
Segmental resection
Composite resection
Comprehensive neck dissections
Radical neck dissection
Modified neck dissection
Selective neck dissections
External-beam radiotherapy
Intensity-modulated radiotherapy
Brachytherapy
Interstitial irradiation
Intraoral cone
Electron-beam therapy
Xerostomia
Dysgeusia
Osseointegrated implants
Mucositis
Sialogogues
Hypogeusia
Ageusia
Dysgeusia

INTRODUCTION

Cancer refers to a variety of malignant neoplasms that occur throughout the body. The term **neoplasm** means "new growth" and describes a rapid growth of the number of cells (**proliferation**) that exceeds normal growth.[1] This overgrowth may be caused by cells that continue proliferation after cessation of the stimuli that initiated the new growth or by cells that do not undergo **apoptosis** (programmed cell death).[1,2] Neoplasms can be either benign or cancerous, depending on whether they invade surrounding or distant tissues. **Carcinomas** are malignant neoplasms derived from epithelial tissue.[1]

Oral cancers are defined in various ways. In this chapter, they will be defined according to the primary anatomic structures. **Oral cancers** affect the oral cavity (mouth) and the **oropharynx,** which is the part of the **pharynx** (throat) located at the back of the mouth. In this chapter, the **oral cavity** will extend from the **vermilion (red) border** of the lips through the mouth to, and including, the **pharyngeal arches.** The arches are formed by the palatoglossus and the palatopharyngeal muscles. Both muscles arise from the **soft palate,** which is the muscular portion of the roof of the mouth located posterior to the root of the tongue. The **palatoglossus** muscle forms the anterior (front) arch on each side of the throat, whereas the **palatopharyngeal** muscle forms the posterior arch.[1] Subdivisions of the oral cavity include the lips, floor of the mouth, buccal mucosa, **palate** (roof of the mouth), and alveolar processes. The oropharynx includes the entire area from the base of the tongue, the pharyngeal wall, the **tonsillar fossae** (the depressions between the pharyngeal arches in which the tonsils are located), and the soft palate.[3] Generally, in this chapter, the term *oral cancer* will include both oral cavity and oropharyngeal cancers, unless otherwise specified.

Squamous cell carcinomas represent more than 90% of cancers of the oropharynx and oral cavity. The etiology of squamous cell carcinomas of the oral cavity and oropharyngeal regions is multifactorial. Salivary gland cancers, including adenoid cystic carcinoma, mucoepidermoid carcinoma, and polymorphous low-grade adenocarcinoma, are present in the oral cavity, among others.[4] The following brief explanation of the biologic basis for cancer formation will be helpful in discussions of preventive modalities.

Cancers are formed when normal cells undergo a sequential, multi-step process from normality to eventual metastatic cancer (cancer that has spread from its site of origin). **Epithelial dysplasia** is a premalignant condition during which cells undergo a combination of cellular and architectural changes. Cell alterations include changes in the size, shape, and number of nuclei, and increased mitosis (cell division) (Figure 5–1 ■). Altered architectural integrity includes formation of rete pegs (elongated ridges of epidermis that point downward), hyperplasia (abnormal increase in the number of cells) of the basilar membrane, and altered maturation.[5] Cell functions that must be disrupted for cancer to occur include (a) growth regulation, (b) apoptosis, (c) differ-entiation, (d) replicative senescence, (e) angiogenesis, (f) DNA repair, (g) tissue remodeling and migration, and (h) immune evasion. **Growth regulation** refers to proliferation beyond the number of cells expected in normal cell division. Apoptosis is programmed cell death, which is the process of removing aging cells or cells with damaged DNA from the body. In cancerous growths, apoptosis is "turned off" so that damaged cells are allowed to replicate (duplicate their genetic material). **Differentiation** involves the degree of alteration of cells from their normal morphology (form) and function. Poorly differentiated neoplasms no longer resemble the cells they derived from originally. Well-differentiated neoplasms retain the original cells' morphology and function (Figure 5–2 ■). **Replicative senescence** is the irreversible *loss* of the cell's ability to stop dividing after a finite number of divisions, which results in faulty cells. **Angiogenesis** is the buildup of vascular tissue needed to sustain cancerous growth. **DNA repair** is the process by which a cell monitors and repairs DNA disruptions before replication to avoid passing faulty DNA material to new cells. Mutation of the p53 gene is observed in head and neck cancers. **Tissue remodeling and migration** refers to the ability to travel beyond the normal borders of the tissue associated with a particular cell (Figure 5–3 ■). **Immune evasion** is a breakdown in the ability to monitor tissues for evidence of cancer.[6]

Some mild forms of epithelial dysplasia can be reversed if preventive measures are taken, such as dietary changes or tobacco and alcohol cessation. The role of the dental professional is critical in the process of recognizing early lesions, and perhaps preventing the transformation to malignancy. These goals are accomplished

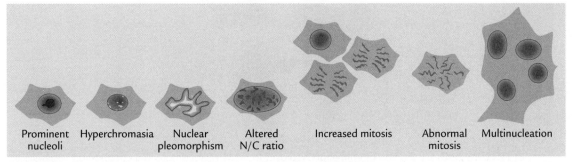

| Prominent nucleoli | Hyperchromasia | Nuclear pleomorphism | Altered N/C ratio | Increased mitosis | Abnormal mitosis | Multinucleation |

■ **FIGURE 5–1**   Cell alterations in epithelial dysplasia. The degree of severity of an epithelial dysplasia is determined, in part, by the frequency and combination of these alterations.
(Reprinted from *Contemporary oral and maxillofacial pathology* [2nd ed.], Sapp, J. P., Eversole, L. R., & Wysocki, G. P. St. Louis: Mosby. © 2004. Reprinted with permission from Elsevier.)

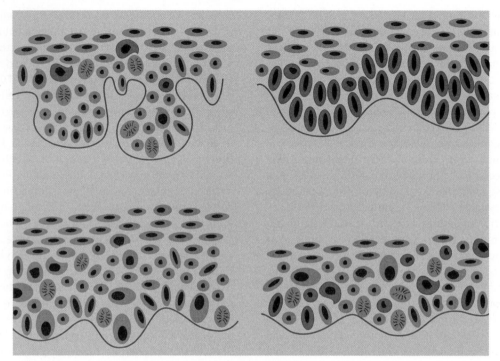

■ FIGURE 5–2 Architectural alterations of the epithelium found in epithelial dysplasia. The degree of severity of the epithelial dysplasia is determined by the extent of severity of these alterations combined with the individual cell abnormalities.
(Reprinted from *Contemporary oral and maxillofacial pathology* [2nd ed.], Sapp, J. P., Eversole, L. R., & Wysocki, G. P. St. Louis: Mosby. © 2004. Reprinted with permission from Elsevier.)

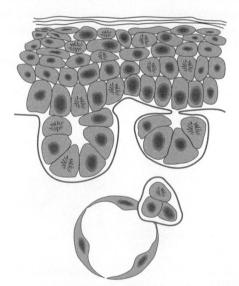

■ FIGURE 5–3 Transition of epithelial dysplasia to invasive squamous cell carcinoma. Malignant cells have penetrated through the basement membrane into the underlying connective tissue, where they are capable of eroding into lymphatic vessels.
(Reprinted from *Contemporary oral and maxillofacial pathology* [2nd ed.], Sapp, J. P., Eversole, L. R., & Wysocki, G. P. St. Louis: Mosby. © 2004. Reprinted with permission from Elsevier.)

by educating patients and assisting them in termination of harmful habits. Because squamous cell carcinomas represent nearly all oral cancers, the remainder of the chapter will refer to this type of cancer.

EPIDEMIOLOGY OF ORAL CANCER

The American Cancer Society estimated 35,310 new cases of oral cavity and pharynx cancers will occur in 2008, with an estimated 7,590 deaths. **Incidence rates** refer to the number of new cases of a disease in a specified population during 1 year per 100,000 individuals. Incidence rates for oral cavity and pharyngeal cancers in men are roughly twice as high as those for women.[4] Estimated incidence rates by gender for 2007 reflected a two-to-one ratio of men to women, with 24,180 new cases expected for men and 10,180 for women.[4] Five-year survival rates for all cancers have demonstrated an increase from 50% in the mid-1970s to 65% in 2001.[4] For all stages of oral cavity and pharynx cancer patients, about 84% will survive 1 year; 5-year and 10-year survival rates are 59% and 48%, respectively.[4] The 1995–2001 Surveillance, Epidemiology, and End Results Program (SEER) data indicate that 5-year survival rates are 59.4% for all stages, 82.1% for localized lesions, 51.3% for regional cancers, and 27.6% for distant cancers of the oral cavity and pharynx.[7] Estimated deaths by gender for 2007 indicate a two-to-one ratio of men to women, with 5,180 deaths expected for men versus 2,370 for women.[4] As the survival rates indicate, **stage** (extent of a cancer in the body[2]) at diagnosis is a critical factor in the expected mortality rate for oral cancer.

As shown in Tables 5–1 ■ and 5–2 ■, oral cancer mortality is disproportionately distributed among ethnic and minority groups. **Mortality rate** refers to the number of deaths in a specified population during 1 year per 100,000 individuals. SEER 1995–2001 data indicate oral cavity and pharynx mortality rates of 3.8 and 1.5 per 100,000 for white men and women, respectively. The mortality rate for African Americans is 6.8 for men and 1.7 for women. Rates for white and African American women are comparable, but the mortality rates for men show a much greater rate for African American males than white males. The gender breakdown in other races ranges from 3.6 and 1.4 for Asian/Pacific Islander men and women, respectively, to 3.2 and 1.4 for American Indian/Alaskan Native men and women, and 2.8 and 0.8 for Hispanic men and women (Tables 5–1 and 5–2).[7]

Reasons for the disproportionate burden of oral cancer on minority populations are complex, and confounding factors make causes difficult to assess. In simplistic terms, confounding factors are two or more factors that can affect a situation, but each factor's individual effect cannot be determined.[1] Lack of access to medical and dental care could contribute to later stage diagnosis.[8] Minority populations are less likely to receive an oral cancer screening by a medical or dental provider. In addition, high-risk individuals are more likely to seek care from a medical rather than a dental provider. A lack of awareness of the signs and symptoms of oral cancer, and the need for regular oral cancer screenings contribute to late diagnosis.[8]

■ **Table 5–1**   Stage Distribution of Oral Cavity and Pharynx Cancer by Race and Gender, 1996–2002

	All Races			*Whites*			*African Americans*		
	Total	*Male*	*Female*	*Total*	*Male*	*Female*	*Total*	*Male*	*Female*
Number of cases	30,031	20,522	9,509	24,344	16,629	7,715	3,061	2,185	876
Percent	100%	100%	100%	100%	100%	100%	100%	100%	100%
Localized	33	30	40	35	32	42	21	17	31
Regional	52	55	46	50	53	44	59	61	52
Distant	10	10	8	9	9	8	15	16	13
Unstaged	5	5	6	5	5	6	5	5	5

Source: Ries, L. A. G., Eisner, M. P., Kosary, C. L., Hankey, B. F., Miller, B. A., Clegg, L., Mariotto, A., Feuer, E. J., & Edwards, B. K., Eds. (2003). *SEER cancer statistics review, 1975–2002.* Bethesda, MD: National Cancer Institute.

■ **Table 5–2** Oral Cavity and Pharynx Cancer 5-Year Survival Rate, 1996–2002, by Stage at Diagnosis, Race, and Gender

	All Races			Whites			African Americans		
	Total	*Male*	*Female*	*Total*	*Male*	*Female*	*Total*	*Male*	*Female*
All stages	58.8	57.6	61.3	60.9	60.6	61.6	39.7	35.6	49.1
Localized	81.3	81.3	81.4	82.1	82.9	80.8	71.1	63.9	79.7
Regional	51.7	51.7	51.4	53.4	54.2	51.3	33.9	32.1	39.1
Distant	26.4	25.4	28.7	26.9	25.6	29.9	21.8	22.6	19.6
Unstaged	45.0	45.4	43.7	45.9	48.5	40.5	30.5	26.6	38.3

Source: Ries, L. A. G., Eisner, M. P., Kosary, C. L., Hankey, B. F., Miller, B. A., Clegg, L., Mariotto, A., Feuer, E. J., & Edwards, B. K., Eds. (2003). *SEER cancer statistics review, 1975–2002*. Bethesda, MD: National Cancer Institute.

RISK FACTORS

The oncology field has started to shift from a treatment-oriented philosophy toward a prevention-oriented philosophy. A similar shift occurred in cardiology, when suspected risk factors were studied sufficiently to determine causal relationships. Educational campaigns directed toward health professionals and the public resulted in well-understood prevention modalities to help overcome cardiac diseases. The important shift toward identifying factors to prevent cancer as further research evolves is a critical one for dental professionals to pursue.[9]

The oral cavity is exposed to a variety of ingested and inhaled agents that may increase the risk of cancer. The multitude of possible contributors to the development of oral carcinoma confounds the difficulty in identifying causative agents. Host susceptibility, environmental factors, and exposure to protective factors all play a role in the development of oral cancer. Primary risk factors for oral cancer include tobacco use, excessive alcohol intake, and increasing age. Tobacco use is the major cause of oral cancer in the United States. The majority of oral cancers occur in individuals older than 40 to 45 years.[7,10,11] However, a recent upswing of cases has been identified in young people with no apparent risk factors.[11,12] **Human papillomavirus infection** is a possible contributor to this phenomenon.[6,12–14] Other risk factors include low intake of fruits and vegetables, excessive sun exposure (lip cancers), and lifestyle issues. It is logical that aging causes changes at the cellular level as a result of pollutants from the environment, habits such as smoking and alcohol consumption, viruses, inadequate nutrition, and chemicals in food and drinks.[15]

Tobacco

Tobacco contributes to an estimated 30% of cancers in the United States. The use of tobacco products accounts for an estimated 75% of *oral* cancers in the United States. Cigarette smoking has been firmly established as a direct causal link of cancer of the oral cavity and pharynx.[16] It has been implicated in causing 75% of oral cavity and pharynx cancer deaths in men in the United States during 1995–1999.[17] An earlier American Cancer Society's 50-state study demonstrated a relative risk of 27.5 and 8.8 among male current and former smokers, respectively, and 5.6 and 2.9 among females, respectively.[18] Currently, the American Cancer Society indicates 90% of oral cancer patients use tobacco. Smokers have a sixfold chance of developing these cancers. In addition, 37% of oral cancer patients who continue to smoke after their cancer is gone will develop second oral cancers, whereas recurrent cancer will occur in 6% of former oral cancer patients who quit.[19] Smokeless tobacco is believed to increase the risk of buccal mucosal, gingival, and labial mucosal cancers by 50 times.[19] Pipe smoking is a contributor to cancer of the lip.[20] In other countries, particularly India, chewing betel or areca nut in a quid called *paan* is associated with a higher risk of oral cancer.[21,22]

Alcohol

Heavy consumers of alcohol who do not use tobacco products have a relative risk of 2.2 for developing oral cancer, regardless of the type of alcohol consumed.[23] The risk for oral cancer development is dose-related, with individuals consuming more than four drinks per day at greatest risk.[24,25] The type of alcohol does not seem to have an effect on the incidence of oral cancer. The American Cancer Society suggests about 75% to 80% of oral cancer patients drink alcohol, and drinkers are 6 times as likely to develop oral cancer.[19] The combination of smoking and alcohol is particularly deadly. Heavy drinkers and smokers have 100 times the risk of developing oral cancer compared with abstainers. The dehydrating influence of alcohol on cell walls provides an avenue for tobacco carcinogens (cancer-producing substances[1]) to enter oral tissues, and is the mechanism of action that contributes to the synergistic effect. In addition, heavy drinkers typically have nutritional deficiencies that lower the body's ability to prevent cancer.[26] When ethanol is metabolized, toxic compounds are released, including acetaldehyde, a recognized carcinogen. Alcohol may decrease retinoic acid, which has a protective function against cancer development. A local toxic effect may produce cellular hyperproliferation.[27] The increased risk associated with the use of tobacco and alcohol products will fade after 10 years of abstinence, lessening the risk to approximately that of any non-drinker and non-smoker.[26]

Age

The 1998–2002 SEER data indicate the median age at diagnosis for cancer of the oral cavity and pharynx for all races and both sexes is 63 years, with 89% of the cases occurring in adults aged 45 years and older.[7] The aging demographical profile of the United States population suggests an increase in oral cancer incidence in coming years. Aging may cause the immune system to become less effective and cause biophysical or biochemical processes that contribute to **carcinogenesis** (production or development of cancer).[11] Although cancer is typically a disease of older populations, several reports in the literature suggest an upturn of cases among young individuals with no apparent risk factors.[28,29] The cause for the increase is unknown.

Race and Ethnicity

The influence of race and ethnicity on incidence of oral cancer is difficult to quantify. There are definite differences in the incidence and mortality rates of various racial groups, but the reason for the differences is unclear. Are they actually related to genetic alterations

of races, or are they associated with lifestyle issues? The genetic code is becoming better understood, and eventual changes in the genetic code that lead to various cancers may become clear. Until then, most researchers attribute the differences to lifestyle and environmental factors.[30] Unraveling the confounding effects of lifestyle variations between racial and ethnic groups is extremely difficult. Brown and others attribute the vast majority of the higher level of esophageal cancer in African American men to alcohol and smoking, but also express concerns that the rate is higher than that expected for alcohol and tobacco alone. They suggest there may be qualitative differences in alcohol consumption, environmental exposure differences, and differences in susceptibility to alcohol and tobacco.[31] Other researchers attribute the major differences in risk variations between whites and African Americans to alcohol and tobacco use, but believe the white population sample had a higher intake of fruits and vegetables and vitamin C, and that the African American sample demonstrated sociodemographic factors associated with increased risk.[32] Minority groups often live in more polluted areas and may be exposed to more environmental carcinogens as a result.[33] Few studies have been done on Latino or Hispanic populations; however, variations in oral and pharyngeal cancer rates occur in Hispanic groups located in different regions of the United States, which suggests behavioral, cultural, genetic, and familial risk factors may be involved. Hispanic populations have lower rates of oral cancer than other racial and ethnic groups. However, in one study, New York City Hispanic men, primarily of Puerto Rican descent, showed much higher incidence and mortality rates than those of Hispanic men and white, non-Hispanic men, in other areas of the country.[34] Further research into the genetic, as well as environmental, factors associated with racial and ethnic groups is necessary to clarify the differences in oral cancer incidence and mortality.

Actinic Radiation (Ultraviolet Light) Exposure

Solar radiation or sun exposure is a known risk factor for cancer of the lip. Typically, the chronic overexposure of ultraviolet radiation from sunlight initially causes **actinic cheilitis,** a demonstrated precancerous lesion, usually occurring on the lower lip.[35] Actinic cheilitis frequently progresses into squamous cell carcinoma. Lip cancer is more prevalent in fair-skinned individuals, particularly men. Reasons for higher incidence in males may be that more men work in outdoor occupations, and the use of cosmetic lipstick may provide some protection for women.[36] Lip cancer is rare in dark-skinned individuals. The rates of lip cancer are decreasing, likely because of an increased awareness of the damage done to skin by exposure to sunlight and increased use of lip balms containing sunscreen.[11]

Potentially Malignant Oral Epithelial Lesions

Leukoplakia, Erythroplakia, and Erythroleukoplakia (Speckled Leukoplakia)

Leukoplakia (white), **erythroplakia** (red), and **erythroleukoplakia** (red and white, or "speckled") lesions are considered premalignant (Figure 5–4 ■). Leukoplakia refers to a white patch on oral mucosa that cannot be wiped or scraped off or classified as any other diagnosis. This term describes a clinical diagnosis only, rather than a histologic one.[37] The risk for malignant transformation is multifaceted. The type of leukoplakia, presence of dysplasia, habits, lifestyle, genetics, and other factors contribute to the possible transformation to malignancy[30] (Figures 5–4 and 5–5 ■). Erythroplakia demonstrates a greater threat for malignant transformation[38] (Figures 5–5a, b, and c; and 5–6 ■). Risk of malignancy varies, but in one study of 257 oral leukoplakia patients, carcinoma developed in 15.7% of the leukoplakic lesions; furthermore, in leukoplakic lesions with dysplasia, 36.4%

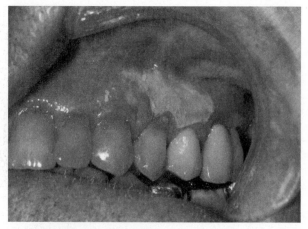

■ **FIGURE 5–4** Leukoplakia.
(Courtesy Dr. Sol Silverman, Jr.)

of the lesions progressed to carcinoma.[39] Lesions with epithelial dysplasia should be surgically excised; however, recurrence is common (Figure 5–7 ■). Lumerman and others determined that only 4 (6.2%) of 65 patients who had surgical excision of epithelial dysplastic lesions developed invasive squamous cell carcinoma, (Figure 5–8 ■) compared with 14 (15.4%) of 91 patients who had no treatment. In addition, 53 (81.6%) of the 65 patients had no recurrence of cancer and 8 (12.3%) had recurrence, whereas only 16 (17.6%) of the 91 non-treatment patients improved without treatment.[40] Discontinuance of any contributing habits such as smokeless tobacco should be encouraged. Researchers[41] have suggested vitamin A and bleomycin as potential **chemopreventive agents** in controlling leukoplakia; these agents reduce the risk of cancer or delay its recurrence.[2] However, additional research is needed.

Oral Lichen Planus

Lichen planus is a chronic dermatologic disease that frequently manifests as lesions of the oral mucosa.[42] Whether oral lichen planus can transform into malignant disease has long been a controversial subject.[43–46] Most of the controversy has stemmed from questions in the diagnosis of oral lichen planus as opposed to other non-oral lichen planus lesions, such as lichenoid contact reactions. Recently, researchers have suggested that a histologic diagnosis is not as critical to the dental practitioner as the need for careful, thorough follow-up examinations. Various researchers have indicated oral lichen planus patients have higher risks of developing oral cancer than the general population. The potential for malignant transformation appears to be small, but oral lichen planus should be regarded as a premalignant condition.[47] Subsequently, clinicians must regularly evaluate and refer for further follow-up, such as biopsy, when indicated.

Human Papillomavirus

Human papillomavirus (HPV) is the most common sexually transmitted disease in the United States. Seventy percent or more of sexually active men and women will become infected with genital HPV.[48] More than eighty types of HPV have been identified, and various parts of the body are affected by different types. HPV-16 and HPV-18 have been linked to oral cancers and 95% of cervical cancers. HPV-16, HPV-18, HPV-31, and HPV-45 are all sexually transmitted. These types do not produce the wart-like lesions typically seen with other types of

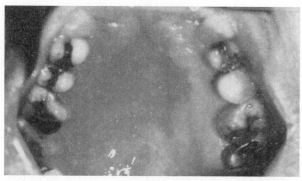

A

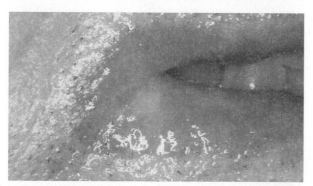

B

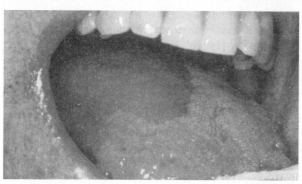

C

■ FIGURE 5–5 Erythoplakia in a 73-year-old man. Biopsy revealed carcinoma in situ of the palate and well-differentiated squamous cell carcinoma of the tongue and labial commissure. **A.** Palate. **B.** Labial commissure (corner of the lip). **C.** Tongue dorsum.
(From Ord, R. A., & Blanchaert, R. H., Jr. [Eds.] [2000]. *Oral cancer: The dentist's role in diagnosis, management, rehabilitation, and prevention*. Carol Stream, IL: Quintessence Publishing Co., Inc. © Quintessence Publishing Co., Inc.)

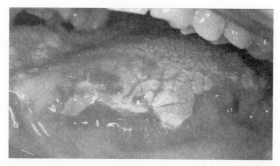

■ FIGURE 5–6 Erythroleukoplakia of the left lateral tongue border. Note the velvety red appearance admixed among the leukoplakic plaques. Biopsy confirmed moderate dysplasia.
(From Ord, R. A., & Blanchaert, R. H., Jr. [Eds.] [2000]. *Oral cancer: The dentist's role in diagnosis, management, rehabilitation, and prevention*. Carol Stream, IL: Quintessence Publishing Co., Inc. © Quintessence Publishing Co., Inc.)

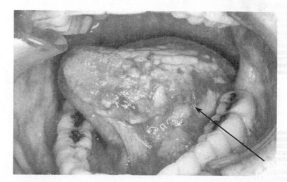

■ FIGURE 5–7 Extensive leukoplakia of the tongue and floor of the mouth in an elderly woman. Pointer shows site of previous tongue biopsy with early focus of carcinoma.
(From Ord, R. A., & Blanchaert, R. H., Jr. [Eds.] [2000]. *Oral cancer: The dentist's role in diagnosis, management, rehabilitation, and prevention*. Carol Stream, IL: Quintessence Publishing Co., Inc. © Quintessence Publishing Co., Inc.)

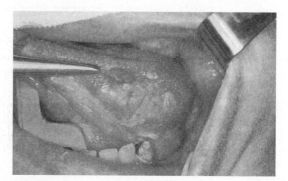

■ FIGURE 5–8 Squamous cell carcinoma, floor of the mouth.
(Courtesy Dr. Sol Silverman, Jr.)

HPV, but may produce cancers that affect the epithelial cells of mucosa and skin.

During the previous decade, squamous cell carcinomas of the tongue and tonsil have increased in Caucasian individuals younger than 45 years.[12] The increase is noteworthy because SEER data from the 1973–2001 time period indicate squamous cell carcinoma in all other sites of oral and pharyngeal cancers remained stable or decreased during the same time period.[49] In Scandinavian countries, oral tongue squamous cell carcinoma incidence increased 5 times among young men and 6 times among young women, compared with an increase of twice the number of new cases in older populations.[12] HPV-16 and HPV-18 infection has been consistently detected in head and neck squamous cell carcinomas, particularly those cases involving the tonsils.[12,50,51] Many oral cancers contain HPV-16, with percentages ranging from 15% to 25%. Because the number of oral cancer lesions that do not contain HPV-16 is large, the link between oral cancer and HPV is unclear at this time.[14]

Immune Deficiency

The most common oral malignancy in HIV-positive individuals is Kaposi's sarcoma. Hairy leukoplakia, although commonly observed in HIV-positive individuals, is not precancerous or dysplastic.[30]

Marijuana

The role of marijuana (cannabis) in the development of oral cancer is uncertain; however, several studies have shown an association of chronic use of cannabis with head and neck carcinoma.[6,21,29,52] Multiple factors may be involved, and the actual risk is unclear. Additional studies are needed to determine if marijuana use is a causative factor or a cofactor with other triggers.

SIGNS AND SYMPTOMS OF ORAL CAVITY OR OROPHARYNGEAL CANCER

A **symptom** is a change from the normal in a body structure, function, or sensation, whereas a **sign** is any abnormality that is discoverable on examination of the patient. A symptom is experienced by the patient; therefore, it is a subjective indication of disease. Because a sign is observable, it is an objective indication of disease.[1] The most common signs and symptoms of oral cancer are listed in Table 5–3 ■.

DETECTION AND DIAGNOSIS OF ORAL CANCER

Health History

A thorough assessment of the patient's present and past habits must be a part of the initial and subsequent patient encounters. Tobacco assessment must include type, amount, frequency, duration (years of smoking), quit attempts including methods used, and current stage of change. (A detailed cessation program is included in Chapter 18.) Alcohol assessment should be included on the health history form and discussed with the patient. Questions similar to the tobacco assessment should be

■ **Table 5–3**   Possible Signs and Symptoms of Oral Cancer

- Presence of mucosal ulcerations that do not resolve within 2 weeks
- Red or white patchy lesions that do not resolve within 2 weeks
- Persistent pain in the mouth
- Persistent lump or thickening in the soft tissues
- Persistent sore throat or a feeling that something is caught in the throat
- Difficult or painful chewing or swallowing
- Difficulty moving the jaw or tongue
- Numbness of the tongue or other area of the mouth
- Swelling of the jaw that causes dentures to fit poorly or become uncomfortable
- Loosening of the teeth or pain around the teeth or jaw
- Hoarseness or change in voice quality
- Ear pain in one ear without hearing loss
- Trismus (difficulty opening the mouth)
- Presence of a neck mass not resolving after antibiotic therapy

asked, including type of alcohol, amount, frequency, duration of use, and quit attempts. A study of dental school health history forms demonstrated only one-third of the forms contained questions about tobacco or alcohol use.[53] Several alcohol screening tools are available, including the Alcohol Use Disorders Identification Test (AUDIT), CAGE, and single-question tools, among many others (Table 5–4 ■). Use of a screening tool may assist the dental professional in determining when to refer patients to their family physician for further evaluation.

A study of 408 patients who visited a walk-in emergency dental clinic used the AUDIT-C screening tool, a 3-question adaptation of the World Health Organization's original 10-question AUDIT questionnaire.[54] Findings indicated one-quarter of the patients had positive results for heavy alcohol use. Because of concerns that dental patients may be offended by questions about their alcohol use, they were asked how they felt about answering the questions. More than 80% of the patients indicated the dentist should feel free to ask about alcohol use; more than 90% felt the dentist should advise them to cut down if drinking were affecting their oral health; and more than 90% indicated they would provide an honest answer if asked how much alcohol they consumed.

■ **Table 5–4**   Alcohol Use Screening Instruments

CAGE
1. Have you ever felt you ought to cut down on your drinking?
2. Have people annoyed you by criticizing your drinking?
3. Have you ever felt bad or guilty about your drinking?
4. Have you ever had a drink first thing in the morning (eye-opener) to steady your nerves or get rid of a hangover?

Positive result is one or more positive responses.

Alcohol Use Disorders Identification Test (AUDIT)
1. How often did you have a drink containing alcohol in the past year?
2. How many drinks containing alcohol did you have on a typical day when you were drinking during the past year?
3. How often did you have six or more drinks on one occasion in the past year?
4. How often during the last year have you found that you were not able to stop drinking once you had started?
5. How often during the last year have you failed to do what was normally expected from you because of drinking?
6. How often during the last year have you needed a first drink in the morning to get yourself going after a heavy drinking session?
7. How often during the last year have you had a feeling of guilt or remorse after drinking?
8. How often during the last year have you been unable to remember what happened the night before because you had been drinking?
9. Have you or someone else been injured as a result of your drinking?
10. Has a relative or friend, or doctor or other health care worker been concerned about your drinking or suggested you cut down?

Each question is scored 0–4 with a cumulative range of 0–40. A score of 8–12 indicates risk of harmful consumption; 13 or more indicates a risk of likely dependence.

AUDIT-C
1. How often did you have a drink containing alcohol in the past year?
2. How many drinks did you have on a typical day when you were drinking in the past year?
3. How often did you have six or more drinks on one occasion during the past year?

Scores follow the same 4-point scale used in the AUDIT system.

Single-Question Tool
1. When was the last time you had more than X drinks in 1 day? (X = 4 for women and 5 for men)

Positive result is any time in the past 3 months.

Source: Vinson, D. C., Galliher, J. M., Reidinger, C., & Kappus, J. A. Reprinted with permission from "Which Approach to Alcohol Screening Should We Use," 2004, *Annals of Family Medicine.* Copyright © 2004 American Academy of Family Physicians. All Rights Reserved.

Even heavy alcohol-consuming patients did not object to answering questions about alcohol use and receiving counseling. In light of this study, dental professionals should be comfortable asking their patients about alcohol use and advising them to quit or cut down.

Oral Cancer Screening/Examination

The topic of oral cancer is seldom mentioned in the popular media,[55,56] and the general public's knowledge of the risk factors, symptoms, and need for an oral cancer screening is low.[57] Health care providers, including dental professionals, have a professional responsibility to provide thorough oral cancer screenings.[58,59] Researchers have emphasized that medical providers have a responsibility to provide oral cancer examinations equal to that of dental providers.[60]

The American Dental Education Association includes oral cancer screenings in their list of competencies for the new dentist; this list was recently published in the *Journal of Dental Education*.[61] The competencies encompass 63 skills divided into several areas, including general skills, information management, currency of skills, practice management, communication, community resources, debt management, diagnosis, treatment planning, and treatment. The list specifically includes "perform head and neck and intraoral examinations" and "obtain medical, dental, psychosocial, and behavioral histories" (p. 850). The inclusion of these competencies, as well as others dealing with integration of multidisciplinary treatment planning, stress the expectation that dentists will perform these skills in their dental practices.

Unfortunately, the reality is that too few practitioners are taking the time to do visual and tactile examinations (examinations performed by touch) that take only 90 seconds.[15] Although the amount of time an oral cancer examination takes varies between providers, it should take only a few minutes, regardless of the provider's expertise level. Performing oral cancer screenings annually on all adult patients is the standard of care for dental professionals and should not be relegated to "as time permits." It is important to remember that the screening involves more than simply a cursory glance at soft tissues. Rather, palpation of lymph nodes in the head and neck region is part of the examination. In **palpation,** the palms and fingers are pressed against the lymph nodes to detect evidence of disease.[1] Some dentists express concerns that patients may consider palpation as inappropriate touching, particularly of the superficial and deep cervical nodes in the sternocleidomastoid muscle area. (This muscle arises from the sternum (breastbone) and the clavicle on each side, runs up the neck and attaches to the skull at the mastoid process and occipital bone.) Patient responses express a different story. In a small study of 61 participants in Utah,[62] 97% (58 study participants) reported they had never had an extraoral examination. Eighty-five percent (51 participants) indicated they felt the examination was worthwhile, a positive experience, and a valuable addition to future dental visits. Forty-seven participants (77%) felt more confident about their care, and 40 participants (66%) felt more relaxed. Carefully explaining the reason for the examination and the procedure of palpating lymph nodes should alleviate patient concerns. Because of the simplicity of the screening and the possibility that it could easily save a patient's life, it should be considered malpractice if not performed on all patients regularly!

Holmes, Dierks, Homer, and Potter found that patients with lesions detected by dental health care providers were diagnosed at an earlier stage of oral cancer than patients whose lesions were detected by primary health care providers. In addition, patients were more likely to start appropriate treatment sooner.[63] This study suggests the importance of the oral cancer screening in a dental setting, as well as the need for additional education of primary health care providers in performing oral cancer screenings.

The steps involved in the examination are included in Table 5–5 ■. Identification of lesions or lumps is critical. If a lesion is found, the patient should be scheduled to return in 14 days for reevaluation. If the lesion is still present, further follow-up is needed.

The American Cancer Society does not recommend the specific frequency of the examination or the populations who should be assessed, but ACS does state that periodic encounters with clinicians for checkups offer the potential for health counseling, cancer screening, and case finding (detection of cancer). These encounters should include performance or referral for conventional tests for cancer screening as appropriate by age and gender. These checkups are also an opportunity for case-finding examinations of the thyroid, testicles, ovaries, *lymph nodes, oral region,* and *skin* [emphasis added]. Also, self-examination techniques or increased

■ **Table 5–5**   Steps in Performing an Oral Cancer Screening

1. Visually assess the patient's head, face, neck, ears, and eyes for absence of symmetry, enlargements, swellings, dry or crusty areas, lesions, and color changes.
2. Palpate lymph nodes to detect changes in size, consistency, and mobility.
3. Observe the lips closed and open. Note the color, texture, and presence of lesions on the upper and lower vermilion borders (area where the skin of the face and lips meet). Palpate the lips for changes in consistency and growths.
4. Assess labial mucosa by pulling the lower lip away from the teeth to observe the labial mucosa and **frena**.[a] Look for changes in color, texture, or swelling.
5. Examine and palpate the buccal mucosa.
6. Examine and palpate the gingiva.
7. Observe the dorsum (upper side) of the tongue for any swelling, ulceration, coating, changes in the pattern of the papillae (small, raised projections), or variation in size, color, or texture. Grasp the tip of the tongue with a piece of gauze and gently pull the tongue out and to the side to allow complete observation of the lateral surface of the right side, then the left. Palpate the tongue to feel for any growths.
8. With the tongue still raised, inspect the floor of the mouth for changes in color, texture, swellings, or ulcerations. Bimanually palpate the sublingual area using the index finger of one hand inside the mouth and the fingertips of the other hand extraorally under the chin.
9. With the patient's head tilted back, observe the hard and soft palate. Use a mouth mirror to intensify the light source. Ask the patient to move the tongue forward and/or down to help to visually assess the oropharynx, including the anterior and posterior **tonsillar pillars**.[b] Look for changes in color, texture, swellings, or ulcerations. Palpate the hard palate, taking care not to stimulate the patient's gag reflex.

[a] **Frena** are folds of labial mucosa that attach the lips to the gingiva.
[b] The **tonsillar pillars** are the thin layers of tissue that run anterior and posterior to the palatal tonsils.

awareness about signs and symptoms of skin cancer, breast cancer, or testicular cancer can be discussed. Health counseling may include guidance about smoking cessation, diet, physical activity, and shared decision making about cancer screening. Whereas in the past the American Cancer Society recommended a cancer-related checkup in a manner that implied a stand-alone examination, the recommendation now stresses that the occasion of a general periodic health examination provides a good opportunity to address examinations and counseling that could lead to early detection (p.19).[64]

Oral cancer screenings should be included in periodic examinations by all health care providers, rather than just by dental professionals. Groups at particularly high risk for oral cancer, including heavy smokers and alcohol abusers, may seek medical care for an unrelated problem. If the medical provider performed an oral cancer screening as part of a medical examination, more oral lesions could be detected. Results from several studies indicate that dental professionals and physicians fail to provide oral cancer examinations for their patients on a consistent basis. Figure 5–9 ■ indicates the most common intraoral areas for squamous cell carcinoma.

Yellowitz and others found that only 54% of 3,200 dentists surveyed knew that the ventral lateral border of the tongue (sides of the underside of the tongue) and the floor of the mouth are the most common sites for oral cancer.[65] National studies indicate less than 15% of adults report having an oral cancer examination within the previous year.[66,67] Clearly, statistics on morbidity and mortality, from comparisons of oral carcinomas diagnosed in early and late stages, indicate that medical and dental professionals must increase their diligence in performing regular, thorough examinations.

Oral cancer can manifest as a variety of appearances. Malignant lesions often mimic other innocuous (harmless) lesions, and misdiagnosis can occur easily in the absence of appropriate follow-up. Readers should consult oral pathology texts and journal articles for further information regarding clinical manifestations of oral cancer.

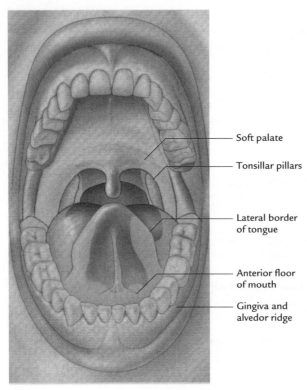

■ FIGURE 5–9   Intraoral area most likely to develop squamous cell carcinoma. Excluding the lip, in order of most likely area for intraoral squamous cell carcinoma to occur, are the lateral borders of the tongue (50%), anterior floor of the mouth (20%), soft palate and tonsillar pillars (15%), gingiva and alveolar ridge (5%).
(Reprinted from *Contemporary oral and maxillofacial pathology* [2nd ed.], Sapp, J. P., Eversole, L. R., & Wysocki, G. P. St. Louis: Mosby. © 2004. Reprinted with permission from Elsevier.)

Screening and Diagnostic Aids

Surgical biopsy (removal of a tissue sample) is the only definitive method available to diagnose oral carcinomas. However, in recent years other aids have become available to assist in determining which lesions should be diagnosed. Because many cases of dysplastic tissue and carcinomas appear innocuous, aids that can assist the dental or medical provider in making a definitive diagnosis and, if necessary, the decision to subject a patient to a surgical biopsy are a welcome addition. Exfoliative cytology, brush biopsy, chemiluminescence, and toluidine blue dye are all currently available tools. Types of biopsies include fine-needle aspiration, punch, and scalpel biopsy. Many other diagnostic tests are currently under study, including molecular tests that analyze DNA and genetic alterations that identify cells as cancerous or normal.[68–73]

Toluidine blue (tolonium chloride)   **Tolonium chloride** is used to aid in early recognition of oral cancers. It is a metachromatic dye that acts as a nuclear stain by binding to DNA; a metachromatic dye stains different components of cells or tissues in different colors, allowing easier examination of tissue samples[1] (Figure 5–10 ■). The reliability of tolonium chloride has been confirmed in several studies.[22,30,74] A large study by Epstein and others found tolonium chloride to be more sensitive than clinical examination alone in detecting carcinoma or **carcinoma in situ** (carcinoma confined to its site of origin). They did not find an excessive number of tests that gave false-positive results, as other researchers had found[74] (Figure 5–11 ■).

Questions remain about the use of toluidine blue. It is absorbed by inflammatory cells as well as dysplastic cells. Because inflammatory cells are often present on the surface of lesions, interpretation can be problematic, which has caused concern for too many false-positive results. This test can be useful to assist in defining the margins of lesions.[22,74] OraTest is a pharmaceutical grade formulation of toluidine blue available from Zila Pharmaceuticals. Contact information is included in the Resources section.

Exfoliative cytology and brush biopsy   **Exfoliative cytology** involves the microscopic examination of cells

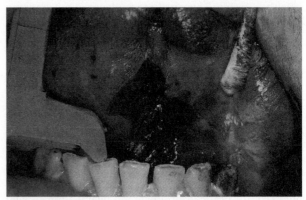

■ FIGURE 5–10   Toluidine blue rinse showing a deeply staining lesion of the floor of the mouth, which was an infiltrating squamous cell carcinoma separate from the tongue cancer in Figure 5–7.
(Reprinted from *Contemporary oral and maxillofacial pathology* [2nd ed.], Sapp, J. P., Eversole, L. R., & Wysocki, G. P. St. Louis: Mosby. © 2004. Reprinted with permission from Elsevier.)

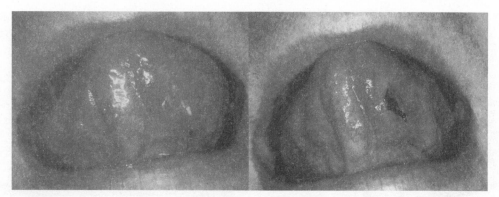

■ **FIGURE 5-11**   Squamous cell carcinoma under the tongue. Appearance of lesion in incandescent light and marked with TBlue[630].
(Courtesy of ViziLite Plus Zila Pharmaceuticals—Pictures provided by Zila, Inc.)

obtained from tissue; the cells are spread on a slide, fixed in place, and then stained. Because more than 90% of oral cancers arise from epithelial tissue, exfoliative cytology is an effective screening aid to determine whether to biopsy a lesion.[30]

Exfoliative cytology is useful for lesions that appear to be innocuous and otherwise would not undergo biopsy. It can often be done when a patient will not agree to a surgical biopsy.

The **oral brush test** is hailed as a new technique that offers a simple, minimally invasive **adjunct** (addition to the principal techniques) to an oral cancer screening; this technique holds great promise in determining lesions that should undergo scalpel biopsy and histologic examination.[70,75–80] The **Brush Test** is used to evaluate common, harmless-appearing, small white and red spots. It is not a replacement for scalpel biopsy, but is used instead to identify potentially precancerous lesions. The Brush Test is performed by the health professional and mailed to a laboratory for computer analysis and evaluation by a pathologist. When performed correctly, the Brush Test reaches all three levels of the stratified squamous epithelium to ensure cells from all three levels are included in the specimen. Researchers are currently evaluating exfoliated cells for molecular markers that will assess the progression of cellular changes and assist in determining treatment modalities.[70]

Chemiluminescence   When a tissue is exposed to a light source with a specific wavelength, it gives off light with a longer wavelength (i.e., fluoresces).[2] This property aids in the detection of cancerous tissues because the fluorescence of normal healthy tissue differs from that of precancerous or cancerous tissues. The change in appearance occurs because their cellular composition causes them to reflect light at different rates. Using a simple handheld device, providers can visually assess oral tissues for abnormalities.[81–84] Chemiluminescent systems provide an adjunct to admittedly faulty direct observation with incandescent light. One study indicated the chemiluminescent technique was better at accentuating white and white/red lesions, rather than red-only lesions.[81] Various types of chemiluminescent devices are available for dental use, including the ViziLite Plus marketed by Zila Pharmaceuticals. The ViziLite Plus system consists of a chemiluminescent device, a 1% acetic acid solution, and swabs containing TBlue[630], a toluidine blue solution (Figure 5–12 ■). Table 5–6 ■ provides instructions for the product's use.

Lesions that should be further evaluated appear distinctly bright white instead of the blue color of normal tissues. The white color is caused by the increased density of nuclear content and mitochondrial matrix found in abnormal cells, which causes the reflection of light. In contrast, when the light is applied to normal epithelium, it absorbs the light and appears dark (Figures 5–13 ■, and 5–14 ■, 5–15 ■).

Multicenter trials in Vancouver, Chicago, and San Francisco with 140 patients demonstrated that use of the ViziLite device increases the clinician's ability to identify lesions that are not seen with conventional lighting. Zila Pharmaceutical representatives are quick to point out that the device is not a *diagnostic* tool, but is instead

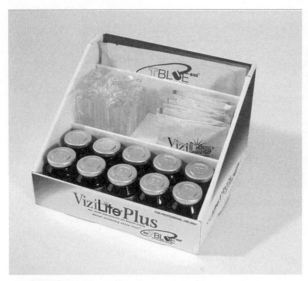

■ **FIGURE 5–12** ViziLite Plus System.
(Courtesy of ViziLite Plus Zila Pharmaceuticals—Pictures provided by Zila, Inc.)

■ **Table 5–6** Instructions for ViziLite Plus

The procedure involves the following steps:
* Patient rinses with a 1% acetic acid solution for 30–60 seconds.
* Activate device by bending the outer capsule to break the inner vial.
* Shake vigorously to mix contents. Insert light stick into open end of retractor and assemble.
* Dim room lighting or use eyewear provided by ViziLite Plus.
* Use the device to visually inspect the oral cavity. The open retractor window should face the tissue being examined.
* Apply the TBlue[630] marking system to lesions visible under ViziLite Plus illumination. Swabs should be applied in sequential order. Swab tubes are labeled 1, 2, and 3.
* Lesions stained with TBlue[630] can be viewed with the ViziLite Plus device. At that point, intraoral photographs can be taken.
* Discard all materials.
* Document any abnormalities on the back of the patient consent form.
* Refer to specialist if suspicious lesion is observed.

Source: Courtesy of ViziLite Plus Zila Pharmaceuticals—Pictures provided by Zila, Inc.

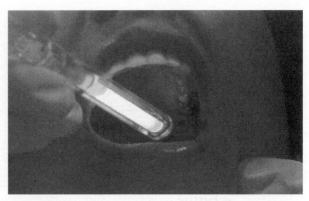

■ **FIGURE 5–13** White light used with ViziLite system. (Courtesy of ViziLite Plus Zila Pharmaceuticals—Pictures provided by Zila, Inc.)

a *screening* device that may help the clinician more easily visualize suspicious lesions.

The VELscope (also called Visually Enhanced Lesion Scope) is a handheld device the clinician uses to observe changes in the appearance of oral tissues (Figure 5–16 ■). Abnormal tissue typically appears as an irregular, dark area that stands out against the otherwise normal, green fluorescence pattern of surrounding healthy tissue (Figure 5–17 ■). The VELscope system does not require the patient to rinse with a solution. A study by Lane and others demonstrated a sensitivity of 98% and specificity of 100% in distinguishing normal tissue from severe dysplasia, carcinoma in situ, and invasive carcinoma.[83] The device has been suggested for use as an oral cancer screening aid, biopsy guide, and tool for distinguishing margins of cancerous tissue[83,84] (Figure 5–18 ■).

Use of imaging tools may assist dental providers in large public health screening events as well as in the more traditional in-office setting. The enhanced ability to visually assess lesions is a major step forward for early detection of lesions.

Biopsy Types

As previously stressed, the *only* way to definitely diagnose oral malignancies is with a biopsy. Different types of biopsies are performed, depending on the size and location of the lesion.

Fine-Needle Aspiration Biopsy
Fine-needle aspiration biopsy is typically performed to differentiate benign and malignant lesions that involve the lymph nodes or salivary glands. Biopsies of this type

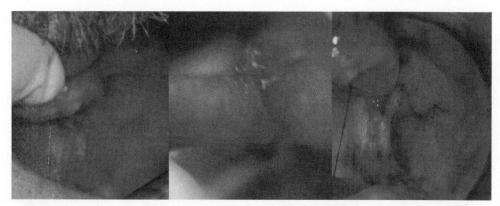

■ FIGURE 5–14   Squamous cell carcinoma in 62-year-old male patient with history of moderate tobacco use. Appearance of lesion in incandescent light, under ViziLite illumination and marked with TBlue.
(Courtesy of ViziLite Plus Zila Pharmaceuticals—Pictures provided by Zila, Inc.)

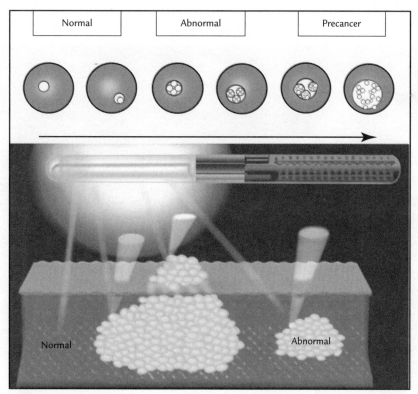

■ FIGURE 5–15   Abnormal cells exhibit a very dense nucleus. White light reflects off dense nuclei in abnormal tissue.
(Courtesy of ViziLite Plus Zila Pharmaceuticals—Pictures provided by Zila, Inc.)

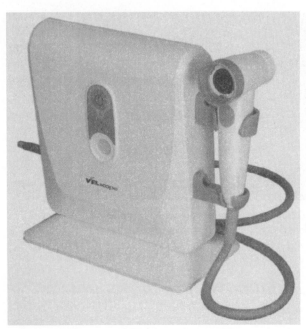

■ FIGURE 5–16 VELscope device.
(Courtesy of VELscope LED Dental, Inc.)

are preferred in those areas because the biopsy does not spread the tumor or disrupt the field for surgical dissection later[30] (Figure 5–19 ■).

Punch Biopsy

Punch biopsy instruments remove a sample of a tissue for evaluation. They are commercially available as disposable devices of various sizes (Figure 5–20 ■).

Scalpel Biopsy

The biopsy specimen should be a representative sample of the lesion. **Incisional biopsy** involves removal of a small piece of tissue, whereas **excisional biopsy** involves removal of the entire lesion. Care must be taken when determining the type of biopsy to perform or whether the patient should be referred to a specialist for biopsy. Incisional biopsy of a small lesion could distort the appearance and consistency of the tissue, interfering with the ability to assess the tissue. According to Silverman, a small lesion that would be altered by biopsy should be seen by the clinician who will ultimately treat the lesion before the biopsy, so that the extent of resection or irradiation can be determined.[30]

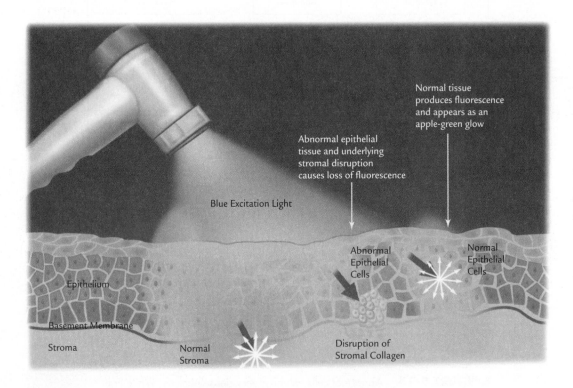

Normal tissue produces fluorescence and appears as an apple-green glow

Abnormal epithelial tissue and underlying stromal disruption causes loss of fluorescence

Blue Excitation Light

Abnormal Epithelial Cells

Normal Epithelial Cells

Epithelium

Basement Membrane

Stroma

Normal Stroma

Disruption of Stromal Collagen

■ FIGURE 5–17 Blue excitation light's effect on normal and abnormal tissues.
(Courtesy of VELscope LED Dental, Inc.)

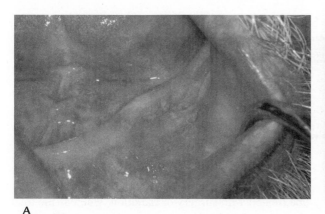

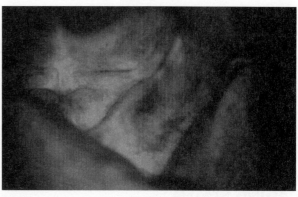

A   B

■ **FIGURE 5–18**   **A.** Area appears to be chronic denture trauma (observed with naked eye). **B.** Intense dark area (observed through Velscope) on the ridge persisted after relief of denture irritation. Biopsy confirmed as severe dysplasia. (Images courtesy of Dr. Edmond Truelove, University of Washington.)

Scar tissue from a previous incisional or excisional biopsy could hamper attempts to identify subsequent cancer in the same area. In addition, cancer cells can sometimes be plunged deep into underlying tissues during the biopsy procedure.

Regardless of the method used to detect changes in epithelial tissues that may be squamous cell carcinoma, the patient should be referred for follow-up and treatment to a cancer center that specializes in head and neck cancers, an **otolaryngologist** (physician who treats head and neck

disorders), or **maxillofacial surgeon** (dental specialist who treats disorders of the mouth, teeth, jaws, and face).

Imaging

Oral cancer is usually detected by clinical examination and confirmed by surgical or fine-needle biopsy. Imaging techniques are then used to provide evidence of the extent of the disease. Imaging may also be used to detect recurrent disease after therapy. Computed tomography and magnetic resonance imaging are the methods currently available for detection of oral cancers.[30,85] Positron emission tomography is being investigated for use in identifying head and neck lesions.[21]

■ **FIGURE 5–19**   Fine-needle aspiration biopsy. Aspiration with a syringe holder, which allows the mass to be stabilized with one hand and aspirated with the other hand.
(From Ord, R. A., & Blanchaert, R. H., Jr. [Eds.] [2000]. *Oral cancer: The dentist's role in diagnosis, management, rehabilitation, and prevention.* Carol Stream, IL: Quintessence Publishing Co., Inc. © Quintessence Publishing Co., Inc.)

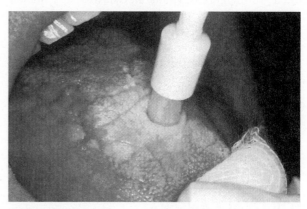

■ **FIGURE 5–20**   Punch biopsy instrument.
(From Ord, R. A., & Blanchaert, R. H., Jr. [Eds.] [2000]. *Oral cancer: The dentist's role in diagnosis, management, rehabilitation, and prevention.* Carol Stream, IL: Quintessence Publishing Co., Inc. © Quintessence Publishing Co., Inc.)

■ **Table 5–7** Grading System for Squamous Cell Carcinoma

Histologic Grade	
GX	Grade cannot be assessed
G1	Well differentiated
G2	Moderately differentiated
G3	Poorly differentiated

PROGNOSIS OF ORAL CANCER: STAGING SYSTEM

The **prognosis,** or forecast of the probable course or outcome,[1] of squamous cell carcinoma is determined by a system of grading (determining the histologic subtype) and staging (determining the clinical extent) of the tumor. Staging is the most important indicator of the two.

Grading is accomplished by determining the degree of differentiation exhibited by the cells and how closely the cells resemble normal tissue structure (Table 5–7 ■). Well-differentiated (grade 1, low-grade) tumors produce keratin, closely resemble the tissue of origin, grow less aggressively, and metastasize later. Tumors that produce little or no keratin but are still recognizable as stratified squamous epithelium are called moderately differentiated or grade 2. Poorly differentiated (high-grade, grade 3) tumors produce no keratin, bear little resemblance to stratified squamous epithelium, lack normal architectural structure, and often grow aggressively and metastasize early in their course.[42]

Staging is based on the size and extent of metastatic spread of the lesion.[42,85,86] The tumor-node-metastasis (TNM) system is used to determine the stage of most cancers (Table 5–8 ■). Three clinical features specify the stage:

- Size, in centimeters, of the tumor (T).
- Involvement of local lymph nodes (N).
- Presence or absence of distant metastasis (M).

TREATMENT OPTIONS FOR ORAL CANCER

Treatment modalities for oral cancer vary, primarily depending on the tumor stage, size, location, relation to the mandible, nodal involvement, and histologic type.[21,42,85,86] Early stage cancer (stages I and II) can be treated with surgery or radiation, whereas the treatment protocol for late stage cancer (stages III and IV) usually includes a combination of surgery, postoperative radiation, and chemotherapy.[3,21,85,86] Photodynamic (laser) therapy has recently been added as a possible option for treating oral cavity cancers. An advantage of this technique is that the area heals without fibrosis (formation of fibrous tissue).[3]

Chemotherapeutic agents are generally not successful in treating oral carcinomas when used as a single modality, and are used as an adjunctive procedure in combination with radiation and surgery.[21,30,85] Smaller intraoral lesions are treated with a single modality, whereas larger lesions or cases that involve lymph nodes require a combination of modalities.[3,21,30,85] Oropharyngeal lesions usually receive radiation therapy. Lip lesions are typically surgically excised with excellent results. Tongue lesions are treated by hemiglossectomy (surgical removal of half of the tongue[1]) followed by radiation therapy. More advanced lesions have a 5-year survival rate of less than 30%.[21] Segmental resection is necessary for alveolar ridge cancers. Radical or modified radical neck dissection is performed when metastasis to local lymph nodes is included. (See the section Surgery later in this chapter for further discussion of operative procedures.)

Radiotherapy may consist of external-beam irradiation, interstitial irradiation or brachytherapy, and intraoral cone or electron-beam therapy.[42] (See the section Radiation Therapy later in this chapter for descriptions of these therapies.)

Considerations Regarding Treatment Options

The oral cavity is a complex structure composed of muscles, nerves, jaws, tongue, and salivary glands. Nutritional intake depends on all of those factors. Los-

■ **Table 5-8**   TNM Staging System for Squamous Cell Carcinoma

Size of Primary Tumor (T)

TX	Primary tumor cannot be assessed
T0	No evidence of primary tumor
T1S	Carcinoma in situ
T1	Tumor 2 cm or less in greatest dimension
T2	Tumor more than 2 cm but not more than 4 cm in greatest dimension
T3	Tumor more than 4 cm in greatest dimension
T4 (lip)	Tumor invades through cortical bone, inferior alveolar nerve, floor of mouth, or skin of face (i.e., chin or nose)
T4a	(In the oral cavity) Tumor invades adjacent structures (e.g., through cortical bone, into maxillary sinus, skin of face, and deep [extrinsic] muscles of tongue [genioglossus,[a] hyoglossus,[b] palatoglossus,[c] and styloglossus[d]])
T4b	Tumor invades masticator space, pterygoid plates, or skull base, and/or encases internal carotid artery

Lymph Node Involvement (N)

NX	Regional lymph nodes cannot be assessed
N0	No regional lymph node metastasis
N1	Single clinically positive ipsilateral (on same side) node less than 3 cm
N2	Metastasis in a single ipsilateral lymph node, 3 cm or less in greatest dimension; or in multiple ipsilateral nodes, none more than 6 cm in greatest dimension; or in bilateral or contralateral nodes, none more than 6 cm in greatest dimension
N2a	Metastasis in single ipsilateral lymph node more than 3 cm but not more than 6 cm in greatest dimension
N2b	Metastasis in multiple ipsilateral lymph nodes, none more than 6 cm in greatest dimension
N2c	Metastasis in bilateral or contralateral lymph nodes, none more than 6 cm in greatest dimension
N3	Metastasis in a lymph node more than 6 cm in greatest dimension

Distant Metastasis (M)

MX	Distant metastasis cannot be assessed
M0	No distant metastasis
M1	Distant metastasis

TNM Staging Categories

Stage	TNM Classification		
0	Tis	N0	M0
I	T1	N0	M0
II	T2	N0	M0
III	T3	N0	M0
	T1	N1	M0
	T2	N1	M0
	T3	N1	M0
IVA	T4a	N0	M0
	T4a	N1	M0
	T1	N2	M0
	T2	N2	M0
	T3	N2	M0
IVB	Any T	N3	M0
	T4b	Any N	M0
IVC	Any T	Any N	M1

[a] The **genioglossus** is located under the tongue; it protrudes and depresses (retracts) the tongue.[1]

[b] The **hyoglossus** is also located under the tongue; it works with the genioglossus to retract the tongue.[1]

[c] The **palatoglossus** is attached to the posterior of the side of the tongue and makes up the anterior pillar of fauces; it raises the back of the tongue to narrow the fauces. The **fauces** is the space between the oral cavity and the pharynx. The soft palate and the base of the tongue form the boundaries of the fauces.[1]

[d] The **styloglossus** is attached to the underside and sides of the tongue. It also aids in retracting the tongue.[1]

Used with the permission of the American Joint Committee on Cancer (AJCC), Chicago, Illinois. The original source for this material is the AJCC Cancer Staging Manual, Sixth Edition (2002) published by Springer-New York. www.springeronline.com.

ing the ability to speak drastically affects a patient's quality of life and ability to socialize. Treatment planning must consider all of the functions performed by the mouth and associated structures. Rehabilitation should be considered before surgical or radiation therapy intervention.

Surgery

Surgical management of malignancies of the oral cavity may involve several approaches, depending on the extent and location of the disease. **Wide local excision** involves the removal of the tumor in soft tissue while leaving a 1-cm to 1.5-cm margin of clinically normal tissue at the periphery (Figure 5–21 ■).

Resection involves removing carcinoma that has invaded bone, leaving a 2-cm margin of radiographically normal bone tissue at the periphery.

Marginal resections involve removal of bone that leaves the inferior border of the mandible intact. **Segmental resection** involves removal of the full height of the mandible. **Composite resection** involves removal of hard and soft tissue, typically the neck nodes, mandible, and soft tissues associated with the primary tumor, as in the tongue or floor of the mouth.

Neck dissections are comprehensive or selective. **Comprehensive neck dissections** include radical neck dissection and modified neck dissection. **Radical neck dissection** removes lymph nodes of the neck, the sternocleidomastoid muscle, the internal jugular vein, and the spinal accessory nerve. **Modified neck dissection** pre-

serves the sternocleidomastoid muscle, or the internal jugular vein, or the spinal accessory nerve. **Selective neck dissections** remove lymph nodes only, preserving the sternocleidomastoid muscle, the internal jugular vein, and the spinal accessory nerve. Weakness in raising the arm above the head and weakness of the lower lip may follow neck dissection.[30] Reconstruction after invasive surgical procedures results in varying degrees of successful restoration of function and appearance, depending on the area. The technique of harvesting flaps from the fibula and radial forearm is frequently used in surgical reconstruction.[42]

Radiation therapy is indicated after surgery if the soft tissue margin is positive, one or more lymph nodes exhibit extracapsular invasion (extension of the tumor outside the lymph node capsule), bone invasion is present, more than one lymph node is positive in the absence of extracapsular invasion, comorbid (existing simultaneously) immunosuppressive disease is present, or perineural invasion (invasion of the sheath surrounding a bundle of nerve fibers[1]) is present.

Radiation Therapy

Computed tomography and/or magnetic resonance imaging, and positron emission tomography scanning are used to identify the lesion and involved structures. Dental panoramic film is used to assess dental status and mandibular involvement. A dental consultation is necessary before any radiotherapy in dentulous or edentulous patients.[42] Teeth that are periodontally involved, mobile teeth, teeth with large carious lesions and periapical

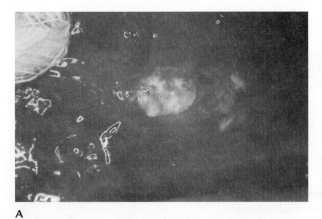
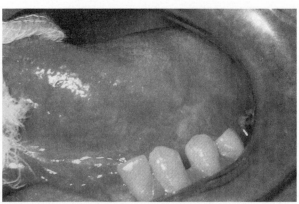

A   B

■ **FIGURE 5–21**   **A.** Leukoplakia of the left lateral tongue border that was confirmed as squamous cell carcinoma. **B.** Appearance of tongue border 9 months after surgical resection.
(From Ord, R. A., & Blanchaert, R. H., Jr. [Eds.] [2000]. *Oral cancer: The dentist's role in diagnosis, management, rehabilitation, and prevention.* Carol Stream, IL: Quintessence Publishing Co., Inc. © Quintessence Publishing Co., Inc.)

pathology, and impacted teeth should be extracted before beginning radiation therapy.

Types of Radiation Therapy

Types of radiation therapy used in oral cancer include primary external-beam radiotherapy, intensity-modulated radiotherapy, brachytherapy or interstitial radiotherapy, and intraoral cone or electron-beam therapy. In **external-beam radiotherapy,** radiation is applied to a tumor from outside the body; immobilization devices are used to minimize damage to areas other than the tumor. Preserving salivary function is an important component. **Intensity-modulated radiotherapy** seeks to treat the tumor and spare more of the normal tissues. **Brachytherapy** delivers high-dose, localized radiation by the implantation of radioactive sources into the tumor.[3,30,42] **Interstitial irradiation** involves the implantation of radioactive sources directly into or around the carcinogenic tissues. **Intraoral cone** or **electron-beam therapy** is the treatment of the skin or mucosal membrane with a non-penetrating beam of electrons.[1]

Radiotherapy may also be palliative to alleviate symptoms of pain or obstruction in patients who cannot undergo curative therapies.

Toxicity and Side Effects of Radiation Therapy

The determinants of toxicity from radiation therapy include the radiation dose and the length of treatment. Complications from irradiation include pain, **xerostomia** (hyposalivation or dry mouth), **dysgeusia** (altered taste perception), cervical caries, epithelial atrophy, focal alopecia (hair loss), focal hyperpigmentation, osteoradionecrosis, and telangiectasias (small enlarged blood vessels near the surface of the skin). Oral candidiasis and mucositis often follow treatment. The threat of osteora-

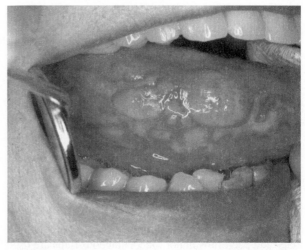

■ **FIGURE 5–23** Mucositis.
(Courtesy Dr. Sol Silverman, Jr.)

dionecrosis (death of bone due to radiation therapy) is possible in any of the mentioned oral cancers [30] (Figures 5–22 ■ and 5–23 ■).

The use of pilocarpine during radiation therapy may help save some salivary function. Use of water, artificial saliva, gum, and so forth may offer some relief. Custom-fitted fluoride trays with a neutral fluoride can significantly reduce cervical caries and will be needed for the remainder of the patient's life.

Osteoradionecrosis remains the major concern, however. Radiation damages bone tissue, and subsequent trauma may result in the loss of varying amounts of bone (Figure 5–24 ■). Meticulous oral hygiene is critical postradiation to minimize the effects of xerostomia and osteoradionecrosis.[30] Nutrition is also

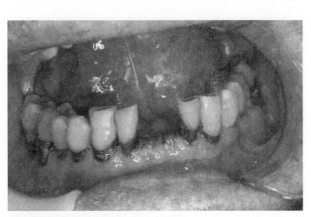

■ **FIGURE 5–22** Radiation-induced caries.
(Courtesy Dr. Sol Silverman, Jr.)

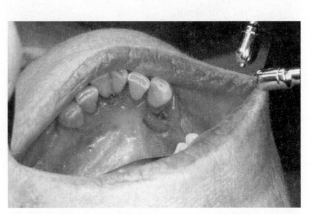

■ **FIGURE 5–24** Osteoradionecrosis.
(Courtesy Dr. Sol Silverman, Jr.)

extremely important, and tooth extraction or other invasive procedures must be avoided if at all possible.[30] Additional information is contained in the section Management of Side Effects from Treatment of Oral Cancer later in this chapter.

Chemotherapy may be used, but clinical trials are conflicting for head and neck cancers and it is not typically used as a single modality. Chemotherapy may be neoadjuvant (before irradiation), concurrent (during irradiation), or adjuvant (after irradiation).[30,85]

Reconstruction

Various methods of reconstruction after surgical removal of the cancerous tumor are used. Deltopectoral flaps and pectoralis major mucocutaneous flaps are used to replace tissues and protect the carotid artery after removal of the sternocleidomastoid muscle. Bone and soft tissue grafts provide good cosmetic appearance and function. **Osseointegrated implants** (implants anchored in the bone) and dentures can be used to replace lost teeth. The fibula can be used to reconstruct the mandible after resection[30,42,85] (Figures 5–25 ■ to 5–29 ■).

Early detection of lesions is critical to allow conservative treatment and to protect the patient's quality of life. Many avenues are available to treat oral cancers, with improved methods constantly being investigated. A

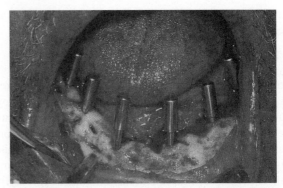

■ FIGURE 5–26   Implant guide pins in place after all holes have been drilled. Alignment is directed slightly lingual because of the relatively larger size of the mandible compared with the maxilla.
(From Ord, R. A., & Blanchaert, R. H., Jr. [Eds.] [2000]. *Oral cancer: The dentist's role in diagnosis, management, rehabilitation, and prevention.* Carol Stream, IL: Quintessence Publishing Co., Inc. © Quintessence Publishing Co., Inc.)

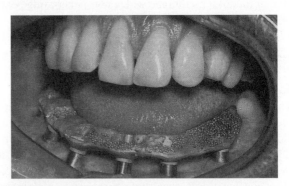

■ FIGURE 5–27   Frame try-in to test fit.
(From Ord, R. A., & Blanchaert, R. H., Jr. [Eds.] [2000]. *Oral cancer: The dentist's role in diagnosis, management, rehabilitation, and prevention.* Carol Stream, IL: Quintessence Publishing Co., Inc. © Quintessence Publishing Co., Inc.)

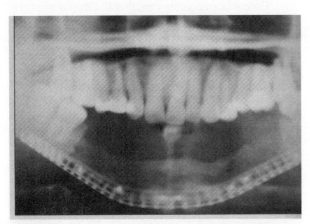

■ FIGURE 5–25   Reconstruction of the mandible immediately after resection for large ameloblastoma. A Timesh titanium basket filled with particulate bone marrow harvested from the ilium (the largest of the three principal bones composing either half of the pelvis).
(From Ord, R. A., & Blanchaert, R. H., Jr. [Eds.] [2000]. *Oral cancer: The dentist's role in diagnosis, management, rehabilitation, and prevention.* Carol Stream, IL: Quintessence Publishing Co., Inc. © Quintessence Publishing Co., Inc.)

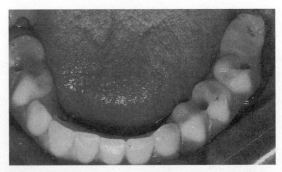

■ FIGURE 5–28   Final prosthesis at the time of delivery.
(From Ord, R. A., & Blanchaert, R. H., Jr. [Eds.] [2000]. *Oral cancer: The dentist's role in diagnosis, management, rehabilitation, and prevention.* Carol Stream, IL: Quintessence Publishing Co., Inc. © Quintessence Publishing Co., Inc.)

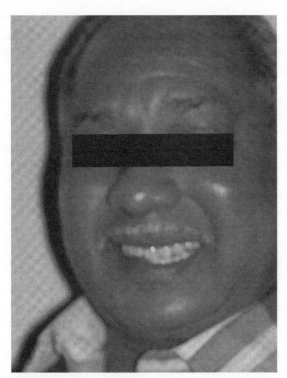

■ FIGURE 5–29   Facial view of patient after placement of the final restoration.
(From Ord, R. A., & Blanchaert, R. H., Jr. [Eds.] [2000]. *Oral cancer: The dentist's role in diagnosis, management, rehabilitation, and prevention.* Carol Stream, IL: Quintessence Publishing Co., Inc. © Quintessence Publishing Co., Inc.)

multidisciplinary team can help oral cancer patients adjust to the aftermath of treatment.

MANAGEMENT OF SIDE EFFECTS FROM TREATMENT OF ORAL CANCER

A variety of complications arise from treatment of oral cancer. The dental professional must be prepared to assist patients in improving their quality of life after treatment. Consultation with other members of the multidisciplinary team is critical. Depending on the type of treatment, side effects vary.

The side effects of cancer therapy are numerous and can be quite debilitating (Table 5–9 ■). Side effects of radiation therapy may be transient (lasting a short time) or lessen with the passage of time, but many are permanent. Cutaneous changes typically manifest as darkened or lightened (vitiligo) skin. Focal alopecia may occur if the hair follicles are in the treatment beam area. Subcutaneous changes may occur, including telangiectasia, fibrosis, and edema (retained fluids, swelling).

Acute **mucositis** (inflammation of a mucous membrane) is a common reaction to cancer therapy, and can become so severe that intake of nutrition is impossible until the condition subsides. Because no curative treatment is available, palliative care is provided. A feeding tube is often inserted temporarily to maintain hydration and nutritional needs. A brief interruption in

■ Table 5–9   Side Effects of Cancer Therapy

Radiation Therapy
Alterations in pigmentation of skin including white patches (vitiligo) or "tanning"
Loss of hair
Subcutaneous changes
    Telangiectasia (spider veins)
    Fibrosis
    Edema (swelling)
Acute mucositis
Xerostomia (hyposalivation or dry mouth) and changes in quality of saliva
Candidiasis (fungal overgrowth)
Hypogeusia, dysgeusia, or ageusia (partial loss, changes in perception, or complete loss of taste, respectively)
Dental caries
Osteoradionecrosis
Soft tissue necrosis (mucosal ulcer)
Chemotherapy
Acute mucositis
Xerostomia and changes in quality of saliva
Hemorrhage
Candidiasis

therapy is necessary when severe mucositis occurs. Patients may require systemic pain relief. Topical solutions such as a mixture of lidocaine, cough syrup, and a coating agent (milk of magnesia, kaolin-pectin), especially if it is chilled, may help in reducing inflammation and discomfort.[87] Systemic prednisone may also help reduce these side effects.[30,88] Systemic narcotics such as morphine may be required.[89] Patients should maintain oral care as much as possible by gently debriding the oral cavity with an ultrasoft toothbrush or wet gauze.[87] Toothbrush bristles may be further softened with warm water[89] if necessary.

Dietary changes to assist in managing xerostomia and mucosal pain may be necessary. Sucking on ice chips or popsicles may help temporarily alleviate pain. Patients should be counseled to avoid hot, spicy, acidic, and rough-textured foods. The use of straws for liquid intake may be suggested. Foods such as applesauce, puddings, custards, gelatins, milk shakes, scrambled eggs, mashed potatoes, and pureed vegetables should be encouraged.[90]

Xerostomia can affect the patient's quality of life because it may make eating or talking difficult and dramatically increase the risk of caries. Various products are available that provide some lubrication, but they are temporary fixes to what can be a major source of discomfort. The dental professional can provide saliva substitutes and encourage the patient to carry water with them at all times. Some saliva substitutes come in the form of chewing gum and lozenges. Sugarless gum or candy may provide some relief. **Sialogogues** (agents that promote flow of saliva, such as pilocarpine, Salagen, and cevimeline) may help stimulate salivary flow in some patients, depending on the amount of damage done to the salivary glands. Avoidance of mouthrinses containing alcohol should be encouraged. Because of the possibility of caries, patients should avoid foods and beverages with high sugar content and must be provided with custom fluoride trays. A mildly flavored neutral sodium fluoride should be dispensed, and the patient should be instructed to use the fluoride at least twice daily.[88–90]

Fungal overgrowth of *Candida albicans* can be severe. The condition is managed with systemic antifungal drugs such as ketoconazole or fluconazole, or topical administration of nystatin or clotrimazole. Topical or systemic pain medication may be necessary.

Taste buds are sensitive to radiation and may be destroyed if they are in the path of the external beam. A partial (**hypogeusia**) or complete (**ageusia**) loss of taste may occur during treatment. **Dysgeusia** (altered taste

perceptions) may also occur. Taste buds will usually regenerate several months after treatment terminates. Zinc supplements may help restore or enhance the ability to taste in some patients.[30,88]

Osteoradionecrosis is a serious complication of head and neck irradiation.[88] As the radiation dose increases, the occurrence of osteoradionecrosis becomes more likely. Bone cells and the accompanying vascular system may be irreversibly damaged, causing sequestrated bone fragments (bone fragments separated from the bone[1]). Jaw resection may be necessary to treat the condition. Hyperbaric oxygen can be effective, but studies regarding its effect are inconclusive.[30]

Soft tissue necrosis may occur in irradiated tissue. The mucosal ulcer is usually self-limiting, but may require surgical intervention. Pain relief will be necessary because the lesions are very painful.[30]

Neurotoxicity is a side effect of some chemotherapeutic agents. It manifests as altered sensation, partial paresthesia (abnormal sensations such as burning, tingling, etc.) of the perioral and intraoral areas affiliated with the trigeminal nerve, or as severe, throbbing pain, particularly in the mandibular molar region. Systemic analgesics, usually narcotics, are required. Residual neuropathy may remain after chemotherapy is completed.[87]

The dental professional must closely follow the cancer therapy of the head and neck cancer patient to ensure caries do not develop and side effects are treated quickly. Treatment coordination with the oncologist and other members of the multidisciplinary team will be required. As the following list shows, this network of health care professionals is extensive:

- Otolaryngologist
- Plastic and reconstructive surgeon
- Oral and maxillofacial surgeon
- Radiation oncologist
- Radiologist
- Dietitian
- Speech language pathologist
- Social worker
- Psychologist
- Physical therapist
- Occupational therapist
- Dentist/maxillofacial prosthodontist
- Dental hygienist
- Facial prosthetics clinician
- Head and neck nurse coordinator/clinical nurse specialist

ROLE OF THE DENTAL TEAM

Table 5–10 ■ summarizes what can dental professionals can do to increase the prevention and early detection of oral cancer. Public awareness is critical. The *Healthy People 2010* objectives[91] call for an increase in the proportion of oral and pharyngeal cancers detected at the earliest stage, and an increase in the proportion of adults who, in the past 12 months, report having had an examination to detect oral and pharyngeal cancers. Through mass media, community efforts, increased vigilance, and advocacy, health care providers can increase public awareness. Health care professionals must become proactive in ensuring they routinely provide thorough oral cancer screenings to all patients at initial and recall appointments.[37] Oral cancer screenings must be offered at sites that are accessible and comfortable for minority populations. Educational programs for health care professionals should train students to perform oral cancer screenings and use diagnostic tools, as well as provide tobacco and alcohol cessation counseling.[8]

Education

The public is woefully uninformed about oral and pharyngeal cancers.[57,92,93] This lack of knowledge is not surprising, considering the paucity of oral cancer educational materials available to them through mass media and print materials.[55,56]

Cruz and others assessed the knowledge of 803 adults in an oral cancer screening program. The researchers found that 311 participants (39%) reported having heard of an oral cancer examination but that only 99 participants (12%) reported ever having one. Three-fourths (608) of the participants knew tobacco was a risk factor for oral cancer, but only one-fourth (204) knew alcohol was a risk factor. Only 204 participants (25%) knew that excessive sunlight was a risk factor for lip cancer.[92] Among the same participants, 77% percent reported their risk for oral cancer was less than or equal to that of others in their gender and age bracket. Interestingly, 31% of the smokers in the group perceived their risk as less than that of other smokers, and 19% perceived their risk as less than that of non-smokers.[94] Other earlier studies found similar results.[57] It is apparent that dental professionals must increase their dissemination of oral cancer information among the general public and individuals in their communities and dental practices.

A variety of materials is available for the education of patients and health care providers through the American Cancer Society, National Oral Health Information Clearinghouse, Oral Cancer Foundation, American Dental Association, American Academy of Otolaryngology, American Association of Oral and Maxillofacial Surgeons, and Support for People with Oral and Head and Neck Cancer, among others. Many of the materials are available free or at minimal cost. See the Resources section at the end of the chapter for suggested Web sites, print, and audiovisual materials.

Dental professionals should obtain and distribute materials to local health departments[95] and other venues including private practices; senior centers; long-term care facilities; drug abuse treatment centers; and schools for nurses, physicians, and physician assistants. Dental professionals should ensure that dental providers are included on health boards and local health consortia. Table 5–10 ■ lists other ways to increase public awareness of oral cancer.

■ **Table 5–10**   Actions the Dental Team Can Take to Increase Awareness

- Provide oral cancer materials to health agencies and community centers.
- Initiate an oral cancer consortium composed of health and social service agencies, educational partners, and community groups.
- Volunteer at health fairs to provide screenings and dispense pamphlets and other information.
- Talk to clients/patients about oral cancer risk factors, prevention, and early detection.
- Perform oral cancer screenings on every patient.
- Provide continuing education programs on oral cancer for other health professionals. Assess clients'/patients' tobacco and alcohol use.
- Initiate tobacco and alcohol cessation programs in practice settings.
- Provide nutritional assessments and nutritional oral cancer prevention strategies.
- Include health promotion strategies in client/patient education.

Public Health Screening for Oral and Pharyngeal Cancers

Oral cancer screenings can be offered as a free public health service for community groups at long-term care facilities, health fairs, senior centers, and other venues. Disposable mouth mirrors and portable headlamps or flashlights make the screenings easy to do in virtually any setting. Including an educational aspect will dispense much-needed information to the public. Location is especially important to reach the most at-risk populations, particularly African American males. Successful programs in African American communities have been staged at barbershops, supermarkets, and local churches in Maryland, Virginia, and Pennsylvania.[96–98] Enlisting the assistance of prominent members in African American communities, such as training barbers and members of the faith community as health ambassadors can help reach those in underserved areas. Using local dental/dental hygiene societies and educational programs can provide expertise in performing screenings and training ambassadors.

Cultural Sensitivity

Paying attention to various cultures is crucial in health promotion activities. Many subcultures in American society have unique views of health and disease. Factors affecting vulnerable populations must be assessed when designing programs. Characteristics such as religious differences, ethnicity, primary language spoken, education, and literacy level affect access to care, response to illness, health-seeking behavior, and trust of Western health providers, among others. Social customs and norms, such as touching, intimate space requirements, acceptable behaviors for gender and age groups, and eye contact, may serve as potential barriers. These concerns must be addressed before initiating health promotion programs.[99]

SUMMARY

Oral and oropharyngeal cancers are life-threatening diseases that can often be prevented through the avoidance of causative agents. Tobacco remains the primary cause of oral cancers. Tobacco acts synergistically with alcohol, so tobacco users who consume excessive amounts of alcohol are particularly at risk. Squamous cell carcinoma makes up more than 90% of oral cancers. Early detection and treatment are critical to prevent morbidity and mortality. Oral cancer strikes a disproportionate number of minority populations and is especially deadly for African American men, who are typically diagnosed at later stages.

Treatment is based on the disease stage at diagnosis, and usually entails surgery and/or radiation, sometimes with the addition of chemotherapy. Side effects can affect quality of life. Surgical interventions may result in disfigurement, and the individual's social, psychological, and physical states are impacted.

Every medical and dental provider has the responsibility to perform annual examinations on patients to screen for lesions. In addition, volunteering at screening events takes little time and provides an excellent public health service, particularly for underserved populations with little access to dental care. Various screening tools are available, including the brush biopsy and chemiluminescent devices. Educating the public and patients about the risk factors as well as signs and symptoms of oral cancer is critical. The public receives little information through mass media, and is unaware of the disease as well as the availability and importance of an oral cancer examination.

REFERENCES

1. *Stedman's concise medical dictionary* (5th ed.). (2005). Baltimore: Lippincott Williams & Wilkins.
2. National Cancer Institute. (n.d.). Dictionary of cancer terms. Retrieved 1/28/07 from http://www.cancer.gov/dictionary/.
3. Smeele, L. (2007). Oral, oropharyngeal, and nasopharyngeal cancer: Intervention approaches. In Ward, E. C., & van As-Brooks, C. J., Eds. *Head and neck cancer: Treatment, rehabilitation and outcomes.* San Diego, CA: Plural Publishing, 87–102.
4. American Cancer Society. (2006). *Cancer facts and figures 2006.* Atlanta: American Cancer Society.
5. Sapp, J. P., Eversole, L. R., & Wysocki, G. P. (2004). Contemporary oral and maxillofacial pathology (2nd ed.). St. Louis: Mosby, 180–95.
6. Saunders, N. A., Coman, W. B., & Guminski, A. D. (2007). Cancer of the head and neck. In Ward, E. C., & van As-Brooks, C. J., Eds. *Head and neck cancer: Treatment, rehabilitation, and outcomes.* San Diego, CA: Plural Publishing, 1–26.
7. Ries, L. A. G., Eisner, M. P., Kosary, C. L., Hankey, B. F., Miller, B. A., Clegg, L., Mariotto, A., Feuer, E. J., &

Edwards, B. K., Eds. (2003). *SEER cancer statistics review, 1975–2002.* Bethesda, MD: National Cancer Institute.

8. Kerr, A. R., Changrani, J. G., Gany, F. M., & Cruz, G. D. (2004). An academic dental center grapples with oral cancer disparities: Current collaboration and future opportunities. *J Dent Educ,* 68(5):531–41.

9. Sabichi, A., Demierre, M., Hawk, E., Lerman, C., & Lippman, S. (2003). Frontiers in cancer prevention research. *Cancer Res,* 63:5649–55.

10. Tabloski, P. A. (2006). *Gerontological nursing.* Upper Saddle River, NJ: Pearson Prentice Hall: 374–78.

11. Oral Cancer Foundation. (2006). *Oral cancer facts.* Retrieved 12/19/06 from http://www.oralcancerfoundation.org/facts/index.htm.

12. Shiboski, C. H., Schmidt, B. L., & Jordan, R. C. K. (2005). Tongue and tonsil carcinoma: Increasing trends in the U.S. population ages 20–44 years. *Cancer,* 103(9):1843–49.

13. Schwartz, S. M., Daling, J. R., Doody, D. R., Wipf, G. C., Carter J. J., Madeleine, M. M., Mao, E., Fitzgibbons, E. D., Huang, S., Beckmann, A. M., McDougall, J. K., & Galloway, D. A. (1998). Oral cancer risk in relation to sexual history and evidence of human papillomavirus infection. *J Natl Cancer Inst,* 90(21):1626–36.

14. Erdmann, J. (2003). Recent studies attempt to clarify relationship between oral cancer and human papillomavirus. *J Natl Cancer Inst,* 95(9):638–39.

15. Silverman, S., Jr. (2001). Demographics and occurrence of oral and pharyngeal cancers: The outcomes, the trends, the challenge. *J Am Dent Assoc,* 132:7S–11S.

16. Shopland, D. R. (1995). Tobacco use and its contribution to early cancer mortality with a special emphasis on cigarette smoking. *Environ Health Perspect,* 103 (Suppl 8):131–42.

17. Schottenfeld, D., & Beebe-Dimmer, J. L. (2005). Advances in cancer epidemiology: Understanding causal mechanisms and the evidence for implementing interventions. *Annu Rev Public Health,* 26:37–60.

18. U.S. Department of Health and Human Services. (1989). *Reducing the health consequences of smoking: 25 years of progress. A report of the surgeon general—1989* (DHHS Publication No. (CDC) 89-8411). Washington, DC: U.S. Department of Health and Human Services.

19. American Cancer Society. (2006). *Oral cavity and oropharyngeal cancer: What are the risk factors for oral cavity and oropharyngeal cancers?* Retrieved 1/12/07 from http://www.cancer.org/docroot/CRI/CRI_2_3x.asp?dt=60.

20. Doll, R. (1996). Cancers weakly related to smoking. *Br Med Bull,* 52(1):35–49.

21. Shaha, A. R., Patel, S., Shasha, D., & Harrison, L. B. (2001). Head and neck cancer. In Lenhard, Jr., R. E.,

Osteen, R. T., & Gansler, T., Eds. *Clinical oncology.* Atlanta, GA: American Cancer Society, 297–329.

22. Sciubba, J. J. (2001). Oral cancer and its detection: History-taking and the diagnostic phase of management. *J Am Dent Assoc,* 132:12S–18S.

23. Thomas, D. B. (1995). Alcohol as a cause for cancer. *Environ Health Perspect,* 103(8):153–60.

24. Nasca, P., & Pastides, H. (2001). *Fundamentals of cancer epidemiology.* Gaithersburg, MD: Aspen.

25. Brouha, X., Tromp, D., Hordijk, G., Winnubst, J., & De Leeuw, R. (2005). Role of alcohol and smoking in diagnostic delay of head and neck cancer patients. *Acta Otolarngol,* 125:552–56.

26. Oral Cancer Foundation. (2006). Alcohol and tobacco. Retrieved 1/13/07 from http://www.oralcancerfoundation.org/facts/alcohol_tobacco.htm.

27. Viswanathan, H., & Wilson, J. A. (2004). Alcohol—the neglected risk factor in head and neck cancer. *Clinical Otolaryngology,* 29:295–300.

28. Oral Cancer Foundation. (2006). Screening the non-high risk oral cancer patient—part 1. Retrieved 1/29/07 from http://www.oralcancerfoundation.org/dental/why_screening_works.htm.

29. Schantz, S. P., & Yu, G. (2002). Head and neck cancer incidence trends in young Americans, 1973–1997, with a special analysis for tongue cancer. *Arch Otolaryngology—Head and Neck Surgery,* 128(3):268–74.

30. Silverman, S., Jr. (2003). *Oral cancer* (5th ed.). Hamilton, Ontario: BC Decker.

31. Brown, L. M., Hoover, R. N., Greenberg, R. S., Schoenberg, J. B., Schwartz, A. G., Swanson, G. M., Liff, J. M., Silverman, D. T., Hayes, R. B., & Pottern, L. M. (1994). Are racial differences in squamous cell esophageal cancer explained by alcohol and tobacco use? *J Natl Cancer Inst,* 86:1340–45.

32. Day, G. L., Blot, W. J., Austin, D. F., Bernstein, L., Greenberg, R. S., Preston-Martin, S., Schoenberg, J. B., Winn, D. M., McLaughlin, J. K., & Fraumeni, J. F., Jr. (1993). Racial differences in risk of oral and pharyngeal cancer: Alcohol, tobacco, and other determinants. *J Natl Cancer Inst,* 85(6):465–73.

33. Walker, B., Figgs, L. W., & Zahm, S. H. (2005). Differences in cancer incidence, mortality, and survival between African Americans and Whites. *Environ Health Perspect,* 103(Suppl 8):275–81.

34. Cruz, G. D., Salazar, C. R., & Morse, D. E. (2006). Oral and pharyngeal cancer incidence and mortality among Hispanics, 1996–2002: The need for ethnoregional studies in cancer research. *Am J Public Health,* 96(12):2194–200.

35. Markopoulos, A., Albanidou-Farmaki, E., & Kayavis, I. Actinic cheilitis: Clinical and pathologic characteristics in 65 cases. *Oral Dis,* 10:212–16.

36. Luna-Ortiz, K., Güemes-Meza, A., Villavicencio-Valencia, V., & Mosqueda-Taylor, A. (2004). Lip cancer experience in Mexico. An 11-year retrospective study. *Oral Oncol,* 40:992–99.

37. Sciubba, J. J. (2001). Oral cancer: The importance of early diagnosis and treatment. *Am J Clin Dermatol,* 2(4): 239–51.

38. Walker, D. M., Boey, G., & McDonald, L. A. (2003). The pathology of oral cancer. *Pathology,* 35(5):376–83.

39. Silverman, S., Jr., Gorsky, M., & Kaugars, G. E. (1996). Leukoplakia, dysplasia, and malignant transformation. *Oral Surg Oral Med Oral Pathol,* 82(3):117.

40. Lumerman, H., Freedman, P., & Kerpel, S. (1995). Oral epithelial dysplasia and development of invasive squamous cell carcinoma. *Oral Surg Oral Med, Oral Pathol Oral Radiol Endod,* 79(3):321–29.

41. Epstein, J. B., & Gorsky, M. (1999). Topical application of vitamin A to oral leukoplakia. *Cancer,* 86(6):921–27.

42. Neville, B. W., Damm, D. D., Allen, C. M., & Bouquot, J. E. (2002). *Oral and maxillofacial pathology* (2nd ed.). Philadelphia: Saunders.

43. Mignogna, M. D., Fedele, S., Russo, L. L., Muzio, L. L., & Bucci, E. (2004). Immune activation and chronic inflammation as the cause of malignancy in oral lichen planus: Is there any evidence? *Oral Oncology,* 40:120–30.

44. Fatahzadeh, M., Rinaggio, J., & Chiodo, T. (2004). Squamous cell carcinoma arising in an oral lichenoid lesion. *J Am Dent Assoc,* 135:754–59.

45. Larsson, A., Warfvinge, G. (2005). Oral lichenoid contact reactions may occasionally transform into malignancy. *Eur J Cancer Prev,* 14(6):525–29.

46. Mignogna, M. D., Fedele, S., & Russo, L. L. (2006). Dysplasis/neoplasia surveillance in oral lichen planus patients: A description of clinical criteria adopted at a single centre and their impact on prognosis. *Oral Oncol,* 42:819–24.

47. Mattsson, U., Jontell, M., & Holmstrup, P. (2002). Oral lichen planus and malignant transformation: Is a recall of patients justified? *Critl Rev Oral Biol Med,* 13(5):390–96.

48. Kerrigan, D., Kelly, J., & Hollen Team. (2006). Understanding cancer and related topics: HPV vaccine to prevent cervical cancer. Retrieved 12/19/06 from http://cancer.gov/cancertopics/understandingcancer.

49. Surveillance, Epidemiology and End Results. SEER Stat database. Incidence – SEER 9 Regs Public-Use, November 2003 submission. Retrieved 11/06 from www.seer.cancer.gov.

50. Chen, R., Aaltonen, L., & Vaheri, A. (2005). Human papillomavirus type 16 in head and neck carcinogenesis. *Rev Med Virol,* 15:351–63.

51. Hemminki, K., Dong, C., & Frisch, M. (2000). Tonsillar and other upper aerodigestive tract cancers among cervical cancer patients and their husbands. *Eur J Cancer Prev,* 9(6):433–37.

52. Zhang, Z., Morgenstern, H., Spitz, M. R., Tashkin, D. P., Yu, G., Marshall, J. R., Hsu, T. C., & Schantz, S. P. (1999). Marijuana use and increased risk of squamous cell carcinoma of the head and neck. *Cancer Epidemiol Biomarkers Prev,* 8:1071–78.

53. Yellowitz, J. A., Goodman, H. S., Horowitz, A. M., & al-Tannir, M. A. (1995). Assessment of alcohol and tobacco use in dental schools' health history forms. *J Dent Educ,* 59(12):1091–96.

54. Miller, P. M., Ravenel, M. C., Shealy, A. E., & Thomas, S. (2006). Alcohol screening in dental patients: The prevalence of hazardous drinking and patients' attitudes about screening and advice. *J Am Dent Assoc,* 137(12):1692–98.

55. Chung, V., Horowitz, A. M., Canto, M. T., & Siriphant, P. (2000). Oral cancer educational materials for the general public: 1998. *J Public Health Dent,* 60(1):49–52.

56. Canto, M. T., Kawaguchi, Y., & Horowitz, A. M. (1998). Coverage and quality of oral cancer information in the popular press: 1987–98. *J Public Health Dent,* 58(3):241–47.

57. Horowitz, A. M., Moon, J., Goodman, H. S., & Yellowitz, J. A. (1998). Maryland adults' knowledge of oral cancer and having oral cancer examinations. *J Public Health Dent,* 58(4):281–87.

58. Horowitz, A. M., Siriphant, P., Sheikh, A., & Child, W. L. (2001). Perspectives of Maryland dentists on oral cancer. *J Am Dent Assoc,* 132:65–72.

59. Horowitz, A. M., Drury, T. F., Goodman, H. S., & Yellowitz, J. A. (2000). Oral pharyngeal cancer prevention and early detection: Dentists' opinions and practices. *J Am Dent Assoc,* 131:453–62.

60. Ahluwalia, K. P., Yellowitz, J. A., Goodman, H. S., & Horowitz, A. M. (1998). An assessment of oral cancer prevention curricula in U.S. medical schools. *J Cancer Educ,* 13(2):90–95.

61. American Dental Education Association. (2002). Competencies for the new dentist. *J Dent Educ,* 66(7):849–51.

62. Johns, S. G. (2001). The extraoral examination from the perspective of the patient. *J Dent Hyg,* 75(4):282–89.

63. Holmes, J. D., Dierks, E. J., Homer, L. D., & Potter, B. E. (2003). Is detection of oral and oropharyngeal squamous cancer by a dental health care provider associated with a lower stage at diagnosis? *J Oral Maxillofac Surg,* 61:285–91.

64. Smith, R. A., Cokkinides, V., & Eyre, H. J. (2006). American Cancer Society guidelines for the early detection of cancer, 2006. *CA Cancer J Clin,* 56(1):11–25.

65. Yellowitz, J. A., Horowitz, A. M., Drury, T. F., & Goodman, H. S. (2000). Survey of U.S. dentists' knowledge

and opinions about oral pharyngeal cancer. *J Am Dent Assoc,* 131:653–61.

66. Centers for Disease Control and Prevention. (1994). MMWR *Morb Mortal Wkly Rep,* 43(11):197–212.

67. Horowitz, A. M., & Nourjah, P. A. (1996). Factors associated with having oral cancer examinations among U.S. adults 40 years of age or older. *J Public Health Dent,* 56:331–35.

68. Johns Hopkins Medical Center. Clinical trials head and neck cancer. Head and Neck Cancer Center. Retrieved 1/18/2007 from http://www.hopkinsmedicine.org/headneckcancer/headnecktrials.html.

69. Kuo, W. P., Whipple, M. E., Jenssen, T., Todd, R., Epstein, J. B., Ohno-Machado, L., Sonis, S. T., & Park, P. J. (2003). Microarrays and clinical dentistry. *J Am Dent Assoc,* 134:456–62.

70. Epstein, J. B., Zhang, L., & Rosin, M. (2002). Advances in the diagnosis of oral premalignant and malignant lesions. *J Can Dent Assoc,* 68(10):617–21.

71. Mager, D. L., Haffajee, A. D., Devlin, P. M., Norris, C. M., Posner, M. R., & Goodson, J. M. (2005). The salivary microbiota as a diagnostic indicator of oral cancer: A descriptive, non-randomized study of cancer-free and oral squamous cell carcinoma subjects. *J Transl Med.* Retrieved 1/3/07 from http://www.translational-medicine.com/content/3/1/27.

72. Partridge, M., Pateromichelakis, S., Phillips, E., Emilion, G. G., A'Hern, R. P., & Langdon, J. D. (2000). A case-control study confirms that microsatellite assay can identify patients at risk of developing oral squamous cell carcinoma within a field of cancerization. *Cancer Res,* 60:3893–98.

73. Wong, D. T. (2006). Salivary diagnostics powered by nanotechnologies, proteomics and genomics. *J Am Dent Assoc,* 137:313–21.

74. Epstein, J. B., Feldman, R., Dolor, R. J., & Porter, S. R. (2003). The utility of tolonium chloride rinse in the diagnosis of recurrent or second primary cancers in patients with prior upper aerodigestive tract cancer. *Head Neck,* 25(11):911–21.

75. Christian, D. C. (2002). Computer-assisted analysis of oral brush biopsies at an oral cancer screening program. *J Am Dent Assoc,* 133:357–62.

76. Svirsky, J. A., Burns, J. C., Carpernter, W. M., Cohen, D. M., Bhattacharyya, I., Fantasia, J. E., Lederman, D. A., Lynch, D. P., Sciubba. J. J., & Zunt, S. L. (2002). Comparison of computer-assisted brush biopsy results with follow up scalpel biopsy and histology. *Gen Dent,* 50(6):500–503.

77. Eisen, D. (2000). The oral brush biopsy: A new reason to screen every patient for oral cancer. *Gen Dent,* 48(1):96–99.

78. Drinnan, A. J. (2000). Screening for oral cancer and precancer—a valuable new technique. *Gen Dent,* 85(3):7–11.

79. Svirsky, J. A., Burns, J. C., Page, D. G., & Abbey, L. M. (2001). Computer-assisted analysis of the oral brush biopsy. *Compendium,* 22(2):99–106.

80. Sciubba, J. J. (1999). Improving detection of precancerous and cancerous oral lesions: Computer-assisted analysis of the oral brush biopsy. *J Am Dent Assoc,* 130:1445–57.

81. Epstein, J. B., Gorsky, M., Lonky, S., Silverman, S., Jr., Epstein, J. D., & Bride, M. (2006). The efficacy of oral lumenoscopy (ViziLite®) in visualizing oral mucosal lesions. *Spec Care Dent,* 26(4):171–74.

82. Ebihara, A., Krasieva, T. B., Liaw, L. L., Fago, S., Messadi, D., Osann, K., & Wilder-Smith, P. (2003). Detection and diagnosis of oral cancer by light-induced fluorescence. *Lasers Surg Med,* 32:17–24.

83. Lane, P., Gilhuly, T., Whitehead, P., Zeng, H., Poh, C., Ng, S., Williams, P. M., Zhang, L., Rosin, M., & MacAulay, C. (2006). Simple device for the direct visualization of oral-cavity tissue fluorescence. *J Biomed Opt,* 11(2):024006-1–024006-7.

84. Westra, W. H., & Sidransky, D. (2006). Fluorescence visualization in oral neoplasia: Shedding light on an old problem. *Clinl Cancer Res,* 12:6594–97.

85. Ord, R. A. (2000). Diagnostic procedures. In Ord, R. A., & Blanchaert, R. H., Jr., *Oral cancer: The dentist's role in diagnosis, management, rehabilitation, and prevention.* Carol Stream, IL: Quintessence, 39–48.

86. National Comprehensive Cancer Network. (2007). Staging guidelines NCCN head and neck cancers. Retrieved 3/1/08 from http://www.nccn.org/professionals/physician_gls/PDF/head-and-neck.pdf.

87. Robbins, M. R. (2000). Oral care of the patient receiving chemotherapy. In Ord, R. A., & Blanchaert, R. H., Jr., Eds. *Oral cancer: The dentist's role in diagnosis, management, rehabilitation, and prevention.* Carol Stream, IL: Quintessence, 133–47.

88. Suntharalingam, M. (2000). Principles and complications of radiation therapy. In Ord, R. A., & Blanchaert, R. H., Jr., Eds. *Oral cancer: The dentist's role in diagnosis, management, rehabilitation, and prevention.* Carol Stream, IL: Quintessence, 111–22.

89. Manne, D. S. (2006). Oral mucositis and xerostomia: Challenging oral health conditions. Part I: Oral mucositis. *Access,* 20(6):34–37.

90. Barker, G. J., Barker, B. F., & Gier, R. E. (2000). *Oral management of the cancer patient* (6th ed.). Kansas City, MO: University of Missouri-Kansas City.

91. U.S. Department of Health and Human Services. (2000). *Healthy people 2010* (2nd ed.). Washington, DC: U.S. Government Printing Office.

92. Cruz, G. D., LeGeros, R. Z., Ostroff, J. S., Hay, J. L., Kenigsverg, H., & Franklin, D. M. (2002). Oral cancer knowledge, risk factors and characteristics of subjects in a large oral cancer screening program. *J Am Dent Assoc,* 133:106471.

93. Horowitz, A. M., Nourjah, P., & Gift, H. C. (1995). U.S. adult knowledge of risk factors and signs of oral cancers: 1990. *J Am Dent Assoc,* 126:39–45.

94. Hay, J. L., Ostroff, J. S., Cruz, G. D., LeGeros, R. Z., Kenigsberg, H., & Franklin, D. M. (2002). Oral cancer risk perception among participants in an oral cancer screening program. *Cancer Epidemiol Biomarkers Prev,* 11:155–58.

95. Maurizio, S. J., Lukes, S. M., & DeMattei, R. D. (2005). An assessment of printed oral cancer materials from local health departments in Illinois. *J Dent Hyg,* 79(1):10.

96. Montgomery County, MD. (2006). Collaborating for change: African American health program annual report 2005. Retrieved 3/1/08 from http://www .montgomerycountymd.gov/hhstmpl.asp?url=/content/hhs/ phs/index.asp#aahip.

97. University of Pittsburg Cancer Institute. (2006). Oral cancer program. Retrieved 1/21/07 from http://www.upci .upmc.edu/report/Clinical/oral/index.html.

98. Virginia Department of Health. (2006). *Virginia department of health partners with barbers to reduce risks of oral cancer.* Retrieved 1/21/07 from http://www.vdh .state.va.us/news/PressReleases/2006/040706OralCancer .asp.

99. Pender, N. J., Murdaugh, C. L., & Parsons, M. A. (2006). *Health promotion in nursing practice* (5th ed.). Upper Saddle River, NJ: Pearson Prentice Hall.

Chapter 6

Dental Trauma

Gary Cuttrell

OBJECTIVES

After studying this chapter, the student will be able to:

1. Define dental trauma.
2. Describe the etiology of dental trauma.
3. Describe the assessment of trauma.
4. List and describe the categories of dental trauma.

KEY TERMS

Anterior
Alveolar ridge
Attachment apparatus
Extra-alveolar time
Dry storage
Dry storage time
Root resorption
Avulsion
Alveolus
Reimplantation
Luxation
Intruded teeth
Extruded teeth
Ischemia
Dentinal tubules
Apices
Resorption
Surface resorption
Root resorption
Extra alveolar time
Cementoblasts
Osteoblasts
Remodeling

(continued)

KEY TERMS (CONTINUED)
Re-contouring
Replacement resorption
Lamina dura
Ankylosis
Labial
Palatal
Mesial
Distal
Pulpal necrosis
Revascularization
Periradicular inflammation
Alveolar fracture

Electric vitality testing
Cold testing
Laser Doppler flowmetry
Perfusion
Tooth germs
Buds
Exfoliate
Apexification
Subluxated
Approximated
Lateral luxation
Abutment teeth

INTRODUCTION

Dental trauma of some form happens to almost everyone. The outcomes are as variable as the injuries themselves. The overwhelming majority involve **anterior** teeth, so injury to these teeth will be the primary focus of this chapter. Research throughout the world has been making steady progress in defining how to increase the successes of preventive measures and therapies rendered to patients with dental trauma. The continued effort in clinical research holds great promise that the outcomes for dental trauma will continue to improve.

Damage to soft tissues, **alveolar ridge,** and dentition require the dental provider to have diagnostic and clinical skills that will minimize permanent damage. This chapter is intended to aid providers in delivering appropriate emergency and follow-up care.

The periodontium is made up of the gingival unit as well as the attachment apparatus and alveolar bone. The **attachment apparatus** consists of the cementum, periodontal ligament, and the alveolar process. These attachment components are involved in traumatic teeth injuries. The periodontal ligament attaches the tooth root to the bony socket (i.e., alveolar process). In addition, the periodontal ligament's specialized cells replace the cementum, periodontal ligament, and alveolar bone. Maintaining the blood supply and health of the periodontal ligament is one of the most important considerations in enabling repair of dentition injuries.[1] Trauma to the attachment apparatus

requires proper diagnosis and assessment to maximize healing. Periodontal ligament healing depends on several factors. These factors include the type of stabilization, the extent of damage, contamination of tissues with toxins from necrotic dental pulp, amount of time the tooth was out of the socket (**extra-alveolar time**), and the storage method used to preserve the tooth (i.e., wet versus dry).[2] **Dry storage** means the tooth is not placed in a fluid or solution to keep the tooth structures moist. The length of time the tooth is stored under dry conditions (**dry storage time**) affects the ability to save the tooth.

Regardless of the patient's age, dental trauma can be emotional and painful. Cost of the repairs can also be a substantial economic burden. Psychologically, children can be especially troubled because of unsightly fractures.[3,4] This embarrassment is not limited to children; it affects all ages when the front teeth are adversely affected. Another burden is the amount of time involved in the healing process and in receiving treatment. Dental trauma's effects include tooth death, **root resorption,** tooth loss, and altered potential to develop permanent teeth.[5]

The term **avulsion** refers to the traumatic removal of a tooth, usually through accidents or sports injuries. An avulsed tooth can be reinserted into the **alveolus** (tooth socket); this procedure is called **reimplantation.** If avulsed teeth are reimplanted more than 15 minutes after avulsion, healing will vary according to the factors listed earlier that affect healing of the periodontal ligament. Even if patients or parents are informed of a poor prognosis, the choice often is to reimplant the avulsed tooth, even when there are better long-term treatment options.[6] Often, the costs of treatments and the final outcome are overruled by the strong desire to restore the tooth. Therefore, clinicians need to understand the outcomes of different types of treatments of dental trauma to guide patients in their decisions.

ETIOLOGY

Many researchers worldwide have studied traumatic dental injuries, and dental providers have developed parameters for treating these injuries. It is reported that about 33% of 5-year-old children have suffered tooth **luxation** (dislocation) of primary teeth. Uncomplicated fracture of a permanent tooth's crown is highly reported among 12-year-old children. Primary dentition trauma peaks at ages 2 to 3 years and corresponds to young children's development of walking skills. Trauma to permanent dentition in boys peaks at 9 to 10 years; active play and sports injuries with falls are the leading causes.[7] Other epidemiologic studies have found that 50% of boys have a dental injury between the ages of 8 and 12 years.[8] The upper central incisors in both primary and permanent teeth are most affected mainly because of their position, followed by the remaining anterior teeth, the upper and lower lateral incisors, and the upper canines.[9]

The acute stage of trauma begins when teeth and supporting structures are subjected to traumatic forces sufficient for injury. Dental injuries include tooth fracture, luxation, intrusive crushing injury, and separation from the attachment apparatus (i.e., avulsion) of the tooth. Two types of tooth displacement are **intruded teeth,** which are pushed inward into the tooth socket, and **extruded teeth,** which are pushed outward from, but not out of, the tooth socket. Intrusive crushing injury involves a much greater inward force. The more severe injuries compromise the vascularization (blood flow) of pulpal and periodontal ligament tissues through obstruction of the blood supply to the tissues. This process is called **ischemia,** and it results in an interrupted blood supply. Wound healing is delayed and complicated by bacteria at the injury site. Bacterial contamination of pulpal tissue occurs through direct exposure to bacteria from the object that caused the injury, from blood clots in the periodontal ligament, or from bacteria brought to the affected area through the blood stream or through the **dentinal tubules** (tubules that extend throughout the surface of dentin).

With appropriate treatment, the periodontal ligament will begin significant healing within 1 to 2 weeks. Pulp tissue may heal within 4 days, but such quick healing usually occurs only for teeth with open **apices.**[7] Limited periodontal ligament damage leads to limited inflammation, and limited inflammation, in turn, leads to healing with new replacement cementum. More severe periodontal ligament damage leads to a severe inflammatory response over a diffuse (wide) area of the root.

Resorption

Resorption refers to the removal of enamel and other tooth components that are composed of calcium salts (calcific), such as dentin and cementum. This process may occur naturally during the shedding of deciduous (primary) teeth; this type of resorption is called **surface resorption.** In dental trauma, the tooth root undergoes resorption. **Root resorption** is classified as either replacement resorption or inflammatory resorption.[10] Replacement resorption is much more common than inflammatory resorption.

The greatest prevalence of resorption is seen in teeth reimplanted after a delay of more than $1^1/_2$ hour. Teeth with dry storage of less than 5 minutes may still have a resorption rate of 36%. Teeth stored dry longer than 30 minutes suffer root resorption at a rate of 90%. The best predictor of overall resorption was total time of dryness prior to storage or reimplantation. The total time the tooth was outside the mouth (**extra-alveolar time**) was the only significant factor in predictors of replacement resorption. After 30 minutes of dry time, root resorption occurs at a high rate. The onset of resorption varies from 102 to 997 days.[10]

Replacement Resorption

Cementoblasts are responsible for depositing cementum on dentin that covers the root. **Osteoblasts** are responsible for producing the alveolar bone that lies under the periodontal ligament. Damage to the periodontal ligament cells and cementum leads to resorption of the root surface through a series of processes. Osteoblasts respond to traumatic injury by producing new bone to repair the alveolar bone. This process is called **remodeling.** The damage to the slow-growing cementoblasts allows osteoblasts to also attach areas of bone directly to the root before the cementoblasts can cover the root with cementum. The direct attachment of bone leads to **re-contouring** of the physiologic bone, with the entire root being replaced by bone. This process is called **replacement resorption.**[11] If the area of damage is large, replacement resorption is irreversible.

Replacement resorption is greater in younger patients because remodeling occurs faster.[10]

Replacement resorption is characterized by the loss of root surface (cementum) accompanied by loss of periodontal ligament space and loss of **lamina dura** (the hard layer lining the tooth alveoli). Consequently, bone is seen to be in direct contact with the root surface. This phenomenon is often referred to as **ankylosis** and may occur in the absence of inflammation.[10]

Cementum, or root, resorption is defined radiographically as the evidence of loss of root substance accompanied by its replacement with bone, such that periodontal ligament space has been lost, but radiolucency is not evident. One clinical test for root resorption is the percussion test, which involves tapping the tooth with a tool and listening for the sound produced by the tooth. A high percussion note indicates resorption. Teeth with no physiologic mobility are another clinical sign of resorption. If there is no radiographic evidence of root resorption but the tooth is clinically ankylosed, replacement resorption has occurred. Resorption of the root may not be visible in x-rays of **labial** or **palatal** tooth surfaces (i.e., surfaces located adjacent to the lips or palate, respectively). Resorption is more commonly visible on the **mesial** or **distal** tooth surfaces.[10]

Inflammatory Resorption

Death of the pulp tissue (**pulpal necrosis**) always occurs after an avulsion injury. Necrotic tissue becomes infected and releases toxins. The wider dentin tubules provide a physiologic path for these inflammatory products to reach the root surface. Inflammatory resorption occurs when surface or replacement resorption involves dentin and the inflammatory toxins of a necrotic, infected pulp. The inflammatory products cause a loss of root surface (cementum), accompanied by the loss of adjacent bone and the formation of an area of radiolucency. In luxation trauma, if **revascularization** (restoration of blood flow) or endodontic procedures on dental pulp and periapical tissues are not successful, necrosis will lead to external inflammatory resorption and rapid loss of the tooth.[11]

Revascularization is possible if the apex of the injured tooth is open, but not if the apex is closed. Limiting inflammation around the root (**periradicular inflammation**) tips the balance toward favorable (cemental resorption) rather than unfavorable (inflammatory resorption) healing.[11]

INITIAL EXAMINATION

Obtaining a complete history of the injury will guide the treatment plan for repair. The soft tissue examination will often help in diagnosing areas of trauma and in planning where to place necessary sutures (fibers used to sew together the tissues) to promote healing. The hard tissue examination involves looking for loosened teeth, fractured teeth, fractured alveolar process, displaced teeth, and missing teeth.[5] Radiographs are always necessary to evaluate the extent of injury to the root and alveolus. If there is extensive soft tissue damage, radiographs may be needed to determine if embedded teeth or tooth fragments are present. Movement of the alveolar process and several teeth together is diagnostic of an **alveolar fracture.**[10] Detection of horizontal root fracture often requires multiple x-rays from different angles to diagnose the fracture.[12] The two main factors of the prognosis include extra-alveolar time and dry storage time. Prolonged drying causes loss of the periodontal ligament and dehydration of the pulp. And prolonged dry storage time is directly related to root resorption. The total extraoral time is the strongest single predictor of which type of resorption will occur.

It appears that contamination, endodontic treatment, or the initial stage of root development does not significantly affect the prognosis.[10] Diagnosis will determine the treatment plan and improve prognosis of the involved teeth. It may be helpful to use a standard checklist during the examination. The checklist will provide good documentation for treatment planning and potential legal questions. It is also a good practice to have pictures as a permanent part of the patient's chart.

It is important at the initial visit to obtain a good history including medical history, prior dental trauma, timing of current trauma, clinical examination of injuries, radiographs, and discussion of treatment options and prognosis of outcomes. The dental provider needs to be aware that a neurologic injury is possible. Closed head or cervical spinal injury should at least be considered if the force was strong enough to fracture, intrude, or avulse a tooth.[13] The patient should be referred to a physician for neurologic evaluation (Table 6–1 ■). Of course, if any doubt exists, emergency transport is appropriate.

Pain control is necessary for the well-being of the patient and often to permit controlled evaluation. The character of the pain will help with assessment of the injury. Pain as a result of temperature change is consistent with pulpal inflammation. Pain related to occlusion may mean that a tooth has been displaced, or that

■ **Table 6–1**   Neurologic Evaluation

A neurologic examination may include the following:
- The history: questions concerning symptoms and condition
- An evaluation of neurologic function
- Diagnostic tests
- Electrodiagnostic tests
- Blood tests
- Other common tests

swelling of periodontal or supporting tissue has occurred. If teeth are mobile, the vascular blood supply may have been disrupted. Extreme tooth mobility leaves little chance that the blood supply has not been damaged, and pulpal necrosis will likely develop.

Electric vitality testing involves placing an electrode on the injured tooth and then passing an electric current through the tooth. The current is increased until the patient feels a sensation in the tooth. This test, however, is of limited use during the acute injury phase, because the normal anatomy is disrupted. Thermal testing may be more useful in the acute phase, but it also may be misleading. A non-traumatized tooth in another area of the mouth should be tested first. This tooth is referred to as a baseline control, because it establishes the level of heat to which a normal tooth responds. A quick response to heat indicates inflammation, which is expected at this stage. No response to heat indicates that pulpal necrosis is highly likely. **Cold testing** is another form of thermal testing; it involves application of ice, cold air, or a vapocoolant (a substance that produces a cooling effect when it evaporates). If the pain stops when the cold is removed, the tooth is normal. A prolonged reaction of pain to cold is diagnostic of pulpal damage that will need further assessment. A follow-up evaluation after a healing period of 7 to 10 days will provide a better assessment. **Laser Doppler flowmetry** provides a real-time measurement of the flow of red blood cells in minute vessels (venules or capillaries) of the circulatory system. This microvascular blood flow is referred to as

perfusion. Researchers have used this technique to provide an objective measurement of pulpal damage, but the cost is currently prohibitive unless the dental office deals with frequent cases of dental trauma.[14]

SOFT TISSUE INJURIES

Soft tissue injuries often are associated with facial trauma. Tears of the gingival tissue and displacement of teeth often are present. Lips commonly have puncture wounds caused by bite injuries when the open mouth is forcibly closed during the accident. Wounds should be rinsed with saline and, if necessary, gently debrided with gauze wetted with mild soapy water to remove foreign material and dead or damaged tissue. This cleaning is often needed to adequately perform the initial examination. Appropriate suturing of tissue is needed for tissue repair and healing. It may be necessary to refer patients to a plastic or oral surgeon if facial or complex suturing is required. It is important to refer patients to their physician to determine if tetanus immunization or booster injections are needed.

CATEGORIES OF TRAUMATIC DENTAL INJURIES

Crown fractures have been classified from class I through IV. Class I involves just the enamel, class II includes enamel and dentin, class III involves enamel, dentin, and pulpal tissues. Class IV is the complete loss of the clinical crown.[15] (Figure 6–1 ■)

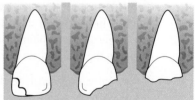
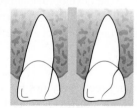

■ **FIGURE 6–1**   Crown fractures.

INJURY TO PRIMARY TEETH

Treatment of pediatric patients may involve behavioral issues, especially with a painful injury. Fortunately, primary teeth allow conservative treatment in most situations. Definitive treatment for pulpal exposures, soft tissue injuries, painful fractures, and necessary extractions are not easily accomplished in the non-cooperative patient. Because children's alveolar bone is softer than adults due to less mineralization and their inability to provide feedback, the extent of the injury may be difficult to diagnose. If injury is suspected, young children may need referral for examination under general anesthesia.

Mobile, non-displaced primary teeth generally heal without treatment (self-heal) and require only reassurances to the child and parents. Displaced primary teeth require assessment of occlusal interferences and pain to decide the appropriate care. Generally, if the primary tooth interferes with the child's bite or endangers the permanent tooth development, the tooth is extracted. If neither condition exists, the tooth is left and allowed to heal. Intruded teeth are assessed for potential endangerment to the permanent tooth, which would require extraction of the primary teeth.

Intruded Primary Teeth

Intrusions of primary central incisors typically do not require treatment. Natural re-eruption of intruded teeth permit a conservative approach helping reduce damage to successor ("permanent" or secondary) teeth.[16] Fortunately, the structures from which permanent teeth are formed (**tooth germs,** or **buds**) are lingual to primary root tips. Intrusions and avulsions of great force would be required to injure the tooth buds; these injuries are more associated with secondary damage to the developing permanent teeth.[9] Children younger than 3 years are more likely to suffer damage to successor permanent teeth, because bone mineralization is incomplete at this age and dental germs are still developing.[9] If, in rare cases, the primary teeth are obviously intruded lingually, it may be necessary to extract the primary tooth to possibly avoid developmental problems with the permanent teeth. Radiographic confirmation should be done before deciding to extract the teeth.

Avulsed Primary Teeth

Many cases of avulsed primary teeth may not be well documented, but studies list these injuries as 7% to 13% of primary tooth trauma.[17] The most frequently avulsed primary teeth are the maxillary incisors at 89%.[18]

Avulsed primary teeth are seldom reimplanted. Many recommend that primary teeth never be replaced,[19,20] because of concern that permanent teeth may be damaged. Damage to the permanent tooth germ occurs 30% of the time after avulsion of primary teeth. Discoloration is the most common damage and occurs more often in children younger than 2 years.[18] Always of concern is the need to use traditional space maintenance appliances to prevent potential loss of arch space. This procedure will require follow-up evaluations by the dentist.

Parents often are concerned about the discoloration of traumatized primary teeth. These teeth often will naturally **exfoliate** (shed enamel crystals) without treatment and need only conservative monitoring. It is important to use other clinical symptoms such as infection to determine if pulpal therapy is necessary.[16,21] Treatment is indicated if any symptoms develop that could affect the development of permanent teeth.

INJURY TO PERMANENT TEETH

Trauma to young permanent teeth may lead to devitalization of the pulp with arrest in root development, resulting in open apices.[22] The open apices are difficult to seal and require apexification procedures. **Apexification** involves placing a root canal dressing, traditionally calcium hydroxide, at the apex, which may induce closure of the root apex.[23] This time-honored treatment requires several months and requires follow-up appointments. A wide range of researches reported successes in healing rates in the 70% to 100% range.[24]

Avulsed Secondary Teeth

Recommendations for reimplanting avulsed teeth with open apices are quite varied. The International Association of Dental Trauma does not recommend reimplanting such teeth. However, the debate as to the proper treatment is still ongoing. Without doubt, the emotional element alone leads to most teeth being reimplanted. If possible, performing endodontic therapy before reimplantation provides a good seal for the open apices and avoids the apexification procedure. This treatment should be completed as aseptically as possible and with minimal trauma to the periodontal ligament on the root surface to yield the best prognosis.[11]

Preservation of Avulsed Teeth

Proper storage of avulsed teeth is essential to the viability of reimplanted teeth if immediate reimplantation is not practical. Although it is known that air drying rapidly reduces the chance of successful reimplantation, proper transport and storage will help maintain the periodontal ligament, thus buying precious time. Matching the osmolality of the storage medium to the tissue fluid will help preserve the periodontal ligament. Research has identified several valid storage media. Hanks balanced salt solution (HBSS), milk, saline, and the patient's own saliva have proved beneficial.[25] Viaspan, a storage medium used for transport of transplant organs has also been effective for avulsed teeth.[26] Viaspan however is expensive and not readily available, and HBSS provides similar results. Milk has proved very effective in preserving the periodontal ligament, but may not be available in many emergency settings owing to the need for refrigeration. Milk substitutes do not need refrigeration and offer an advantage over natural whole milk. Of the different milk substitutes studied, whole milk and the reconstituted baby formulation Enfamil were within the physiologic pH range (6.6–7.8) for periodontal ligament cells and within the physiologic osmolarity range (230–400).[25] Although other milk substitutes were within the physiologic osmolarity range, they were not as effective as storage media, probably because their pH values were outside the physiologic range.[25] Tap water often is used for storage because of its ready availability, but it is a very poor storage media. In fact, water's low osmolality results in cell death of the periodontal ligament.[25,27] Storage of avulsed teeth on ice is a low alternative if none of the approved storage media is available. Although time of reimplantation of avulsed teeth is critical, allied health and lay people would do well to learn proper storage to increase survival in the hands of dental professionals. There are commercial products that offer proper storage media and containers for avulsed teeth.[28,29] It seems that, unless immediate reimplantation or storage in an acceptable media is available, avulsed teeth have poor survival rates.

Preservation of Periodontal Ligament

Preserving the periodontal ligament is a race to minimize the inflammation that occurs when avulsion damages the ligament and to minimize the pulpal infection that follows damage of the vascular bed.[11] Inflammatory resorption follows in **subluxated** (partially dislocated) and luxated teeth when pulp necrosis develops, but is controlled with timely endodontic treatment.[30] Although it is well-known that reimplantation in less than 15 minutes provides the greatest chances of survival, proper storage and handling of avulsed teeth increase the survival rate after they are implanted.[31] Splinting materials and fixation with slight mobility will aid reorientation of the periodontal membrane fibers and help preserve the periodontal ligament.[32]

Case reports of reimplanted teeth after prolonged air drying (18 hours) indicate that their appearance can be improved and their functionality restored; nevertheless, long-term root resorption leads to a poor prognosis.[33]

Clinical Steps for Reimplantation

Final clinical steps involve removal of any obstructions in the socket. Obstructions may include collapsed alveolar bone or the coagulum of the clot (i.e., the soft, insoluble mass of the clot). Coagulum may be gently rinsed out with saline. A blunt instrument can be used to reposition the socket bone to allow replacement of the avulsed tooth.[11]

Splinting

Semirigid or flexible splints show less root resorption and improved periodontal ligament healing compared with rigid fixation.[34] Rigid fixation time of less than 2 weeks reduces the chance of ankylosis.[35,36] A semirigid (physiologic) splint to reposition the teeth is placed for 7 to 10 days. The splint should not impinge on the gingiva and cannot interfere with occlusion. If the injury involved fractures of the alveolar ridge, splint placement is necessarily increased up to 8 weeks, even though the chances of tooth ankylosis are increased. Radiographs are needed to verify splint placement and the course of healing.[11]

Healing of the Pulp

Pulp healing in permanent teeth varies with the degree of trauma to the crown and periodontal ligament. Crown fractures with no luxation heal 99% with no apparent long-term effects.[37] Crown fractures with luxation result in pulpal necrosis in 25% of cases, whereas 70% heal with no apparent long-term effects. The pulpal necrosis is associated with periodontal ligament damage, emphasizing that the primary factor in pulp healing is related to compromised circulation that occurs with luxation.[38]

Fractured Secondary Teeth

Fractured anterior coronal fragments are often saved and presented to the dentist after injury. If there is a good fit of the fragment, it is possible to use a reattachment process that involves an acid-etch bonding treatment. (See Chapter 13 for discussion of etching processes.) Fragment retention provides an alternative to conventional resin composite restorations but weakness of the bonding junction may lead to poor long-term results.[39]

Displaced Secondary Teeth

Displaced teeth incur injury to the periodontal ligament, the pulp, and the bone in the alveolar sockets. Dental professionals must decide which treatments give the teeth the best chance to heal. The act of repositioning, in itself, often requires force that can lead to more injury. In cases of young teeth still in formation, the pulp has the ability to heal and complete tooth development. The edges of significantly displaced alveolar bone will need to be **approximated** (put close together) to encourage bony healing and to provide a better foundation for gingival repair. Repositioning the periodontal ligament portions of the bony socket and root from avulsed and severely displaced teeth provides a good chance for healing. Repositioning of the ligament in some categories of injury is still under investigation; therefore, discretion should be taken in selecting a clinical treatment. Displacement of teeth to the side of the socket (**lateral luxation**) may be better treated with spontaneous repositioning for young patients and orthodontic repositioning for patients older than 12 years.[40] An extra-alveolar time of 60 minutes makes survival of the periodontal ligament cells unlikely.[10]

Intruded Secondary Teeth

Intrusion injury accounts for 3% of permanent teeth injuries; its prognosis for healing is directly related to the stage of root development. Apical diameters less than 0.7 mm have a higher probability of developing necrosis than apical diameters greater than 1.2 mm.[40] Treatment of intruded secondary teeth follow three general recommendations: (1) spontaneous re-eruption, (2) immediate surgical repositioning and fixation, and (3) orthodontic repositioning.[40] An intruded tooth with mature root formation and closed apices has the best prognosis if repositioning occurs within 90 minutes of the injury, followed by timely pulpal therapy to prevent a necrotic pulp.[41] Necrotic pulps trigger inflammatory root resorption, which leads to tooth loss.[42]

PUBLIC EDUCATION ON DENTAL TRAUMA

More than 60% of avulsion injuries occur at home or school.[43] Availability of emergency kits on-site, and to emergency personnel, would help prevent dry storage or use of inappropriate storage media, and would help to ensure better healing results. Provision of regular and frequent information for educators and health care providers is necessary to ensure the best treatment. The correct protocols to increase the survivability and viability of traumatized teeth are simple, but they often are not followed, because often the information about their use has been forgotten. Proper medical and dental treatments, such as evaluation for tetanus injections, neurologic examinations, and proper storage and stabilization of injured tooth structures, provide safe and effective treatment for this common emergency.[27] It is important to let the public know that dry storage of avulsed teeth results in irreversible injury to the periodontal membrane and usually leads to loss of the tooth, making it a long-term temporary solution.[27] Surveys of school children have shown them to be better versed in emergency treatments for other body parts. Lack of basic knowledge for emergency treatment of avulsed teeth reduces the chance of a favorable prognosis.[44] Education of teachers, parents, and students in the basic management of dental trauma should be encouraged to improve outcomes.[45] Educational programs need reinforcement so that the public retains the knowledge needed to properly handle dental traumas.[46]

RESEARCH ON DENTAL TRAUMA

Carl E. Misch has looked at life expectancies of both fixed prosthodontic (cemented) bridge work and removable prosthodontic (non-cemented) bridge work appliances; he found that, since 1993, dental implants have had the highest survival rate for single-tooth implants than for any other method of tooth replacement.[47] Misch acknowledges that the longevity of implant crowns needs a longer history before such a blanket statement can be made. Use of implants requires, as stated, a clinical judgment of **abutment teeth** (teeth used to support fixed or removable prosthodontic appliances) and the risks associated with their potential loss. Implants with a high success rate (i.e., above the ninetieth percentile) should be strongly considered in some categories of traumatic dental injury replacement. Further research and evaluation of success rates in traumatic dental injuries and treatments need to consider the best initial treatment options. This investigation should look at total costs and final outcomes for patient function and esthetics. Of course, implants are an option for only patients of an age that allow implants as a valid choice.

The Cochrane Collaboration, an international organization that prepares, maintains, and disseminates systematic reviews of health care interventions, offers an electronic resource for locating high-quality information.

The Cochrane Library focuses primarily on systematic reviews of controlled trials of therapeutic interventions. Two Cochrane protocols provide guidance in the research of dental trauma. The first deals with "Interventions for treating traumatized permanent front teeth: Root fracture."[48] The second protocol deals with "Interventions for treating traumatized permanent front teeth: Luxated (dislodged) teeth."[49] Continued research in all categories is providing guidelines for more defined and appropriate treatment for dental trauma.

SUMMARY

Maintaining a viable, functioning tooth is the desirable outcome after traumatic dental injuries. When this outcome is not possible, timing and restorative options need to be addressed. If the tooth is lost immediately or has a poor prognosis, the patient needs to be aware of options to restore function and esthetics. These options range from removable and fixed prosthodontics to dental implants. All of these procedures are acceptable restorative options. The newest option for dental implants has shown very good results, has become a reliable choice, and has inherent benefits. As evidenced by worldwide articles dealing with dental trauma, this subject will continue to be studied, because dental trauma is one of the common accidents that occur in everyday life.

REFERENCES

1. Roberson, T. M., Heymann, H. O., & Swift, Jr., E. J. (2006). *Sturdevant's art and science of operative dentistry* (5th ed.) 38–39.
2. Von Arx, T., Filippi, A., & Lussi, A. (2001). Comparison of a new dental trauma splint device (TTS) with three commonly used splinting techniques. *Dent Traumatol,* 17:272.
3. Slack G. L., & Jones, J. M. (1955). Psychological effect of fractured incisors*, Br Dent J* 99:386–88.
4. Cortes, M. I., Marcenes, W., & Shelham, A. (2002). Impact of traumatic injuries to the permanent teeth on the oral health-related quality of life in 12- to 14-year old children. *Community Dent Oral Epidemiol,* 30:193–98.
5. Douglass, A. B., & Douglass, J. M. (2003). Common dental emergencies. *Am Fam Phys,* 67(3):515.
6. Nguyen, P.-M. T., Kenny, D. J., & Barrett, E. J. (2004). Socio-economic burden of permanent incisor replantation on children and parents. *Dent Traumatol,* 20:124–29.
7. Andreasen, J. O., Andreasen, F. M., Bakland, L. K., & Flores, M. T. (2003). *Traumatic dental injuries: A manual*

8. (2nd ed.). Blackwell Munksgaard, Blackwell Publishing Professional, 2121 State Avenue, Ames Iowa 50014-8300, USA, 8–11.
8. Flores, M. T., Andreasen, J. O., & Bakland, L. K. (2001). Guidelines for the evaluation and management of traumatic dental injuries. *Dent Traumatol,* 17:193–96.
9. Sennhenn-Kirchner, S., & Jacobs, H.-G. (2006). Traumatic injuries to the primary dentition and effect of the permanent successors—A clinical follow-up study. (Abstract). *Dent Traumatol,* 22(5):1.
10. Boyd, D. J., Kinirons, M. J., & Gregg, T. A. (2000). A prospective study of factors affecting survival of replanted permanent incisors in children. *Int J Paediatr Dent,* 10:200–204.
11. Trope, M. (2002). Clinical management of the avulsed tooth: Present strategies and future directions. *Dent Traumatol,* 18:1–11
12. Bramante, C. M., Menezes, R., Moraes, I. G., Bernardinelli, N., Garcia, R. B., & Letra, A. (2006). Use of MTA and intracanal post reinforcement in a horizontally fractured tooth: A case report. *Dent Traumatol,* 10(1111):277.
13. Davis, J. J., & Vogel L. (1995). Neurological assessment of the child with head trauma. *J Dent Child* 62: 93–96.
14. Mesaros, S. V., & Trope, M. (1997). Revascularization of traumatized teeth assessed by laser Doppler flowmetry. *Endod Dent Traumatol,* 13:24–30.
15. Ellis, R. G., & Davey, L. W. (1970). *The classification and treatment of injuries to the teeth of children,* (5th ed.). St. Louis, MO: Mosby.
16. Spinas, E., Melis, A., & Savasta, A. (2006). Therapeutic approach to intrusive luxation injuries in primary dentition. A clinical follow-up study. (Abstract). *Eur J Paediatr Dent* 7(4):179–86.
17. Andreasen, J. O., & Andreasen, F. M. (1994). *Textbook and color atlas of traumatic injuries to the teeth* (3rd ed.). Copenhagen, Denmark: Blackwell Munksgaard: 1994:219-425,750.
18. Christophersen, P., Freund, M., & Harild, L. (2005). Avulsion of primary teeth and sequelae on permanent successors. *Dent Traumatol,* 21:321–23.
19. McTigue, D. J. (2000). Diagnosis and management of dental injuries in children. *Pediatr Clin North Am,* 47:1067–84
20. Flores, M. T., Andreasen, J. O., & Bakland, L. K. (2001). Guidelines for the evaluation and management of traumatic dental injuries. *Dent Traumatol,* 17:49–52.
21. Holan, G., & Fuks, A. B. (1996). The diagnostic value of coronal dark-gray discoloration in primary teeth following traumatic injuries. *Pediatr Dent,* 18:224–27
22. Andreasen, J. O. (1970). Etiology and pathogenesis of traumatic dental injuries. A clinical study of 1,298 cases. *J Dent Res,* 78:339–42.

23. Ghose, L. J., Baghdady, V. S., & Hikmat, B. Y. M. (1987). Apexification of immature apices of pulpless permanent anterior teeth with calcium hydroxide. *J Endod,* 13:285–90.

24. Pradhan, D. P., Chawla, H. S., Gauba, K., & Goyal, A. (2006). Comparative evaluation of endodontic management of teeth with unformed apices with mineral trioxide aggregate and calcium hydroxide. *J Dent Child,* 73(2):79–84.

25. Pearson, R. M., Liewehr, F. R., West, L. A., Patton, W. R., McPherson, J. C., & Runner, R. R. (2003). Human periodontal ligament cell viability in milk and milk substitutes. *Am Assoc Endod* 29(3):184–86.

26. Trope, M., & Friedman, S. (1992). Periodontal healing of replanted dog teeth stored in Viaspan, milk and Hanks' balanced salt solution. *Endo Dent Traumatol,* 8:183–88.

27. Andersson, L., Al-Asfour, A., & Al-Jame, Q. (2006). Knowledge of first-aid measure of avulsion and replantation of teeth: An interview of 221 Kuwaiti schoolchildren. *Dent Traumatol,* 22:57, 60, 558

28. Emergency Medical Treatment Toothsaver (EMT Toothsaver). Phoenix, AZ: SmartPractice.

29. Emmanouil, S., Regan, J. D., Kramer, P. R., Witherspoon, D. E., & Opperman, L. A. (2004). Survival of human periodontal ligaments for transport of avulsed teeth. *Dent Traumatol,* 20:21–28.

30. Qin, J., Ge, L., & Bai, R. (2002). Use of a removable splint in the treatment of subluxated, luxated and root fractured anterior permanent teeth in children. *Dent Traumatol,* 18(2):81–85.

31. Krasner, P., & Person, P. (1992). Preserving avulsed teeth for replantation. *J Am Dent Assoc* 123(11):80–88.

32. Oikarinen, K. (1990). Tooth splinting: A review of the literature and consideration of the versatility of a wire-composite splint. *Endod Dent Traumatol,* 6:237–50.

33. Cho, S. Y., & Cheng, A. C. (2002). Replantation of an avulsed incisor after prolonged dry storage: A case report. *J Can Dent Assoc* 68(5):297–300.

34. Berude, J. A., Hicks, M. L., Sauber, J. J., & Li, S. J. (1988). Resorption after physiological and rigid splinting of replanted permanent incisors in monkeys. *J. Endod* 14:592–600.

35. Nasjleti, C. E., Castelli, W. A., & Caffesse, R. G. (1982). The effect of different splinting times on replantation of teeth in monkeys. *Oral Surg* 53:557–66.

36. Von Arx, T., Filippi, A., & Lussi, A. (2001). Comparison of a new dental trauma splint device (TTS) with three commonly used splinting techniques. *Dent Traumatol,* 17:267.

37. Robertson, A., Andreasen, F. M., Andreasen, J. O., & Noren, J. G. (2000). Long-term prognosis of crown-frac-tured permanent incisors. The effect of stage of root development and associated luxation injury. *Int J Paediatr Dent,* 123(3):191.

38. Andreasen, F. M., Noren, J. G., & Andreasen, J. O., Engelhardtsen, S., & Lindh-Strombert, U. (2006). Long-term survival fragment bonding in the treatment of fractured crowns: A multicenter clinical study. The Cochrane Library, Issue 4. Retrieved from The Cochrane Central Register of Controlled Trials (Central) database.

39. Andreasen, J. O., Andreasen, F. M., Bakland, L. K., & Flores, M. T. (2003). *Traumatic dental injuries: A manual* (2nd ed.) Blackwell Munksgaard, Blackwell Publishing Professional, 2121 State Avenue, Ames, Iowa 50014-8300, USA, 14.

40. Gungor, H. C., Cengiz, S. B., & Altay, N. (2006). Immediate surgical repositioning following intrusive luxation: A case report and review of the literature. *Dent Traumatol,* 10(1111):340–43.

41. Kenny, D. J., Barrett, E. J., & Casas, M. J. (2003). Avulsions and intrusions: The controversial displacement injuries. *J Can Dent Assoc* 69:308–13.

42. Hedegard, B., & Stalhone, I. (1973). A study of traumatized permanent teeth in children aged 7–15 years. Part I. *Swed Dent J,* 66:431–38

43. Loh, T., Sae-Lim, V., Yian, T. B., & Liang, S. (2006). Dental therapists' experience in the immediate management of traumatized teeth. *Dent Traumatol,* 22:66–70.

44. Kinoshita, S., Kojima, R., Taguchi, Y., & Noda, T. (2002). Tooth replantation after traumatic avulsion: A report of 10 cases. *Dent Traumatol,* 18:153–56.

45. Kahabuka, F. K., Willemsen, W., Wan't Hof, M., & Burgerskijk, R. (2006). The effect of a single educational input given to school teachers on patient's correct handling after dental trauma. The Cochrane Library, Issue 3. Retrieved from Cochrane Central Register of Controlled Trials database.

46. Misch, C. E. (2005). *Dental implant prosthetics* (1st ed.). St Louis, MO: Mosby, 2–3.

47. Guyatt, G., & Rennie, D. (Eds). (2005). *Users' guide to the medical literature* (5th ed.). American Medical Association Press, 32.

48. Al-Hennawi., D., Day, P. F., & Duggal, M. S. (2005). Interventions for treating traumatized permanent front teeth: Root fracture. (Protocol). *Cochrane Database Syst Rev,* Issue 3. Art. No.: CD005408. DOI: 10.1002/14651858.CD005408.

49. Belmonte, F. M., Abrao, C. V., Day, P. F., Macedo, C. R., Saconato, H., & Trevisani, V. F. M. (2006). Interventions for treating traumatized permanent front teeth: luxated (dislodged) teeth.

Chapter 7

Host Defense Mechanisms in the Oral Cavity

Beth E. McKinney

OBJECTIVES

After reading this chapter, the student should be able to:

1. List the four host defense mechanisms operational in the oral cavity.
2. Describe how the epithelium functions as a microbial barrier in the mouth.
3. Describe how an ideal dentition functions as a defense mechanism.
4. Describe the cycle of enamel demineralization and remineralization.
5. Apply the knowledge of host defense mechanisms to practicing a medical model of dental care.
6. Identify early and late colonizers in bacterial plaque, and discuss their roles in the disease process.
7. Explain the significance of plaque pH.
8. Differentiate between cellular and humoral immunity.
9. Describe the role of granulocytes in host defense.
10. Describe the importance of oral health in promoting systemic health.
11. Identify the major salivary glands.
12. List the protective functions of saliva.
13. Describe the antimicrobial properties of saliva.
14. Define xerostomia and name two possible causes.
15. Recognize xerostomia in patients.
16. Prescribe appropriate therapies for a patient with compromised salivary function.
17. Discuss the functions of the immunoglobulins.

KEY TERMS

Infection
Proliferation
Gastrointestinal tract
Cellular
Humoral
Immunoglobulins
Keratin
Vasoconstriction
Pulpal polyps
Granulomas
Herpetic
Saliva
Acquired (salivary) pellicle
Cellular immunity
Humoral immunity
Precursors
Tonsils
Complement system
Candida albicans
Granulocytes
Leukocyte adhesion disorder
Beta-defensin peptides
LL-37
Plunc

(continued)

KEY TERMS (CONTINUED)

Homeostasis

Exocrine glands

Parotid gland

Amylase

Submandibular gland

Sublingual gland

Palatal salivary glands

Lingual salivary glands

Buccal salivary glands

Labial salivary glands

Whole saliva

Unstimulated saliva

Viscosity

Saliva substitutes

Stimulated saliva flow

Sialorrhea

Ptyalism

Sialoliths

Histadine

Statherin

Bacteriostatic

Salivary peroxidase

Hypothiocyanate

Lactoperoxidase

Salivary mucins

Immunoglobulin M

Immunoglobulin G

Immunoglobulin A

Immunoglobulin D

Immunoglobulin E

Job syndrome

INTRODUCTION

Colonization of the human body by bacteria is the normal, universal—and even preferred—state of affairs. The entire body is vastly populated by billions of tiny microbes whose eradication is neither possible nor desirable. Typically, human beings and microbes coexist peacefully and in many cases have forged mutually beneficial relationships. **Infection** is the state in which disease is caused because of the failure of the host's protective mechanisms and the **proliferation** of pathogenic microbes. Fortunately, it is only an occasional outcome.

This chapter will provide an overview of host defense mechanisms in the oral cavity and is not a substitute for a course in immunology. The reader who finds this subject intriguing is referred to the medical literature that teaches pathophysiology and the study of clinical disease processes. Unfortunately, this topic has not generated much interest in past dental and dental hygiene educational curriculums. However, discussions of this subject have started, and as genetic research continues to advance, the prevention of disease by the mediation of the body's own defense systems will no doubt receive intense investigation.

The mouth is the gateway for food and drink destined for the **gastrointestinal tract.** It is also the structure with which we communicate most frequently (i.e., it handles speech). As such, the mouth is constantly exposed to the outside environment and potential invasion by microbial pathogens. To ensure the safety of the body from infection, a number of defensive systems exist: (1) anatomic barriers, (2) normal oral flora, (3) the immune system, and (4) saliva.

Anatomic barriers include the epithelium and an ideal dentition. Normal oral flora includes bacteria that discourage colonization by pathogenic microbes. The immune system includes **cellular** and **humoral** components; the latter are found in body fluids. The saliva is a mucosal secretion and contains **immunoglobulins.**

ANATOMIC BARRIERS: THE GREAT WALL OF MESENCHYME

The skin is the largest organ in the human body. Epithelium is a formidable barrier to microbial invasion. Microbes cannot cause infection without first getting past this anatomic barrier. Until breached, no infection can occur. As long as the epithelium is intact, most microbes find this barrier exceedingly difficult to penetrate. Like personal protective equipment worn for patient care, an intact epithelium is an excellent protective mechanism for the oral cavity. Like a torn latex glove, cuts, scrapes, and abrasions all provide possible routes of entry for a pathogen. Minute insults to the oral epithelium occur with disturbing regularity; a patient with a floss cut, pizza burn, or tortilla chip scrape is a good example.

The epithelium in the oral cavity does not differ appreciably from the rest of the body, except for the fact that it is always wet. The majority of oral epithelium is keratinized. **Keratin** is a fibrous, sulfur-containing protein, which cannot be penetrated, even by gastric acid. (Pills that must be absorbed intact in the intestines are often coated with keratin so that they will not dissolve in the stomach.) The junctional epithelium at the bottom of the gingival sulcus/crevice lacks any keratin at all and is perhaps the oral site most susceptible to invasion by microorganisms.

Mucosal epithelium in the mouth is more highly vascularized than the skin on the hand. Because of the increased blood perfusion, any injury to the barrier is immediately met with the blood's defensive components. Healing time in the oral cavity can then occur more rapidly. Conversely, activities such as smoking cause a decrease in the diameter of capillaries (**vasoconstriction**) in the oral tissues, leading to exacerbation of periodontal disease where it exists.

The epithelial barrier is such a good defense mechanism that the body will often go to great lengths to recreate one when it is lost. For example, **pulpal polyps** (Figure 7–1 ■) are made of granulomatous tissue, which occasionally forms in large carious lesions that have invaded the pulp.[1] **Granulomas** are an inflammatory response to foreign substances that have invaded a body tissue. A large number of different types of immune cells and fibroblasts form the granuloma as they surround the foreign substance.[2] Typically granulomas are not painful.

During infancy, the oral environment is relatively un-colonized by microbes. At the presence of the first tooth, the microbial tenants of the oral cavity undergo a vast change. This change can be significant, not to mention pathologic, if the baby's caregivers happen to have active dental caries, untreated periodontal disease, or an active oral **herpetic** lesion, all of which are easily transmissible to the baby. As humans age, achievement and maintenance of an ideal anatomic dentition afford maximum protection against microbial dental infection. In other words, esthetically pleasing teeth are not just the goal of models and actors. Possession of twenty-eight teeth in class 1 occlusion and with healthy interdental papillae is the oral anatomic condition most naturally resistant to microbial onslaught. Restorations with overhangs, lack of interdental papillae, periodontal pockets, or drifting or crowded teeth are all examples of anatomic situations that give microbial pathogens an advantage in colonization of the tooth structure, thereby contributing to dental disease.

An ideal dentition also includes the anatomic barrier of tooth enamel. Tooth enamel is the hardest substance in the human body, harder even than cortical bone. Enamel is more mineralized than bone or dentin. It is estimated that enamel is composed of approximately 96% mineral by weight and is therefore highly inorganic. The inorganic phase of enamel is based on the mineral hydroxyapatite, which is made up mainly of calcium, phosphate, and hydroxyl ions. After teeth are fully erupted, the hydroxyl group is often substituted by fluoride, giving additional protection against caries. When the substitution occurs, the enamel is composed of fluorapatite.

Tooth enamel is constantly undergoing a process of demineralization and remineralization. Demineralization occurs with exposure to the acids found in foods, beverages, and the stomach, and to acids produced by bacteria in plaque. Remineralization is the repair of the enamel rods after prolonged exposure to an acidic environment. When teeth erupt, they are anatomically complete, but histologically incomplete and immature. After eruption, the missing ions are supplied from the saliva, a process termed posteruptive maturation. For this reason, partially erupted first permanent molars are particularly susceptible to developing occlusal caries. In addition, newly improved glass ionomer products have been developed to

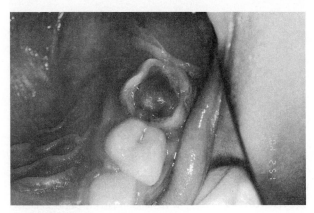

■ **FIGURE 7–1**   Pulpal polyps.

seal such teeth when a dry environment cannot be achieved. Without specific knowledge of the caries process, the development of a caries lesion is likely to be seen as a continuous process resulting in the ever-increasing loss of tooth mineral until a clinically discernible hole in the tooth structure is present. This conception is incorrect. The process of demineralization is not irreversible or inevitably progressive. If damage has not progressed beyond a still yet to be defined point, lost mineral can be replaced. As dentistry moves more from a surgical model towards a medical model, emphasis is on enamel repair during the early stages of the caries process. Although dentistry has typically focused on the surgical treatment of caries, the practice of dental hygiene with its more preventive approach is ideal for adopting a medical model that focuses on the reversal of the caries process by alternative interventions.

Backer-Dirks, in a long-term study, noted that more than 50% of the proximal lesions seen at the initial examination did not progress, indicating an arrestment phenomenon due to remineralization.[3] Additional support for remineralization is derived from the frequent observations of teeth that are acid-etched prior to placement of pit-and-fissure sealants. For those etched areas not covered with the resin, the chalky white appearance disappears over a period of a few days, and the enamel regains its initial translucent, glossy appearance.

Remineralizing conditions in the mouth are usually fairly constant. For example, the local pH may be lowered to the point at which enamel demineralization occurs from ingestion of acidic foods, or from the production of acid by bacteria after ingestion of carbohydrates, particularly refined foods. If the insults are brief and widely separated in time, remineralizing conditions can be restored in the intervening periods and the slight damage repaired. On the other hand, frequent or protracted periods of acid exposure, with insufficient time intervals for remineralization, ultimately lead to the development of overt caries. Recent developments in oral hygiene products have remineralization as a goal. Toothpastes and chewing gums are being formulated with bioavailable calcium and phosphate ions in a milk-derived protein called Recaldent.

Saliva, which will be discussed in greater detail later in the chapter, is an important factor in remineralization. Individual capacity for salivary remineralization varies depending on both the quantity and quality of saliva. Throughout life, minerals from the saliva are used to repair acid-damaged tooth structure. This repair process can range from an almost immediate replacement of daily ion losses from the enamel surface, to a slow repair (under proper conditions) of more extensive subsurface (white spot) lesions.

Fluoride has a major influence on both demineralization and remineralization.[4] Only small concentrations of fluoride are needed to inhibit demineralization or to enhance remineralization. As little as 0.1 ppm fluoride can reduce the amount of enamel dissolution in vitro (i.e., under artificial conditions in a laboratory). The presence of fluoride at the remineralizing site can accelerate re-hardening by a factor of up to fivefold. Fluoride enhances tooth mineralization both through systemic routes and topical applications. In the mouth, fluoride can come from a variety of sources:

- Short-term contact with fluoridated drinking water.
- The continual low fluoride output of the salivary glands.
- The bound fluoride in the plaque, which is released when the pH drops to around 5.5.
- The fluoride contained in the mature enamel layer after demineralization.
- Dental restorations such as glass ionomers, which release fluoride.
- Topical fluoride applications in forms ranging from toothpaste to varnishes.

The reader is referred to Chapter 12 for a more complete discussion of the uses, types, and benefits of fluoride.

Figure 7–2 ■ is a photograph of a 76-year-old woman who has healthy dentition, healthy periodontium, and excellent occlusion. People with normal immune function and regular preventive dental care can maintain

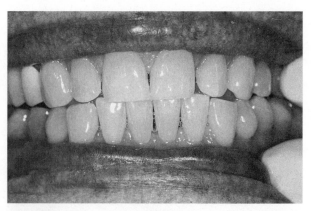

■ **FIGURE 7–2** Healthy dentition, healthy periodontium, and excellent occlusion.

healthy, esthetically pleasing teeth for a lifetime. Dentures are neither a natural, nor inevitable, part of the aging process. Caries and periodontitis are disease states, not naturally occurring conditions.

NORMAL ORAL FLORA

The formation of supragingival dental plaque begins with the **acquired (salivary) pellicle,** which is an acellular protein layer of saliva components adsorbed onto the surface of the enamel. The bacteria colonize on this pellicle. The pellicle plus the bacteria and the gel they create constitute a biofilm (dental plaque).[5] For several hours after a prophylaxis or toothbrushing has removed the biofilm, there is a steady change in the quantity and composition of the pellicle as new proteins are added from the saliva. The more the plaque matures, the denser it becomes and the more it retains acid against the tooth. In subgingival plaque, a sample of only a cubic millimeter may contain as many as a hundred million organisms. In a healthy sulcus, loose gram-positive cocci such as *Streptococcus gordonii* and *Streptococcus oralis* predominate. In periodontal pockets the bacterial population becomes predominately colonized by gram-negative anaerobes.[6] Later colonizers responsible for the disease process include *Porphyromonas gingivalis* and *Actinobacillus actinomycetemcomitans.* In the periodontal pocket, bacteria are shielded from salivary flow. Bacteria with limited attachment ability are contained within the walls of the gingival pocket.

The most variable factor in the pathogenicity of plaque colonies is the makeup of the microbial population.[7] Not all bacteria are bad. Some species discourage the attachment of other more pathogenic species, whereas others serve as a bridge.[8] Early colonizers include *Streptococcus mitis* and *Streptococcus sanguis.* *Veillonella,* when present, metabolizes lactic acid generated by the later colonizers *Streptococcus mutans* and *Lactobacillus,* which are responsible for caries formation. This action decreases the amount of acid available to demineralize tooth structure. Several studies indicate that the presence of *Veillonella* decreases caries risk. It becomes evident that the varieties, metabolic characteristics, and interrelationships of the bacteria are important in determining whether disease will occur.

The pH of plaque can drop to as low as 4.0 on the Stephan curve after use of a glucose mouth rinse.[9] Damage control from acid in the plaque is achieved by dilution and chemical buffering, and by increasing the protective ions (mainly, calcium, phosphate, and fluoride) in the vicinity of the teeth.[10] The water content of the saliva and plaque aid greatly in diluting the acid and in transporting acid into the main flow of saliva where it is further diluted and swallowed. Saliva acts as a strong buffer for the acidic plaque. This higher adsorption capacity for fluoride in the plaque also increases bicarbonates, phosphates, and ammonia concentrations derived from the saliva. These neutralizing actions serve as a brake in the rapidity and extent to which the pH can drop during periods of acidogenesis.

Each individual has a different potential for modifying the drop and recovery of the pH represented by the person's individual Stephan curve. For example, if a group of individuals are given a glucose mouthrinse, each person demonstrates a different, but reproducible, pH pattern. Once the pH begins to drop, the salivary buffers help to shorten the time that the pH is at its lowest and most damaging level.

Figure 7–3 ■ depicts the complicated arrangement of the community known as bacterial plaque. The early colonizers represented here are desirable organisms to have in an environment that can never be sterile. It is the later colonizers that cause disease. The goal of preventive dentistry then is not the eradication of all microorganisms, but the selective encouragment of the right mix.

THE IMMUNE SYSTEM IN THE ORAL CAVITY

The body's immune system has several components, all of which are active in the oral cavity. These components all monitor the body and distinguish it from anything that is foreign. Anything deemed not to belong is attacked. This process can be good in the case of a flu virus or a parasite; conversely, this process is bad in the case of a transplanted organ. Most significant for this discussion, in periodontal disease, the immune system causes as much or more tissue damage than the bacteria.

The lymph system is composed of two parts: cellular and humoral immunity. **Cellular immunity** is carried out by T cells from the thymus; **humoral immunity** is carried out by B cells from the bone marrow.[11] The cells from which T cells are formed (**precursors**) also originate in the bone marrow; however, the thymus is where they become fully functional. From the thymus, the T cells migrate to the lymph nodes, spleen, and blood. Both parts of the lymph system are involved in defending the body against bacteria and viruses. The

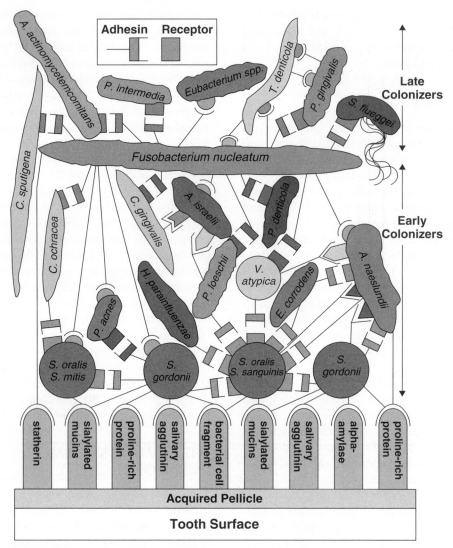

■ **FIGURE 7–3** Complicated arrangement of the community known as bacterial plaque.
(Kolenbrander, P. D., Palmer, R. F., et al. Bacterial Interactions and Successions During Plaque Development.
Periodontology 2000. Vol. 42, 2006. 47–79. Reprinted with permission of Wiley-Blackwell Publishing.)

tonsils contain a large proportion of B cells. Another part of the immune system is the **complement system,** which is composed of about 20 proteins whose primary function is to lyse foreign cells.

Candida albicans (Figure 7–4 ■) is a yeast organism that resides in very small quantities on human mucosa. It is kept from proliferation by saliva, normal oral flora, and T lymphocytes.[12] When there is a defect in any or all of these defense mechanisms, the candida organism can proliferate and cause infection as seen here in this patient with AIDS. If candida is also present in the blood and spreads throughout the body, it can be fatal.

The blood also has a myeloid (bone marrow) system of **granulocytes** (mature granular leukocytes) whose function is to find and attack foreign invaders. Granulocytes include eosinophils, neutrophils, basophils, and macrophages.[13] The main access that phagocytic cells and their antibacterial products have to the oral cavity is through the gingival sulcus/crevice and the tonsils. Polymorphonuclear leukocytes are the first neutrophils found in the gingival sulcus/crevice in response to plaque bacteria. They are able to migrate through the junctional epithelium to the site of infection. About 500 leukocytes per second are estimated to emigrate from the tissues,

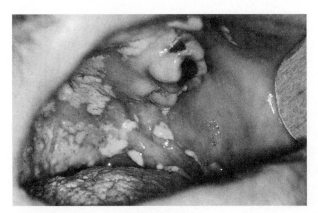

■ **FIGURE 7–4**   *Candida albicans.*

through the gingival sulcus/crevice into the oral cavity. Because lymphocytes secrete a number of toxic substances, they destroy not only foreign cells but also the body's own cells over a period of time. Some of these secretions include interleukins, cytokines, collagenase, C-reactive protein, and tumor necrosis factor. As this army of cells indicates, the development of periodontal disease is a complicated process.

Leukocyte adhesion disorder (LAD) is a rare genetic disease of the white blood cells. The leukocytes cannot migrate to sites of infection. One of the first signs of this disorder is severe periodontal disease in a child. Figure 7–5 ■ shows a 5-year-old child with LAD, with severe bone loss around all of her primary teeth. It is untreatable by current methodologies. Typically, people with LAD die from infection by early adulthood. New gene therapies may hold some promise in treating this disorder.

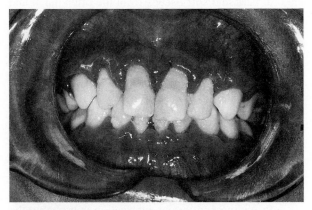

■ **FIGURE 7–5**   Child with LAD, aged 5 years, with severe bone loss around all of her primary teeth.

A new area of research is human **beta-defensin peptides;** to date, three have been identified (hBD-1, 2, and 3).[10,14–16] These peptides have been found in the mucosa, the salivary glands, and the gingiva. They have a broad spectrum of antimicrobial activity and offer little opportunity for bacteria to develop resistance. Another antimicrobial peptide, designated **LL-37,** has been found in human neutrophils, skin, gingiva, and junctional epithelium. Peptides are believed to play important roles in the immune defense mechanism. Another category of **PLUNC** (palate, lung, and nasal epithelium clone) proteins, only recently identified, seem to act as sensors for gram-negative bacteria in the oral cavity.[17] These three categories of newly found proteins appear to play more of a role in periodontal disease than in the caries process.[18] Immunoglobulins are also part of the body's immune system.

SALIVA AND ITS ROLE IN PROMOTING ORAL HOMEOSTASIS

The importance of saliva as a host defense mechanism cannot be understated. The same watery fluid that used to make placement of the perfect sealant on a second molar so difficult is actually filled with a wide variety of antimicrobial properties. The defense functions of the saliva are part of the body's ability to maintain **homeostasis,** that is, the ability to remain in balance and successfully resistant to challenges by chemical and bacterial agents.[19] Disease ensues only when the bacterial challenge exceeds the body's defense capabilities and/or a person lacks commitment to self-care. Saliva helps modulate and augment the previously described major body defense systems in the protection of oral tissues.

Salivary Glands

The salivary glands are **exocrine glands,** meaning their secretion (saliva) leaves the glands to bathe the oral cavity. Saliva is derived mainly from the major salivary glands—the parotid, submandibular, and sublingual glands. Of these, the **parotid gland** secretes a serous watery fluid that contains electrolytes, but is relatively low in organic substances. The parotid gland secretes the majority of the sodium bicarbonate that is essential in neutralizing acids produced by cariogenic bacteria in the dental plaque and the majority of the enzyme **amylase,** which initiates intraoral digestion of carbohydrates.[20] The **submandibular gland** secretes a mixed serous and mucous fluid, whereas the **sublingual gland**

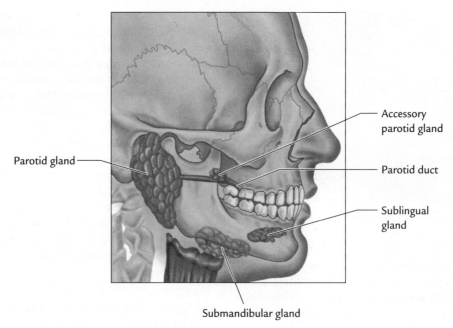

Parotid gland

Accessory parotid gland

Parotid duct

Sublingual gland

Submandibular gland

■ **FIGURE 7–6** Salivary gland.

has a greater proportion of mucous output than the other major glands. The minor glands (Figure 7–6 ■), which include **palatal, lingual, buccal,** and **labial salivary glands,** empty onto the mucous membrane in many locations on the palate, under the tongue, and on the inner sides of the cheeks and lips. These minor glands are mainly mucus-secreting glands that lubricate these surfaces, and allow for improved mastication and passage of food into the esophagus.[21] The minor salivary glands also contribute fluoride that bathes the teeth and enhances caries resistance.[22–24]

Pure saliva produced by the oral glands is sterile, until it is discharged into the mouth. When the fluids from all major and minor glands mix with each other, this secretion becomes known as **whole saliva.** Whole saliva is further altered by the presence of particles of food, tissue fluid, sloughed epithelial cells, and lysed bacteria (bacteria whose cellular components have disintegrated from the action of enzymes, antibodies, or complement). It becomes even more complex with the inclusion of living cells and their metabolic products such as bacteria and leucocytes; the latter are derived from the gingival sulci/crevices and tonsils.

The protective functions of saliva can be divided into five categories (1) lubrication, (2) flushing/rinsing, (3) chemical, (4) antimicrobial (including antibacterial,

antifungal, and antiviral), and (5) maintenance of supersaturation of calcium and phosphate ions bathing the enamel, and helping to buffer demineralization and aid remineralization of tooth structures.[25,26]

The salivary defensive system functions continuously, but its secretion becomes greatest and most active during food ingestion. The lowest flow rate is during sleep. This is one reason why early childhood caries, caused by a baby sleeping with a bottle containing milk or other sugary substances, occurs so rapidly.

A very thin microscopic layer of mucus protects the oral hard and soft tissues from the often harsh and abrasive foods during mastication. The moistening of food by saliva facilitates chewing and swallowing. Speech is enhanced by the reduced friction between the dry tongue and soft tissues. Conversely, xerostomia results in a greatly increased risk of caries. Chewing, swallowing, and speaking are all adversely affected by xerostomia. In addition to changes in taste, a chronic burning often occurs. When this condition persists, it is termed "burning mouth syndrome." In someone who has xerostomia, mild candidiasis, tooth erosion, and caries are often found even in the presence of good oral hygiene and dietary habits.

Providing continuous lubrication is probably the most important defensive function of the salivary glands.

It is the fluid that transports the buffering agents, the antimicrobials, and the demineralization and remineralization properties of saliva. In addition, the fluid output of the glands is essential for (1) diluting acids, (2) flushing food particles embedded around the teeth, (3) clearing refined carbohydrates, and (4) physically removing any free-floating bacteria.[26]

The composition of saliva varies, depending on whether it is stimulated or unstimulated. During the day, submandibular glands secrete the greatest proportion of **unstimulated saliva.** The flow rate of resting saliva for all three glands is very low and is about one-tenth of that during stimulated flow. Approximately two-thirds of the resting saliva is derived from the submandibular glands; one-quarter is from the parotids; and approximately one-twentieth is from the sublingual glands. The minor salivary glands secrete almost one-tenth of the total amount of saliva. The customary unstimulated flow rate of the salivary glands is subject to a circadian rhythm, with the highest flow in mid-afternoon and the lowest around 4:00 A.M.

Upon moderate stimulation, the submandibular and parotid glands secrete approximately equal amounts of saliva, whereas at full stimulation the parotid has the greatest output. When salivary flow is stimulated by chewing gum, 1 to 2 ml of whole saliva per minute can be expected. The minimum level of stimulated salivary flow necessary to maintain oral health is unknown, but when the flow is below 1 ml per minute, occurrence of xerostomia is a cause for concern. Once the flow rate is below 0.7 ml per minute, a diagnosis of xerostomia may be rendered. In the course of a single day, up to 1 liter of saliva is secreted into the oral cavity.

The total amount of saliva secreted varies considerably between and within individuals, depending on the environmental factors. Seasonal variations occur, with flow being lower in warm weather and higher in cold. Salivary flow is greater during standing than sitting, and greater when one is lying down. These postural changes parallel changes in systemic blood pressure. Recent product developments in dental health have led to the creation of kits designed to assess salivary quantity and quality. These materials are currently available and can assess the saliva's **viscosity** (ability to flow), pH, flow rate, and buffering capacity. Currently, these tests are not commonly used by private general dental practitioners. In addition, the test data are rarely routinely collected as part of an oral examination and recorded in a patient record. Although the importance of the presence of adequate saliva is known, very few treatments are available once a salivary problem is diagnosed. Even the treatments that currently exist, such as **saliva substitutes** and drugs like cevimeline, are poor substitutes for the real thing.

Stimulated saliva flow results from physiologic, psychologic, pharmacologic, and disease effects.[27,28] Examples of physical stimulation are the simple acts of chewing food and gum. Psychologic stimulation can be evoked by the same anticipation experienced by Pavlov's now famous dogs. Saliva can also be stimulated by the use of cholinergic drugs that increase exocrine gland secretions, such as pilocarpine or cevimeline. Under certain conditions, saliva flow can be abnormally high—a condition termed **sialorrhea** (or **ptyalism**), which is manifested by drooling. Ptyalism can occur with forms of mental impairment and some neurologic conditions, and occasionally during pregnancy.

The suppression of salivary flow is more serious. This condition also can result from physiologic, pharmacologic, and/or disease effects. The dry mouth sensation that accompanies panic is an example of a physiologic response. More than 350 pharmaceuticals are known to cause varying degrees of xerostomia.[29,30] Disease states of the glands include **sialoliths** (stones) within the gland ducts, resulting in obstruction of saliva flow, Sjögren syndrome, or postradiation exposure of the glands during cancer therapy.[30,31]

Sjögren syndrome is an autoimmune disease that typically affects older women. Its primary oral symptom is xerostomia (Figure 7–7 ■). People with xerostomia are at high risk for the development of caries, including caries in unusual places, such as the incisal edges of teeth. Treatment includes drugs such as cevimeline, saliva substitutes,

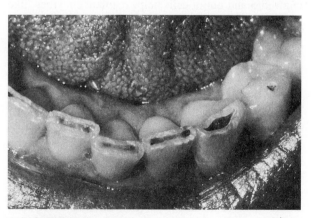

■ **FIGURE 7–7**   Xerostomia as seen in a patient with Sjögren's syndrome.

and lots of fluoride. Even with treatment, individuals with compromised salivary glands are usually affected for life.

Organic Components of Saliva

In addition to the secretion of different proportions of electrolytes, salivary glands secrete organic molecules that can be categorized into five major groups: amylase, mucins, phosphoproteins, glycoproteins, and immunoglobulins. Two of the families of small salivary proteins—**histadine** and **statherin**—deserve specific mention, because they help control the status of calcium and phosphate in the saliva. These proteins prevent fallout of the calcium and phosphate that maintain supersaturation in relation to hydroxyapatite. They prevent a rapid drop in saliva pH and aid in its quicker recovery. In addition, they both are antifungal and **bacteriostatic** (i.e., capable of inhibiting bacterial growth without destroying the bacteria).

The salivary glands also produce various enzymes. **Salivary peroxidase** reacts with saliva to form the antimicrobial compound **hypothiocyanate,** which inhibits the capability of the bacteria to fully use glucose. **Lactoperoxidase** strongly adheres to hydroxyapatite as a component of the acquired pellicle, and can influence the qualitative and quantitative characteristics of the microbial population of dental plaque.

Salivary Mucins

Salivary mucins are glycoproteins secreted by the salivary glands.[32] The pellicle that covers enamel is rich in mucins, which help clear carbohydrates from the mouth and protect against caries. Mucins also help modulate calcium channel activity in the mouth, thereby assisting in the maintenance of tissue integrity. The passage of calcium into and out of cells helps regulate enzymes, like zinc, that are responsible for tissue repair. It is believed that the presence of salivary mucins and their ability to modulate this activity enhance the repair process in oral soft tissues.

Immunoglobulins

There are five categories of immunoglobulins in the human body: immunoglobulin M (IgM), immunoglobulin G (IgG), immunoglobulin A (IgA), immunoglobulin D (IgD), and immunoglobulin E (IgE). Immunoglobulins are antibodies made of protein. They, too, defend the body against all types of infection and, sometimes, even when there is no infection (i.e., allergic reactions). Although dentistry is primarily concerned with only one of the immunoglobulins, a brief review of all of them

may be helpful in obtaining a basic understanding of their functions.

Immunoglobulin M is located on B cells and is found circulating in the blood. It is the largest of the immunoglobulins and, as such, cannot easily exit the circulatory system. It is the earliest of the group to appear at the site of infection. Its presence in a blood test indicates recent infection. It is also the main immunoglobulin that reacts when someone is given the wrong type of blood during a transfusion. IgM is the first immunoglobulin to be found in a fetus.

Immunoglobulin G has four subtypes. It is the most abundant of the immunoglobulins, and is found in both blood and other tissue liquids. Immunoglobulin G is effective against bacteria, viruses, and fungi. It is the only immunoglobulin that can pass through the placenta. This immunoglobulin is also responsible for food allergies, and is found in egg yolks (in birds it is called IgY).

Immunoglobulin A has two subtypes: serum IgA and secretory IgA (Figure 7–8 ■). Dentistry is most concerned with secretory IgA. All exocrine gland secretions are rich in IgA, and it can be found not only in tears and saliva, but also in vaginal fluid and colostrum. Secretory IgA initiates the inflammatory process. It prevents both bacteria and viruses from adhering to mucous membranes. IgA deficiency is the most common type of

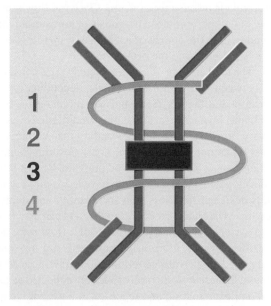

■ **FIGURE 7–8** Immunoglobulin A.
Retrieved October 2, 2007, from http://www.wikepedia.com

immunoglobulin deficiency and is seen in autoimmune diseases like rheumatoid arthritis and lupus.

Immunoglobulin D occurs in the smallest concentrations. Little is known about it, but it is closely linked to IgM and is found on B cells. Its function largely remains a mystery.

Immunoglobulin E is found in only mammals and it is widespread throughout the body. It can be found in blood, tissue fluid, and exocrine gland secretions. It can be found attached to leukocytes, basophils, eosinophils, macrophages, and platelets. It is the major defense against parasitic infections, and may also play a role in the defense against cancer cells. This immunoglobulin is responsible for most allergic reactions and for anaphylaxis (a systemic allergic reaction that can be fatal). New allergy therapies that specifically target IgE are being developed.

Job syndrome is also known as "hyper-IgE syndrome;" this rare disorder is characterized by an overabundant production of IgE. Its symptoms are recurrent staphylococcal infections of the skin, lung infections, and some changes in the bone (e.g., scoliosis, or lateral curvature of the spine). The disorder was named for the skin infections that were thought to resemble those suffered by the biblical character Job. This syndrome also has an interesting dental component. The primary dentition does not exfoliate, which can result in two very crowded sets of teeth being present at the same time. Treatment includes chronic antibiotic use for the skin infections and very carefully timed extraction of the primary dentition.

SUMMARY

The oral cavity is intricately connected to the rest of the body. It serves as the entrance to the digestive system and, as such, is never a sterile environment. The oral cavity has a number of host defense mechanisms that operate to prevent infection. Some, like saliva, are unique to the oral environment. Others, like cellular and humoral immunity, operate throughout the entire body. Oral disease, just like any other disease, occurs when the challenge posed by pathogens exceeds the body's capability for defense and repair. In the case of dental caries, the defense and self-repair mechanisms of the body operate continuously in the saliva, the plaque, and the enamel. In the case of periodontal disease, the immune system also plays a large part, providing protection as well as causing its own damage. In the case of

soft tissue infections (e.g., candidiasis), the epithelial barrier, normal oral flora, and saliva play the largest roles in preventing infection. These natural oral defense mechanisms are not dependent on the frailties of human knowledge, motivation, memory, or technique.

As is readily apparent to even the most inexperienced dentist or dental hygiene clinician, the maintenance of a healthy mouth is not an easy task. All the host protective mechanisms available in the oral cavity are often inadequate for the job. Personal self-care, such as toothbrushing and flossing, is a necessity. The level of self-care needed to achieve and maintain health differs for every individual, depending, in part, on how strong or compromised the person's host defenses are. Regular professional dental care is also usually required to maintain a healthy mouth. This care may include everything from appropriately timed professional prophylaxes to orthodontics to correction of malocclusion. The host defense mechanisms in the oral cavity, together with delivery of modern dental care, make dental disease a preventable and highly treatable disorder.

REFERENCES

1. Jontell, M., Okiji, T., Dahlgren, U., & Bergenholtz, G. (1998). Immune defense mechanisms of the dental pulp. *Crit Rev Oral Biol Med,* 9:179–200.
2. *Stedman's medical dictionary.* (2006). Baltimore, MD: Lippincott Williams & Wilkins.
3. Backer-Dirks, O. (1970). Posteruptive changes in dental enamel. *J Dent Res,* 4:131–48.
4. Tenouvo, J. (1997). Salivary parameters of relevance for assessing caries activity in individuals and populations. *Community Dent Oral Epidemiol,* 25:82–86.
5. Kolenbrander, P., & Palmer, R. (2004). Human oral bacterial biofilms. In Ghannoum, M., & O'Toole, G. A., Eds. *Microbial biofilms.* Washington, DC: ASM Press, 85–117.
6. Laforce, F., Hopkins, J., Trow, R., & Wang, W. (1976). Human oral defenses against gram-negative rods. *Am Rev Respir Dis,* 114:929–35.
7. Kolenbrander, P., Palmer, R., Rickard, A., Jakubovics, N., Chalmers, N., & Diaz, P. (2006). Bacterial interactions and successions during plaque development. *Periodontology 2000,* 42:47–79.
8. Kolenbrander, P., Andersen, R., Blehert, D., Egland, P., Foster, J., & Palmer, R. (2002). Communication among oral bacteria. *Microbiol Molec Biol Rev,* 66:486–505.
9. Edgar, W. M., Higham, S. M., & Manning, R. H. (1994). Saliva stimulation and caries prevention. *Adv Dent Res,* 8:239–45.

10. Dale, B., Kimball, J., Krisanaprakornkit, S., Roberts, F., Robinovitch, M., O'Neal, R., Valore, E., Ganz, T., Anderson, G., & Weinberg, A. (2001). Localized antimicrobial peptide expression in human gingiva. *J Periodontal Res,* 36:285–94.

11. Lehner, T. (1972). Cell-mediated immune responses in oral disease: A review. *J Oral Pathol,* 1:39–58.

12. Lilly, E., Shetty, K., Leigh, J., Cheeks, C., & Fidel, P. (2005). Oral epithelial cell antifungal activity: Approaches to evaluate a broad range of clinical conditions. *Med Mycol,* 43:517–23.

13. Merrell, W., Cripps, A., & Clancy, R. (1980). An overview of immunology with special reference to oral disease. *Aust Dent J,* 25:84–92.

14. Dale, B., & Fredericks, L. (2005). Antimicrobial peptides in the oral environment: Expression and function in health and disease. *Curr Issues Mol Biol,* 7:119–33.

15. Dunsche, A., Acil, Y., Dommisch, H., Siebert, R., Schroder, J., & Jepsen, S. (2002). The novel human beta-defensin-3 is widely expressed in oral tissues. *Eur J Oral Sci,* 110:121–24.

16. Dunsche, A., Acil, Y., Siebert, R., Harder, J., Schroder, J., & Jepsen, S. (2001). Expression profile of human defensins and antimicrobial proteins in oral tissues. *J Oral Pathol Med,* 30:154–58.

17. Bingle, C., & Gorr, S. (2004). Host defense in oral and airway epithelia: Chromosome 20 contributes a new protein family. *Int J Biochem Cell Biol,* 36:2144–52.

18. Bissell, J., Joly, S., Johnson, G., Organ, C., Dawson, D., McCray, P., & Guthmiller, J. (2004). Expression of beta-defensins in gingival health and in periodontal disease. *J Oral Pathol Med,* 33:278–85.

19. Tandler, B., Gresick, E. W., Nagoto, T., & Philliss, C. J. (2001). Secretion by striated ducts of mammalian major glands: A review of ultrastructural, functional and evolutionary perspective. *Anat Rec,* 264:125–45.

20. Bardow, A., Madson, J., & Nautofte, B. (2000). The bicarbonate concentration in human saliva does not exceed the plasma level under normal physiological conditions. *Clin Investig,* 42:45–53.

21. Pedersen, A. M., Bardow, A., Jensen, S. B., & Nauntofte, B. (2002). Saliva and gastrointestinal functions of taste, mastication, swallowing and digestion. *Oral Dis,* 8:117–29.

22. Boros, I., Kesler, P., & Zelles, T. (1999). Study of saliva secretion and the salivary fluoride concentration of the human minor labial glands by a new method. *Arch Oral Biol,* 44 (Suppl. 1):511–14.

23. Feruson, D. B. (1999). The flow rate and composition of human labial gland saliva. *Arch Oral Biol,* 44 (Suppl.):1511–14.

24. Lagerof, F., & Oliveby A. (1994). Caries-protective factors in saliva. *Adv Dent Res,* 8:229–38.

25. Dowd, F. J. (1995). Saliva and dental caries. *Dent Clin North Am,* 43:579–97.

26. Lageroff, F. (1998). Saliva: Natural protection against caries. *Rev Belge Med Dent,* 337–481.

27. Chausau, S., Becker, A., Chausau, G., & Sharpiro, J. (2002). Stimulated parotid saliva flow rates in patients with Down syndrome. *Spec Care Dentist,* 103:378–83.

28. Sommers, M. (2003). Response of the body to immunologic challenge. In Price, S., & Wilson, L., Eds. *Pathophysiology: Clinical concepts of disease process* (6th ed.). St. Louis: C.V. Mosby.

29. Bergdhal, M., & Bergdhal, J. (2000). Low unstimulated salivary flow and subjective oral dryness; association with medication, anxiety, depression and stress. *J Dent Res,* 27:18.

30. Salerno, S., Cannizzaro, F., Lo Castro, A., Loinbardo, F., Barress, B., Speciale, R., & Lagalla, R. (2002). Interventional treatment of sialoliths in main salivary glands. *Radiol Med* (Torino), 13:378–83.

31. Stern, Y., Feinmesser, R., Collins, M., Shotts, S. R., & Cotton, R. T. (2002). Bilateral submandibular gland excision and parotid duct ligation for treatment of sialorrhea in children: Long term results. *Arch Otolaryngol Head Neck Surg,* 128:801–803.

32. Slomianyk, B., Murty, V., Piotrowski, J., & Slomiany, A. (1996). Salivary mucins in oral mucosal defense. *Gen Pharmacl,* 27:761–71.

Chapter **8**

Toothbrushes and Toothbrushing Methods

Elaine Sanchez Dils

OBJECTIVES

After studying this chapter, the student will be able to:

1. Describe the history of the toothbrush.
2. Describe manual toothbrush designs including size, shape, and texture.
3. Demonstrate toothbrushing methods and techniques.
4. Describe the rationale for each toothbrushing method.
5. Describe design, methods, and uses of powered toothbrushes.
6. Describe toothbrush efficiency and safety evaluations.
7. Recommend appropriate toothbrushing time and frequency.
8. Determine appropriate time for toothbrush replacement.
9. Demonstrate brush care for dentures, orthodontic appliances, and tongues.

KEY TERMS

Toothbrush
Filaments
Toothbrushing
Power toothbrush
Battery-powered brushes
Efficacy
Sonic-powered toothbrushes
Manual toothbrush
Head
Bristles
Handle
Tufts
Toe
Heel
Shank
Concave
Convex
Multilevel profiles
Flat
Texture
Firmness
Stiffness
Hardness

(continued)

KEY TERMS (CONTINUED)

Angled filaments
End rounding
Bass method
Rolling technique
Stillman method
Charters technique
Orthodontic appliances
Fones method
Leonard technique
Horizontal technique
Smith method
Scrub toothbrushing technique
Modified brushing technique
Mechanical brush
Sonic toothbrush
Ionic toothbrushes

Oscillation movement
Reciprocation
Rotational movements
Category
Direct source
Pulsation-type head
Disclosing agents
Disclosants
Toothbrush abrasion
Full dentures
Denture brush
Clasp brush
Fungiform
Papillae
Fissured tongue
Halitosis
Tongue cleaners

INTRODUCTION

Soft, microbial dental plaque continually forms on the tooth surfaces, and is the primary agent in the development of dental caries and periodontal diseases. If plaque biofilm is completely removed with self-care procedures, dental caries and periodontal diseases can be prevented. Unfortunately, the majority of the population is unable, uninstructed, or unwilling to spend the time to adequately remove plaque from all tooth surfaces. Plaque deposits can be removed either mechanically or chemically. The focus of this chapter is the mechanical removal of plaque, using toothbrushes and toothbrushing techniques. Incidentally, the **toothbrush** is the most commonly used instrument in plaque removal.

THE HISTORY OF THE TOOTHBRUSH

The exact origin of mechanical devices for cleaning teeth is unknown. However, since ancient times, individuals have chewed twigs from plants with high aromatic properties. Chewing these twigs freshened breath and spread out fibers at the tips of the twig, which were then used for cleaning the teeth. In Arabic countries before the emergence of Islam, individuals used a piece of the root of the arak tree, because the root fibers stood out like bristles; this device

was called a *siwak.* These chew sticks not only helped to physically clean teeth but also helped to prevent plaque development, because the fibers contained antibacterial oils and tannins.[1] To this day the siwak and other chew twigs are used throughout the world to remove plaque.

During the Tang dynasty (618–907 A.D.) the Chinese invented a toothbrush with a handle and bristles. They used hog bristles similar to those in some contemporary brushes. In 1780 in England, William Addis manufactured "the first modern toothbrush."[2,3] This brush had a bone handle and holes for placement of natural hog bristles. In the early 1900s, celluloid began replacing the bone handle. This change came about during World War I, when bone and hog bristles were in short supply. As a result of this supply issue, nylon bristles were introduced. Initially, nylon bristles were copies of natural bristles in length and thickness; however, they were stiffer than the natural bristles. They did not have the hollow stem of natural bristles; therefore, they did not allow water absorption. Other advantages of nylon bristles, or **filaments,** were the ability to form the bristles in various diameters and shapes, and to round the bristle ends to be gentler on gingival tissues.

For various reasons, **toothbrushing** spread throughout the world. In the seventh century, Mohammed made rules about oral hygiene; specifically, he made it a religious obligation. In 1916, Dr. Alfred C. Fones, founder of dental hygiene, wrote a textbook, *Mouth Hygiene,* which specifically directed dental hygienists to teach specific toothbrushing methods to schoolchildren (Figure 8–1 ■). In 1919, the American Academy of Periodontology developed guidelines for both toothbrush design and brushing techniques.[4]

In 1939, the first **power toothbrush** was developed in Switzerland. This brush had a power cord and was introduced in the United States in the 1960s by Squibb under the name Broxodent.[5] This product was a great success. Soon afterwards **battery-powered brushes** were developed and marketed. Unfortunately, problems with these battery-powered products, including short "working times" and mechanical breakdowns, were encountered. The enthusiasm for the powered toothbrush declined, and was recommended mainly for those with dexterity problems and developmental disabilities.[5]

In the 1980s, powered toothbrushes were revitalized with the introduction of the InterPlak. Compared with manual toothbrushes, powered toothbrushes have shown an increased **efficacy** (ability to produce a desired effect); this result was consistent in published studies.[3,6–10] Since then, **sonic-powered toothbrushes** have been developed, and studies continue to report that they remove more plaque compared with manual toothbrushes. Most recently, battery-powered, disposable toothbrushes have been introduced.

MANUAL TOOTHBRUSH DESIGNS

Manual toothbrushes vary in size, shape, texture, and design (Table 8–1 ■, Figure 8–2 ■).[11] A **manual toothbrush** consists of a **head** with **bristles** and a **handle.** When the bristles are bunched together, they form **tufts.** The head is arbitrarily divided into the **toe,** which is at the extreme end of the head, and the **heel,** which is closest to the handle (Figure 8–3 ■). The **shank** is a constriction that usually occurs between the handle and the head. The handled is grasped by the hand during brushing.[4] Toothbrushes are manufactured in different sizes—large, medium, and small—to adapt better to the oral anatomy of different individuals.[11,12] Toothbrushes also differ in their defined hardness or texture being classified as hard, medium, soft, or extra soft. Extra soft and soft toothbrush bristles are preferred, because hard bristles damage teeth by causing abrasion of the tooth surface.

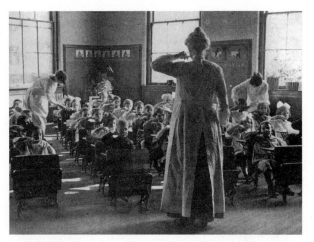

■ **FIGURE 8–1** Fones School of Dental Hygiene instructors and students during a toothbrush drill, circa early 1900s.
(Courtesy of Fones School of Dental Hygiene, University of Bridgeport, CT)

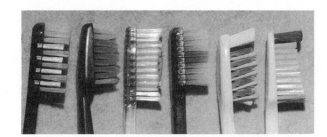

■ **FIGURE 8–2** Lateral profiles of selected toothbrushes.

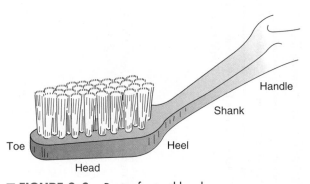

■ **FIGURE 8–3** Parts of a toothbrush.

■ Table 8–1 *Manual Toothbrushes*

Toothbrush Brand	Commercial Name	Handle Design	Sizes Available	Bristle Design	Bristle Type	Unique Features
Biotene (Laclede Inc)	**Biotene Supersoft Toothbrush**	Wide, ergonomic grip	One size	Soft, gentle	Soft, gentle	Gentle bristles massage & clean without irritating dry, sensitive gum tissue, large, extra wide comfort grip provides extra control while brushing
Colgate	**360® Whole Mouth Clean Brush**	Ergonomic, cushioned thumb grip	Compact head	Tapered with raised cleaning tip	Soft	Raised cleaning tip for access to posterior areas; soft, textured cheek & tongue cleaner for gentle, effective bacteria removal; soft rubber polishing cups for gentle stain removal
	360 Sensitive	Ergonomic, cushioned thumb grip	Compact head	Ultra soft bristles with raised cleaning tip	Ultra soft	Softer bristles, removes plaque efficiently
	Wave	Ergonomic, contoured handle with no-slip grip	Compact, ultra compact, & full heads	Multiheight, curved bristles	Soft, Wave Sensitive	Curved handle for better control & reinforcing good brushing technique, unique bristle trim to effectively remove plaque & bacteria
GlaxoSmithKline *Aquafresh*™	**Extreme Clean®**	Soft rubber grip	Standard head	Angled tip	Soft, medium	Combination of bristles & gentle rubber wipers; flexible head, neck, & tip
	XTensive™	Soft rubber grip	Standard head	Multi-angled & multilength, angled tip	Soft, medium	Multilength bristles, flexible head & neck
	Max-Active®	Thicker, ergonomic rubber grip	Standard head	Multi-angled & multilength, angled tip	Soft, medium	Comfort handle; multi-angled bristles; flexible tip, head, & neck
	Direct®	Soft rubber grip	Standard head	Flat	Soft, medium	Flexible neck

(continued)

Toothbrush Brand	Commercial Name	Handle Design	Sizes Available	Bristle Design	Bristle Type	Unique Features
	Dragon Tales™	Thick, soft rubber grip	Child sized	Flat	Extra soft	Character cap, stand-up feet, flexible neck, small angled head
Nimbus®	Microfine	Ergonomic, 2 component	Regular, compact, & child head	2 level multi-tuft	Single end tapered	Provides access to sulcular areas via tapered bristle
Oral-B	Pulsar Pro-health	Rubber grip handle with front & back thumb stops for firmer grip & extra control	35 and 40 soft	Carefully polished end-round bristles are gentle on teeth & gums, power tip bristles are extra long to help brush hard-to-reach areas	Soft gentle bristles, MicroPulse bristles (elastomeric bristles) with textured cleaning pads that grip the surface of the teeth & sweep away food & plaque	Pivoting action penetrates deep between teeth; pulsing action lifts up & sweeps away food & plaque; split head technology adjusts to the contours of teeth to enhance reach and provide great mouth feel
	CrossAction	Ergonomic nonslip handle to accommodate 5 basic toothbrush grips	35 and 40 soft	Carefully polished end-round bristles are gentle on teeth & gums, power tip bristles are extra long to help brush hard-to-reach areas	CrissCross bristles angled in opposing directions to lift out & sweep away plaque; blue indicator bristles fade to signal that toothbrush needs to be replaced	See bristle design & type
	Advantage Plus	Nonslip universal thumb & finger grip; squeezable, easy-to-grasp handle	35 and 40 soft	Carefully polished end-round bristles are gentle on teeth & gums, power tip bristles are extra long to help brush hard-to-reach areas	Blue indicator bristles fade to signal toothbrush needs to be replaced, gum massaging bristles are outer angled to gently massage & stimulate gums & clean along the gumline	See bristle design & type
PHB	Rx Ultra Suave	Slender & wide	Adult, child	.003 Dupont Tynex	Ultra soft	For tender tissue concerns, comes with protective cover

(continued)

■ **Table 8–1** *(continued)*

Toothbrush Brand	Commercial Name	Handle Design	Sizes Available	Bristle Design	Bristle Type	Unique Features
	Infant Brush	Oval	1 size	.005 Dupont Tynex	Soft	Introduces infants & toddlers to dental care
	Finger Brush	Fits over finger tip	1 size	Molded in brush		
POH	#1 Staggered	Straight, translucent or opaque	Adult	3 row, alternating, 18 tuft	Soft, Dupont Tynex, .007, end rounded & polished	For deep fissures, grooves, & depressions; shape memory handle
	#2 Ortho	Straight, translucent	Adult	2 row, in line, 12 tuft	Soft, Dupont Tynex, .007, end rounded & polished	Bristles get between brackets & wires, shape memory handle
	#3 Regular	Straight, translucent	Adult	3 row, in line, 20 tuft	Soft, Dupont Tynex, .007, end rounded & polished	Original Bass layout, shape memory handle
Pro-Dentec®	Pro-DenRx™		Pro-30, Pro-35, Pro-40	Blue Sweeptip™, gum sweeping bristles	Extra soft (.007) end rounded for gentleness	Cleans hard-to-reach back teeth; thin to help access hard-to-reach areas; removes plaque between teeth and along gumline; 3 sizes; free imprinting
	Kids Kare™		Pro-20		Extra soft (.007) end rounded for gentleness	Cleans hard-to-reach back teeth; thin to help access hard-to-reach areas; removes plaque between teeth and along gumline; 4 styles; free imprinting
Soladey	Soladey-2	Standard, narrow with titanium dioxide rod for ionic action	Standard, 1 size	Standard, small head	Standard medium	Ionic toothbrush, reduces bacteria, can remove stain, no toothpaste or batteries needed
	Soladey-Eco	Standard, wide grip handle with titanium dioxide rod in handle for ionic action	Standard, 1 size	Standard, small head	Standard medium	Ionic toothbrush, reduces bacteria, can remove stain, no toothpaste or batteries needed *(continued)*

Toothbrush Brand	Commercial Name	Handle Design	Sizes Available	Bristle Design	Bristle Type	Unique Features
Sunstar Butler SUN STAR™ BUTLER	**GUM® MicroTip**	Clear handle, rubber thumb grip	Compact, full	Dome Trim® bristles	Sensitive, soft	Interdental-cut bristle trim, microfeathered inside bristle rows
	GUM Technique™	Ergonomic, 4-sided handle	Compact, full	Dome Trim® bristles	Sensitive, soft	4 angled thumb pads encourage brushing at a 45° angle
	GUM Kids Technique™	Ergonomic, 4-sided handle with ribs on all sides, fun designs on handle	Compact	Dome Trim® bristles	Ultra soft	4 angled thumb pads encourage brushing at a 45° angle
	GUM SuperTip	Front & back textured rubber thumb grip	Compact, full, subcompact	Raised inner bristles, Super Tip bristles for hard to reach areas	Sensitive, soft	Multilevel trim design
	GUM Crayola Suction Cup/Games Brushes	Easy to hold in kid-sized hands	Age 3–5, 5–9	Flat trim	Ultra soft	Suction cup reduces counter clutter, kids play a different game with each handle
	GUM End Tuft Brush	Comfortable rubber thumb grip	Compact, full	Tapered trim, 3 rows, 7 tufts	Soft	Small head addresses furcations, implants, distal of the last molar & other hard-to-reach areas
TePe	**Super Nova**	Ergonomic handle with thumb pad, long neck, & small head	Compact, adult	2 levels for interdental access	Extra soft	Interdental access for effective cleaning
Tess	**Signature**	Straight handle/tapered head	Adult, junior, and preschool	Flat bristle trim	Soft or extra soft Dupont Tynex nylon	14 handle colors, custom imprinting available
	Concept Curve	Contoured angled handle	Adult compact head	Flat bristle trim	Soft or extra soft Dupont Tynex nylon	5 pearlescent handle colors, custom imprinting available
	Accent	Clear angled handle with rubber grip	Adult compact head	Multilevel bristles	Soft Dupont Tynex nylon	Custom imprinting available

(continued)

■ **Table 8–1** (continued)

Toothbrush Brand	Commercial Name	Handle Design	Sizes Available	Bristle Design	Bristle Type	Unique Features
Ultradent	**Opalescence Smile-brush**	Nonslip, grip handle	One size	Top bristles angled for hard-to-reach areas, outer bristles gently massage & clean gums	Soft filament bristles with rounded ends	Ergonomic handle, flexible neck, soft filament bristles with rounded ends, available in 4 colors
Vista Dental Products VISTA™	**Vista Breeze**™	Contra-angle design	Adult full & compact, youth, & junior	Block pattern bristle design on a diamond-shaped head	Soft DuPont bristles	Extremely affordable take-home item, available in 5 bright colors
	Vista Spring™ **Soft**	Ergonomic, flexible handle with soft rubber grip	Adult	Angled, v-shaped bristle pattern on an oval angle head provides access to hard-to-reach areas	Extra soft DuPont bristles	Flexible zone in the neck relieves pressure on sensitive teeth & gums during brushing; individually wrapped; convenient dispenser box; custom printing available
	Vista Spring™ **Firm**	Ergonomic flexible handle with soft rubber grip	Adult	Angled, v-shaped bristle pattern on an oval angle head provides access to hard-to-reach areas	Extra soft DuPont bristles	Flexible zone in the neck relieves pressure on sensitive teeth & gums during brushing

Source: Toothbrush focus. *Dimensions of Dental Hygiene.* 2007; 5(5): 24–25

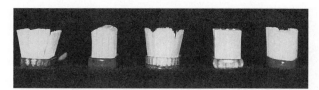

■ **FIGURE 8–4**   Cross-sectional profile of five tooth-brushes: Butler GUM; Colgate Total; Oral-B; Reach.

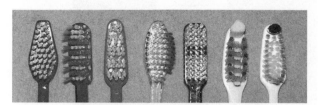

■ **FIGURE 8–5**   Overhead appearance of selected toothbrushes, from left to right: Reach Advanced Design; Aquafresh; Colgate Plus; Crest Complete; Jordan V.

More recently, toothbrush heads have been altered to vary bristle lengths and placement in attempts to better reach interproximal areas (Figures 8–4 ■ and 8–5 ■). Handles have also been ergonomically designed to accommodate multiple dexterity levels, that is, to work efficiently and safely without causing stress to hand muscles or damage to the gingiva.

TOOTHBRUSH PROFILES

When viewed from the side, toothbrushes have four basic lateral profiles: concave, convex, flat, and multileveled rippled or scalloped. The **concave** shape, with shorter bristles in the middle of the head, may be most useful for increased cleaning of facial tooth surfaces. **Convex** shapes, with longer bristles in the middle of the head, appear more useful for improved cleaning of lingual surfaces.[11] In laboratory and clinical studies, toothbrushes with **multilevel profiles** were consistently more effective than **flat** profiles in which the bristles are the same length, especially when interproximal efficacy was evaluated.[6,13–16]

NYLON VERSUS NATURAL BRISTLES

The nylon bristle is superior to the natural hog bristle in several aspects. Nylon bristles flex as many as 10 times more often than natural bristles before breaking; they do not split or abrade and are easier to clean. The shape and stiffness of nylon bristles can be standardized. Natural bristle diameters vary greatly in each filament. This can lead to wide variations in the resulting texture.

BRISTLE SHAPE AND TEXTURE

Nylon bristles can be manufactured in various dimensions that influence their shape and texture. *Texture* is defined as bristle resistance to pressure and is referred to as **firmness, stiffness,** or **hardness.** A thinner diameter filament allows the bristle to be softer and more resilient. The usual range of diameters for adult toothbrush bristles is 0.007 to 0.015 inches. The shorter a filament, the stiffer and less flexible it will be. In addition, an increase in the number of bristles within a tuft will make the tuft feel stiffer. **Angled filaments** remove direct pressure from the tooth and gingiva, and therefore appear to be more flexible.[4] Factors such as temperature, uptake of water, and frequency of use also influence the bristle texture.

End rounding is a term used to describe the heat treatment in which each filament end is sealed and rounded[4] (Figure 8–6 ■). Originally, individual toothbrush bristles were cut bluntly and often had sharp ends. In 1948, Bass reported that these bristle tips could damage the soft tissues and that rounded, tapered, or smooth bristle tips were less abrasive.[17] Although Bass's research was not performed according to strict research protocol, his findings have remained undisputed for more than 40 years. To this day, end-rounded tips are recommended for the safety of hard and soft oral tissues.

HANDLE DESIGNS

Most toothbrushes have some type of plastic handle. The plastic allows the handle to be durable while being resistant to water. Plastic is also inexpensive and easily manipulated for an attractive design.[4] Handle design and length may provide comfort and compliance during toothbrushing (Figure 8–7 ■). These factors have been documented to improve the quality of toothbrushing, particularly in children whose dexterity may not be highly developed.[6,7] The most important aspects of a toothbrush handle are that it is easy to hold and does not slip or rotate during use, and that it does not have sharp corners or projections. An offset, curve, or twist in the shank may help to adapt the brush into hard-to-reach areas of the mouth.[4]

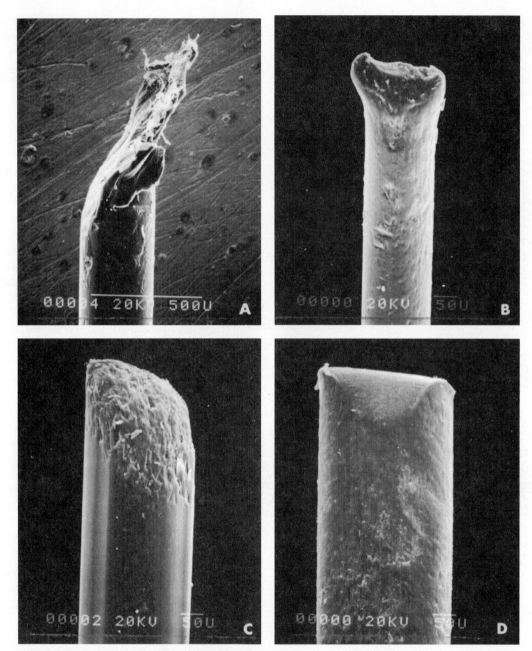

■ **FIGURE 8–6** End rounding of toothbrush bristle.
(Courtesy of K. K. Park, B. A. Matis, A. G. Christen, Indiana University Dental School.)

MANUAL TOOTHBRUSHING METHODS

The purposes of toothbrushing include (1) removal of plaque biofilm and disturbance of its re-formation; (2) removal of food, debris, and stain from the oral cavity; (3) stimulation of the gingival tissues; and (4) applica-

tion of a dentifrice containing specific ingredients to address caries, periodontal disease, or sensitivity.

During the last 50 years, many toothbrushing methods have been introduced, and most are identified by an individual's name, such as Bass, Stillman, or Fones, or by a term indicating a primary action to be followed, such

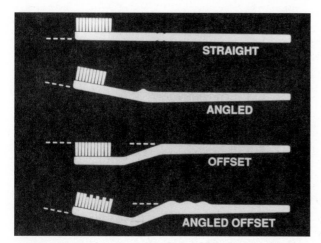

■ FIGURE 8–7 *Four basic shapes of toothbrush handles.*
(Courtesy of J Clin Dent)

as "roll" or "scrub" (Table 8–2 ■). The most natural brushing methods used by patients are a reciprocating horizontal scrub technique, a rotary motion such as the Fones technique, or a simple up-and-down motion over the maxillary and mandibular teeth, the Leonard technique.[18–20] All of these techniques are able to adequately clean the facial, lingual, and to some extent, the occlusal surfaces of the teeth; all however are relatively ineffective in cleaning interproximal areas. Only the Bass technique is effective in cleaning the sulcus.

Bass Method

The **Bass method** is acceptable for all patients. This method is effective at removing plaque at the gingival margin and directly below it. The toothbrush bristles are angled apically at a 45-degree angle to the long axis of the tooth. The filaments are then gently placed subgingivally into the sulcus. With very light pressure, the brush is jiggled with very short horizontal strokes, while keeping the bristles in the sulcus. After several vibrations, the bristles are removed from the sulcus, and the brush is repositioned on the next 2 or 3 teeth (Figure 8–8 ■).

Rolling Method

The **rolling technique** is most appropriate for children whose dexterity is not sufficient to master the Bass technique. The bristles are positioned apically along the long

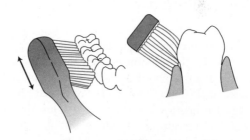

■ FIGURE 8–8 Bass technique.

■ Table 8–2 Manual Toothbrushing Methods

Technique	Bristle Position	Brushing Motion	Effect Claimed
Bass	At 45 degrees, with tips in sulcus	Vibratory, horizontal jiggle	Subgingival cleansing, gingival stimulation
Rolling	Apically against attached gingiva	Sweep in arc toward occlusal surface	Supragingival cleansing, gingival stimulation
Stillman	Against apical part of gingiva and cervical part of tooth	Vibratory, pulsing strokes	Gingival stimulation
Charters	At 45 degrees to tooth	Circular, vibratory strokes	Gingival stimulation, inter-proximal cleansing
Fones	At 90 degrees to tooth	Large circles over teeth and gingiva	Supragingival cleansing, gingival stimulation
Leonard	At 90 degrees to tooth	Vertical strokes	Supragingival cleansing, gingival stimulation
Horizontal	At 90 degrees to tooth	Horizontal strokes	Supragingival cleansing, gingival stimulation
Smith	At occlusal surface	Sweep toward gingiva	Supragingival cleansing
Modified (in combination with an above method)		Sweep toward occlusal surface	Supragingival cleansing

axis of the tooth. The edge of the brush head should be touching the facial or lingual aspect of the tooth. Then with light pressure the bristles are rolled against the tooth from the apical position toward the occlusal plane. This motion is repeated several times; then the brush is repositioned on the next teeth, with bristles overlaping a portion of the teeth previously cleaned. The heel or toe of the brush is used on the lingual aspect of the anterior teeth (Figure 8–9 ■).

Stillman Method

The **Stillman method** was originated to massage and stimulate the gingiva while cleansing the cervical areas. The bristles are positioned apically along the long axis of the tooth. The edge of the brush head should be touching the facial or lingual aspect of the tooth. A slight blanching effect should be seen; then the brush is slightly rotated at a 45-degree angle and vibrated over the crown (Figure 8–10 ■).

Charters Method

The **Charters technique** is effective for cleaning around devices used to correct improper contact of opposing teeth (**orthodontic appliances**), and plaque under abutment teeth of a fixed bridge. The bristles are placed at a 45-degree angle toward the occlusal or incisal surface of the tooth. The bristles should touch at the junction of the free gingival margin and tooth. A circular vibratory motion is then activated (Figure 8–11 ■).

Fones Method

The **Fones method** is not to be used by adults, but may be a easy technique for young children to learn. The teeth are clenched, and the brush is placed inside the cheeks. The brush is moved in a circular motion over both maxillary and manibular teeth. In the anterior region, the teeth are placed in an edge-to-edge position and the circular

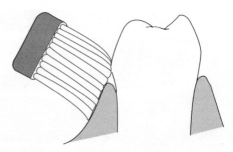

■ **FIGURE 8–10** Stillman toothbrushing technique seen diagrammatically.

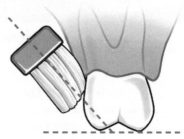

■ **FIGURE 8–11** Charters toothbrushing technique.

motion is continued. On the lingual aspect, an in-and-out stroke is used against all surfaces. This technique can be damaging if done too vigorously (Figure 8–12 ■).

Leonard Method

In the **Leonard technique,** the toothbrush is placed at a 90-degree angle to the long axis of the tooth. The teeth are held in an edge-to-edge position. Next, the toothbrush is moved in a vertical, vigorous motion up and down the teeth. The maxillary and mandibular teeth are brushed separately (Figure 8–13 ■).

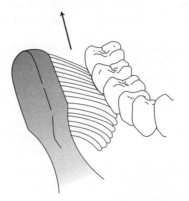

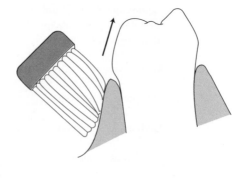

■ **FIGURE 8–9** Rolling stroke toothbrushing technique.

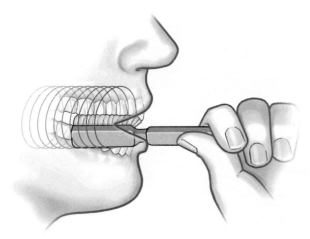

■ **FIGURE 8–12**   Fones toothbrushing technique: Circulatory motion extending from maxillary to mandibular teeth.

Horizontal Method

In the **horizontal technique,** the teeth are placed edge to edge, while the brush maintains a 90-degree angle to the long axis of the tooth. The brush is then moved in a horizontal stroke. This technique is known to cause excessive toothbrush abrasion (Figure 8–14 ■).

Smith Method

The **Smith method** is a physiologic technique, which follows the pattern that food follows when it is in the mouth during mastication. The bristles are positioned directly onto the occlusal surface. The brush is then moved back and forth with the bristles reaching from the occlusal surface to the gingiva. Smith also recommends a few gentle horizontal strokes to clean the sulcus areas near furcations (Figure 8–15 ■).

Scrub Toothbrushing Method

The **scrub toothbrushing technique** is a combination of horizontal, vertical, and circular strokes. It also incorporates vibration movements in certain areas. Care should be taken with this technique to avoid excessive pressure (Figure 8–16 ■).

Modified Brushing Methods

In attempts to enhance brushing of the entire facial and lingual tooth surfaces, the original techniques have been modified. The **modified brushing technique** integrates a rolling stroke after use of the vibratory motion. The position of the brush is maintained after the completion of the original method's stroke. The bristles are then rolled coronally over the gingiva and teeth. During this rolling motion, care should be taken that some of the filaments reach the interdental areas.

POWERED TOOTHBRUSHES
Design

Powered toothbrushes were first advertised in *Harper's Weekly* in February 1886,[8] but did not become a factor in the U.S. marketplace until Broxadent was introduced in the 1960s. Since then, the design of the power toothbrush

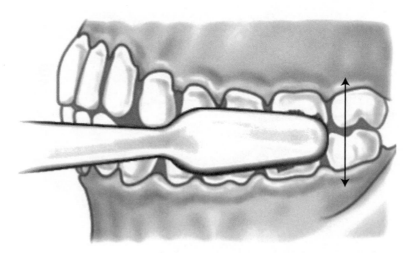

■ **FIGURE 8–13**   Leonard toothbrushing technique.

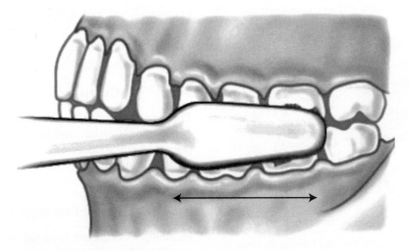

■ **FIGURE 8-14** Horizontal toothbrushing technique.

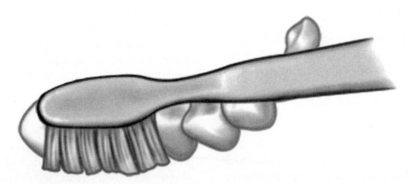

■ **FIGURE 8-15** Smith toothbrushing technique.

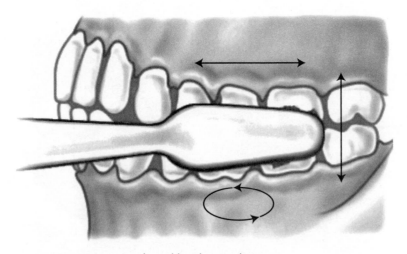

■ **FIGURE 8-16** Scrub toothbrushing technique.

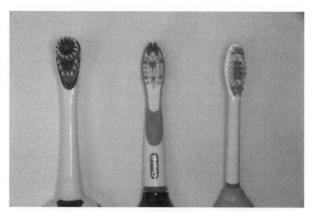

■ **FIGURE 8–17**   Selected power toothbrushes, from left to right: Crest SpinBrush; Oral-B Sonic Complete; Sonicare Elite.

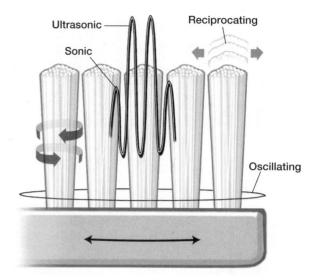

■ **FIGURE 8–18**   Movements of power-assisted toothbrushes.

has changed significantly (Figure 8–17 ■). Today the power toothbrushes can be categorized as mechanical, sonic, or ionic (Table 8–3 ■). A **mechanical brush** literally uses the motion of the bristles to remove the plaque and debris. The **sonic toothbrush** emits sound waves in addition to the movement of the filaments. The vibration is said to help loosen the plaque and food particles for removal. Lastly, the **ionic toothbrushes** are believed to temporarily reverse the negative ionic charge of a tooth to a positive charge. A portion of the toothbrush, that is also positively charged, is thought to attract the plaque and food particles away from the tooth, allowing bristles to brush the loosened particles away.

The main patterns of movements in the modern power toothbrushes are oscillation, reciprocation, and rotational. The **oscillation movement** takes the bristles in a consistent back-and-forth movement. Next, **reciprocation** moves the bristles up and down or back and forth. Lastly, **rotational movements** are circular. The **category** of sonic power toothbrushes refers to the speed at which the bristles move (Figure 8–18 ■).

Power toothbrushes also have varied power sources. A **direct source** brush has a cord that can be plugged into an electrical outlet. Although this type of brush will never slow because of a lack of power, the cord could interfere with the toothbrushing technique. Battery-powered brushes, as well as rechargeable battery-powered brushes, are also available. The battery-powered brushes' initial cost is low, but the cost of battery replacement could add up. In addition, the batteries may corrode if they come in contact with

water. With the rechargeable style, the charger may be bulky and must accompany the toothbrush. Some brushes come with a switch that the patient must hold down while the toothbrush is in operation. This brush could cause difficulty for patients who have dexterity problems.

The speed of a powered toothbrush varies widely. The typical reciprocating brushes movements can range from 3,800 to 7,600 per minute. In comparison, the action of a **pulsation-type head** can produce approximately 40,000 pulses per minute.

Powered Toothbrush Methods and Uses

Most powered toothbrush manufacturers do not recommend a specific brushing method. However, some guidelines for using a power brush are available. It is recommended that the brush be positioned slightly differently for each surface of the tooth. Each tooth and corresponding gingival areas should be brushed separately, always with light, steady pressure. The bristles of a powered toothbrush should never bend.[4]

Powered toothbrushes can be beneficial for a variety of reasons. These brushes have been found helpful for parents who brush their children's teeth. Powered toothbrushes are especially helpful for people who are physically handicapped, developmentally disabled, elderly, or arthritic, or who have dexterity issues. These brushes are also highly recommended for patients who require a larger handle, because powered models are easier to grasp.

■ Table 8-3 Toothbrushes

While every attempt is made to be as comprehensive as possible, there may be inadvertent omissions of toothbrushes.

Toothbrush Brand	Commercial Name	Handle Design	Sizes Available	Bristle Design	Bristle Type	Unique Features
Colgate	Power Toothbrushes	Ergonomic	Motion, motion whitening	Dual action head	Soft	Replaceable dual action brush head, curved neck, motion whitening has soft polishers to help remove stains
	Kids' Power Toothbrushes	Ergonomic	One size, different characters for children over 3	Oscillating head	Extra soft	Oscillating head cleans teeth & gently sweeps away plaque, slimmer handle for easy grip
HydraBrush	HydraBrush Express	Ergonomic profile, streamlined	2 brush head sizes	Completely surrounds teeth, correct approach angle automatic	Ultra soft, standard soft, nylon/Tynex	8 microheads provide automated Bass technique
	HydraBrush Dentifrice Delivery System	Ergonomic profile, streamlined	2 brush head sizes	Completely surrounds teeth, correct approach angle automatic with 4 water jets/nozzles	Ultra soft, standard soft, nylon/Tynex	8 microheads provide automated Bass technique for brushing & water flossing
Oral-B	Triumph®	Curved handle for ergonomics & comfort	Professional model available	FlossAction™ & ProWhite™ brush heads leverage oscillating-rotating technology	MicroPulse™ bristles for hard-to-reach approximal areas	Onboard computer that provides positive feedback & guidance for patients
	Sonic Complete®	Advanced ergonomic handle	Professional model 3-mode version	Angled, CrissCross, Indicator bristles	Soft, cushioned head with nylon bristles	3 customized cleaning & massaging modes
	Vitality™	Rubberized ergonomic grip provides comfort & control	Precision clean, Sensitive clean, & Sonic models available	Choose between oscillating-rotating, sensitive (extra soft), & sonic	Brush specific, all with indicator bristles	Benefits of Oral-B rechargeable power for under $20
Philips Oral Healthcare **Sonicare**™	Sonicare Elite e9000 Series	Ergonomic, tapered handle	2 brush heads: standard & compact	Nylon	Extra soft	2 brush head sizes, 2 cleaning modes, programmable Quadpacer, slim angled neck

(continued)

While every attempt is made to be as comprehensive as possible, there may be inadvertent omissions of toothbrushes.

Toothbrush Brand	Commercial Name	Handle Design	Sizes Available	Bristle Design	Bristle Type	Unique Features
Pro-Dentec®	Rota-dent One Step®	Like a hygiene hand-piece		Hollow brush head, short tip brush head, long tip brush head	.003 Tynex microfilaments, 5,000 microfilaments per head	Microfilament brush tips designed to reach underneath gums & in between teeth, lifetime warranty, 90,000 filament sweeps per second
Sunstar Butler SUN STAR™ BUTLER	GUM® Pulse® Rotapower®	Comfortable, ergonomic	23 tufts on circular head	Oscillating bristle action	Ultra soft	Battery operated, requires no recharging
	GUM Sesame Street®	Comfortable, designed for small hands, ergonomic	23 tufts on circular head	Oscillating bristle action	Ultra soft	Available characters: Big Bird, Cookie Monster, Elmo; battery operated no recharging; collectible character stand
Ultreo™ Ultreo™	Ultreo Ultrasound Toothbrush	Slim-waisted, ergonomically designed handle fits comfortably in the hand for easy maneuvering	One size	Precisely tuned sonic action bristles with power tip create bubbles & clean on contact	Combination of soft & extra soft bristles	Ultrasound waveguide channels ultrasound energy to activate & transform inactive bubbles into pulsating bubbles that can remove plaque bacteria
Waterpik Inc	Sensonic® Professional Toothbrush	Lightweight, ergonomic handle with soft, no-slip grip	One	2 color-coded, contoured, compact brush heads, 1 interdental brush head	Extra soft, nylon	Sonic technology, recharge indicator light on handle, 2 brush speeds for customized brushing & enhanced compliance, 2-minute timer with 30 second interval indicator, available only through dental offices

Source: Toothbrush focus. *Dimensions of Dental Hygiene.* 2007; 5(5): 24–25

TOOTHBRUSH EFFICIENCY AND SAFETY EVALUATIONS

Published testing methods are now available to evaluate both safety and efficacy of manual and powered toothbrushes. Differences between products can be determined and, in several areas, are predictive of clinical results. The areas that are evaluated are listed in Table 8–4 ■. These tests can be predictive of the products' ability to remove clinical plaque and can report clinical differences between toothbrush designs.[6,7,16] Even with these evaluation methods, clinical advantages of various toothbrush-head configurations for removing dental plaque and debris (i.e., cleaning efficacy) have been difficult to substantiate. This problem is attributed to the wide variations in how patients brush their teeth, such as the amount of toothbrushing time, type of motion, and amount of applied pressure. The shape and number of teeth also vary among patients. Published studies on the clinical superiority of newly designed manual or powered toothbrush have been inconsistent.

TOOTHBRUSHING TIME AND FREQUENCY

For many years, dental providers advised patients to brush their teeth after every meal. Research has indicated that, if plaque is completely removed every other day, no harmful effects will occur in the oral cavity.[21] On the other hand, very few individuals completely remove plaque; therefore, frequent brushing is still extremely important and recommended. These repeated brushings will maximize sulcular cleaning as a measure to control periodontal disease, as well as introduce more frequent use of fluoride dentifrices to control caries. In areas with periodontal pockets, even more frequent oral hygiene procedures are indicated.

Thorough toothbrushing requires a different amount of time for each individual, depending on such factors as the tendency to accumulate plaque and debris; the person's psychomotor skills; and the adequacy of clearance of foods, bacteria, and debris by the saliva. Often a compromise is made by suggesting 5 to 10 strokes in each area or by advocating the use of a timer. A person should be encouraged to brush for up to 2 minutes and to use a timing device. In addition, many power toothbrushes are designed with built-in timers that signal the patient when to move to another area of the mouth; the timers shut off when the designated number of minutes has passed.

A routine brushing pattern should also be established to avoid exclusion of any area. One systematic pattern is to begin with the distal surface of the most posterior tooth, and to continue brushing the surfaces around the maxillary (upper) arch until the last molar on the other side of the arch has been reached. The mandibular (lower) arch is then brushed in a similar manner. It is important to explain to the patient that the bristles should always overlap previously cleaned teeth.

Patients tend to apportion more time and effort on the facial areas of the anterior teeth.[22] Often, right-handed people do not brush the right side of the arch as well as the left side; left-handed people similarly neglect the left side of the arch.

CLINICAL ASSESSMENTS OF TOOTHBRUSHING

Whatever techniques are recommended, the main purpose of toothbrushing is to remove dental plaque from the teeth and the gingival crevice, without damaging the teeth and surrounding structures. Disclosing agents provide a means of evaluating the thoroughness of cleaning the teeth.[23,24]

Disclosing agents, or **disclosants,** may be in either a liquid or a tablet form. They allow the patient to see plaque in the mouth before or after brushing. These agents can give patients a literal road map to remove the plaque. The chewable tablet or the liquid disclosant should be swished around in the mouth for 15 to 30

■ **Table 8–4**   Toothbrush Laboratory Testing Procedures

- Abrasion
- Depth of deposit removal
- Distal surface cleaning
- Gingival margin cleaning
- Efficacy of interproximal access
- Polishing
- Removal of smooth surface (area) deposit
- Stain removal
- Efficacy of subgingival access

seconds and then expectorated. Home use of disclosants by the patient can be encouraged to permit self-evaluation of the effectiveness of plaque-control programs.

Toothbrush abrasion, or the wearing away of oral tissues as a result of toothbrushing, can occur from the use of highly abrasive dentifrices, too-firm brush bristles, incorrect brushing methods, or excessive pressure during brushing. Common abrasion locations are on the facial surfaces of the teeth and on the cervical areas of exposed root surfaces. Measures to reduce progression of the abrasion include use of soft-bristled brushes, changes in brush angulation, use of less-abrasive dentifrices, and application of less pressure during brushing.

TOOTHBRUSH REPLACEMENT

Toothbrush wear (e.g., splayed, bent, or broken bristles) is influenced more by the brushing method than by the length of time or number of toothbrushings per day.[25] The average life of a manual toothbrush is 2 to 3 months. This estimate can vary greatly depending on brushing habits. It is also sound advice for patients to have several toothbrushes, and to rotate the use of these brushes to ensure use of a dry brush. Toothbrushes can become contaminated. Drying the toothbrush gives a less favorable environment for the contaminants to survive. In addition to regular replacement, replacement after contagious illness is imperative.

DENTURES AND REMOVABLE ORTHODONTIC APPLIANCES

Patients with full dentures can meet their oral hygiene needs by using a soft nylon brush for the oral tissues and a denture brush to clean all areas of the denture. The denture brush, used with a non-abrasive cleaner, should reach into the recessed alveolar ridge area of the denture to ensure proper cleaning (Figure 8–19 ■). Patients should brush oral tissues at least once a day using gentle vibration and long, straight strokes from the posterior to anterior mouth regions.[24]

Patients with removable partial dentures and removable orthodontic appliances need at least two toothbrushes. One brush is needed for the natural teeth and another for the appliance. Brushing clasps, wires, and other metal parts can wear out a regular toothbrush. A clasp brush is 2 to 3 inches long, narrow, and tapered, and is usually found on the side of a denture brush. Special attention is needed to carefully clean all plaque biofilm from the clasps.

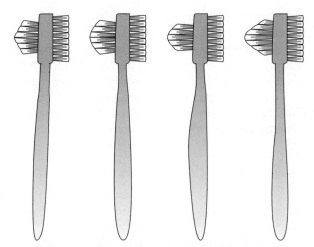

■ **FIGURE 8–19**   Denture brushes with clasp brush.

TONGUE BRUSHING

The tongue is anatomically perfect for harboring bacteria. The fungiform (mushroom-shaped) papillae create elevations and depressions in the tongue, which can house debris and microorganisms. A patient with a fissured tongue (deep grooves on the tongue surface) is more prone to accumulate bacterial plaque and debris. The tongue can transmit organisms during toothbrushing, and infection or reinfection of a periodontal pocket. Interestingly, halitosis (oral malodor, or bad breath) most often originates on the tongue. For these reasons, the tongue, especially those with fissuring or prominent papilla, should be regularly cleaned.

The brushing of the tongue helps reduce the debris, plaque, and number of oral microorganisms. Appropriate technique involves placing the head of the toothbrush near the middle of the tongue, with the bristles pointed toward the throat. Then the tongue is extruded, and the brush is swept forward. This motion is repeated six to eight times across the entire tongue. Using a dentifrice on the brush helps the cleansing action.[26]

Commercial tongue cleaners, made of plastic or a flexible metal, are also available. They are curved so they can be placed over the tongue without touching the teeth. These instruments are swept over the dorsum of the tongue to remove bacterial plaque and debris.

THE AMERICAN DENTAL ASSOCIATION ACCEPTANCE PROGRAM

The American Dental Association (ADA) acceptance program is a voluntary program for evaluation of toothbrushes. Companies may submit their toothbrushes and, if the brushes meet the ADA criteria, the company may use the ADA Seal of Acceptance, as a marketing tool, on their toothbrush package and in advertisements. The ADA recently was named in a lawsuit filed against toothbrush manufacturers for failing to adequately warn people about the possible dangers of brushing with a hard-bristled toothbrush.[27] As always, dental providers should recommend products that they have thoroughly researched.

SUMMARY

A toothbrush is the primary instrument used for oral hygiene care. There are many different types of toothbrushes. There are manual and power toothbrushes, with each having various designs of the handle, head, and bristles. These variations all have unique benefits.

The several different toothbrushing methods remove plaque most efficiently, depending on the patient and the anatomy of the oral cavity. Any method that is taught should be effective and used routinely, and should not damage hard or soft tissues, or cause excessive tooth wear. In initiating effective toothbrushing, it is necessary to (1) select the appropriate toothbrush(es) for the patient; (2) create individual goals for toothbrushing and explain the need for good oral hygiene; (3) teach a technique or combination of brushing methods necessary to meet established goals; and (4) assess and refine toothbrushing techniques as a part of the total oral hygiene program.

REFERENCES

1. Hattab, F. N. (1997). Meswak: The natural toothbrush. *J Clin Dent,* 8:125–29.
2. Golding, P. S. (1982). The development of the toothbrush. A short history of tooth cleansing. *Dent Health* (London), 21:25–27.
3. Smith, C. (2000). Toothbrush technology—Even the Pharaohs brushed their teeth. *J Dent Technol,* 17:26, 27.
4. Wilkins, E. (2005). *Clinical practice of the dental hygienist* (9th ed.). Baltimore, MD: Lippincott Williams & Wilkins.
5. Penick, C. (2004). Power toothbrushes: A critical review. *Int J Dent Hygiene* 2:40–44.
6. Saxer, U. P., & Yankell, S. L. (1997). Impact of improved toothbrushes on dental diseases. I. *Quintessence Int,* 28:513–25.
7. Saxer, U. P., & Yankell, S. L. (1997). Impact of improved toothbrushes on dental diseases. II. *Quintessence Int,* 28:573–93.
8. Ring, M. E. (1985). *Dentistry: An illustrated history.* St. Louis: C.V. Mosbyo, 1–319.
9. Boyd, R. L. (1997). Clinical and laboratory evaluation of powered electric toothbrushes: Review of the literature. *J Clin Dent,* 8:67–71.
10. Warren, P. R., Smith, R. T., Cugini, M., & Chater, B. V. (2000). A practice-based study of a power toothbrush: Assessment of effectiveness and acceptance. *JADA,* 131:389–94.
11. Yankell, S. L., & Emling, R. C. (1978). Understanding dental products: What you should know and what your patient should know. *Univ Pa Cont Dent Educ,* 1:1–43.
12. Mintel, T. E., & Crawford, J. (1992). The search for a superior toothbrush design technology. *J Clin Dent,* 3:C1–C4.
13. Volpe, A. R., Emling, R. C., & Yankell, S. L. (1992). The toothbrush—A new dimension in design, engineering and clinical evaluation. *J Clin Dent,* 3:S29–S32.
14. Volpenhein, D. W., Handel, S. E., Hughes, T. J., & Wild, J. (1996). A comparative evaluation of the in vitro penetration performance of the improved Crest Complete toothbrush versus the current Crest Complete toothbrush, the Colgate Precision toothbrush and the Oral-B P40 toothbrush. *J Clin Dent,* 7:21–25.
15. Saxer, U. P., & Yankell, S. L. (1997). A review of laboratory methods to determine toothbrush safety and efficacy. *J Clin Dent,* 8:114–19.
16. Beals, D., Ngo, T., Feng, Y., Cook, D., Grau, D. J., & Weber, D. A. (2000). Development and laboratory evaluation of a new toothbrush with a novel brush head design. *Am J Dent,* 13:5A–14A.
17. Bass, C. C. (1948). The optimum characteristics of toothbrushes for personal oral hygiene. *Dent Items Int,* 70:697–718.
18. Tsamtsouris, A., White, C. E., & Clark, E. R. (1979). The effect of instruction and supervised tooth brushing on the reduction of dental plaque in kindergarten children. *J Dent Child,* 465:204–209.
19. Home care of the mouth. (1934). In Fones, A. C., Ed. *Mouth hygiene* (4th ed.). Philadelphia: Lea & Febiger, 294–315.
20. Leonard, H. J. (1939). Conservative treatment of periodontoclasia. *JADA,* 26:1308–18.
21. Lang, K. P., Cumming, B. R., & Löe, H. (1973). Tooth brushing frequency as it relates to plaque development and gingival health. *J Periodontol,* 44:396–405.
22. Tsamtsouris, A. (1978). Effectiveness of tooth brushing. *J Pedod,* 2:296–303.
23. Carranza, F. A., & Newman, M. G., Eds. (1996). *Clinical periodontology* (8th ed.) Philadelphia: W.B. Saunders, 1–1033.
24. Wilkins, E. M. (1994). *Clinical practice of the dental hygienist* (7th ed.). Philadelphia: Lea & Febiger, 1–893.
25. Craig, T. T., & Montague, J. L. (1976). Family oral health survey. *J Am Dent Assoc,* 92:326–32.
26. Christen, A. G., & Swanson, Jr., B. Z. (1978). Oral hygiene: A history of tongue scraping and brushing. *J Am Dent Assoc,* 96:215–19.
27. Toothbrush abrasion spurs suit. (1998). *The Albuquerque Journal.*

Chapter 9

Dentifrices, Mouthrinses, and Chewing Gums

Meg Horst Zayan

OBJECTIVES

After studying this chapter, the student should be able to:

1. Differentiate between a cosmetic and a therapeutic dentifrice, mouthrinse, and chewing gum.
2. Explain the three phases of research necessary when applying to investigate a new drug.
3. Discuss how approval or non-approval of a new product by the Food and Drug Administration (FDA) differs from acceptance or rejection by the American Dental Association (ADA).
4. List and define the purpose of each dentifrice ingredient including percentage quantities.
5. Explain the various reasons that the same abrasive material in toothpaste can cause differing levels of abrasion on tooth structure.
6. Define the three types and amounts of fluoride compounds commonly used in dentifrices.
7. Identify the agents used in dentifrices to produce anticaries, anti-calculus, whitening, and antihypersensitivity effects.
8. Explain the active ingredients in anti-plaque and anti-gingivitis mouthrinses sold over the counter and as a prescription item.
9. Describe the advantages and disadvantages of mouthrinses containing alcohol.
10. Describe the benefits of chewing gum and the ingredients used to help reduce oral disease.

KEY TERMS

Therapeutic
Dentifrices
Mouthrinses
Chewing gums
Hypersensitivity
Chlorhexidine
Dose
Efficacy
Chemotherapeutic agents
Ingestion
Dentifrice
Therapeutic dentifrice
Cosmetic toothpaste
Pump dispenser
Dual-chamber pump dispenser
Extrinsic stains
Intrinsic stains
Amelogenesis
Fluorosis
Dentifrice abrasiveness
Calcium carbonate
Sodium monofluorophosphate
Phosphate abrasives
Silicas

(continued)

KEY TERMS (CONTINUED)

Polishing agents

Toothbrush abrasion

Humectants

Preservatives

Thickening

Binding agents

Sodium lauryl sulfate

Noncariogenic

Chemical plaque control

Manual plaque-control

Stannous fluoride

Triclosan

Soluble pyrophosphates

Tooth root

Obturation

Fluoride varnish

Potassium nitrate

Desensitization agent

Dentin–pulpal interface

Occluding

Sclerosing

Carbamide peroxide

Hydrogen peroxide

Therapeutic mouthrinses

Zinc sulfate

Alcohol

Organoleptic assessment

Mucoadhesion

Chlorhexidine

Substantivity

Essential oil

Irrigator

Aerosol-generating procedures

Cetylpyridinium chloride

Fluoride mouthrinses

INTRODUCTION

Dentifrices and mouthrinses are major products for routinely administering effective cosmetic and **therapeutic** agents in the mouth. **Dentifrices** are substances used to clean the teeth. **Mouthrinses** are used to flush food debris from the oral cavity, freshen breath, or if fluoridated, to deposit fluoride on the teeth. These products are the most widely used by consumers, generating the largest sales of all dental products. **Chewing gums** are a newer category of products with cosmetic claims and the ability to deliver therapeutic compounds.

Dentifrices and mouthrinses differ considerably. Dentifrices are complex and difficult to formulate. Tremendous innovations have occurred in the past 25 years in the appearance and packaging of dentifrices. The contemporary consumer is faced with many alternatives in appearance (pastes, gels, stripes) and packaging (conventional tubes, stand-up tubes, pumps), as well as products marketed specifically for children and adults. In addition, numerous claims are made for dentifrices including the prevention or reduction of calculus formation, dental

caries, plaque, gingivitis, **hypersensitivity,** and the ability to whiten teeth. Because the public routinely uses dentifrices one to three times per day, they may be the most beneficial dental products. Some of this benefit may be lost when patients rinse immediately after brushing, because rinsing decreases the concentration or reservoir of the active agent in the oral cavity.

Mouthrinses are available in liquid form, the traditional method for stabilizing and delivering many pharmaceutically active agents. Mouthrinses are considered by consumers to have primarily cosmetic benefits (i.e., breath freshening); therefore, mouthrinses are not used as frequently or routinely as dentifrices in the daily oral-hygiene regimen. The Food and Drug Administration (FDA) has approved products that contain **chlorhexidine,** a therapeutic agent in mouthrinses as prescription-only products.

Chewing gums have the potential to be used by the consumer for periods of 5 to 20 minutes several times a day, until the flavor of the product dissipates. This product form enables delivery of a cosmetic or therapeutic agent for a longer time than with dentifrices or mouthrinses. In addition to prolonged delivery of an agent, chewing gums stimulate salivary flow, which can provide a buffer effect and also ensure removal of debris from occlusal and inter-proximal sites. To ensure safety and avoid harmful gas-trointestinal effects, active agents delivered by chewing gums must be safe for swallowing at the **dose** delivered in one use, or contained in the entire product sold in one package.

SAFETY AND EFFICACY

Caution is needed before introducing a new therapeutic product to the market. Some of the concerns surrounding new products are: Will the active agent disrupt the "nor-mal" bacterial balance of the mouth? Should the search for an ideal agent focus on depressing or eliminating spe-cific disease-related organisms or a broad spectrum of organisms? Should a product be used to preserve a dis-ease-free state, while risking possible development of drug resistance? Regardless of the apparent effectiveness of any new product in the laboratory or in controlled clin-ical studies, the public safety of the product is paramount, because it will have widespread availability and will be used unsupervised by consumers.

Various processes exist by which oral-care agents are evaluated and regulated in the United States to ensure standards for safety and **efficacy** standards.[1] These stan-dards apply not only to prescription medications but also to over-the-counter (OTC) drugs. There are two govern-ment levels of regulation of oral **chemotherapeutic agents** (chemical substances or drugs). The government levels include the Food and Drug Administration (FDA) and the Federal Trade Commission (FTC). The FTC reg-ulates advertising of OTC and prescription drugs to pro-tect consumers against false claims as to the uses, effectiveness, and safety of these drugs.

The United States Pharmacopoeia Convention (USP) is an independent public health organization. It establishes public standards for prescription and OTC drugs available in the United States. Federal law requires that these drugs meet the USP public standards. Other groups that review these agents include consumer advo-cacy organizations and review panels for advertising stan-dards. One voluntary reviewer is the Council on Scientific Affairs (CSA) of the American Dental Association (ADA). Interestingly, each of the major television net-works also has an in-house review committee.

The FDA conducts an ongoing review of all OTC products. One aim of regulation is to protect the patient–consumer from useless or harmful products. All approval or disapproval decisions by the FDA have the force of law. The stages of FDA approval include (1) the manufacturer's preclinical research and development (animal testing, laboratory testing, and toxicity evalua-tion); (2) FDA review of manufacturing information on the drug product, which is submitted as part of an inves-tigational new drug (IND) application; and (3) clinical research conducted by the manufacturer after approval of the IND application. The investigative process usually includes three phases: In phase 1, the study is limited in scope and uses 20 to 80 subjects to determine the safe dose for humans.[2] For dental products, this phase usu-ally involves taking agents into the body through the mouth (**ingestion**) or exaggerated (three or four times per day) topical applications to the surface of oral mucosa or teeth, or both. Phase 2 usually involves sev-eral hundred subjects to demonstrate the initial clini-cal efficacy of the drug, and to define a dose range that is safe and efficacious. Phase 3 generally includes expanded controlled and uncontrolled trials with "final" formulas to demonstrate long-term safety and efficacy. These trials range from 3 to 6 months for plaque and gingivitis studies, to 2 or 3 years for caries studies. Gen-erally, phase 3 studies involve several hundred to sev-eral thousand people. After the investigation process is completed, the company submits a new drug applica-tion (NDA), which contains data on the results from the trials. After the FDA reviews and approves the NDA, marketing may begin, but post-marketing surveillance of the product is mandatory.

Over the years, the FDA has requested that manu-facturers of OTC products submit a listing of the active (i.e., therapeutic) and inactive ingredients in their prod-ucts as a basis for helping to codify regulations govern-ing OTC sales. The requirement that all inactive ingredients be listed alphabetically on the product label is among the many FDA recommendations to provide better control of OTC oral therapeutic products.[3] Active ingredients, as well as inactive agents, should be in no higher concentrations than necessary for the intended purpose. In addition, the indicated objective of the active agent(s) must be on the label. Furthermore, FDA would consider the inclusion of the name of an active agent(s) without stating the proposed benefits as misleading. Proof must exist to substantiate any claim for a specific thera-peutic benefit. For example, if a dentifrice has not been subjected to laboratory or clinical trials, but its label lists "decay-fighting fluorides" without listing the proposed benefits of the fluorides, the product manufacturer cannot claim that the dentifrice is anticariogenic. The manufacturer can claim only that the product contains fluoride. It is possible that the fluoride in the untested dentifrice might not be compatible with other dentifrice ingredients, or that the fluoride may not be released in an active ionic form and therefore be totally ineffective.

Recommendations also apply to packaging and labeling guidelines, which help to regulate advertising. For example, the recommendations suggest that all containers for OTC therapeutic dentifrices, rinses, and gels containing fluoride have the following information on the label:

- Identification of the product, such as "anticaries dentifrice."
- The product's use, such as "aids in the prevention of dental caries."
- A warning, such as, "Do not swallow. Developing teeth of children under 6 years of age may become permanently discolored if excessive amounts of fluoride are repeatedly swallowed."
- Directions for product use, such as "Adults and children 6 years of age or older should brush teeth thoroughly at least twice daily, or as directed by a dentist or physician."

In April 1997, the FDA issued a labeling requirement for fluoride toothpaste: "Keep out of reach of children under 6 years of age. If you accidentally swallow more than used for brushing, seek professional help or contact a poison control center immediately." This recommendation may be an exaggerated response, because most experts believe that neither an adult nor a child could absorb enough fluoride to cause a serious problem.

After years of ignoring claims of anti-gingivitis efficacy for various OTC dentifrices and rinses, in 1988 the FDA advised manufacturers of such products that they must either cease making such claims or substantiate (verify) them. In 1990 the FDA published its call for data stating:

> The Food and Drug Administration is announcing a call for data for ingredients containing products bearing antiplaque and antiplaque related claims, such as "for the reduction or prevention of plaque, tartar, calculus, film, sticky deposits, bacterial buildup and gingivitis." The agency will review the submitted data to determine whether these products

are generally regarded as safe and effective and not misbranded for the label uses. This notice also describes the Attorney General's enforcement of policy governing the marketing of over-the-counter (OTC) drug products bearing antiplaque and antiplaque related claims during the pendency of this review. This request is part of the ongoing review of OTC drug products conducted by the FDA.[4]

Then in 2003, the FDA published its call for rulemaking, stating "The Food and Drug Administration issued an advanced notice of proposed rulemaking that would establish conditions under which OTC drug products for the reduction or prevention of dental plaque and gingivits are generally recognized as safe and effective and not misbranded. This notice is based on the recommendations of the Dental Plaque Subcommittee of the Non Prescription Drugs Advisory Committee (NDAC) and is part of the FDA's ongoing review of OTC drug products."[5]

In addition to the FDA's regulation of OTC products, the American Dental Association's Council on Scientific Affairs (CSA) reviews dental products on a *voluntary* basis. A product does not need to undergo review by ADA; in fact, the major reason products go under the review process is to carry the ADA Seal of Acceptance, which helps advertise the product to the public. The CSA is directed to study, evaluate, and disseminate information with regard to dental therapeutic agents, their adjuncts, and dental cosmetic agents that are offered to the public or to the profession.[1] The most important activity of the CSA in meeting this charge is its acceptance program. Unlike the FDA review process, the primary review responsibilities for the acceptance program are conducted by consulting dental professionals who are appointed by the CSA but are not employees of the ADA. If the product is considered safe and effective after extensive clinical and laboratory research, the Seal of Acceptance is granted and can be used by the manufacturer in marketing the product. Studies have shown that seven of ten consumers recognize this seal.[6] It is important to realize that the ADA is a professional, private organization that does not have regulations comparable to those of the FDA.

DENTIFRICES

According to the dictionary, the term dentifrice is derived from *dens* (tooth) and *fricare* (to rub). A simple, contemporary definition of a **dentifrice** is a mixture used on the tooth in conjunction with a toothbrush.

Dentifrices are marketed as toothpastes and gels, and to a lesser extent, as toothpowders. Some dentifrices are sold as liquid gels, liquid pastes, stripes, and with breath strips. All are sold as either therapeutic or cosmetic products. A **therapeutic dentifrice** must reduce some disease-related process in the mouth. Usually the actual or alleged therapeutic effect is to reduce caries incidence, gingivitis, plaque, or tooth sensitivity. The purpose of a **cosmetic toothpaste** is to clean and polish the teeth. The sales appeal of either product, however, is strongly linked to its flavor and foaming action.

In 1970, the dentifrice market amounted to an estimated $355 million. By 1988 it had increased to $1 billion, in 1996 to $1.5 billion, in 2000 to $1.9 billion, and in 2005 to $2.1 billion (Figure 9–1 ■).[7] Simply, the dentifrice market is rapidly increasing as consumers place an increased value on oral health, esthetics, and prevention of tooth decay.

Packaging

The development of the toothbrush in 1857 provided the stimulus to market commercial dentifrices. Toothpowders were popular because boxes and cans from which they could be dispensed already existed. The formulas consisted of little more than water, soap, and flavor.

Toothpastes began to appear on the market following the development of lead tubes for packaging. The change to plastic packaging during World War II simultaneously caused the following effects:

- Eliminated the possibility of the user ingesting lead.

- Reduced the possibility of incompatibility of the tube and paste components.
- Aided the expelling of the paste by squeezing.
- Permitted an easier and more economic production of tubes.
- Provided a good surface for the printing of decorative designs and information.

The initial plastic tubes were permeable, which allowed the liquids in the dentifrices to seep through pores in the plastic and through the packaging. As a result the flavors were lost. This problem has been resolved with the use of new plastic materials and the use of laminated or layered packaging materials.

In 1984, Colgate introduced the plastic **pump dispenser** to the market. Separate color compartments used to dispense "striped" products were introduced in Stripe dentifrice by Lever Brothers, and are now used in Aquafresh (GlaxoSmithKline Consumer Healthcare, L.P.) and Colgate Total Stripe (Colgate-Palmolive Co.). Chesebrough-Pond's introduced a **dual-chamber pump dispenser** to keep the peroxide and baking soda components of their dentifrice, Mentadent, separate until immediately before use; then they are delivered together on the toothbrush.

Of the variety of packaging, plastic tubes dominate the market with consumers having the option of a gel or a paste dentifrice. GlaxoSmithKline introduced Sensodyne Fresh Impact, which provides a combination of paste and gel. And Church & Dwight Co., Inc., recently marketed Arm & Hammer Advance White dentifrice in a new liquid gel.

Dentifrice Ingredients

Dentifrices were originally developed to provide a cosmetic effect and deliver a pleasant taste. They are effective in removing **extrinsic stains,** those that occur on the surface of the tooth. These stains, which are often the end products of bacterial metabolism, range in color from green to yellow to black. Stains may also result from smoking, foods, coffee, tea, cola-containing drinks, and red wines. OTC dentifrices do not remove **intrinsic stains,** which are a result of altered formation or maturation of dental enamel (**amelogenesis**). Examples are the white-to-brown color changes seen in **fluorosis** (mottling on teeth caused by ingestion of excessive amounts of fluoride) or the grayish-blue appearance of enamel after ingestion of tetracycline. Dentifrices and other OTC

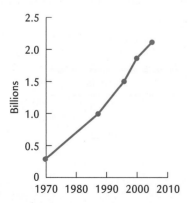

■ **FIGURE 9–1**   Rapid sevenfold increase in toothpaste sales over the past 30 years, including 2005.

products are also ineffective in altering the yellowing color of teeth seen with physiologic aging and in altering the hues of tooth color produced by differing shades of dentin. Therefore, they can only claim to "make your teeth their whitest or brightest;" they cannot state, "Makes your teeth whiter or tooth color lighter."

Toothpastes contain several or all of the ingredients listed in Table 9–1 ■. Gel dentifrices contain the same components as toothpastes, except that gels have a higher proportion of the thickening agents. Both tooth gels and toothpastes are equally effective in plaque removal and in delivering active ingredients.

Abrasives

The degree of **dentifrice abrasiveness** depends on the inherent hardness of the abrasive, size of the abrasive particle, and the shape of the particle. Several other variables can affect the abrasive potential of the dentifrice: the brushing technique, the pressure on the brush, the hardness of the bristles, the direction of the strokes, and the number of strokes. Results for the abrasive tested alone can differ from those for the same abrasive tested as part of a dentifrice formula. The salivary characteristics of individuals may also affect dentifrice abrasiveness.

The most common types of abrasives used are carbonates, phosphates, and silicas. Carbonates include calcium carbonate (chalk) and sodium carbonate (baking soda). **Calcium carbonate** is an economical and highly effective abrasive, although the calcium ion limits the amount of soluble fluoride in toothpaste up to 7 ppm. When the combination of fluoride and calcium carbonate is desired, it is recommended that **sodium monofluorophosphate** be used. Sodium fluoride, which provides soluble fluoride is compatible with sodium bicarbonate.

Phosphate abrasives include calcium pyrophosphate and dicalcium phosphate dihydrate. These phosphates are effective in having the teeth feel clean and white. **Silicas,** such as silicon oxides, mechanically cleanse the tooth, are chemically inert, and do not react with other dentifrice ingredients. They are currently the most commonly used abrasive found in dentifrices. Aluminum oxides and perlites have also been introduced into dentifrice formulas, with additional efficacy claims.[8–12]

Abrasiveness Testing

Standard laboratory testing for abrasiveness uses a machine with several brushes.[13] The length of the reciprocating stroke, number of strokes, and pressure of the brush can be adjusted. According to the experimental objectives, enamel, dentin, or cementum is brushed, and the amount of calcium or phosphorus in the resultant slurry is analyzed. A more accurate method has been developed in which extracted teeth are irradiated to activate some of the tooth phosphorus to become radioactive phosphorus. After brushing of the root surfaces of sound canines and molars, the amount of radioactive phosphorus removed is measured. This method may provide a more accurate assessment of abrasiveness compared with classical chemical analyses. Results are referenced against the amount of tooth substance removed by the use of the control abrasive (calcium pyrophosphate).[14]

Abrasives usually do not damage enamel, but they may dull the tooth luster. To compensate for this, polishing agents are added to the dentifrice formulation. These **polishing agents** are usually small-sized particles of aluminum, calcium, tin, magnesium, or zirconium compounds. Typically, the manufacturer blends the abrasives and the polishing agents to form an abrasive system.

■ **Table 9–1** Toothpaste Constituents

Ingredient	*Percentage*
Abrasives	20–40
Water	20–40
Humectants	20–40
Foaming agent (soap or detergent)	1–2
Binding agent	Up to 2
Flavoring agent	Up to 2
Sweetening agent	Up to 2
Therapeutic agent	Up to 5
Coloring or preservative	<1

Agents, such as chalk or silica, may have both polishing and abrasive effects. Smaller particles (1 mm) have a polishing action, and larger particles (20 mm) have an abrasive action.

In selecting a dentifrice, the abrasiveness and polishing characteristics should meet individual needs. The majority of the population does not accumulate visible stain when engaged in their own style of personal oral hygiene. For these individuals, a dentifrice with high polishing and low abrasion should be recommended. For other individuals, an additional amount of abrasive is needed to control accumulating stain. As the abrasive level increases, greater care must be taken to perfect brushing techniques so as to avoid self-inflicted injury to the teeth or soft tissues. Such injuries can result from excessive pressure, hard bristles, and prolonged brushing.

When **toothbrush abrasion** damage does occur, it usually appears as a V-shaped notch in the cementum apical to the cementoenamel junction (Figure 9–2 ■). This area is vulnerable because enamel is about 20 times harder than dentin or cementum. More serious defects usually occur in older individuals who maintain a very high level of oral hygiene.

Humectants

Toothpaste consisting of only a toothpowder and water results in a product with several undesirable properties. Over time, the solids in the paste tend to settle out of

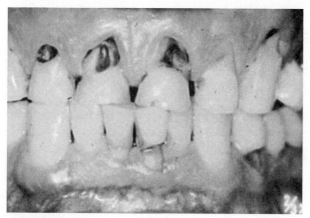

■ FIGURE 9–2   V-shaped notches in central incisors resulting from use of a dentifrice with a harsh abrasive system.
(Courtesy of Dr. B. Baker, University of Texas Dental School, San Antonio.)

solution and the water evaporates. This process may result in caking of the remaining dentifrice. Until the 1930s, most toothpaste had a short shelf life because of this problem. Once the tube was opened, the first expelled paste was liquid, but the last paste in the tube was either impossible to expel or too hard to use. To solve this problem, **humectants** were added to maintain the moisture and prevent hardening. Commonly used humectants are sorbitol, mannitol, glycerol, and propylene glycol. These humectants are nontoxic, but mold or bacterial growth can occur in their presence. For this reason, **preservatives** such as sodium benzoate are added to prevent their growth.

Humectants help maintain the consistency of toothpaste, but despite their presence, the solids tend to settle out of the paste. To counteract this, **thickening** or **binding agents** are added to the formula. Gums, such as gum tragacanth, were first used. These were followed by colloids derived from seaweed, such as carrageenan. These, in turn, were replaced by synthetic celluloses. These celluloses, in low concentrations, are also often used as humectants; in higher concentrations they function as gelling agents in the formulation of gel dentifrices. At high concentrations (>40%), humectants also act as preservatives.

Soaps and Detergents

Because toothpastes were originally manufactured to keep the teeth clean, soap was the logical cleansing agent. As the toothbrush bristles dislodge food debris and plaque biofilm, the foaming or sudsing action of the soap aids in the removal of the loosened material. However, soaps have several disadvantages: They can be irritating to the mucous membrane, their flavor is difficult to mask and often causes nausea, and many times soaps are incompatible with other ingredients, such as calcium.

When detergents appeared on the market, soaps largely disappeared from dentifrices. Today, **sodium lauryl sulfate** (SLS) is the most widely used detergent. It is stable, possesses some antibacterial properties, and has a low surface tension, which facilitates the flow of the dentifrice over the teeth. Sodium lauryl sulfate is active at a neutral pH, has a flavor that is easy to mask, and is compatible with the current dentifrice ingredients. Rantanen and others have suggested that some dentifrices containing SLS may cause mucosal irritation in humans.[15] Low-SLS dentifrices that claim a lower incidence of oral ulcers have been marketed.

Flavoring and Sweetening Agents

Flavor, along with smell, color, and consistency of a product, are important characteristics that lead to public acceptance of a dentifrice. If dentifrices did not possess these characteristics, they would probably be poorly accepted. For taste acceptance, the flavor must be pleasant, provide an immediate taste sensation, and be relatively long lasting. Usually synthetic flavors are blended to provide the desired taste. Spearmint, peppermint, wintergreen, cinnamon, and the most recently introduced flavor, vanilla give toothpaste a pleasant taste, aroma, and refreshing aftertaste. It is difficult to formulate a flavor that is universally acceptable, because people have different color and taste preferences. Some manufacturers use essential oils such as thymol, menthol, and so forth, which may provide a "medicinal" taste to the product. In addition, these oils may impart antibacterial effects, as will be discussed later in this chapter.

Sweetening Agents

In early toothpaste formulations, sugar, honey, and other sweeteners were used. Because these materials can be broken down in the mouth to produce acids and lower plaque pH, they may increase caries. They have been replaced with saccharin, cyclamate, sorbitol, and mannitol as primary **noncariogenic** sweetening agents. Sorbitol and mannitol serve a dual role as sweetening agents and humectants. Glycerin, which also serves as a humectant, adds to the sweet taste. A new sweetener in some dentifrices is xylitol. In laboratory studies, it is not metabolized by bacteria to produce acid. In human studies, where it was placed in chewing gums and food, xylitol was noncariogenic. In addition, it demonstrated an anti-caries capability by facilitating the remineralization of incipient carious lesions.

Baking-Soda Dentifrices

Baking soda (sodium bicarbonate) has had a long history of use as an oral-hygiene aid. Church and Dwight, a manufacturer of baking soda, and also the manufacturer of the original baking-soda toothpaste, reinforces that dentists and hygienists recommend brushing with baking soda for healthier teeth and gums. In a series of papers published in 1998, anti-plaque, gingivitis reduction, stain-removal, and odor-reducing efficacy were documented for sodium bicarbonate–containing dentifrices.[16]

Some dental providers also have suggested the mixture of baking soda with peroxide as an alternative to the use of commercial dentifrices. Many patients attribute benefit to the routine use of these products. It was inevitable that these products would be incorporated into toothpastes. All contain hydrated silica, which is compatible with fluoride. Baking-soda dentifrices actually contain only a small amount of baking soda, in addition to the standard fluoride-compatible abrasives.

Methods of Controlling Plaque and Gingivitis

The most intriguing method of controlling plaque and gingivitis is the concept of **chemical plaque control,** in which chemical compounds are used to supplement the usual brushing, flossing, and use of auxiliary aids employed in mechanical plaque control. Anti-plaque agents can act directly on the plaque bacteria or can disrupt different components of plaque to permit easier and more complete removal during toothbrushing and flossing. This opportunity to use chemistry to enhance oral-hygiene procedures is important, because **manual plaque-control** methods can be difficult to teach and monitor, tedious to perform, time-consuming, and impossible to accomplish by some physically and mentally handicapped persons. In addition, non-motivated individuals will not use manual methods.

The present chemical plaque-control agents should not be considered a panacea, or cure for all plaque problems, because these agents have not been proven to be a total substitute for routine oral-hygiene measures. Excessive emphasis on chemical control may encourage some patients to de-emphasize proven oral-hygiene methods.

At the present time, an agent (or agents) that have fluoride's ability to control caries is being sought to control plaque and gingivitis, and to prevent periodontitis. The properties of an ideal form of such an agent are listed in Table 9–2 ■. Colgate Total brands contain triclosan and Colgate Pro-Health uses a combination of sodium hexametophosphate, a whitening and anti-calculus agent, and stabilized stannous fluoride. Triclosan will be discussed later in this chapter.

Therapeutic Dentifrices

The most commonly used therapeutic agent added to dentifrices is fluoride, which aids in the control of caries. In 1960, the Council on Dental Therapeutics of the American Dental Association classified Crest toothpaste with stannous fluoride as a caries prophylactic dentifrice on the basis of several studies that indicated its

■ **Table 9–2**   Properties of an Ideal Agent to Control Gingivitis

- High, immediate antimicrobial activity
- Broad-spectrum efficacy against bacteria and yeasts
- Chemical stability in formulations and in the oral cavity
- Substantivity (ability to stick) to oral tissues, and to be released over time in an active form
- Toxicologic and ecologic safety
- No topical adverse reactions (staining, burning)
- No taste or aftertaste problems
- No inhibition of taste perception
- No systemic toxicity
- No change in oral or gastrointestinal flora
- Neither carcinogenic nor teratogenic
- No adverse reactions
- Compatibility with dentifrice or mouthwash formulations

effectiveness. For the first time, a therapeutic dentifrice was awarded the Seal of Provisional Acceptance. In 1964, on the basis of further new and favorable data, the classification was upgraded to full acceptance.[17]

The original level of fluoride in OTC dentifrices and gels was restricted to 1,000 to 1,100 ppm fluoride and a total of no more than 120 mg of fluoride in the tube, with a requirement that the package include a safety closure. Most dentifrices today still contain 1,000 ppm. Therapeutic toothpastes, dispensed on prescription, could contain up to 260 mg or 4,950 ppm of fluoride in a tube.

The following fluorides are generally recognized as effective and safe for OTC sales: 0.22% sodium fluoride (NaF) at a level of 1,100 ppm, 0.76% sodium monofluorophosphate (MFP) at a level of 1,000 ppm, and 0.4% stannous fluoride (SnF_2) at a level of 1,000 ppm. Fluoride levels were increased to 1,500 ppm sodium monofluorophosphate in OTC Extra Strength Aim. A prescription dentifrice, Colgate PreviDent 5,000, contains 5,000 ppm of fluoride.

One baking soda–peroxide–fluoride dentifrice (Mentadent) contains a combination of 0.75% stable peroxide gel in conjunction with baking soda, and 1,100 ppm of sodium fluoride. The materials are packaged in a two-chamber pump to permit the baking soda and peroxide components to be mixed with the fluoride at the time of delivery.

Multiple clinical studies of fluoride dentifrices containing NaF, MFP, or SnF_2 in the presence of compatible abrasives and stable formulations have been submitted to and been accepted by the ADA. The ADA, therefore, awards the Seal of Acceptance to fluoride dentifrices solely on the basis of laboratory data—if the experimental design protocol is identical or similar to that of previous ADA-accepted products.[18] Not all fluoride-containing dentifrices have demonstrated anticaries activity. The level of active fluoride must be adequate and must be maintained over the shelf life of the dentifrice.

A combination of calcium-phosphate in dentifrices with fluoride is also gaining momentum in today's market. It is speculated that dentifrices containing calcium phosphate help prevent the formation of dental caries and also rapidly remineralize demineralized tooth structure. Calcium phosphate encourages the remineralization of enamel by rapidly hydrolyzing to form apatite. The addition of calcium and phosphate ions to a fluoride dentifrice may improve the ability of enamel to resist caries initiation and subsequent progression of a lesion.[19–21]

Stannous Salts

Stannous fluoride (SnF_2), specifically the stannous ion, has reported activity against caries, plaque, and gingivitis.[22] Although SnF_2 has a long record as an anticaries agent, long-term stability in dentifrices and mouthrinses has been questioned. Recently, the development and subsequent laboratory and clinical efficacy of a stabilized SnF_2 dentifrice was marketed in the United States by Procter & Gamble as Crest Pro-Health. This product combines a stabilized stannous fluoride (0.454%) and sodium hexametaphospate. Superior efficacy has been shown for Crest Pro-Health in antimicrobial, plaque acidogenicity, gingivitis or gingival bleeding, and calculus control.[23] Other clinical studies compared the antigingivitis benefits of standard sodium fluoride dentifrices with the benefits of triclosan-containing dentifrices containing pyrophosphate/copolymer. Results demonstrated superior benefits for the stabilized 0.454% stannous fluoride/sodium hexametaphosphate dentifrice in reducing gingivitis compared with the triclosan/copolymer dentifrice.[24] These studies support the strong retention and lasting antimicrobial efficacy of high stabilized stannous fluoride/sodium hexametaphosphate dentifrices.

Triclosan

Triclosan is a broad-spectrum antibacterial agent, marketed by its manufacturer, Ciba-Geigy, for use in oral products under the trade name Irgacare. Triclosan is effective against a wide variety of bacteria and is widely used as an antibacterial agent in OTC consumer products in the United States, including deodorant soaps and antibacterial skin scrubs. It has also been shown to be a useful antibacterial agent in oral products. A review of the available pharmacologic and toxicologic information concluded that triclosan can be considered safe for use in dentifrice and mouthrinse products.[25]

Many dentifrices and mouthrinses containing triclosan are marketed in Europe. In the United States, Colgate Total developed by Colgate-Palmolive, contains triclosan, a patented copolymer, "Gantrez," and fluoride. Colgate Total has undergone extensive safety and clinical efficacy testing, and was approved in 1997 by the FDA as the first dentifrice *to help prevent gingivitis, plaque, and caries* [emphasis added].[25–27] In 2001, a 2-year study on Colgate Total documented long-term anticaries efficacy.[28] Additional research supports that a triclosan dentifrice inhibits plaque regrowth and provides anti-calculus activity, thereby reducing gingival inflammation.[29]

Dentifrice products containing a zinc citrate and triclosan combination have also received attention. Clinical evaluation has shown this combination to be effective in reducing acid production and plaque formation, and in preventing gingivitis. Summaries of the zinc citrate–triclosan studies have been published.[30–32] This combination is not currently marketed in the United States.

Anti-calculus Dentifrices

Calculus-control dentifrice formulations are designed to interrupt the process of mineralization of plaque to calculus. Plaque has a bacterial matrix that mineralizes because of the supersaturation of saliva with calcium and phosphate ions. Crystal growth inhibitors may be added to dentifrices to provide a reduction in calculus formation.

In the late 1970s, anti-calculus dentifrices began to appear on the market without any evidence of effectiveness.[33] In 1985, Procter & Gamble supplemented their existing Crest anti-cariogenic toothpaste with a similar anticaries formula that also contained a combination of tetrasodium phosphate and disodium dihydrogen pyrophosphate. These **soluble pyrophosphates** are crystal growth inhibitors, which retard the formation of calculus.[34] This combination has been demonstrated in clinical studies to significantly reduce the amount of calculus formed, compared with a control dentifrice. The dentifrice was marketed as Crest Tartar Control. A recent addition to the list of available products is a dentifrice with both a whitening and an anti-calculus claim.[35] The product, Colgate Tartar Control Plus Whitening Fluoride Toothpaste, contains tetrasodium pyrophosphate, sodium tripolyphosphate, a copolymer, and NaF. GlaxoSmithKline's Aquafresh Whitening with Tartar Protection Toothpaste contains the same active ingredients.

Antihypersensitivity Products

Many patients experience pain when exposed areas of the **tooth root,** especially at the cementoenamel junction, are subjected to heat or cold. Treatment for this sensitivity includes the stimulation of secondary dentin, blocking of the pulpal neural response, **obturation** (closure) of dentinal tubules, and coagulation or precipitation of tubular fluids. In coagulation the fluid in the tubules becomes thicker, whereas in precipitation the minerals in the fluid separate from the fluid and form a deposit. Both mechanisms help to close the tubules. Antihypersensitivity agents include potassium oxalate strontium chloride, sodium citrate, and potassium nitrate. Most recently, the FDA approved **fluoride varnish** as an agent to treat hypersensitivity; this agent is a thin resin that contains fluoride and is brushed onto tooth surfaces.

Potassium nitrate is a commonly used, FDA-approved OTC **desensitization agent,** that is, it reduces the reaction of nerves in the teeth to stimuli such as heat and cold. Potassium nitrate is known to desensitize the nerve by penetrating through the length of the dentinal tubules and to depolarize sensory nerve endings located at the **dentin–pulpal interface.** These actions interrupt the transmission of pain signals to the brain.[36] OTC dentifrices include Sensodyne Fresh Mint Toothpaste (GlaxoSmithKline), Crest Sensitivity Protection Fluoride Toothpaste (Procter & Gamble), Colgate Sensitive Maximum Strength Toothpaste (Colgate Palmolive), and Orajel Sensitive Pain Relieving Toothpaste for

Adults (Del Laboratories, Inc.). Most dentifrices containing potassium nitrate also contain fluoride. Prior to the development of potassium nitrate as a desensitizing agent, the **occluding** (blocking) or **sclerosing** (hardening) of exposed dentinal tubules was the primary method used to control hypersensitivity. Strontium chloride, potassium oxylate, potassium nitrate, and sodium citrate are examples of OTC agents used to occlude the exposed dentinal tubules.[37]

Whiteners

Considerable controversy surrounds the use of stain removers and tooth whiteners. Products are being marketed for professional or in-home use by patients. The cosmetic benefits of these dentifrices remain important to patients and the OTC sales of these products continue to increase. Many claims for efficacy and safety are under review by agencies and government panels.

Surveys reveal a growing U.S. market share for dentifrices claiming "whitening" or "stain control" properties. These dentifrices control stain via physical methods (abrasives) and chemical mechanisms (surface-active agents or bleaching/oxidizing agents). Although the public perceives these products as more abrasive than ordinary toothpastes, their abrasiveness is usually intermediate among the products tested.

Dentifrices marketed with tooth-whitener claims are available as a toothpaste or gel, or are used in a two- or three-step treatment "process." These products usually contain hydrogen peroxide or carbamide peroxide as their bleaching or whitening ingredient. **Carbamide peroxide** breaks down to form urea and hydrogen peroxide. **Hydrogen peroxide,** in turn, forms a free radical that contains oxygen, which is the active bleaching molecule. Home-bleaching products may contain other chemicals to aid in the delivery of the bleaching agent. Glycerin or propylene glycol is commonly added to thicken the solution and prolong contact with the tooth surface. In the two- or three-step products, agents can be delivered to the teeth via a custom-made tray or by toothbrushing.

MOUTHRINSES

Freshening bad breath has been the traditional purpose of mouthrinses. However, mouthrinses can be cosmetic, therapeutic, or both. Cosmetic benefits include a pleasant taste and sensation, a decrease in microorganisms, and halitosis control. Therapeutic benefits include a

reduction in bacterial plaque, gingivitis, and dental caries. **Therapeutic mouthrinses** are available over the counter and by prescription. Mouthrinses are often used daily by patients; therefore, it is important that patients understand proper usage of mouthrinses to achieve successful outcomes. When antimicrobial mouthrinses are used daily along with brushing and flossing, they are most effective in reducing plaque and gingivitis.[38]

The claimed active ingredients of mouthrinses include quaternary ammonium compounds, phenolic compounds, sanguinarine, and chlorhexidine. Ammonium compound and sanguinarine mouthrinses have not shown consistent efficacy and therefore are not recommended as part of an anti-plaque/anti-gingivitis self-care program. As with dentifrices, commercial sales of cosmetic rinses have been related to taste, color, smell, and the pleasant sensation that follows use. The pleasant sensation is often enhanced by the addition of astringents. Commonly used astringents are alum, zinc stearate, zinc citrate, and acetic or citric acids. **Zinc sulfate** has been added to mouthrinses as a claimed anti-plaque ingredient.

Alcohol in mouthrinses is used as a solvent, a taste enhancer, and an agent providing an aftertaste. The alcohol content of commercial rinses, ranging up to 27%, may constitute a danger for children, especially those from 2 to 3 years of age. According to the American Association of Poison Control (AAPC), 5 to 10 ounces of a mouthrinse containing alcohol can be lethal for a child weighing 26 pounds. Between 2000 and 2005, the AAPC's poison-control centers logged more than 90,000 reports of exposures to mouthrinses containing alcohol; 24,000 cases concerned persons younger than 6 years of age, 16,000 were between the ages of 6–19 years, and 52,000 were older than 19 years of age. Of these exposures, 9 died and another 258 had major outcomes of permanent injuries.[39] The American Academy of Pediatrics recommends that OTC liquid preparations be limited to 5% ethanol, that safety closures be required, and that the packaged volume be kept to a reasonable minimum to prevent the potential for lethal ingestion.[40]

The Council on Scientific Affairs of the American Dental Association requires child-resistant caps on all alcohol-containing mouthrinses that bear the ADA Seal of Acceptance. The council also requires manufacturers of ADA-accepted mouthrinses that contain more than 5% alcohol to include the following statement on the label: "Warning: Keep out of reach of children. Do not swallow. Contains alcohol. Use only as directed." The attorneys general of 29 states have petitioned the

U.S. Consumer Products Safety Commission to require child safety caps on bottles of mouthwash that contain more than 5% alcohol.

Although some research links alcohol-containing rinses to oral cancer, numerous published studies support the safety of these mouthrinses. The ADA reports that mouthrinses containing alcohol are considered safe and effective.

Cosmetic Mouthrinses: Halitosis

Bacterial proliferation and plaque accumulation on the surface of the tongue are major factors contributing to halitosis. Ninety percent of halitosis originates from the oral cavity and 10% from systemic or non-oral causes.[41] The effects of this oral malodor can cause patients to become insecure in social situations and self-conscious during daily living. The seriousness of this condition elicits many patient requests for treatment and for validation that mouthrinses claiming to aid in malodor, actually do so.

The effect of most breath-freshening claims is caused by flavors and has no effect after 3 to 5 hours. These mouthrinses mask odors and provide little antibacterial function. They usually contain a flavoring agent that provides a pleasant taste, an astringent that refreshes the mouth, ethyl alcohol, which acts as a solvent and a taste enhancer, water, and an active ingredient to reduce the number of microorganisms.[42] Antibacterial components such as chlorhexidine, sanguinarine, cetylpyridinium chloride, triclosan, essential oils, phenolic compounds, quaternary ammonium compounds, benzalkonium chloride hydrogen peroxide, sodium bicarbonate, zinc ions, and combinations of these components have all been considered to reduce halitosis.

A study performed by Borden and others tested the effects of four mouthrinses on halitosis. Results showed that all four mouthrinses were effective in reducing oral malodor within 4 hours after a single use.[43] Another study tested the effectiveness of mouthrinses containing an antibacterial agent to reduce malodor when used alone, and in conjunction with tongue brushing and toothbrushing. Results showed that, although a reduction in halitosis was evident for mouthrinses used as a sole treatment, the reduction was significantly higher with the combination of mouthrinses and tongue brushing and toothbrushing.[44]

Zinc chloride found in some mouthrinses has gained momentum in its efficacy claims for reducing malodor in patients with good oral health. Studies report that zinc chloride is effective in neutralizing volatile sulfur compounds (VSC) and killing the gram-negative bacteria responsible for VSC formation for greater than 3 hours. A combination of zinc chloride, thymol, and eucalyptus oil found in BreathRx products has also been reported to be effective in reducing halitosis.[45–47]

A quantitative assessment of bad breath, including the smelling of exhaled air (**organoleptic assessment**), identifying the oral cavity as the source, and measuring VSC is effective in verifying product claims for treating halitosis. In diagnosing and treating complaints of bad breath, the clinician should consider psychologic as well as physical factors.[48]

Xerostomia Mouthrinses

Many people experience dry mouth (xerostomia) traceable to several possible causes, such as damage to the salivary glands after radiation therapy for head and neck cancer, Sjögren syndrome, and drug usage such as antihistamines, anticholinergics, antihypertensives, diuretics, narcotics, anticonvulsants, and anti-anxiety and tranquilizing drugs, especially the tricyclic antidepressants. In such cases the oral mucous membrane is continually dry and uncomfortable. Artificial salivas have been developed to ameliorate the dryness (i.e., make it more tolerable); these products are used ad libitum (as desired) by the patient to moisten the mucous membrane. Several moisturizing agents are also available to xerostomia patients.[49]

Because xerostomia is correlated with an increased caries incidence, the rinses usually contain fluoride as well as chemical compounds, such as carboxymethylcellulose, calcium, and phosphorous, in concentrations that closely parallel those of saliva. The rinses that contain fluoride may, in reality, be remineralizing solutions.

Two commonly used xerostomia mouthrinses are Oasis Mouthwash by Sensodyne and Biotène Mouthwash. Oasis Mouthwash claims to moisturize the mouth owing to its mucoadhesive formula, to lock in moisture owing to a xanthum gum polymer and carboxymethyl cellulose compound, and to help protect the mouth from dryness owing to a glycerin coating of the mucosal surface. A study reported in 2006 states that Oasis Mouthwash's **mucoadhesion** formula (i.e., its ability to adhere to mucosa) helps manage symptoms up to 2 hours. The recommended usage is to rinse with the mouthwash in the morning and at bedtime as part of a daily oral care regimen.[50] Biotène Mouthwash is a combination of natural salivary enzymes (glucose oxidase, lactoperoxidase, and lysozyme) and protein. It claims to boost and replenish the natural defenses of saliva, while killing harmful bacteria and maintaining health bacteria. The recommended usage is to swish 1 tablespoon (15 ml) of the mouthwash for 30 seconds, two to three times per day.

Therapeutic Mouthrinse Agents

Chlorhexidine Gluconate

The FDA has approved prescription plaque-control rinses containing 0.12% chlorhexidine. Directions call for a twice-daily, 60-second rinse with one-half ounce of such solutions. Chlorhexidine has proved to be one of the most effective anti-plaque agents to date.[51,52] **Chlorhexidine** is a cationic compound that binds to the hydroxyapatite of tooth enamel, the pellicle, plaque bacteria, the extracellular polysaccharide of the plaque, and especially to the mucous membrane. The chlorhexidine adsorbed to the hydroxyapatite is believed to inhibit bacterial colonization and prevent pellicle formation.[53,54] After binding, the agent is slowly released in an active form over 8 to 12 hours. This ability of the oral tissues to adsorb an active agent and to permit its slow release in active form over a prolonged period is known as **substantivity.** As the substantivity of an anti-plaque agent decreases, the frequency of use needs to be increased.

The use of chlorhexidine in periodontal therapy is often recommended for some patients. It has not proved beneficial as the sole method of treating periodontitis with deep pockets, but chlorhexidine irrigation following root planing (smoothing of root surfaces), prophylaxis, or periodontal surgery may be effective in helping to control inflammation and subgingival plaque.[55,56]

In some countries, such as the United States, chlorhexidine products are available only by prescription. In others, such as the United Kingdom, they are available over the counter. Although chlorhexidine is quite effective, it is not active against all relevant anaerobic bacteria. A high minimal concentration is necessary for efficacy.

Some side effects are associated with chlorhexidine use; staining of the teeth, tongue, and tooth-colored restorations is the most common effect. Occasionally altered taste sensation, irritation of the oral mucosa, and burning sensation are reported.[57] Chlorhexidine is inactivated by most dentifrice surfactants; therefore, it is not included in dentifrices. Also, because of this inactivation, it is critical for dental professionals to alert patients not to use chlorhexidine mouthrinses within 30 minutes before or after regular toothbrushing.

Although chlorhexidine may be more effective than any other current anti-plaque agent and has a definite role in preventive and control dental procedures, it is not a "magic bullet." Its side effects and inadequate activity range somewhat limit its use.

Essential Oils

It is reported that **essential oil** mouthrinses are effective in controlling plaque and gingivitis because the oil alters the bacterial cell wall.[58–60] The active ingredients (essential oils) used in these mouthrinses include a combination of thymol, menthol, eucalyptol, and methyl salicylate in a hydroalcoholic vehicle containing 21.6% to 26.9% alcohol.[61] Although the safety of essential oils is well established,[62–66] some patients may have difficulty tolerating the burning sensation associated with the alcohol content. In addition, slight extrinsic staining has been reported with the use of essential oils rinses, which is a possible transient (short-term) side effect of any antimicrobial agent. Essential oil mouthrinses are indicated for patients who are in need of and compliant with anti-plaque/anti-gingivitis mouthrinses. They may not be indicated for patients who belong to religious organizations that prohibit the use of alcohol in any form; patients in orthodontic devices (e.g., braces); or patients who have a chemical dependency, diabetes, or xerostomia.[67]

Listerine Antiseptic was the first OTC anti-plaque and anti-gingivitis mouthrinse to be approved by the ADA in 1988.[68] Patients are advised to rinse twice daily with one-half ounce of Listerine for 30 seconds, in addition to their usual oral-hygiene regimen. Listerine has been used as a mouthrinse for more than 110 years. The original formula contains 26.9% alcohol. Flavor variations of the original product include Cool Mint, Natural Citrus, and Freshburst Listerine Antiseptics; these products, which contain 21.6% alcohol, also received the ADA seal.

Microorganisms do not develop a resistance to the antibacterial effects of essential oils, such as clove oil (eugenol) and thyme oil (thymol).[69] In long-term clinical trials, Listerine has been shown to reduce both plaque accumulation and severity of gingivitis by up to 34%.[70] Microbial sampling of plaque in these trials has demonstrated no undesirable shifts in the composition of the microbial flora.

As with chlorhexidine, just rinsing with an essential oil mouthrinse is unlikely to be effective in treating periodontitis, because the solution does not reach the depths of the periodontal pockets. Irrigation studies, using irrigator tips designed to deliver solutions subgingivally, suggest that Listerine and Peridex may have some value as adjuncts to mechanical therapy. These studies involved the use of an **irrigator,** a device that uses water to flush debris from surfaces of the teeth and the gingival sulcus.

For the dental professional, it may be important for patients to use a mouthrinse prior to **aerosol-generating procedures.** Unless the dental professional uses an effective dry-field technique, in a 30-second period, the bacterial aerosol generated by an ultrasonic scaler, which removes calculus, an air-powered tooth polisher, or a slow-speed or high-speed turbine can be roughly equivalent to the patient sneezing in the dental provider's face.[71–74] A study by Wyler and coworkers found that even a preliminary rinse of the mouth with water temporarily reduced the bacterial aerosol population by 61%, brushing alone by 85%, and use of an antibacterial mouthrinse by 97%.[75] Fine and coworkers, using a simulated office-visit model, showed that pre-procedural use of an antimicrobial mouthrinse (Listerine) resulted in a 93.6% reduction in the number of viable bacteria in a dental aerosol produced by ultrasonic scaling.[76]

Quaternary Ammonium Compounds (Cetylpyridinium Chloride)

The most common quaternary ammonium compound used in mouthrinses is **cetylpyridinium chloride** (CPC). This compound is a clinically studied bactericidal agent that interacts with the bacterial cell membrane and, through cellular pressure, weakens and disrupts the membrane to effectively kill bacteria. It has been shown to reduce plaque and gingivitis for up to 12 hours, and to reduce plaque biofilm and gingivitis by 14% to 24%.[77–79] Crest Pro-Health Rinse by Procter & Gamble uses this bactericidal agent and markets their product as an anti-gingivitis/anti-plaque alcohol-free mouthrinse that contains CPC. Its recommended usage is to swish 20 ml of Crest Pro-Health Rinse twice daily, 30 seconds at each use, for the product to provide all the benefits indicated. Because of the absence of alcohol content, this product claims to have little-to-no burning sensation and may have some benefit in reducing halitosis. Other mouthrinses that fall under this category include Scope, Cepacol, Clear Choice, and Rembrandt.

Fluoride Rinses

Fluoride mouthrinses are effective in the reduction of the incidence of dental caries. They are intended for daily or weekly use, depending on their categorization as low-concentration/high-frequency or high-concentration/low-frequency rinses. Some low-concentration mouthrinses are available over the counter, whereas most others require a prescription. The active agents in fluoride mouthrinse products are NaF, acidulated phosphofluorides, or SnF. Their concentration for daily use is 0.05% (250 ppm); for weekly use the concentration of each agent is 0.2% (900 ppm), 0.44% (440 ppm), and 0.63% (250 ppm), respectively. The dose directions are 5 ml (1 teaspoon) of product to be used once daily or 10 ml of product to be used once weekly. The rinse is to be swished for 60 seconds and then expectorated. For stannous fluoride, the daily rinse concentration is diluted with water to produce a 0.1% concentration. Stannous fluoride and acidulated phosphofluoride mouthrinses are *not* recommended for weekly usage.

Published long-term clinical studies have consistently shown the anticaries effectiveness of fluoride mouthrinses to be equal or superior to fluoride dentifrices. It is found that the fluoride in mouthrinses is retained in dental plaque and saliva to help prevent dental caries.[80] Studies report a 30% to 40% average reduction in the incidence of dental caries for fluoride mouthrinse users. Their use is recommended for persons in fluoridated and non-fluoridated communities.

Fluoride mouthrinses are highly indicated for patients who have a history of moderate-to-rampant caries, who are undergoing orthodontia or who wear prosthetic appliances (e.g., dentures or bridges) that aid in adherence of plaque biofilm. Moreover, patients with inadequate oral-hygiene habits, patients with dentition areas of demineralization or root exposure/sensitivity, and patients experiencing xerostomia should also use these mouthrinses. Fluoride mouthrinses are not recommended for children under 6 years of age or those who have difficulty swishing and expectorating. Because of the alcohol content found in some fluoride mouthrinses, they may not be recommended for persons unable to tolerate alcohol content.[81]

CHEWING GUM

Because gum chewing is pleasurable, people normally chew for longer periods of time than they spend brushing their teeth. Likewise, gum may complement toothbrushing by reaching many of the tooth surfaces commonly missed during brushing. The average American fails to contact approximately 40% of tooth surfaces during toothbrushing, especially the posterior teeth and lingual surfaces. Regular toothbrushing removes only about 35% to 40% of dental plaque on tooth surfaces. In addition, chewing gum is especially advantageous during the course of the day when toothbrushing is not possible or convenient.

Beneficial effects of gum chewing include increased saliva production, resulting in the mechanical removal of dental plaque and debris.[82–84] Studies have shown that chewing sugared or sugar-free gum is an effective means of reducing plaque accumulation, and that gum chewing can also effectively reduce established plaque on many tooth surfaces.

In the United States, there has been an increase in published research devoted solely to chewing gum and its potential oral health benefits. The interest of researchers in effective gum additives, coupled with the acceptance and use of chewing-gum products by the general public, makes this a new and potentially important category to be considered by dental professionals. Globally, chewing gum is the fastest-growing sector of the confectionary market, ahead of both chocolate and sweets.[82] The attraction is influenced through the marketing appeal of sugar-free gums, gums that whiten or strengthen teeth, and gums that help in mental concentration or act as a snack substitute between meals. Adults are particularly interested in the product appeal.[85]

During gum chewing, salivary flow rates increase, especially in the first few minutes, because of both mechanical and gustatory (taste) stimulation. Increased salivary stimulation can continue for periods of 5 to 20 minutes, usually until the flavor in the product dissipates. However, even with unflavored chewing gum, saliva flow, as evidenced by swallowing rates, increases over the baseline.[86] The beneficial effects of additional saliva in the mouth include increased plaque biofilm calcium levels, and increased buffer capacity and mineral supersaturation; the latter two effects help regulate or increase plaque pH.[87] In addition, increased saliva flow can assist in loosening and removing debris from occlusal or interproximal sites, and can be beneficial to xerostomia patients.

The focus of chewing gum research to date has been on "sugar-free" products, which contain polyol sweeteners such as sorbitol or xylitol.[88] These sweeteners are not broken down by plaque or oral microorganisms to produce acid.[89] Plaque pH studies have documented reduction of plaque acidity and maintenance of plaque neutrality both during and, with xylitol, for periods of 2 to 3 weeks after gum chewing.[90] In addition, gums containing xylitol have shown anticaries activity in several long-term studies.[89] Xylitol is considered non-acidogenic and not fermentable by bacteria responsible for caries production. It is recommended that 6 grams to 10 grams of xylitol gum be chewed daily, three to five times per day, for 5 minutes at each session.[91]

Sorbitol, although effective, is not as effective as xylitol. When compared with sugar-sweetened gum, sorbitol-sweetened gum had low carcinogenicity when it was chewed no more than three times per day, and xylitol-sweetened gum was non-cariogenic in all of the protocols tested.[92] During a 3-year clinical study, dental caries was significantly reduced during chewing of a sorbitol-based chewing gum after meals.[93] It can be concluded that sorbitol is slowly fermented through anaerobic metabolism by *Streptococcus mutans,* whereas xylitol is not fermented at all.[94]

Studies have shown that a commercial chewing gum containing 5% sodium bicarbonate (Arm and Hammer Dental Care) is capable of removing significant amounts of plaque and reducing gingivitis when used as an adjunct to regular toothbrushing. Stain removal is also of interest to the consumer.[95] Studies simulating a realistic situation (twice-daily brushing and unsupervised use of a baking soda chewing gum) demonstrated reduction in stain after 4 weeks.[95]

Consumers have relied on chewing-gum products for "fresh breath." A recent report on reducing VSC associated with oral malodor and organoleptic scores indicates that the products tested are effective primarily as masking agents (flavor) and for the mechanical role of cleaning tooth surfaces. Reduced malodor levels were obtained during initial use of the products, but decreased to baseline levels at the 3-hour assessment times.[96]

Reynolds has proposed the introduction of casein phosphopeptide (CPP) to chewing gum as a mechanism to remineralize early carious lesions.[97] Trident Advantage gum, with Recaldent, makes use of this technology through the addition of CPP and amorphous calcium phosphate (ACP). Two studies compared remineralization of enamel with sugar-free gum containing CPP–ACP to equivalent gum not containing these agents.[98,99] Superior results were obtained in the gum containing CPP–ACP. An overview of selected agents added to chewing gums in the United States is presented in Table 9–3 ■.

Compounds such as chlorhexidine and fluorides delivered to the oral cavity through a gum would appear to be useful. Compared with dentifrices that contain abrasives, and mouthrinses that contain water and alcohol vehicles, the gum product would contain a minimum of potentially interfering agents. Gum would also provide

■ **Table 9–3**   Examples of Agents Added to Chewing Gums

Agent	Purpose/Claim	U.S. Example(s)
Aspirin	Pain relief	Aspergum
Caffeine	Increase alertness	Stay Alert
Calcium carbonate	Neutralize stomach acid	Chooz
Casein phosphopeptide–amorphous calcium phosphate	Remineralize and strengthen teeth	Trident White
Chlorhexidine	Anti-plaque, anti-gingivitis	None
Dimenhydrinate	Motion sickness	None
Fluoride	Anticaries	None
Sodium bicarbonate	Freshen breath	Dental Care
	Whiten teeth	Trident Advantage
	Reduce plaque	
Xylitol	Anticaries	Trident
		BreathRx Theragum
		Theragum

a sustained time of release and availability in the oral cavity. In addition, the active agents would be available at occlusal sites, which are prime areas for plaque growth and pit-and-fissure decay. Neither of these agents is available in the United States and research in this area is limited. However, some studies done outside of the United States show some level of significance in caries decline with the use of chlorhexidine and fluoride added to chewing gum.[100,101] One study reported increased staining on baseline-stained teeth with chlorhexidine chewing gum.[102] Because chewing-gum products are often in the mouth several times a day, the concentration of ingredients released, especially fluoride, must be safe for swallowing.

SUMMARY

The self-use of dentifrices and mouthrinses is proving to be an important preventive dental health measure. Dentifrices, mouthrinses, and chewing gums can be categorized as either cosmetic or therapeutic. Cosmetic products have traditionally been used to remove debris, provide a pleasant "mouth feel," and temporarily reduce halitosis. To improve their products' marketability, manufacturers have added flavors, stripes, sprinkles, and colors to dentifrices and mouthrinses. Recently, other ingredients have also been added to temporarily depress the oral bacterial population, or to prevent or moderate some disease process in the mouth.

The widespread use of therapeutic fluoride dentifrices and mouthrinses is credited with helping to reduce the worldwide prevalence of dental decay. Other agents are now being used to target other oral-health problems.

The FDA has developed rigid guidelines for testing the safety and efficacy of products before their introduction on the market. Part of the function of the regulatory process is to differentiate between products whose potential risks are sufficiently low to allow them to be sold over the counter, and those whose possible hazards justify restriction to prescription use.

Although the ADA considers anti-plaque, anti-calculus, and breath-freshening claims as cosmetic, they will review data and allow manufacturers to make these statements, if they are coupled with a disease-related activity (e.g., prevents gingivitis or caries). Toothpastes containing potassium nitrate, strontium chloride, and sodium citrate have antihypersensitivity properties; other toothpastes with tetrasodium phosphate and disodium dihydrogen pyrophosphate retard the formation of calculus. Chlorhexidine is a highly effective anti-plaque and anti-gingivitis agent, but it has significant side effects and may be dispensed by prescription only. Listerine, which contains essential oils, has been popular for over a century, and has demonstrated the same properties but not the side effects of chlorhexidine.

Chewing gum products are a new dental category in which manufacturers are making claims for cosmetic and therapeutic effectiveness. At this time, the FDA has not approved any chewing gum products for dental therapeutic claims.

REFERENCES

1. Trummel C. (1994). Regulation of oral chemotherapeutic products in the United States. *J Dent Res,* 73:704–708.

2. United States Department of Health and Human Services, Food and Drug Administration, Center for Drug Evaluation and Research. (2008). Drug Applications—Phase 1 Clinical Studies, Phase 2 Clinical Studies, Phase 3 Clinical Studies. Retrieved February 13, 2008. http://www.fda.gov/cder/about/smallbiz/definitions.htm.

3. United States Department of Health and Human Services, Food and Drug Administration, Center for Drug Evaluation and Research. (1998). Guidelines for industry, national uniformity for non prescription drugs—Ingredient listing for OTC drugs. Retrieved November 26, 2007, from http://www.fda.gov/cder/guidance/index.htm.

4. U.S. Food and Drug Administration. (September 9, 1990). Over-the-counter dental and oral health care drug products for antiplaque use; safety and efficacy review. *Fed Reg,* 55:38560–62.

5. U.S. Food and Drug Administration. (May 29, 2003). Oral health care drug products for over-the-counter human use; antigingivitis/antiplaque drug products. Establishment of a monograph. *Fed Reg,* 68:32232–34. Retrieved November 26, 2007, from http://www.fda.gov/OHRMS/DOCKETS/98fr/03-12783.pdf.

6. American Dental Association. (2006). What is the ADA Seal of Acceptance? *J Am Dent Assoc,* 137:267.

7. ACNielsen Study Finds 43 Brands Have Billion Dollar Global Presence October 31, 2001. Retrieved February 13, from http://www2.acnielsen.com/news/2001103.shtml.

8. Matheson, J. R., Cox, T. F., Baylor, N., Joiner, A., Patil, R., Karad, V., Ketkar, V., & Bijlani, N.S. (2004). Effect of toothpaste with natural calcium carbonate/perlite on extrinsic tooth stain. *Int Dent J.* 2004; 54(5 Suppl 1):321–5.

9. White, D. J. (2001). Development of an improved whitening dentifrice based upon "stain-specific soft silica" technology. *J Clin Dent,* 12:25–29.

10. Hefferren, J. & Li, N. (2005). Dentifrice abrasives: Heroes or villains? Cleveland, OH: Academy of Dental Therapeutics and Stomatology. Retrieved November 26, 2007, from http://www.ineedce.com/pdf_files/adts_dentifrice_abrasives.pdf.

11. Volpe, A. R., Petrone, M. E., Principe, M., & DeVizio, W. (2002). The efficacy of a dentifrice with caries, plaque, gingivitis, tooth whitening and oral malodor benefits. *J Clin Dent,* 13:55–58.

12. Joiner, A. (2006). Review of the extrinsic stain removal and enamel/dentine abrasion by a calcium carbonate and perlite containing whitening toothpaste. *Int Dent J,* 56:175–80.

13. Richmond, R., MacFarlane T. V., & McCord, J. F. (2004). An evaluation of the surface changes in PMMA biomaterial formulations as a result of toothbrush/dentifrice abrasion. *Dent Mater,* 20:124–32.

14. Hefferren, J. J. (1976). A laboratory method for assessment of dentifrice. *J Dent Res,* 55:563–753.

15. Rantanen, I., Jutila, K., Nicander, I., Tenovuo, J., & Soderling, E. (2003). The effects of two sodium lauryl sulphate containing toothpastes with and without betaine on human oral mucosa in vivo. *Swed Dent J,* 27:31–34.

16. Hefferren, J. J. (1998). Historical view of dentifrice functionality methods. *J Clin Dent,* 9:53–56.

17. American Dental Association. (1964). Council on Dental Therapeutics. American dental reclassification of Crest toothpaste. *J Am Dent Assoc,* 69:195–96.

18. American Dental Association. (2005). Council on Scientific Affairs. Acceptance program guidelines: Fluoride-containing dentifrices. Chicago, IL: American Dental Association.

19. Charig, A., Winston, A., & Flickinger M. (2004). Enamel mineralization by calcium-containing-bicarbonate toothpastes: Assessment by various techniques. *Compend Contin Educ Dent,* 25 (9 Suppl 1):14–24.

20. Tung, F. S., & Eichmiller, M. C. (2004). Amorphous calcium phosphates for tooth mineralization. *Compend Contin Educ Dent,* 25 (9 Suppl 1):9–13.

21. Reynolds, E. C. (1997). Remineralization of enamel subsurface lesions by casein phosphopeptide-stabilized calcium phosphate solutions. 1. *J Dent Res,* 76(9):1587–95.

22. Tinanoff, N. (1995). Progress regarding the use of stannous fluoride in clinical dentistry. *J Clin Dent,* 6:37–40.

23. White, D. J., Kozak, K. M., Gibb, R., Dunavent, J., Klukowska, M., & Sagel, P. A. (2006). A 24-hour dental plaque prevention study with stannous fluoride dentifrice containing hexametaphosphate. *J Contemp Dent Pract,* 7:1–11.

24. Archila, L., Bartizek, R. D., Winston, J. L., McClanahan, S. E., & He, T. (2004). The comparative efficacy of stabilized stannous fluoride/sodium hexametaphosphate dentifrice and sodium fluoride/triclosan/copolymer dentifrice for the control of gingivitis: A 6-month randomized clinical study. *J Periodontol,* 75:1592–99.

25. DeSalva, S., King, B., & Lin, Y. (1989). Triclosan: A safety profile. *Am J Dent,* 2:185–96.

26. Panagakos, F. S., Volpe, A. R., Petrone, M. E., DeVizio, W., Davies, R. M., & Proskin, H. M. (2005). A review of comprehensive advanced oral antibacterial/anti-inflammatory technology of the clinical benefits of a triclosan/copolymer/fluoride dentifrice. *J Clin Dent,* 16 (Suppl 1-19).

27. Volpe, A. R., Petrone, M. E., DeVizio, W., Davies, R. M., & Proskin, H. M. (1996). A review of plaque, gingivitis, calculus and caries clinical efficacy studies with a fluoride

dentifrice containing triclosan and PVM/MA copolymer. *J Clin Dent,* 7:S1–S14.

28. Mann, J., Vered, Y., Babayof, I., Sintas, J., Petrone, M. E., Volpe, A. R., & Proskin H. M. (2001). The comparative anticaries efficacy of a dentifrice containing 0.3% Triclosan and 2.0% copolymer in a 0.243% sodium fluoride/silica base and a dentifrice containing 0.243% sodium fluoride/silica base: A two-year coronal caries clinical trial on adults in Israel. *J Clin Dent,* 12:71–76.

29. McClanahan, S. F., Bollmer, B. W., Court, L. K., McClary, J. M., Majeti, S., Crisanti, M. M., Beiswanger, B. B., & Mau, M. S. (2000). Plaque regrowth effects of a Triclosan/pyrophosphate dentifrice in a 4-day non-brushing model. *J Clin Dent,* 11:107–13.

30. Adams, S. E., Theobald, A. J., Jones, N. M., Brading, M. G., Cox, T. F., Mendez, A., Chesters, D. M., Gillam, D. G., Hall, C., & Holt, J. (2003). The effect of toothpaste containing 2% zinc citrate and 0.3% triclosan on bacterial viability and plaque growth in vivo compared to a toothpaste containing 0.3% triclosan and 2% copolymer. *Int Dent J,* 53:398–403.

31. Adams, S. E., Lloyd, A. M., Naeeni, M. A., Coope, Y. L., & Holt, J. S. (2003). The effect of toothpaste containing 2% zinc citrate/0.3% Triclosan on the glycolysis of plaque bacteria ex vivo after food intake. *Int Dent J,* 53:391–97.

32. Brading, M. G., Cromwell, V. J., Jones, N. M., Baldek, J. D., & Marquis, R. E. (2003). Antimicrobial efficacy and mode of action studies on a new zinc/triclosan formulation. *Int Dent J,* 53:363–70.

33. American Dental Association. (1979). *Therapeutics* (38th ed.). Chicago: American Dental Association, 345–46.

34. Zacherl, W. A., Pfeiffer, H. J., & Swancar, J. R. (1985). The effect of soluble pyrophosphates on dental calculus in adults. *J Am Dent Assoc,* 110:737–38.

35. Volpe, A., Manhold, J., Lobene, R., & Yankell, S. (2000). Influences of directed research and clinical observation on the development of a tartar control whitening dentifrice. *J Clin Dent,* 11:63–67.

36. Jacobsen, L., & Bruce, G. (2001). Clinical dentin hypersensitivity: Understanding the causes and prescribing a treatment. *J Contemp Dent Pract,* 2:1–8.

37. Haywood, V. B., Cordero, R., Wright, K., Gendreau, L., Rupp, R., Kotler, M., Littlejohn, S., Fabyanski, J., Smith S. (2005). Brushing with a potassium nitrate dentifrice to reduce bleaching sensitivity. *J Clin Dent,* 16:17–22.

38. Silverman, S., & Wilder, R. (2006). Antimicrobial mouthrinses as part of a comprehensive oral care regimen. Safety and compliance factors. *J Am Dent Assoc,* 137:22S–26S.

39. American Association of Poison Control. 2000–2005 Annual AAPCC TESS Reports. Retrieved February 13, 2008 from http://www.aapcc.org/annual.htm.

40. American Academy of Pediatrics, Committee on Drugs. (1984). Ethanol in liquid preparations intended for children. *Pediatrics,* 73:405.

41. Farrell S., Bake, R. A., Somogyi-Mann, M., Witt, J. J., & Gerlach, R. W. (2006). Oral malodor reduction by a combination of chemotherapeutic and mechanical treatments. *Clin Oral Invest,* 10:157–63.

42. Darby, M. L., & Walsh, M. M. (2003). *Dental hygiene theory and practice* (2nd ed.). Philadelphia: W.B. Saunders.

43. Borden, L. C., Chaves, E. S., Bowman, J. P., Fath, B. M., & Hollar, G. L. (2002). The effect of four mouthrinses on malodor. *Compend Contin Educ Dent,* 23:531–36.

44. Loesche, W. J. (2003). Microbiology and treatment of halitosis. *Curr Infect Dis Rep,* 5:220–25.

45. Codipilly, D. P., Kaufman, H. W., & Kleinberg, I. (2004). Use of novel group of oral malodor measurements to evaluate an anti-oral malodor mouthrinse (TriOral^{TM}) in humans. *J Clin Dent,* 15:98–104.

46. Pedersen, E. J. (2003). *U.S. Patent No. 660,7711.* Mouth hygienic composition in the treatment of halitosis. Washington, DC: U.S. Patent and Trademark Office. Retrieved November 26, 2007, from http://www.patentstorm.us/patents/6607711-description.html.

47. Loesche, W. J. (1999). The effects of antimicrobial mouthrinses on oral malodor and their status relative to U.S. Food and Drug Administration regulation. *Quintessence Int,* 30:311–18.

48. Eli, I., Baht, R., Koriat, H., & Rosenberg, S. W. (2001). Self perception of breath odor. *J Am Dent Assoc,* 132:621–26.

49. Haveman, C. W., & Redding, S. W. (1998). Dental management and treatment of xerostomia patients. *Texas Dent J,* 115:43–56.

50. Corcoran, R. A. (2006). Evaluation of a combined polymer system for use in relieving the symptoms of xerostomia. *J Clin Dent,* 17 (Spec Iss):34–38.

51. Lorenz, K., Bruhn, G., Heumann, C., Netuschil, L., Brecx, M., & Hoffman, T. (2006). Effect of two new chlorhexidine mouthrinses on the development of dental plaque, gingivitis, and discoloration. A randomized, investigator blind, placebo-controlled, 3-week experimental gingivitis study. *J Clin Periodontol,* 33:561–67.

52. Kolahi, J., & Soolari, A. (2006). Rinsing with chlorhexidine gluconate solution after brushing and flossing teeth: A systematic review of effectiveness. *Quintessence Int,* 37:605–12.

53. Turesky, S., Warner, V., Lin, P. S., & Saloway, B. (1977). Prolongation of antibacterial activity of chlorhexidine adsorbed to teeth. *J Periodontol,* 48:646–49.

54. Drisko, C. (2000). Trends in surgical and nonsurgical periodontal treatment, *Periodontol 2000,* 2001;25:77–88.

55. Faveri, M., Gursky, L. C., Feres, M., Shibli, J. A., Salvador, S. L., & deFiqueiredo, L. C. (2006). Scaling and root planing and chlorhexidine mouthrinses in the treatment of chronic periodontitis: A randomized, placebo controlled clinical trial. *J Clin Periodontol,* 33:819–28.

56. Moghadam, B. K. H., Drisko, C. L., & Gier, R. E. (1991). Chlorhexidine mouthwash-induced fixed drug eruption. *Oral Surg Oral Med Oral Pathol,* 71:431–34.

57. Gurgan, C. A., Zaim, E., Bakirsoy, I., & Soykan, E. (2006). Short term effects of 0.2% alcohol-free chlorhexidine mouthrinse used as an adjunct to non-surgical periodontal treatment: A double blind clinical study. *J Periodontol,* 77:370–84.

58. von Fraunhofer, J. A., Kelley, J. I., DePaola, L. G., & Miller, T. F. (2006). The effect of a mouthrinse containing essential oils on dental restorative materials. *Gen Dent,* 54:403–407.

59. Sekino, S., & Ramberg, P. (2005). The effect of a mouthrinse containing phenolic compounds on plaque formation and developing gingivitis. *J Clin Periodontol,* 32:1083–88.

60. Charles, C., Sharma, N., Galustians, H., McGuire, A., & Vincent, J. (2001). Comparative efficacy of an antiseptic mouthrinse and an antiplaque/antigingivitis dentifrice. A six-month trial. *J Am Dent Assoc,* 132:670–75.

61. U.S. Department of Health and Human Services. (2003). Oral health care drug products for over-the-counter human use; antigingivitis/antiplaque drug products; establishment of a monograph; proposed rules. *Fed Reg,* 68:32231–87. (Codified at 21 CFR pr 356).

62. Charles, C. H., Mostler, K. M., Bartels, L. L., & Mankodi, S. M. (2004). Comparative antiplaque and antigingivitis effectiveness of a chlorhexidine and an essential oil mouthrinse: 6-month clinical trial. *J Clin Periodontol,* 31:878–84.

63. Sharma, N., Charles, C. H., Lynch, M. C., Qaqish, J., McGuire, J. A., Galustians, J. G., & Kumar, L. D. (2004). Adjunctive benefit of an essential oil-containing mouthrinse in reducing plaque and gingivitis in patients who brush and floss regularly: A six-month study. *J Am Dent Assoc,* 135:496–504.

64. Bauroth, K., Charles, C. H., Mankodi, S. M., Simmons K., Zhao, Q., Kumar, L. D. (2003). The efficacy of an essential oil antiseptic mouthrinse vs. dental floss in controlling interproximal gingivitis: A comparative study. *J Am Dent Assoc.,* 134:359–65.

65. Sharma, N. C., Charles, C. H., Qaqish, J. G., Galustians, H. J., Zhao, Q., Kumar, L. D. (2002). Comparative effectiveness of an essential oil mouthrinse and dental floss in controlling interproximal gingivitis and plaque. *Am J Dent,* 15:351–55.

66. Charles, C. H., Sharma, N. C., Galustians, H. J., Qaqish, J., McGuire, J. A., Vincent, J. W. et al. (2001). Comparative efficacy of an antiseptic mouthrinse and an antiplaque/antigingivitis dentifrice. A six-month clinical trial. *J Am Dent Assoc,* 132:670–75.

67. Stilley, K. R. (2002). Chemotherapeutics. In Daniel, S. J., & Harfst, S. A., Eds. Dental hygiene: *Concepts, Cases, and Competencies.* St. Louis: C.V. Mosby, 418.

68. American Dental Association. (1988). Council on Dental Therapeutics accepts Listerine. *J Am Dent Assoc,* 117:515–17.

69. Meeker, H. G., & Linke, H. A. B. (1988). The antibacterial action of eugenol, thyme oil, and related essential oils used in dentistry. *Compend Contin Educ Dent,* 9:32–40.

70. Menaker, L., Weatherford, T. W., Pitts, G., Ross, N. M., & Lamm, R. (1979). The effects of Listerine antiseptic on dental plaque. *Ala J Med Sci,* 16:71–77.

71. Miller, R. L., & Micik, R. E. (1978). Air pollution and its control in the dental office. *Dent Clin North Am,* 22:453–76.

72. Klyn, S. L., Cummings, D. E., Richardson, B. W., & Davis, R. D. (2001). Reduction of bacteria-containing spray produced during ultrasonic scaling. *Gen Dent,* 49:648–52.

73. Harrell, S. K., Barnes, J. B., & Rivera-Hidalgo, F. (1996). Reduction of aerosols produced by ultrasonic scalers. *J Periodontol,* 67:28–32.

74. Logothetis, D. D., & Martinez-Welles, J. M. (1995). Reducing bacterial aerosol contamination with a chlorhexidine gluconate pre-rinse. *J Am Dent Assoc,* 126:1634–39.

75. Wyler, D., Miller, R., & Micik, R. (1990). Efficacy of self-administered preoperative oral hygiene procedures in reducing the concentration of bacteria in aerosols generated during dental procedures. *J Dent Res,* 50:509.

76. Fine, D., Yip, J., Furgang, D., Barnett, M. L., Olshan, A. M., & Vincent, J. (1993). Reducing bacteria in dental aerosols: Pre-procedural use of an antiseptic mouthrinse. *J Am Dent Assoc,* 124:56–58.

77. Stookey, G. K., Beiswanger, B., Mau, M., Isaacs, R. L., Witt, J. J., & Gibb, R. (2005). A 6-month clinical study assessing the safety and efficacy of two cetylpyridinium chloride mouthrinses. *Am J Dent,* 18 (Spec Iss):24A–28A.

78. Kozak, K. M., Gibb, R., Dunavent, J., & White, D.J. (2005). Efficacy of a high bioavailable cetylpyridinium chloride mouthrinse over a 24-hour period: A plaque imaging study. *Am J Dent,* 18 (Spec No.):18A–23A.

79. Blenman, T. V., Morrison, K. L., Tsay, G. J., Medina, A. L., & Gerlach, R. W. (2005). Practice implications with an alcohol-free, 0.07% cetylpyridinium chloride mouthrinse. *Am J Dent,* 18 (Spec No.):29A–34A.

80. Centers for Disease Control. (2001). Fluoride OTC rinses. *MMWR Rec Rep,* 50 (RR14):1–42.

81. Wilkins, E. M. (2005). *Clinical practice of the dental hygienist* (9th ed.). Baltimore, MD: Lippincott Williams & Wilkins, 558–60.

82. Dawes, C., & Kubienec, K. (2004). The effects of prolonged gum chewing on salivary flow rate and composition. *Arch Oral Biol,* 49:665–69.

83. Polland, K. E., Higgins, F., & Orchardson, R. (2003). Salivary flow rate and pH during prolonged gum chewing in humans. *J Oral Rehabil,* 30:861–65.

84. Itthagarun, A., & Wei, S. H. (1997). Chewing gum and saliva in oral health. *J Clin Dent,* 8:159–62.

85. Press Release Cadbury Schweppes. 30 Oct. 06: Cadbury Schweppes enters UK Chewing Gum Market. Revised 5/5/08. http://www.cadburyschweppes.com/EN/Media-Centre/PressReleases/uk_gum_launch.htm.

86. Yankell, S. L., & Emling, R. C. (1999). Clinical effects on plaque pH, pCa and swallowing rates from chewing a flavored or unflavored chewing gum. *J Clin Dent,* 10:86–88.

87. Koparol, E., Ertugrul, F., & Sabah, E. (2000). Effect of gum chewing on plaque acidogenicity. *J Clin Pediatric Dent,* 24:129–32.

88. Edgar, W. M. (1999). A role for sugar free gum in oral health. *J Clin Dent,* 10:89–93.

89. Gutkowski, S. (2005). X marks the spot. *Contemp Oral Hygiene,* 5:10–13.

90. Edgar, W. M. (1998). Sugar substitutes, chewing gum and dental caries—A review. *Br Dent J,* 184:29–32.

91. Beebe, S. (2006). The expanding utility of xylitol. *Dimensions,* 10:34–36.

92. Burt, B. A. (2006). The use of sorbitol- and xylitol-sweetened chewing gum in caries control *J Am Dent Assoc,* 137:190–96.

93. Hildebrandt, G. H., & Sparks, B. S. (2000). Maintaining mutans streptococci suppression with xylitol chewing gum, *J Am Dent Assoc,* 131:909–16.

94. Beiswanger, B. B., Boneta, A. E., Mau, M. S., Katz, B. P., Proskin, H. M., & Stookey, G. K. (1998). The effect of chewing sugar-free gum after meals on clinical caries incidence. *J Am Dent Assoc,* 129:1623–26.

95. Kleber. C. J., Putt, M. S., Milleman, J. L., Davidson, K. R., & Proskin, H. M. An evaluation of sodium bicarbonate chewing gum in reducing dental plaque and gingivitis in conjunction with regular toothbrushing., *Compend Contin Educ Dent,* 2001 Jul;22(7A):4–12.

96. Reingewirtz, Y., Girault, O., Reingewirtz, N., Senger, B., & Tanenbaum, H. (1999). Mechanical effects and volatile sulfur compound-reducing effects of chewing gums: Comparison between test and base gums and a control group. *Quintessence Int,* 30:319–23.

97. Reynolds, E. C., Black, C. L., Cai, F., Cross, K. J., Eakins, D., Huq, N. L., Morgan, M. V., Nowicki, A., Perich, J. W., Riley, P. F., Shen, P., Talbo, G., & Webber, F. (1999). Advances in enamel remineralization: Casein phosphopeptide-amorphous calcium phosphate. *J Clin Dent,* 10:86–88.

98. Iijima, Y., Cai, F., Shen, P., Walker, G., Reynolds, C., & Reynolds, E. C. (2004). Acid resistance of enamel subsurface lesions remineralized by a sugar-free chewing gum containing casein phosphopeptide-amorphous calcium phosphate. *Caries Res,* 38:551–56.

99. Shen, P., Cai, F., Nowicki, A., Vincent, J., & Reynolds, E. C. (2001). Remineralization of enamel subsurface lesions by sugar-free chewing gum containing casein phosphopeptide-amorphous calcium phosphate. *J Dent Res,* 80:2066–70.

100. Thorild, I., Lindau, B., & Twetman, S. (2006). Caries in 4-year-old children after maternal chewing of gums containing combinations of xylitol, sorbitol, chlorhexidine, and fluoride. *Eur Arch Paediatr Dent,* 7:241–45.

101. Thorild, I., Lindau, B., & Twetman, S. (2004). Salivary mutan streptococci and dental caries in three-year-old children after maternal exposure to chewing gums containing combinations of xylitol, sorbitol, chlorhexidine, and fluoride. *Acta Odontol Scand,* 62:245–50.

102. Thorild, I., Lindau, B., & Twetman, S. (2003). Effect of maternal use of chewing gums containing xylitol, chlorhexidine, or fluoride on mutans streptococci colonization in the mothers' infant children. *Oral Health Prev Dent,* 1:53–57.

Chapter 10

Self-Care Measures to Supplement Toothbrushing

Christine French Beatty
Nahid Nikpour

OBJECTIVES

After studying this chapter, the student should be able to:

1. Describe the reasons why supplemental oral health self-care is needed to complement toothbrushing.
2. Identify factors, in addition to oral conditions, that influence selection of supplemental oral hygiene devices and techniques.
3. Identify the process of developing an oral health self-care plan.
4. State the purposes, indications, contraindications, techniques, advantages, and limitations of various oral hygiene devices.
5. Justify the purpose and describe techniques for the use of mouthrinses and oral irrigators.
6. Describe proper oral hygiene self-care for dental implants, removable partial dentures and full dentures.

KEY TERMS

Process of care model
Comprehensive oral assessment
Re-care
Evidence-based principles
Self-care
Oral self-care
Oral health self-care
Co-discovery
Virulence
Oral cleanliness
Dental floss
Embrasure
Pontics
Rotated teeth
Waxed dental tape
Polytetrafluoroethylene
Variable-thickness floss
Spool method of flossing
Loop method of flossing
Clefting
Bacterial endocarditis
Bacteremias
Dental floss holder
Dental floss threader

(continued)

KEY TERMS (CONTINUED)

Automated flossers
Lingual brackets
Interproximal brushes
Interdental brushes
Diastemas
Medicament
Uni-tuft brush
Single-tuft
End-tuft brush
Nares
Burnishing
Rubber
Plastic tips
Rubber tip stimulators
White knitting yarn
Synergistic
Bulimia
Irrigation devices
Periodontopathic

Cannula
Oral malodor
Halitosis
Putrefaction
Fungiform
Filiform
Terminal sulcus
Endosseous implants
Peri-implantitis
Stomatitis
Candidiasis
Alkaline peroxide
Alkaline hypochlorite
Commercial acid cleansers
Proteolytic enzymes
Household bleach
Vinegar
Antimicrobial mouthwash
Microwave radiation

INTRODUCTION

It has long been recognized that the plaque biofilm that forms and remains on tooth surfaces is the primary etiologic factor in the development of both dental caries and periodontal diseases.[1–5] Patients need to understand that prevention and maintenance of periodontal disease and caries depends on effective daily removal and control of this plaque biofilm.[6–10] Studies have documented that long-term maintenance of a high level of oral hygiene results in a greatly reduced incidence of tooth mortality, dental caries, and periodontal diseases.[11] In addition, because other medical conditions are affected by periodontal diseases, failure to practice adequate oral hygiene can have adverse effects on overall health.[7,12–14]

Although toothbrushing is effective in cleaning the buccal, lingual, and occlusal surfaces, it leaves the proximal surfaces essentially untouched.[10] Limitations of the toothbrush in removing plaque from the proximal surfaces and other hard-to-reach areas indicate a need to recommend supplemental measures.[15] Regular interproximal plaque removal is recommended for the following reasons:

- Incomplete plaque removal can increase the rate and growth of new plaque.[16]
- Plaque re-growth occurs first in the interproximal areas.[17,18]
- Allowing plaque to remain on some tooth surfaces can facilitate development of a complex microflora on other clean surfaces.[9,19]
- Individuals who clean interproximally on a daily basis have less plaque and calculus.[6]
- Gingivitis, periodontitis, and caries occur more frequently in interproximal areas.[10]
- Interproximal plaque removal is beneficial for preventing gingival and periodontal infections, as well as for reducing or eliminating diseases in these tissues.[1]
- Daily effective interproximal plaque removal can facilitate prevention of caries.[20]

The dentition or periodontal tissues can be altered as a result of disease, repair, or from architectural tissue changes after therapy. When alterations occur, a device and/or technique must be introduced to accommodate them. Although it has been shown that removal of supragingival plaque influences the subgingival plaque composition, plaque removal efforts should also extend as far subgingivally as possible.[9,19]

The **Process of Care Model** is useful when determining the most appropriate products and practices for supplemental oral self-care[21] (Table 10–1 ■). The model consists of five phases: assessment, diagnosis, planning, implementation, and evaluation. Discussion of the application of the model to oral self-care follows.

The oral health professional must carefully assess a patient's numerous oral health and disease risk factors to personalize recommendations for the most effective supplemental measures. Having an understanding of risk for oral diseases is critical to being able to make decisions about treatment, prevention, and control of these conditions.[22] Identifying risk factors in the patient that relate to the development, progression, and maintenance of dental caries, periodontal diseases, and other oral conditions is an essential aspect of patient care. These risk factors include current oral self-care practices, and past and current oral health status in relation to all oral diseases and conditions.

The importance of this assessment phase cannot be overemphasized. Self-care recommendations must be individualized on the basis of results of an assessment.[10] Table 10–2 ■ presents the components of a **comprehensive oral assessment** that should be considered when making self-care recommendations. Researchers have found that oral health practitioners vary in their assignment of risk scores for oral diseases. The use of a computerized tool to assign these risk scores has

been suggested to reduce the extent of variation, and to increase the uniformity and accuracy of clinical decision making.[23]

During the diagnosis and planning phases of the Process of Care Model, appropriate preventive oral self-care practices and products to address the risks are jointly determined with the individual.[6] Involvement of the client in this decision-making process will increase the level of commitment and success of behavioral changes.[24,25] During the implementation phase of the model, the oral health professional can then apply individualized, theory-based, and evidence-based educational and motivational strategies to facilitate behavioral change. This process should be accomplished during the appointments required for therapy.[10,26–30] Ensuring that recommended self-care plans are personalized and consistent with the lifestyle of the individual will increase the potential for long-term compliance. Monitoring and reinforcing at regular intervals will also increase compliance with recommendations.[10,30] The self-care plan is documented in the dental chart and modified as needed at subsequent **re-care** (follow-up) visits on the basis of the evaluation results. This type of documentation allows for continuity of care.

The evaluation phase of the Process of Care Model focuses on outcomes to determine whether modifications to the oral hygiene strategies are indicated. The evaluation process is continuous over the patient's lifespan, because the dentition and soft tissues may become altered with time, and the patient's abilities and dexterity change. Continuation or change of a self-care plan is based on outcomes such as current condition of the soft and hard tissues, and changes made to the modifiable risk factors.[7] Involvement of the individual in these decisions will help to ensure long-term commitment to the oral self-care plan.[31]

■ **Table 10–1** Phases of the Process of Care Model

Phases	Activities
Assessment	Data of general and oral health status are systematically collected.
Diagnosis	Data are analyzed to formulate a diagnosis.
Planning	The evidence-based plan is derived and prioritized on the basis of mutually congruent goals.
Implementation	Preventive procedures to promote/maintain oral health and therapeutic procedures to control disease are implemented to achieve oral health goals.
Evaluation	Attainment of oral health goals is mutually analyzed, and new care plan components are determined as necessary.

■ **Table 10–2** Components of a Comprehensive Oral Assessment

Medical History
- Medical conditions
- Medications
- Allergies
- Physical/mental challenges
- Lifestyle, living circumstances, and social factors
- Mental health

Dental History
- Chief complaint
- Past periodontal treatment
- Past caries experience
- Exposure to fluoride
- Previous records and radiographs

Clinical examination
- Intraoral/extraoral soft tissues
- TMJ
- Teeth and missing teeth
- Restorations
- Tooth mobility
- Tooth position
- Occlusal and interdental relationships
- Parafunctional habits[a]
- Periodontal soft tissues
- Probing depths, CAL, and bleeding on probing
- Recession
- Mucogingival relationships
- Furcation involvement
- Hard and soft tissue trauma/lesions
- Flow and quality of saliva

Radiographs
- Caries
- Overhanging restorations and open margins
- Periodontal structures
- Furcation involvement
- Other pathology

Deposits
- Plaque
- Calculus

Current self-care practices
- Current self-care practices including products and devices
- Current use of fluorides or other therapeutic agents
- Lifestyle (diet, tobacco, etc.)

Learning and compliance factors
- Coordination, dexterity and ability
- Motivation and readiness
- Comprehension

TMJ, temporomandibular joint; CAL, clinical attachment loss.
[a]Parafunctional habit is the habitual use of a body part for other than the most common use, such as grinding teeth.

Recommending oral self-care products to boost office productivity is a commonly suggested approach.[32] However, this practice does not consider the principles of evidence-based practice.[33,34] According to **evidence-based principles,** recommendations for a self-care plan should be based on the best available scientific evidence; the needs, values, and desires of the patient; and the professional judgment and clinical expertise of the oral health care practitioner.

There is frequently a gap between the published evidence and the evidence used by practitioners to make clinical decisions.[35] As researchers learn more about oral diseases, risk factors, and ways to prevent and control these diseases, providers will need to adjust their recommendations to match the new knowledge. The provider needs to continually learn to become aware of new evidence in relation to oral diseases, the efficacy and safety of self-care products, and procedures to prevent oral diseases. Development of a self-care plan should follow a systematic approach that incorporates prescribed techniques based on sound evidence so as to enhance plaque removal and reduction of risk without causing trauma to the hard and soft oral tissues. Moreover, the American Dental Association has a seal of approval program that can be used when evaluating products for patients.[36]

This chapter will discuss various supplemental self-care aids for oral hygiene (Table 10–3 ■), their application (Table 10–4 ■), evidence of their effectiveness, and their potential for trauma. This information is for the practitioner's consideration in developing supplemental self-care recommendations. This discussion includes self-care aids for interdental cleaning, as well as a general discussion of self-care for patients with malodor, implants, and dentures.

■ **Table 10–3**   Supplemental Self-Care Aid

- Dental floss
- Dental floss holder
- Dental floss threader
- Automated flosser
- Interproximal brush
- Uni-tuft brush
- Toothpick
- Toothpick holder
- Wooden or plastic triangular stick
- Rubber or plastic tip
- Yarn
- Pipe cleaner
- Gauze strip
- Tongue cleaners

■ **Table 10–4**   Application of Interproximal Supplemental Aids

- Proximal surfaces
- Hard-to-reach areas
- Rotated teeth
- Malaligned teeth
- Partially erupted teeth
- Irregular tooth morphology
- Embrasure spaces
- Isolated teeth[a]
- Furcations
- Orthodontic appliances
- Implants
- Fixed prosthetic appliances

[a]An isolated tooth occurs when the teeth that normally surround the tooth are missing.

ORAL HEALTH SELF-CARE

Self-care includes all activities and decisions made by an individual in relation to the prevention, diagnosis, and treatment of personal ill health, and the maintenance or control of chronic conditions. This concept, as applied to care of the oral cavity, is referred to as **oral self-care** or **oral health self-care.** The term is used in place of earlier terms such as *personal plaque control* and *oral physiotherapy* to emphasize the client's responsibility for their preventive oral health decisions and practices. One primary purpose of oral health self-care is to prevent or arrest periodontal diseases and caries by reducing plaque accumulation.[1,2] Less-than-optimal oral self-care is regarded as a major risk factor for oral diseases. To determine the most appropriate oral self-care practices for each individual, the oral health professional must complete a risk assessment that is based on the results of a comprehensive assessment, as discussed previously (Table 10–2).

On the basis of the assessment, an oral health self-care plan should be recommended before initiating therapy for treatment of disease. It is adjusted as needed after therapy, according to the results of evaluation. A one-size-fits-all approach to making recommendations to patients regarding their oral self-care plan does not work. There is no universally accepted oral hygiene method, practice, device, or frequency of cleaning.[10] Critical thinking must be applied to develop an individualized, appropriate oral hygiene regimen based on the dictates of the oral condition, personal preferences, abilities, dexterity, and lifestyle of the individual.[37]

Once the oral health self-care plan has been developed, adequate instruction in the use of any recommended method or device must be provided. Selecting the right device, minimizing the number of recommended devices, simplifying the instructions, and providing effective strategies to motivate the patient will help promote successful implementation of, and increase compliance with, the oral self-care plan. Instructions should include the strategies of co-discovery, observation, explanation, demonstration, and request for a return demonstration to assess understanding.[31] **Co-discovery** is the process in which the oral care professional explains diagnostic methods and results to the patient during dental examinations; this sharing of information allows the patient and professional to learn about the patient's oral condition at the same time. In addition, reasons for noncompliance should be explored so they can be addressed in an attempt to overcome them.[25]

FREQUENCY OF SELF-CARE

Although mechanical plaque removal is important to the prevention of dental caries, it appears that only a very high level of personal mechanical plaque removal impacts the dental caries rate. This level is difficult for the average person to sustain.[10] Also, it is not known at what developmental stage plaque becomes cariogenic. Fluorides and appropriate dietary control should be emphasized, in addition to interproximal plaque removal, for optimal effect on the caries rate of proximal surfaces.[16] According to a study correlating caries with daily flossing, it seems advisable to remove interproximal plaque at least once every 24 hours for caries prevention.[10,20] More frequent toothbrushing with a fluoride dentifrice will provide greater protection.

Research has shown that effective oral hygiene every 48 hours is compatible with gingival health.[10] With more daily attempts at plaque removal, however, it is more probable that the additive efforts will maximize the removal of plaque. Intervals that exceed 48 hours between removal of plaque biofilm will likely result in development of gingivitis.[17] For those with existing gingival inflammation or periodontal infection, plaque removal every 48 hours is not frequent enough.[6] It has been shown that colonization and maturation of plaque occurs more rapidly in the presence of inflammation.[38] Therefore, to control gingivitis versus preventing its onset, patients should practice the meticulous removal of plaque biofilm from all surfaces at least on a daily basis. Another factor in the decision of frequency is the patient's susceptibility to gingivitis and periodontitis. Susceptible patients require more frequent cleaning to prevent inflammation.

Because the ideal frequency of interproximal plaque removal has not been identified, individual factors such as the amount of inflammation, susceptibility to caries, gingivitis, and periodontitis, plaque removal efficiency, and accumulation and **virulence** (relative power and degree of pathogenicity) of plaque must be considered in the recommendation of frequency. The frequency should be between 12 and 48 hours depending on these factors.[39] Determining the risk factors that increase susceptibility to caries and periodontal diseases can identify which individuals need consistent interproximal cleaning, and at what frequency. Regardless of the disease of interest, the frequency of mechanical plaque removal for self-care must be tailored to the patient. **Oral cleanliness,** defined as all surfaces of all teeth being plaque-free, can be achieved by most patients who adhere to the traditional recommendation of brushing twice a day and flossing once a day.[10]

The length of time that should be devoted to self-care is also not consistent. How much time is needed will depend on the degree of susceptibility, the extent of periodontal breakdown, the condition of the teeth and restorations, the patient's dexterity and motor skills, and the presence of obstacles to self-care.[40]

DENTAL FLOSS

Dental floss is best indicated for plaque and debris removal from a type I **embrasure** (space formed by the contour and position of adjacent teeth). In a type I embrasure, the papilla fills the interproximal space and the teeth are in contact. For type II and III embrasures (Figure 10–1 ■), devices other than floss may be more effective in removing plaque from proximal surfaces.[39] Effective use of dental floss accomplishes the following objectives:

1. Removes plaque and debris that adheres to proximal surfaces of the teeth and restorations, orthodontic appliances, undersurfaces of fixed prostheses and **pontics** (artificial teeth set in a bridge), and implant abutments.[41–50]
2. Helps to control bleeding even before scaling and root planing has been initiated.[51]
3. Prevents the formation of calculus.[52]
4. Aids the clinician in identifying the presence of interproximal calculus deposits, overhanging restorations, or interproximal carious lesions.

5. May arrest or prevent interproximal carious lesions.[20,53]
6. Reduces gingival bleeding and inflammation.[41,51]
7. Reduces malodor.[41]
8. May be used as a vehicle for the application of polishing or chemotherapeutic agents to interproximal and subgingival areas.[54,55]

Not all interproximal contact areas, whether natural or restored, have the same configuration (contour). Consequently, several types of dental floss are available to accommodate these differences. Dental floss varies from thin unwaxed varieties to thicker waxed tapes, and include variable-thickness floss. Unwaxed floss is frequently recommended because it is thin and slips easily through tight contact areas. Thin silk floss has the advantage of "squeaking" when the proximal surface is clean. However, unwaxed floss can fray or tear if used around heavy calculus deposits, defective and overhanging restorations, or **rotated teeth** (teeth whose long axis is not in the normal occlusal position), which may discourage continued use. In these situations, shred-resistant, lightly waxed, or waxed floss are recommended. Various types of floss are presented in Table 10–5 ■ and Figure 10–2 ■.

Waxed dental tape, unlike round dental floss, is broad and flat, and may be effective in an interproximal space that does not have tight contact points. Tape is preferred if used with dentifrice for interproximal stain removal. Some types of unwaxed floss, such as those made of **polytetrafluoroethylene** (PTFE, Teflon-like), are stronger and more shred-resistant. Patients who have

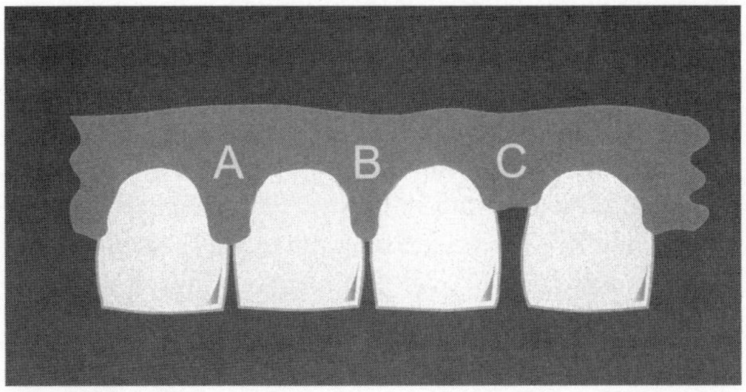

■ **FIGURE 10–1** Embrasure types. **A.** Type I—papilla fills interproximal space. **B.** Type II—slight to moderate recession of papilla. **C.** Type III—extensive recession or complete loss of papilla.

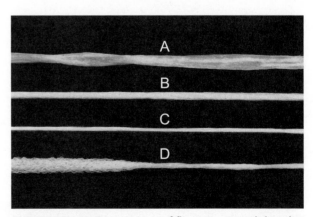

■ **FIGURE 10–2** Varieties of floss. **A.** Waxed dental tape. **B.** Waxed dental floss. **C.** Unwaxed round floss. **D.** Variable-thickness floss.

■ **Table 10–5**   Comparison of Various Types of Dental Floss

Type of Floss	Indications	Advantages	Disadvantages
Waxed dental tape (broad/flat)	Embrasure: II & III Loose contact Large surface areas Can use with dentifrice	Tear resistance More control	Difficult to use in tight contacts
Waxed dental floss	Embrasure: I Around rough tooth surfaces & restorations	Strength and durability Shred resistance Ease of insertion Prevents tissue trauma	Patient discomfort due to thickness
Unwaxed round floss	Embrasure: I Tight contacts	Slips in easily	Tears easily on contact with calculus and defective restorations Patient discouragement
Tufted Super floss (stiff end) Variable thickness	Embrasure: II & III Fixed bridge (stiff end) Exposed furcation Orthodontic appliances Implant prosthesis	Covers greater surface area Stiff end Easier insertion Ease of reaching hard-to-access areas Easier to use than floss threaders	Requires coordination Catches on rough surfaces
Colored floss	Visualization of plaque and debris Use by beginner Use by those with weak eyesight	Motivational and educational Increases compliance	NA
Flavored floss	More appealing Lack of motivation	Motivational Easy to see	NA
Impregnated floss/tape, containing fluoride, baking soda, herbal extracts, abrasives, or antimicrobials	Caries control Therapeutic effect on gingiva	Ease of application to hard-to-access areas	Abrasiveness of some agents Efficacy not well documented

NA, not applicable.

tight contacts or rough proximal tooth surfaces and rough restorations have been shown to prefer PTFE floss.[56]

Another variety of dental floss is **variable-thickness floss,** which has increments of soft tufts alternating with standard floss. The standard floss can be passed through the contacts, and the tufts can be used to clean larger proximal surface areas. Variable-thickness floss may be recommended for use in cleaning implant abutments, areas with open contacts, wide embrasures, or sites where recession and bone loss permit access to furcations. Another type of tufted floss is a thicker mesh that stretches for easy insertion. It is also useful to remove plaque from the distal aspect of the most distal tooth in all quadrants. Some tufted floss has a stiff end to allow for threading under bridges, beneath tight contact areas, under pontics, through exposed furcations, and around

orthodontic wires (Figure 10–3 ■) without having to use floss threaders.

Some brands of dental floss and tape are colored and/or flavored. In addition to increased appeal, color provides a visual contrast to plaque and oral debris, thus enabling one to see what is being removed and possibly increasing the motivation to floss. One study indicated a user preference for waxed over unwaxed floss and mint-flavored waxed floss over plain waxed floss.[57]

Various agents have been impregnated into dental floss, and have the potential to help prevent and control oral diseases. Examples of these include floss treated with baking soda, fluoride, herbal extracts, antimicrobial agents, or abrasives for whitening. In studies conducted in Sweden, use of floss with a chlorhexidine gel has been shown to reduce caries incidence in children.[54] A study with fluoride

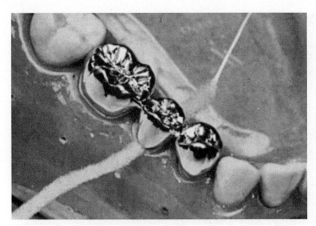

■ **FIGURE 10–3**   Variable-thickness floss with stiff end used to clean under the pontic and on the proximal surfaces of abutments of a fixed bridge.
(Courtesy of Dr. Linda S. Scheirton, Creighton University, Omaha, NE.)

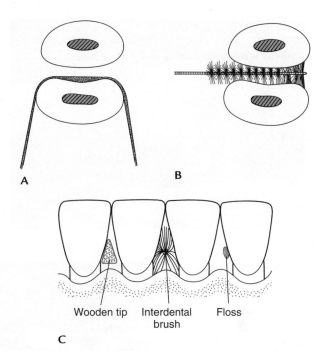

Wooden tip   Interdental   Floss
brush

C

■ **FIGURE 10–4**   Surface coverage comparison of different interdental aids. **A.** Floss adapted to a mesial surface of a maxillary molar shows its inability to fully cover the concave surface. **B.** Interproximal brush in the same area shows how it adapts into the concave surface. **C.** Compares access of a wooden triangular stick, an interdental brush, and dental floss in an open embrasure.
(From The Clinical Practice of Dental Hygiene. Copyright © 2005 by Lippincott Williams & Wilkins.)

impregnated dental floss demonstrated 10 times higher fluoride concentration of the saliva in the treated interproximal sites, which lasted up to 60 minutes for some sites.[55]

Clinical trials have shown no significant differences in the plaque removal efficacy of various types of floss, including the cleansing ability of unwaxed floss compared with waxed floss.[42,57–62] Wax residue has not been found on tooth surfaces cleaned with waxed floss.[63] In addition, no clear differences have been demonstrated in comfort and ease of use of different types of floss.[60] Study participants have expressed varying preferences in different studies, sometimes for waxed floss, sometimes for tape, and sometimes for polytetrafluoroethylene (Glide) floss.[56–64] One study found that a difference in force is required to use the thicker floss types.[59] The issues of preference and force could affect flossing frequency. Because the evidence does not identify a best type of floss, recommendations should be based on the patient's specific oral conditions, preference, and ability.

A limitation of flossing is its inability to conform to, or take the same shape as, a concave proximal root surface such as the mesial surface of the maxillary premolar. When these surfaces are exposed, other interproximal devices should be considered as supplements to clean those surfaces more effectively (Figure 10–4 ■). These aids are discussed in a later section of this chapter.

Dental Flossing Methods

Two frequently used flossing methods are the spool method and the circle, or loop, method. Both facilitate control of the floss and ease of handling. The spool method is particularly suited for teenagers and adults who have acquired the necessary neuromuscular coordination required to use floss. The loop method is suited for children as well as adults with less nimble hands or physical limitations caused by conditions such as poor muscular coordination or arthritis. Flossing is a complex skill. Therefore, until children develop adequate dexterity, usually around the age of 10 to 12 years, their attempts at flossing will be ineffective, and an adult should perform flossing on the child.[65] Younger children whose teeth still exhibit primate spaces with no interproximal contacts will not require flossing.

In the **spool method of flossing,** a piece of floss approximately 18 inches long is used. The bulk of the floss is lightly wound around the middle finger. Space should be left between wraps to avoid impairing circulation to the fingers (Figure 10–5A ■). The rest of the floss is similarly wound around the same finger of the opposite hand. This finger can wind, or take up, the

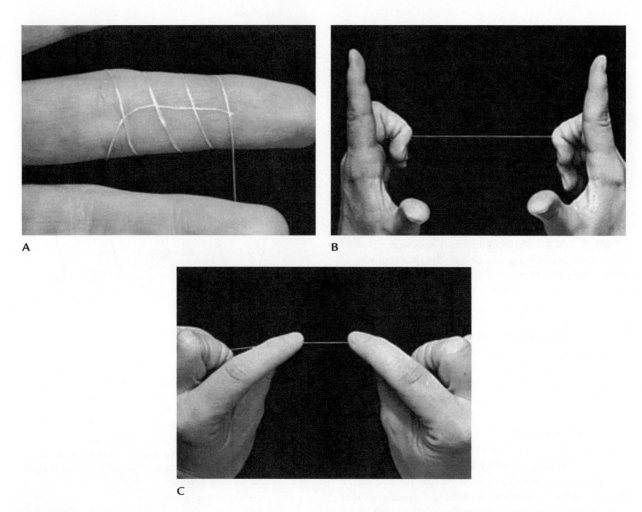

A

B

C

■ **FIGURE 10–5**   Spool method of flossing. **A.** Floss is lightly wound and spaced around the middle finger of each hand. **B.** The last three fingers are clenched, pulling the floss taut and leaving the index finger and the thumb of each hand free. **C.** The floss is held with the index finger and thumb of each hand by grasping a section three-quarters to 1 in. long between the hands.
(Courtesy of Dr. Linda S. Scheirton, Creighton University, Omaha, NE.)

floss as it becomes soiled or frayed to permit access to an unused portion. The last three fingers are clenched and the hands are moved apart, pulling the floss taut, thus leaving the thumb and index finger of each hand free (Figure 10–5B ■). The floss is then secured with the index finger and thumb of each hand by grasping a section three-quarters to 1 inch in length between the hands (Figure 10–5C ■). Once in the mouth, the floss is guided with the index fingers to floss the mandibular teeth, or with the thumbs to floss the maxillary teeth.

In the **loop method of flossing,** the ends of the 18-inch piece of floss are tied in a knot. All of the fingers, but not the thumbs, of the two hands are placed close to one another within the loop (Figure 10–6 ■). In both flossing methods, the same basic procedures are followed. The thumb and index finger of each hand are used in various combinations to guide the floss between the teeth.

When inserting floss, it is gently eased between the teeth with a seesaw motion at the contact point. The gentle seesaw motion flattens the floss, making it possible to ease through the contact point and prevent snapping it through, thus avoiding trauma to the interdental papilla (Figure 10–7A ■). Once past the contact point, the floss is adapted to each interproximal surface by creating a C-shape (Figure 10–7B ■). The floss is then directed apically into the sulcus and back to the contact area (up and

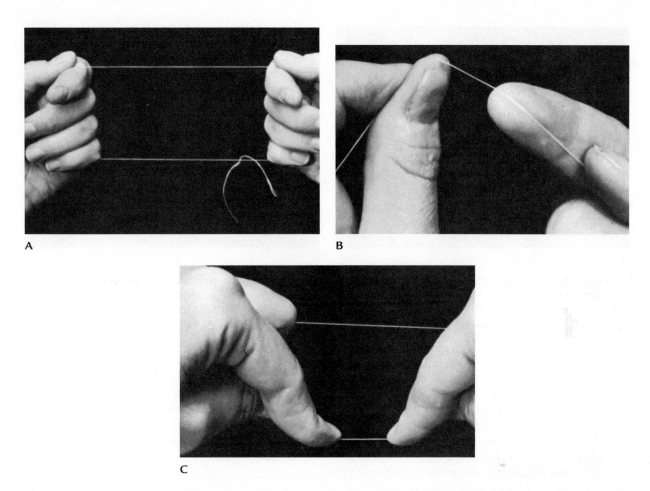

■ FIGURE 10–6   Loop method of flossing. **A.** All fingers except the thumbs are placed within the loop for easy maneuverability. **B.** For the mandibular teeth, the floss is guided with the two index fingers. **C.** For the maxillary teeth, the floss is guided with two thumbs or one thumb and one index finger.
(Courtesy of Dr. Linda S. Scheirton, Creighton University, Omaha, NE.)

down against the side of the tooth) several times or until the tooth surface is clean. This stroke must be gentle to avoid damaging the sulcular area and causing floss cuts. The number of strokes required depends on the thickness of the plaque. If floss is used daily, fewer strokes are required. Also, the use of Teflon-type floss may require more strokes to "grab" the plaque for complete removal. The procedure is repeated on the adjacent tooth in the proximal area; care is used to prevent damage to the papilla while readapting the floss to the adjacent tooth. A clean, unused portion should be used for each interproximal area to prevent fraying as well as for sanitary purposes.

In general, flossing is best performed by cleaning each tooth in succession, including the distal surface of the last tooth in each quadrant. The individual should be assisted with problem areas and encouraged to use whichever method produces the best results.

Criteria for evaluation are based on the efficacy of plaque removal and safety of the flossing method. Because adequate flossing will result in reduction of gingival inflammation and bleeding as well as less calculus formation, these results are cues available for evaluation. Incorrect flossing can often be detected through clinical observation of the technique (Figure 10–8 ■).

Significant damage from flossing has been reported.[66–69] Signs that suggest incorrect use of dental floss include gingival cuts, soft tissue **clefting** (formation of a V-shaped slit in the gingival that extends apically from the gingival margin) and cervical wear on interproximal root surfaces (Figure 10–9 ■). If flossing

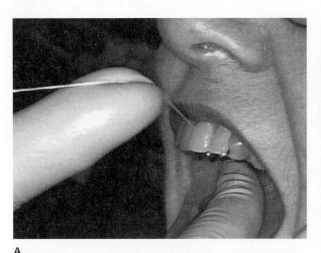

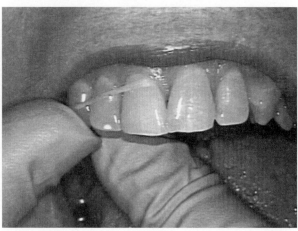

A   B

■ **FIGURE 10–7**   Flossing technique. **A.** The floss is gently inserted between the teeth with a back-and-forth sawing motion at the contact point, after which **B.** the floss is adapted to each proximal surface by creating a C-shape, directed apically into the sulcus. Then the floss is slid down to the contact area with pressure against the proximal surface, repeating several times or until the surface is clean.

trauma is evident, further instruction should be given until the individual has become adept.

It is important to note that a flossing habit has traditionally been difficult for people to embrace. In reality, only a very small proportion of individuals practice daily flossing. Findings have ranged from 2% to 33% of the population.[52,70–76] Floss may be superior to other interproximal cleaning methods, but for those who have not or will not adopt a flossing behavior, another interproximal device may be more effective than no interproximal cleaning.[77] A less-effective device used on a regular basis is superior to sporadic use of a more-effective device. A frank discussion of the patient's willingness to floss or use another interdental device will aid in the discussion of alternatives.

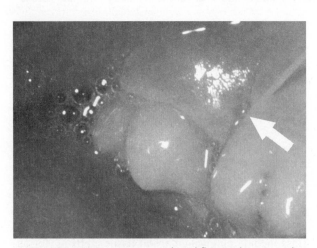

■ **FIGURE 10–8**   Improper dental floss technique with potential for gingival "floss-cuts" (arrow). Floss should adapt to the proximal surface in a C-shape without cutting into the gingiva.

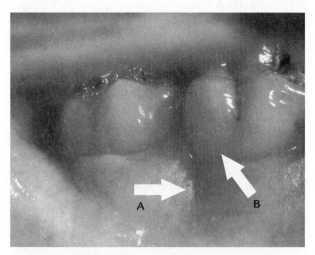

■ **FIGURE 10–9**   Flossing damage. **A.** Gingival "floss cut" (arrow) created by failure to adapt floss to interproximal surface in a C-shape. **B.** Groove created on mesial aspect of tooth (arrow) caused by movement of floss in buccolingual (horizontal) rather than apico-occlusal (vertical) direction.

Sometimes individuals agree to adopt a behavior, because this is what the clinician wants to hear. Axelsson has referred to this reaction as a "hasty affirmative in a moment of suddenly inspired courage."[78]

Although the occurrence is uncommon, **bacterial endocarditis** (bacteria-induced inflammation or infection of the heart and its valves) has been reported in susceptible individuals who have gingivitis or periodontitis and floss only sporadically.[79,80] One study demonstrated that patients who delayed flossing from 1 to 4 days developed **bacteremias** (presence of bacteria in the blood) 86% of the time.[81] Susceptible patients should be made aware of this risk and counseled to floss or practice interproximal plaque removal in some other manner.[80,82]

Despite low compliance, flossing should be encouraged. Research has shown that non-flossers do not believe they can floss effectively and easily, yet they are able to develop the skill with practice.[83] Other studies have demonstrated that continual re-instruction and reinforcement are needed to help patients maintain the flossing habit.[84,85] The individual's participation in selecting an interproximal cleaning device and planning a regimen is crucial to improving and/or enhancing compliance.[31,86] Proper instruction and practice allows most motivated adults to master either the spool or loop method of flossing. In some circumstances, the use of a floss holder, floss threader, variable-thickness floss, or pre-cut floss strands with a stiff end may be more effective. Sometimes, other alternatives are needed; these will be discussed later in this chapter.

Dental Floss Holder

The **dental floss holder** is a device that holds floss and eliminates the need for placing fingers in the mouth. It is recommended for individuals with:

- Physical disabilities[87]
- Poor manual dexterity[88]
- Large hands[88]
- Limited mouth opening[88]
- A strong gag reflex[89]
- Low motivation for traditional flossing[90]

The floss holder may also be helpful when one person is assisting another with flossing.

Several studies have demonstrated that the use of a floss holder was equivalent to finger flossing in reducing plaque, inflammation, and bleeding, with no significant trauma found as a result of its use.[88–92] In these same studies, a significant majority of individuals preferred the floss holder over finger-manipulated flossing. It has been suggested that the use of a floss holder may be more effective in establishing a regular flossing habit in non-flossers, and should be considered when individuals experience difficulty with manual flossing.[91]

In one study, individuals tended to prefer the technique they learned first, whether it was finger flossing or the use of a floss holder.[89] Dental students included in another study had a preference for finger flossing.[88] Results of these studies suggest that dental professionals may have a preference for finger flossing because they have an established finger-flossing habit and because they have high manual dexterity. As a result, they may resist recommending floss holders. Because the use of a floss holder requires thorough instruction to use it effectively and safely, it is important that dental professionals consider this option to help non-flossing patients become flossers.

A variety of different floss-holder designs are available (Figure 10–10 ■). Most commonly, they consist of a yoke-like device with a 3/4- to 1-inch space between the two prongs of the yoke. The floss is secured tightly between the two prongs, and the handle is grasped to guide the floss during use. The width and length of the handle are important features to consider when recommending the use of a floss holder to those with limited gripping abilities.[87] Most floss holders require that floss be strung around various parts of the holder before each use. This assembly mechanism allows for re-threading of the floss whenever the working portion becomes soiled or begins to fray. Some devices have a floss reservoir in the handle. This improvement allows for ease of threading and advancing the floss while maintaining the proper tautness.

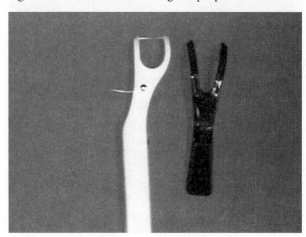

■ **FIGURE 10–10**   A variety of floss holders.

Several brands of pre-threaded, one-time-use floss holders are available (Figure 10–11 ■). They require minimal dexterity and control the floss tension, factors that may help improve compliance. However, the expense of disposable floss aids may reduce compliance. One study of a disposable floss aid found equivalent plaque, inflammation, and bleeding reduction compared with finger flossing, with no significant gingival trauma. Participants had a slight preference for the disposable floss aid compared with using regular floss.[93]

Use of a floss holder involves inserting the floss interproximally, and applying the same technique used for finger-manipulated flossing. Once through the contact point, the floss and holder are pushed distally to clean the mesial surface of a tooth or pulled mesially to clean the distal surface (Figure 10–12 ■). This pulling or pushing motion makes the floss conform to the tooth convexities, thus allowing the floss to slide apically into the sulcus. The floss is then activated in the same manner as with finger-manipulated flossing, by moving the floss in the direction of the long axis of the tooth.

Strict attention should be given to achieving the desired floss tension during assembly of the floss holder. To ensure tautness, the user can force the prongs together while securing the floss. The most persistent problems with the yoke-like devices are the difficulties in loading and threading the floss, and maintaining tension of the floss between the prongs, as well as the decreased ability to adapt the floss into a C-shape around the proximal surface. Any device recommended should allow for ease

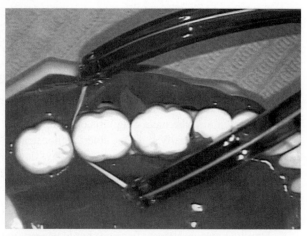

■ **FIGURE 10–12** Correct use of a floss holder on the distal surface of a second molar. Floss is taut, and the holder is pulled forward to adapt the floss to the distal surface in a C-shape. Then the floss is slid up and down to floss the surface in the usual manner.

of threading, maintenance of proper tautness, and easy manipulation by the user.

Dental Floss Threader

A **dental floss threader** is a plastic loop into which a length of floss is inserted, similar to threading a needle. The threader is used to carry the floss interproximally in the following circumstances:

- Through embrasure areas under contact points that are too tight for floss insertion.
- Between the proximal surface and gingiva of abutment teeth of fixed prostheses.
- Under pontics.
- Around orthodontic appliances.
- Between splinted teeth.

Care should be taken to prevent trauma by not forcing the stiff end of the floss threader into the gingival tissues. When cleaning under a fixed bridge, the floss threader is inserted from the facial aspect and pulled completely through to the lingual aspect until the floss is against the abutment or pontic (Figure 10–13A ■). The floss may then be disengaged from the threader. The floss is adapted to one abutment tooth surface in the area of the embrasure (Figure 10–13B ■) and then moved in the direction of the long axis of the tooth to remove plaque from the

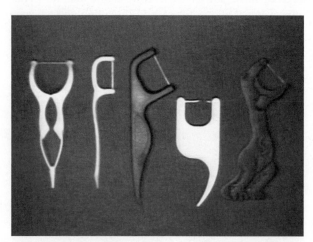

■ **FIGURE 10–11** A variety of pre-threaded floss holders for one-time use.

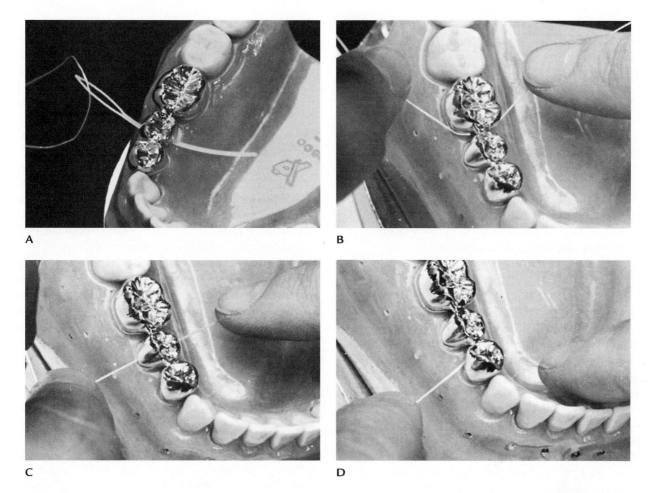

■ **FIGURE 10–13**   Flossing under a fixed bridge **A.** The floss threader is inserted under the pontic from the facial aspect and pulled completely through to the lingual. **B.** The floss is adapted in a C-shape to one abutment proximal tooth surface to floss that surface in the normal manner. **C.** The floss is glided under the pontic. **D.** The floss is adapted to the opposite abutment proximal tooth surface with a C-shape to floss that surface in the usual manner.
(Courtesy of Dr. Linda S. Scheirton, Creighton University, Omaha, NE.)

proximal surface. It is important to glide the floss through the space between the pontic and the gingiva to clean the underside of the pontic (Figure 10–13C ■). After cleaning the underside of the pontic, it is necessary to slide the floss to the opposite proximal surface (Figure 10–13D ■). Removal of the floss from between the abutment and pontic is accomplished by pulling it out from the facial aspect.

OTHER INTERDENTAL AIDS

Because periodontal diseases and dental caries develop most frequently in the interdental and proximal areas, it is important to select effective devices to remove plaque from the proximal tooth surfaces. Dental floss has been recognized as an effective device for cleaning the interdental areas.[10,15,39] However, low patient compliance and limited effectiveness of floss in open embrasure spaces and exposed root concavities has led to a search for alternative interproximal aids to supplement toothbrushing.[74,94–97]

Toothbrushing and flossing are the standard means of plaque removal for a healthy dentition.[98,99] However, clinical attachment loss as a result of disease or trauma and difficult-to-reach sites will likely require selected aids as a supplement to toothbrushing and flossing. Because clinical attachment loss results in root exposure, the surface becomes concave, limiting the effectiveness of dental floss.

Despite the fact that effective toothbrushing leaves 30% of tooth surfaces untouched, and removes only about 50% of plaque present on the teeth, only 2% to 32% of people floss regularly, regardless of how often they are instructed.[16,70–75,100,101] Patient compliance with manual flossing is low, because it is a complex and time-consuming task that requires a great deal of coordination, manual dexterity, and motivation.[15] People get discouraged about flossing, because it is technique-sensitive, is difficult to learn, can turn the fingertips blue, requires concentration, and demands the use of two hands. Others think it must be done first thing in the morning or last thing at night, when they have little time and energy for it.

The selection of an alternative aid must be based on the patient's periodontal condition, ability, and preference.[101–104] Although it is notable to help non-flossers find ways to supplement toothbrushing, it is also important to understand that, in some cases, use of an alternative aid instead of flossing may compromise the patient's oral hygiene and ultimately their future oral health. Also, many aids have the potential to cause trauma to soft and hard tissues. Hence, evidence-based decisions should be made concerning the selection of aids, and they should be recommended with caution. In addition, patients should be fully informed of any risks associated with their oral hygiene practices.

The number of aids that are recommended should be limited to two or three to avoid overwhelming the patient. Research indicates that patients will use only this many aids no matter how many are recommended.[30,105]

A thorough assessment is important to determine which aids might be most useful. In addition, careful instruction, monitoring, and reinforcement are required for successful application of supplemental aids. Although these aids may be easier to use than dental floss, all aids require dexterity, time, and motivation.[10]

Automated Flosser

Because of poor compliance with flossing, **automated flossers** have been developed in an attempt to find a device to replace floss and provide effective interproximal plaque removal without causing trauma. These automated cleaners are marketed as power flossers for patients who are unable or unwilling to floss.[106] Because automated flossers are more convenient to use, can be used with one hand, and require less manual dexterity,[103]

they may be helpful for individuals who are handicapped or have dexterity issues. Numerous studies with various designs have indicated that power flossers are comparable to dental floss in their ability to remove plaque, and improve gingivitis and bleeding, with no significant pathology resulting from their use.[88,95,103,107–110,111] Studies showed that patients preferred the use of an automatic flosser compared with dental floss, which is likely to increase compliance with its use.[107,109,111]

It is especially difficult to clean around permanent orthodontic appliances. In one study, the use of an automated interdental cleaning device was compared with manual flossing in patients with **lingual brackets,** and was found to be as effective as meticulous flossing. Participants preferred the use of the automatic flosser.[111]

Various automated flosser designs have been developed. Two major units currently available in the United States have been tested for efficacy and safety. The Waterpik Power Flosser has a single nylon filament tip that moves at 10,000 linear strokes per minute (Figure 10–14 ■).[109,111] The tip spins rapidly in the interproximal space to clean the proximal surfaces. This design can be used when it is not possible to pass floss through the contact of adjacent teeth to reach the interdental space. The Oral B Hummingbird[95] has a "flossette," which is similar in appearance and use to a very small floss holder (Figure 10–15 ■). The user guides the floss into the interproximal space. When the device is turned on, the floss moves side to side, and in an orbital motion.[112] Results of investigations with both

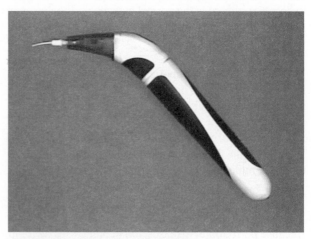

■ **FIGURE 10–14** Automated floss holder with a single nylon filament tip (WaterPik).

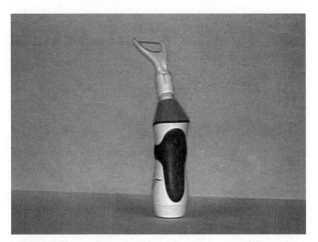

■ **FIGURE 10–15**   Hummingbird automated flosser. (Courtesy of Mark McIntyre, Oral-B.)

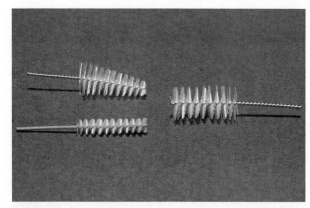

■ **FIGURE 10–17**   Replaceable interproximal brush inserts in varying sizes and shapes.

designs have shown that they safely clean the proximal surfaces supragingivally and subgingivally, and control gingivitis and bleeding as effectively as dental floss.

Interproximal Brush

Interproximal brushes, also known as **interdental brushes,** are manufactured in different sizes and designs (Figure 10–16 ■). The brush consists of a plastic handle and a small tapered or cylindric filamentous brush tip (Figure 10–17 ■) that is either attached to the handle (non-replaceable) or inserted into the handle (replaceable). Some designs have a straight handle, and others have an angled handle. The angled handle provides

better access to difficult-to-reach areas. The core of the brush that holds the bristles is made of plastic, wire, or nylon-coated wire.[113]

Interdental brushes are recommended for interproximal areas where the papilla is missing or shortened (type II & III embrasures) and root concavities[114] (Figure 10–18 ■). The interproximal brush can also be used to effectively clean around orthodontic appliances (Figure 10–19 ■), space maintainers, small **diastemas** (spaces between adjacent teeth), class IV furcations (Figure 10–20 ■), fixed prostheses (Figure 10–21 ■), splints, and dental implants, when spaces are large enough to easily receive the device. Caution should be

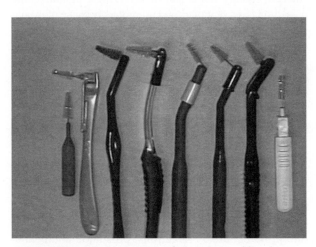

■ **FIGURE 10–16**   Variety of interproximal brushes.

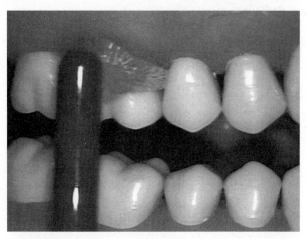

■ **FIGURE 10–18**   Interproximal brush in an open embrasure space with the brush following the contour of the gingiva.

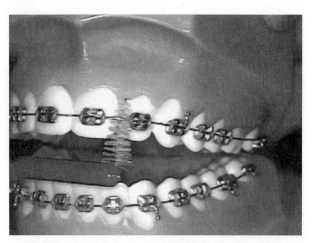

■ **FIGURE 10–19** Interproximal brush applied to orthodontic appliances.

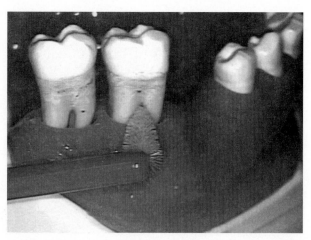

■ **FIGURE 10–20** Interproximal brush directed into an open furcation.

exercised to prevent damage to the tooth or soft tissues from the firm wire or plastic core of the brush. Only brushes with a plastic or nylon-coated core should be used around implant abutments to prevent scratching of the titanium surface.[115]

The brush tip should be moistened and inserted at an angle following the contour of the gingiva.[116] A buccolingual movement is used to remove plaque and debris. The type of embrasure determines the selection of the design and size of the interdental brush. The recommended brush tip should be slightly larger than the inter-

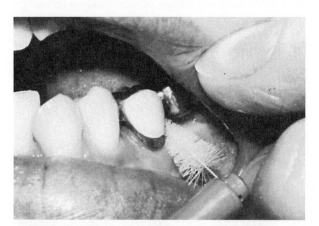

■ **FIGURE 10–21** Interproximal brush inserted between the abutment and pontic of a fixed prosthesis at an angle approximating the gingival contour. Brush can be inserted under the pontic if space allows.
(Courtesy of Dr. Linda S. Scheirton, Creighton University, Omaha, NE.)

proximal space, and should provide equal coverage on each proximal surface to adequately clean the two adjacent proximal surfaces.

Numerous studies have demonstrated the efficacy of interproximal brushes in removing plaque and reducing bleeding.[117–120] In open embrasures, these brushes are superior to other interdental devices, including dental floss, because the bristles fill the space and reach the surfaces within the root concavities. In one investigation, the interproximal brush removed plaque more effectively than waxed dental floss from interproximal surfaces in type III embrasure spaces. The interdental brush removed plaque from the distal and mesial surfaces of exposed root surfaces equally, but dental floss left more plaque on the mesial surfaces of molars and premolars because of mesial root concavities.[121] A more recent study showed that interproximal brushes, regardless of their shape, removed plaque better than dental floss from proximal surfaces of open embrasure spaces.[15] Another study found that use of the interproximal brush resulted in improved periodontal health, even before scaling and root planing.[51] Yet another study demonstrated that, with proper instruction, an interproximal brush, combined with dental floss, was more effective than a power flosser.[102]

A powered interproximal brush is available; its design is similar to interproximal brushes that have a handle. Upon activation, several end-rounded, 0.006-diameter bristle tufts oscillate to remove plaque from interproximal areas, furcations, prosthetic abutments, and implants. Studies have demonstrated that use of an automated interproximal brush with these characteristics was safe and effective in reducing gingivitis and removing plaque from accessible proximal surfaces.[122–124]

Interdental brushes can be used for delivery of antimicrobial, fluoride, and desensitizing agents by inserting the brush tip into the **medicament** (medicine or remedy) and applying it into the hard-to-access areas.[15] The use of antimicrobial agents in this manner can improve gingival health. However, in one study, researchers demonstrated that biofilm removal with the interdental brush had a greater effect on the reduction of gingivitis and bleeding than the added antimicrobial.[124]

Uni-Tuft Brush

The **uni-tuft brush,** also called **single-tuft** or **end-tuft brush,** consists of a small group of tufted bristles that are flat or tapered, and are attached to a straight or angled handle[113] (Figure 10–22 ■). The handles of some uni-tuft brushes can be bent by softening them in very hot or boiling water. An angled handle will allow easier access to hard-to-reach areas.[97] Uni-tuft brushes can be used as an alternative to floss for removal of plaque from specific sites, including the lingual surfaces of mandibular teeth, type III embrasures, distal surface of the most posterior teeth (Figure 10–23 ■), orthodontic appliances, crowded or misaligned teeth, and proximal surfaces of teeth adjacent to edentulous spaces. This device can be adapted to clean under and around dental appliances, including implant abutments and prostheses, and in

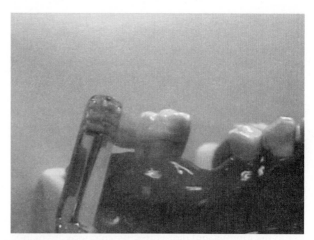

■ **FIGURE 10–23**   Adaptation of a uni-tuft brush against the distal surface of the last molar.

exposed furcations, as long as the space allows safe insertion of the device.[15]

The Sulcabrush (Figure 10–24 ■) is a specific, double-headed uni-tuft brush; the brush heads are on opposite ends of the handle and are at opposite angles. The brush heads are more finely tapered to provide better access to lingual surfaces at the gingival margin, in smaller embrasure spaces, and around crowded teeth.

Application starts by placing the brush into the embrasure space, furcation, or other appropriate area with gentle pressure. A combination of rotary motion and sulcular strokes with moderate pressure will result in effective cleaning.[71,116]

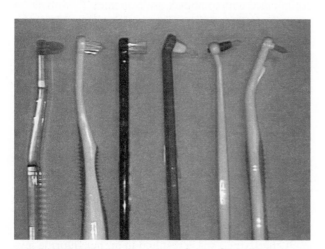

■ **FIGURE 10–22**   A variety of uni-tuft brushes.

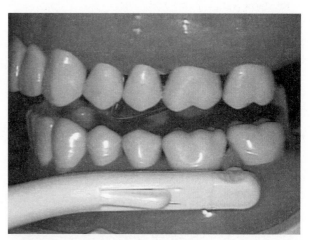

■ **FIGURE 10–24**   Application of Sulcabrush interproximally.

Toothpick

A historical review of toothpick use suggests that toothpicks are one of the earliest and most persistent means of picking the teeth.[125] The toothpick may date back to the days of the cave people, who probably used sticks to pick food from between the teeth.[126] Use of the toothpick is described by Shakespeare, and writings about table manners in the 1600s include references to the use of toothpicks.[127] Throughout history, toothpicks have been made from bronze, copper, gold, iron, silver, ivory, bone, bird claws, quills, straw, tortoise shell, whiskers, and carved wood.[125,128] Today, toothpicks are made of wood and are either round or rectangular. Round toothpicks are gentler to the gingiva and more effective in removing plaque biofilm.[129] Current recommendations to use toothpicks refer to round toothpicks.

Because improper use can result in damage to the oral tissues, proper use of the toothpick is an important aspect of oral hygiene self-care instruction. Oral injuries caused by improper use of toothpicks include splintering in the gingiva, trauma to and blunting (loss) of the interdental papilla (Figure 10–25 ■), recession, and grooves produced by abrasion at the cementoenamel junction (Figure 10–26 ■).[125,126,128] Toothpick injuries in the United States have been documented by the Centers for Disease Control and Prevention and the Consumer Products Safety Commission.[125,128] Injuries that have caused serious medical conditions and even death include young children poking the eyeball and ear; lodging of the toothpick in the esophagus, posterior **nares**

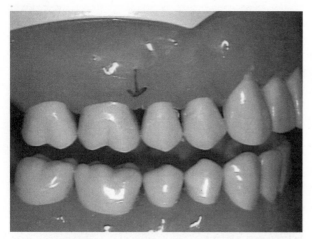

■ **FIGURE 10–25** Gingival trauma (blunting of the interdental papilla) caused by improper use of a tooth pick.

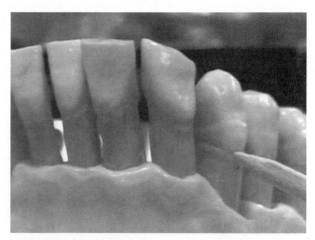

■ **FIGURE 10–26** Abrasion at the cementoenamel junction caused by improper use of a toothpick.

(openings between nasal cavity and nasopharynx), and gastrointestinal tract travel to distant sites in the body. Patients who use toothpicks should be made aware of the need for precaution to prevent serious injuries to themselves and others.

Consistent use of the toothpick can result in firm, resilient tissue. Effectiveness of toothpicks to remove plaque depends on the ability to make contact of the toothpick surface with the tooth surface. Therefore, it is more effective in smaller surface areas[129] and from the buccal aspect compared with the lingual.[77] Toothpick material with low surface hardness and high strength have been demonstrated to improve efficacy.[128] Toothpicks are generally considered easier to manipulate than floss, and compliance with toothpick use is greater.[105] Motivation is a primary factor in the success of the toothpick versus floss.[77] The proper technique for toothpick use is described in Table 10–6 ■.

Toothpicks have been suggested as a means of delivering antimicrobials and fluoride to the interproximal areas. Several studies that tested the effect of impregnating toothpicks with fluoride for caries control have shown positive results.[55,130,131] These studies have demonstrated that fluoride concentrations varied from 5 to 25 ppm, and fluoride release varied for different brands. One minute of treatment with a fluoridated toothpick resulted in 10 times higher fluoride levels in the approximal areas, which lasted up to 60 minutes after treatment. Use of a fresh toothpick in each approximal space resulted in higher fluoride levels than use of the same toothpick throughout the

■ **Table 10–6**   Technique for Proper Toothpick Use

- Premoisten the toothpick with saliva to soften the wood.
- Place the blunt tip of the toothpick at a right angle to the buccal and lingual surfaces.
- Place it at less than a 45-degree angle to extend just below the gingival margin.
- Pull or push it across the buccal or lingual surfaces from one interproximal space to the next.
- As the tip becomes frayed from use, use it as a small cleaning "brush" to rub the tooth surfaces.
- Interproximally, angle the toothpick horizontally, and use the sides of the toothpick to clean the approximal surfaces on either side of the interdental papilla.
- Use care with subgingival insertion, and refrain from vigorous interproximal use to avoid damage to the soft and hard oral tissues.

mouth. Use of fluoride-impregnated toothpicks three times a day inhibited further demineralization, lowered counts of microorganisms in plaque, and resulted in less depth of carious lesions in the dentin.

Other studies have found conflicting results concerning the value of toothpicks as a mechanism to deliver fluroide and antimicrobials. One study showed a limited reduction of dental plaque from a 1% chlorhexidine gel delivered by toothpick to the interproximals areas.[132] In another study toothpicks impregnated with chlorhexidine or fluoride showed no effect on plaque pH.[133] Further research is indicated in this area.

Toothpick Holder

Although a toothpick may be manipulated by hand, its effectiveness is improved by inserting it into a toothpick holder. This handle holds the toothpick securely at the proper angle in order to increase access and enhance proper adaptation of the toothpick in hard-to-reach areas. Using the toothpick in this way especially increases its effectiveness from the lingual aspect.[134] Use of the toothpick in the toothpick holder has been demonstrated to reduce gingival bleeding in non-surgically treated, plaque-induced gingivitis, and in patients with slight chronic periodontitis at a level equivalent to the use of floss.[135] However, it is important to remember that, as previously discussed, the toothpick has a greater potential to cause gingival recession, papillary blunting, and abrasion of the tooth surface, even when it is mounted in a toothpick holder.

A variety of toothpick holders are available commercially (Figure 10–27 ■). The toothpick is inserted into an adjustable plastic contra-angled handle, and the projecting end of the toothpick is broken off by snapping it in a downward direction. The broken end leaves a stem to prevent the tip from disengaging from the holder during use. The toothpick can be positioned at an acute angle (angle less than 90 degrees) on one end to access lingual surfaces, and at an obtuse angle (angle greater than 90 degrees but less than 180 degrees) on the other end to adapt to buccal surfaces (Figure 10–28 ■).

The use of the toothpick holder is indicated in the following circumstances:

- Removing biofilm along the gingival margin and within the gingival sulci or periodontal pockets (Figure 10–29 ■).
- Cleaning small concave proximal surfaces.
- Cleaning exposed furcation areas that are still in contact with underlying bone.
- Cleaning around orthodontic appliances and fixed prostheses.
- Applying chemotherapeutic agents, such as **burnishing** fluoride into the tooth surface to treat hypersensitivity, or delivering chlorhexidine into the gingival sulcus.

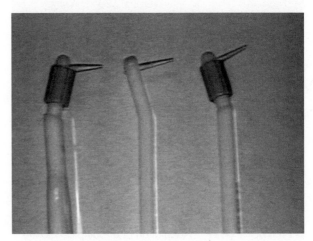

■ **FIGURE 10–27**   A variety of toothpick holders.

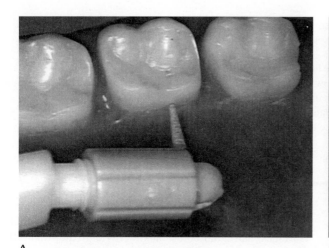

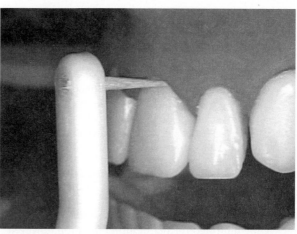

A   B

■ **FIGURE 10–28   A.** Adaptation of a toothpick to the lingual surfaces at the gingival margin of posterior teeth.
B. Adaptation of a toothpick to the facial surfaces at the gingival margin of anterior teeth.

Wooden or Plastic Triangular Stick

A modern adaptation of the toothpick is the triangular-shaped wooden or plastic stick.[134] (Figure 10–30 ■). Interproximal cleaning can be aided with these triangular sticks. Wooden sticks are made of balsa or birch wood, and are more pliable than plastic sticks. Wooden picks have another advantage over plastic picks; the wooden tip can be softened in the mouth by moistening with saliva. A softer, more pliable stick can be adapted more easily to the proximal surface for more effective cleaning, and has

less potential for gingival damage over time. These sticks are triangular in cross section (Figure 10–31 ■) to slide easily between the teeth, to conform to the shape of the embrasure space, and to reduce potential tissue trauma.

Triangular wood and plastic sticks should be used for only type II or III embrasures where the papilla does not completely fill the embrasure space.[71] The patient should be instructed in the correct use of these triangular sticks to prevent gingival damage caused by inappropriate use.[116] Instructions for use of the triangular

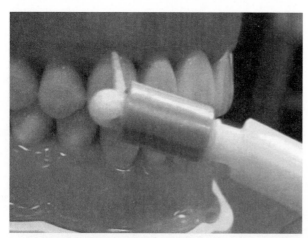

■ **FIGURE 10–29**   Adaptation of a toothpick into the gingival sulcus or periodontal pocket.

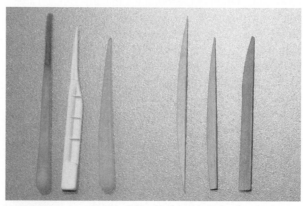

■ **FIGURE 10–30**   Variety of wooden and plastic triangular sticks. The three sticks at the left are plastic, and the one on the far left has a flocked design. The three sticks at the right are wooden. Note the balsa wood composition of the wooden stick on the far right compared with the other two of birch wood.

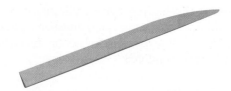

■ FIGURE 10–31 Cross-sectional drawing of a triangular wood stick.

wood stick are described in Table 10–7 ■ and illustrated in Figure 10–32 ■. In contrast to wood sticks, plastic sticks can be washed thoroughly and re-used.

Using triangular wood or plastic sticks to reduce biofilm accumulations has demonstrated a reduction in inflammation and bleeding sites.[134,136,137] These picks have been shown to reduce inflammation more in the coronal regions of the interproximal pocket than in the apical regions, and more from the buccal aspect than the lingual.[3] Wood triangular sticks have been shown to remove biofilm 2 to 3 mm subgingivally by depressing the papilla.[134] Triangular wood picks are not as effective as dental floss for biofilm removal from the lingual interproximal areas, but are more effective and less damaging to the tissues than round toothpicks.[77,129] Because wooden picks are more pliable than plastic, they may cause less gingival damage over time.

Rubber or Plastic Tip

Rubber or **plastic tips,** sometimes referred to as **rubber tip stimulators,** consist of a conical, flexible rubber or

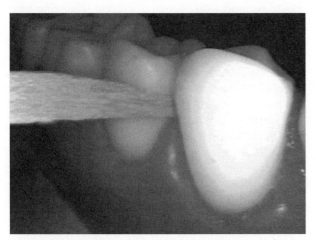

■ FIGURE 10–32 Placement of wooden triangular stick interproximally with the flat portion against the gingiva.

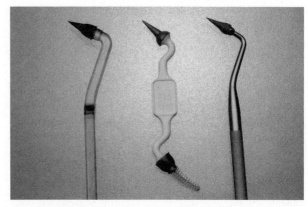

■ FIGURE 10–33 Variety of rubber tips.

plastic tip attached to a handle (Figure 10–33 ■). The tips made from plastic tend to be too rigid and may damage the gingiva.[116] Rubber tips are used primarily for gingival massage and recontouring of gingival papilla after periodontal therapy. Although a possible role for the rubber tip stimulator to increase gingival circulation, keratinization, and epithelial thickening has been proposed, the overall improvement in gingival health resulting from its use is more likely due to effective removal of plaque biofilm.[114]

■ Table 10–7 Directions for Use of a Triangular Wood Stick

- Moisten the end of the triangular wood stick to soften it.
- Insert the triangular wood stick interproximally from the buccal aspect.
- Place the flat surface, or base of the triangle, on the interdental papilla.
- Use a finger rest to help prevent applying too much pressure of the tip of the stick against the gingiva.
- Press against the interdental papilla to flatten it slightly.
- Angle the tip of the stick slightly coronally or incisally.
- Move the triangular wood stick in a buccolingual direction.
- Apply approximately four burnishing strokes with moderate pressure on each side of the embrasure.
- Discard the stick when the wood becomes splayed to prevent splinters from being forced into the gingiva. Splaying will likely occur after use in one quadrant or arch.
- Plastic sticks can be thoroughly washed and re-used.

Rubber tips can also be used to remove plaque and debris from exposed furcation areas, type II and III embrasure spaces, and along the gingival margin. The rubber tip is not recommended for type I embrasures and healthy gingival contour. The tip is inserted interproximally into an open embrasure space at a 90-degree angle. The side of the rubber tip should rest on the gingiva and against the exposed proximal tooth surfaces (Figure 10–34 ■). A buccolingual or small circular motion against the proximal surfaces is applied from both the lingual and labial aspects. The tip can also be used on the buccal and lingual surfaces by placing it on the tooth surface, slightly beneath the gingival margin, and tracing it along the contour of the gingival margin.[96]

The efficacy of the rubber tip stimulator in removing plaque biofilm and improving overall gingival health has been questioned because of conflicting information and lack of evidence.[114] In one study, an automated rubber tip was compared with the use of dental floss. Results indicated that the tip was as effective as dental floss in reducing gingival and bleeding index scores, although dental floss resulted in slightly less plaque re-growth. No evidence of gingival irritation or abrasion was found from the application of this tip, but it is important to note that it was a short-term study. Participants reported a preference for the use of the rubber tip compared with dental floss.[107] This powered rubber tip device, however, is no longer on the market. Aggressive application of the stimulator with heavy pressure can traumatize and destroy the soft tissues.[71] The use of the rubber tip should be limited and closely monitored.

Knitting Yarn

In areas where the papilla has receded and the embrasure is open, **white knitting yarn,** with no dyes, can be used in place of floss for interproximal cleaning. Synthetic knitting yarn is recommended because wool yarn leaves microfibers that could irritate soft tissues.[116] The increased width of the yarn provides more surface coverage and access to a shallow root concavity.[97]

Knitting yarn can be used around the abutment of a fixed appliance and under pontics when the space is large enough. It is also useful in open interproximal spaces, on the distal surface of the most posterior teeth, in exposed furcations, and around malpositioned teeth or separated teeth.[114] When access is limited, a floss threader may be used to insert the yarn into the embrasure (Figure 10–35 ■). Once the yarn has been drawn through, the technique is the same as for dental floss, with care taken not to traumatize the tissue. Because of its diameter, knitting yarn will not fit into the submarginal space.

Pipe Cleaner

Pipe cleaners have been suggested for use in class III embrasures and class IV furcations.[113] The metal core makes insertion easier in open spaces, but pipe cleaners should be used with caution to prevent damaging hard and soft tissues. Because of the metal core, pipe cleaners should never be used with implants to prevent scratching the titanium.[115]

Pipe cleaners are cut into 3-inch lengths, and a section is inserted into the embrasure space or furcation area. The pipe cleaner is wrapped around the proximal or inner root surfaces, and moved back and forth or buccolingually in a "shoeshine" motion[71] (Figure 10–36 ■). Similar to knitting yarn, because of their diameter, pipe cleaners cannot be inserted into the sulcus.

Gauze Strip

A gauze strip can be used for cleaning the proximal surfaces of teeth adjacent to edentulous areas, teeth that are widely spaced, or implant abutments. Gauze strips have also been recommended to clean the distal surface of the

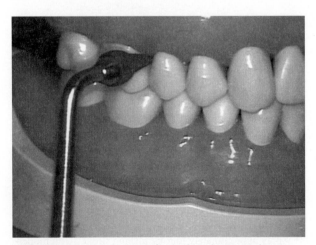

■ **FIGURE 10–34** Use of interdental tip stimulator to remove plaque, with the stimulator inserted interproximally into an open embrasure space at a 90-degree angle to the long axis of the tooth. It is traced along the gingival margin or moved in a buccolingual direction to clean the surfaces.

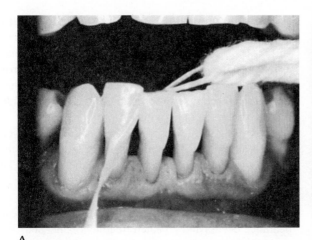
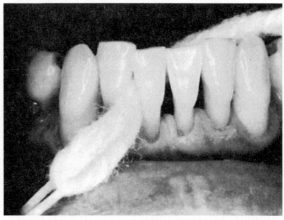

A

B

■ **FIGURE 10–35**   Use of knitting yarn in a wide, open embrasure. **A.** Yarn is looped through dental floss and inserted through the contact point. **B.** Yarn is drawn through the embrasure.
(Courtesy of Dr. Linda S. Scheirton, Creighton University, Omaha, NE.)

most posterior teeth in the mouth and for dental implant abutments.[116]

A 1-inch-wide gauze bandage is cut into lengths of 6 to 8 inches and folded in half or in thirds. The lengthwise edge of the gauze is positioned with the fold toward the gingiva, and the edges folded inward to avoid gingival irritation. The gauze is adapted by wrapping it around the exposed proximal surface to the facial and lingual line angles of the tooth in a C-shape. A buccolingual shoeshine stroke is used to loosen and remove plaque and debris (Figure 10–37 ■). Knitting yarn, pipe cleaners, and gauze strips are less popular with the advent of variable thickness floss, but their use may be indicated when variable thickness floss is unavailable or not affordable.

Rinsing

Vigorous rinsing of the mouth can aid in the removal of food debris and materia alba. The technique involves forcefully pushing the water back and forth through the

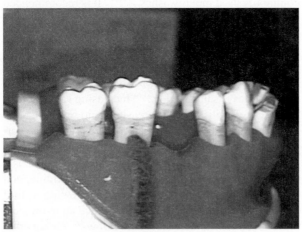

■ **FIGURE 10–36**   Application of pipe cleaner in a type III furcation.

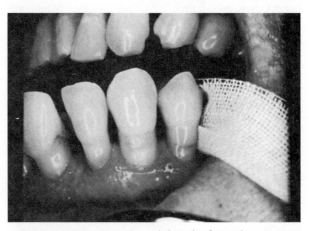

■ **FIGURE 10–37**   A 6-inch length of 1-inch gauze bandage folded in half with the folded edge adjacent to the gingiva for adaptation.
(Courtesy of Dr. Linda S. Scheirton, Creighton University, Omaha, NE.)

interproximal areas of clenched teeth, using the muscles of the tongue, lips, and cheeks to force the water, and using as much pressure as possible.[138] It has traditionally been recommended to help return the mouth to a neutral pH after the acid production that results from ingestion of fermentable carbohydrates, for the purpose of preventing dental caries.[139] Although some continue to recommend mouthrinsing with water after consumption of fermentable carbohydrates, national guidelines for dental caries prevention[139–145] do not include water mouthrinsing as a strategy. The 1990 National Health Interview Survey asked the public to rank the effectiveness of procedures that were known to prevent dental caries. Rinsing with water was not included on that list.[146]

Research has demonstrated no effect of water rinsing on the number of bacteria present in plaque.[147,148] Studies have shown that any effect of water rinsing on bacterial counts is short term, which reduces its effectiveness in caries prevention.[149,150] On the other hand, various studies have shown long-lasting effects from supervised and unsupervised rinsing with chemotherapeutic agents versus water as an adjunct to oral hygiene.[76,147,151–160]

The American Academy of Periodontology (AAP) states that the use of antimicrobial agents to help reduce bacterial plaque may be beneficial for the prevention and treatment of gingivitis in some patients.[6] The use of antimicrobial rinsing is included as an adjunct to oral hygiene measures in the AAP parameters for the treatment of plaque-induced gingivitis, slight-to-moderate chronic periodontitis, refractory periodontitis, necrotizing diseases, and in periodontal maintenance, when oral hygiene is only partially effective.[7] However, these rinses are not recommended to take the place of oral hygiene measures.

The provider should be aware of the active ingredients and products that have been approved for rinsing. The active ingredients in one approved rinse are thymol, menthol, eucalyptol, and methyl salicylate. Active ingredients of the other two are chlorhexidine digluconate and triclosan.[6] In addition, it is important to be aware of inactive ingredients, such as alcohol, that may be contraindicated for certain individuals.[161]

Effects of rinsing with antimicrobials include reduced supragingival plaque, lower bacterial counts throughout the mouth, less papillary bleeding, and fewer bacteria on the dorsum of the tongue.[162–164] These antimicrobial effects include control of bacteria associated with both dental caries and gingivitis.[144,160,164] In fact, daily

rinsing with an antimicrobial was shown to result in greater plaque reduction than flossing on visible tooth surfaces.[117,158,159] Antimicrobial rinsing has been used as part of a full-mouth disinfection approach to improve oral tissue health.[164,165] Rinsing with 15 ml of chlorhexidine for 30 seconds twice a day is the recommended protocol to control gingivitis.[166]

Rinsing with chlorhexidine twice daily for 1 week every 3 months has been suggested for oral disinfection to control dental caries in high-risk patients.[167,168] The idea is to kill bacteria in waves.[100] The reason for the quarterly repetition is that, although *Streptococcus mutans* is significantly reduced by this procedure, reappearance occurs and repeated treatment is needed.[169] A combined rinsing with chlorhexidine and fluoride has been shown to be more effective than rinsing with either compound by itself, because their effect is **synergistic,** that is, their combined effects are greater than their individual effects.[22,170] It is important to stress to patients that rinsing with antimicrobials is recommended as an adjunct to toothbrushing and interdental cleaning, not as a substitute.[164]

Water rinsing is recommended for special circumstances. To neutralize the mouth acids in radiation therapy patients, Wilkins has recommended rinsing throughout the day with saline and baking soda or with plain water and baking soda followed by plain water.[161] Water rinsing has been shown to effectively prevent the occurrence or decrease the severity of chemotherapy-induced oral mucositis in some studies, whereas other studies have demonstrated superior results in controlling mucositis with antimicrobial rinses such as iodine and commonly used mouthwashes.[171–173] It is recommended that patients with **bulimia** rinse with plain water or bicarbonate of soda in water immediately after vomiting.[161,174] During wearing of orthodontic appliances, rinsing is recommended after eating to rinse away food particles.[175]

One of the protective factors in the prevention of dental caries is salivary flow.[176] Increasing salivary flow may be accomplished by increasing fluid intake. Chewing increases salivary flow,[177] and chewing gum after eating has especially been shown to stimulate salivary flow.[178,179] Chewing gum has also been suggested as a vehicle for agents such as fluoride, chlorhexidine, and calcium phosphate to prevent caries. Chewing xylitol gum for 5 minutes after a meal will have an antimicrobial effect and will increase salivary flow.[180] Eating other foods that stimulate salivary flow, such as cheese and sugar substitutes, has also been recommended.[177] Patients should be counseled to chew only sugar-free gum as a means of stimulationg salivary flow to prevent dental caries.

The plaque pH and the dynamic balance between demineralization and remineralization determine the outcome of dental caries development.[179] The level of fluoride in the saliva affects the amount of fluoride absorbed by the plaque, and will in turn affect the demineralization/remineralization process.[181]

Dental caries prevention can be enhanced by stimulating saliva, using fluorides, and controlling bacteria with antimicrobials. Besides the use of fluorides, rinsing with chlorhexidine has been shown to be the most effective antimicrobial to prevent dental caries. The effectiveness of water rinsing to control dental caries is not supported by research results.

Irrigation

Irrigation devices are a means of irrigating specific areas of the mouth, whereas rinsing is a means of flushing the entire mouth. The advantage of irrigation is that periodontal lesions are most common interdentally, and rinsing does not reach these areas of limited access.[160] Irrigation with an antimicrobial agent has consistently achieved better results than rinsing with an antimicrobial agent.[182] There is inadequate evidence to compare the value of supragingival irrigation with water to rinsing with an antimicrobial in the reduction of gingival inflammation.[183]

Irrigation is recommended as an adjunct to daily oral hygiene, including toothbrushing, dental floss, and other aids as needed.[183] It is not the best method to disrupt or remove biofilm, is not effective without toothbrushing, and should not be used as a substitute for mechanical plaque removal.[184] Irrigation is also considered an adjunct to periodic professional instrumentation for a patient who is in periodontal maintenance.[182] The primary effects on the periodontal apparatus result from scaling and root planing.[6,160] Irrigation does not prevent the repopulation of the pocket by pathogenic bacteria nor increase significantly the intervals between maintenance visits.[185]

Home irrigation is not indicated for those who have effective oral hygiene and have no gingival inflammation.[183] Results of a study with patients undergoing non-surgical periodontal therapy indicated that, if good oral hygiene was practiced after the therapy, there was no difference between outcomes with and without irrigation

with water or an antimicrobial.[186] However, individuals with inconsistent or ineffective interproximal cleaning, fixed orthodontic appliances, crowns, fixed bridges, implants, and malodor may benefit from a home irrigation self-care regimen.[183,184,187–189] In some cases, irrigation has been suggested as an alternative to local delivery of antibiotics, to reduce the risk of bacterial resistance that may occur with local antibiotic therapy.[190] Oral irrigation may also be helpful for individuals who have their jaws temporarily wired together for stabilization after surgery or have head and neck trauma. Just like other self-care measures, the benefits are derived only if self-care is practiced routinely.[160]

The action of irrigation is the disruption of loosely attached or unattached supragingival and subgingival plaque, and removal of food debris. The action is twofold. Loosely attached microflora are disrupted when the pulsating fluid makes initial contact. There is a secondary flushing action as the irrigant is deflected from the tooth surface. The microflora is disrupted both qualitatively and quantitatively. Gingivitis reduction is a result of the alteration of subgingival microflora, rather than a reduction in the amount of plaque.[191–193]

A home-irrigation device that provides a pulsating stream of fluid versus a continuous stream is preferred.[194] With a pulsating stream of water, compression and interpulse decompression occur, allowing contaminants to escape and avoiding injury to soft tissues.[183,191] With a continuous flow, there is constant tissue compression, which hinders the escape of contaminants.

Use of Antimicrobials

Some studies have demonstrated that supragingival irrigation with water in addition to toothbrushing removes plaque, and reduces bleeding and gingival inflammation.[191,192,195] Other studies have found that irrigation with an antimicrobial instead of water increases the effectiveness of home-irrigating devices[196–203] by significantly reducing the subgingival **periodontopathic** microflora (microflora capable of causing diseases in the periodontium and supporting structures of the teeth). On the basis of a comprehensive systematic review of the literature, the AAP has confirmed that supragingival irrigation with antimicrobials is superior to water irrigation in the treatment of gingivitis, because water irrigation showed limited reduction of pathogen counts.[183,197] The American Association of Orthodontists recommends irrigation with an antimicrobial to reduce the level of bacteria during orthodontic treatment.[189] Oral irrigation has been shown to be superior to rinsing for the delivery of antimicrobials to control subgingival flora.[199]

Chlorhexidine is the most researched antimicrobial used for irrigation.[183] Dilution of chlorhexidine to concentrations of 0.02%, 0.04%, 0.06%, and 0.1% has decreased plaque and gingival inflammation, while controlling the staining that occurs with the use of chlorhexidine.[182,183,198] Even with these lower concentrations, greater volumes of medicaments were delivered with jet irrigation than with rinsing at the normal 0.12% concentration.[183]

Irrigation with povidone-iodine has been used successfully to disinfect periodontal pockets and reduce total counts of periodontal pathogens.[197] This agent is suggested by the AAP for pocket disinfection and control of necrotizing ulcerative periodontitis.[6] An herbal-based mouthrinse used for subgingival irrigation showed reduction in gingivitis and bleeding.[204] Other irrigants that have been tested include stannous fluoride, Listerine antiseptic, acetylsalicylic acid (aspirin), hydrogen peroxide, and sodium hypochlorite (household bleach).

Effects of Irrigation

Supragingival irrigation improves and prevents gingivitis, but has no significant effect on periodontitis.[183] It reduces the subgingival periodontal pathogens and reduces bleeding.[160] The fluid penetrates subgingivally 3 mm, or half the probing depth, which explains why irrigation reduces gingivitis even though plaque is not eliminated.[160] Any reduction of pocket depth that may result from irrigation is related to a reduction in inflammation and subsequent gingival shrinkage. Irrigation does not improve attachment levels of the junctional epithelium.[160] Because supragingival irrigation also penetrates subgingivally, it may be as effective as subgingival irrigation in preventing the recolonization of a subgingival microflora after thorough instrumentation of the pockets.[160]

Supragingival irrigation does not project into deep pockets, and has limited effect on the subgingival microflora in deep pockets. This failure to reach the base of the pocket may explain why supragingival irrigation is more effective against gingivitis than periodontitis.[160] Irrigation has been shown to reduce proinflammatory cytokines (interleukin 1-β and prostaglandin E_2) in the gingival crevice. These cytokines lead to bone resorption when periodontal diseases are present.[205]

Home subgingival irrigation has been used to deliver medicaments further into the gingival sulcus.[206,207] Several studies demonstrated additional reductions in gingivitis and bleeding when an antimicrobial agent is used

subgingivally.[193,199] A soft latex-free rubber tip (Pik Pocket by Waterpik) was tested for subgingival irrigation to deliver the antimicrobial into the pocket.[208] When the tip was placed 1 mm subgingivally, the mean pocket penetration was 90% for 4-mm to 6-mm pockets and 64% for pockets of 7 mm or deeper; rinsing showed only 21% pocket penetration. Subgingival irrigation with this tip was reported to be comfortable to the patients. Subgingival irrigation requires a good deal of dexterity combined with compliance for successful results.[209]

Irrigation Tips and Units

Various irrigation tips are available (Figure 10–38 ■). The standard tip is designed for supragingival use. The tip is directed at the tooth at a 90-degree angle, at or coronal to the gingival margin. The gingival margin is followed, stopping at each interproximal area for 5 to 6 seconds. This process is done from both the buccal and lingual aspects.[210] For supragingival irrigation, a force of 80 to 90 psi (pounds per square inch) can be tolerated without damage to the tissues.[183] Supragingival irrigation has been used successfully in maintenance patients and is easy to master.[183]

For subgingival irrigation, a syringe or **cannula** (small tube) is used. Rubber-tipped cannulas can be angled into the gingival sulcus about 2 mm, allowing a focused lavage (washing or irrigation), which adds to the depth of penetration. A cannula-type tip yields results equivalent to those of a syringe.[183] A latex-free tip should be recommended. Cannula tips have not been tested for safety and efficacy.[210] They require high dexterity and

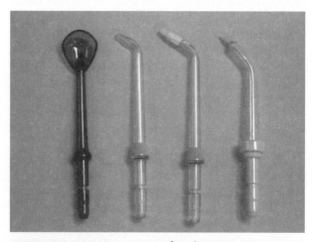

■ **FIGURE 10–38** Variety of oral irrigator tips.

should be limited to individuals with adequate skill.[183] After periodontal therapy, the recommended protocol, or procedure, is subgingival irrigation for at least 28 days, to be followed by reevaluation at 2 to 3 months.[166] Use of the cannula-type tip requires commitment on the part of the patient, and compliance may be an issue.[183,210] Patient motivation is required to increase compliance with the addition of irrigation to other daily oral hygiene measures.[164]

Various irrigation unit designs are available (Figure 10–39 ■). Although there is not much difference among the brands, results with one brand do not necessarily translate to effectiveness with another brand.[211] Evidence-based practice demands review of clinical evidence for a particular brand before recommending it.

New designs have been developed and tested. Studies of a new unit with a magnetic device showed that magnetized water more effectively reduced calculus formation.[212,213] Compared with irrigation using non-magnetized water, irrigation with magnetized water showed no significant effect on bleeding or gingivitis. Another new high-pressure water irrigator was tested. For the first time, results showed the removal of established plaque, as well as a reduction of gingival and interproximal plaque; the latter effects were demonstrated previously with pulsed irrigators. The high-pressure water irrigator resulted in less gingival abrasions than an electric toothbrush.[214] A novel oral irrigator that incorporates micro-bubbles of air into the water system reduced gingivitis, bleeding, and plaque, compared with manual brushing, but the difference was not statistically significant.[215]

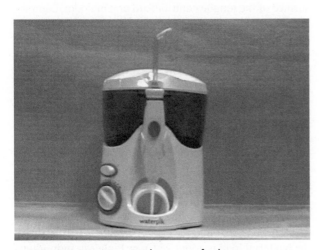

■ **FIGURE 10–39**   Oral irrigator for home use.

Irrigation-Induced Bacteremias

The potential for irrigation to induce bacteremias has been studied, but it does not appear to be hazardous to healthy patients, because routine oral hygiene has been shown to create bacteremia.[81,82,206,216] Oral irrigators used inappropriately by individuals with poor oral hygiene have induced bacteremias, but the relationship to bacterial endocarditis is unclear.[82,183,217]

There is less risk of bacterial endocarditis from irrigation of a healthy mouth, because the microbial load is higher in the presence of inflammation.[183,216] It has been suggested that the risk of bacteremia from brushing is greater in individuals with poor oral hygiene, and that the use of irrigation to reduce subgingival pathogens could be instrumental in reducing the incidence of bacteremia.[210] However, the AAP suggests that supragingival and subgingival irrigation should be recommended with caution to patients who require premedication before periodontal therapy, because there is no specific information on the degree of risk for bacteremia from irrigation in this population.[183]

ORAL MALODOR AND THE TONGUE

Oral malodor, also referred to as bad breath and **halitosis,** is defined as an unpleasant breath emanating from the oral cavity, regardless of its origin.[218] Oral malodor has been a common problem among different human populations since ancient times.[219] Hippocrates prescribed an antidote for malodor in 400 B.C. In general, about 95% of the world population is affected. The National Institute of Dental and Craniofacial Research reported that 25% of Americans have chronic oral malodor.[220]

Although it occurs in the oral cavity, the originating source of malodor can be the oral cavity; nasal, nasopharyngeal, sinus, or oropharyngeal areas; respiratory tract; systemic or gastrointestinal diseases or disorders; odiferous (odor-causing) foods; or medicines.[221] Xerostomia contributes to malodor because it prevents oral clearance. The oral cavity has been identified as the major origin for the development of malodor.[222] About 85% to 90% of malodor originates from the oral cavity, and about 50% of this problem is associated with tongue residues.[223] A thorough physical examination can rule out a systemic disorder.

Usually odors in the oral cavity occur when sulfur-containing proteins and peptides are hydrolyzed by gram-negative bacteria in an alkaline environment.[221] **Putrefaction** refers to a combination of protein hydrolysis by the bacteria and catabolism of the basic amino acids. The end result of putrefaction is malodor-producing volatile sulfur compounds (VSC).[218] Odiferous sulfur-containing end products created by this process include hydrogen sulfide, methylmercaptans, and dimethyl sulfide.

A study reported 8 times higher VSC in patients with periodontal disease.[224] These VSC have been associated with the progression of periodontal disease by increasing the permeability of the mucosal membrane, which allows for invasion of bacteria into the tissue. The wound-healing process can be delayed or disturbed by these compounds because they interfere with the synthesis of DNA and protein.[221] A shift from a predominantly gram-positive to a gram-negative and anaerobic bacterial population is associated with the production of VSC and odor production.

Local factors such as reduced salivary flow and a rise in oral pH accelerates this shift. Research studies have demonstrated that a pH at or above neutral favors the formation of malodor, whereas an acid pH inhibits malodor.[225] Because the pH of plaque is at its highest in the morning, the alkalinity of the oral cavity leads to the production of unpleasant morning breath.[226]

The tongue surface provides a niche for periodontal pathogens.[227] In addition, inconsistent or ineffective interproximal plaque removal can provide a recess for gram-negative bacteria to degrade sulfur-containing amino acids, resulting in malodor[228] The presence of periodontal disease may also be a contributing factor to malodor because the inflammatory process creates substrates that stimulate bacterial growth.[221] The putrefaction process and its concomitant odor occur more rapidly when bacterial accumulations are high.[226] Because periodontitis and gingivitis are associated with malodor, for some people, management of periodontal disease is an important aspect in the control of malodor.[224,229,230]

People with excellent oral health can be affected by halitosis, because the dorsum of the posterior section of the tongue is the major site for development of malodor (Figure 10–40 ■). This area does not benefit from the natural washing effects of the oral cavity. Therefore, applications of tongue cleaners become important to control malodor and maintain oral health.[222]

Treatment considerations can include professional debridement and irrigation of soft tissues as needed, control of gram-negative bacteria, increasing salivary flow, neutralizing VSC, and removal of plaque. This process requires thorough oral hygiene, including tongue hygiene.[221,228] Regular intraoral rinsing with chemotherapeutic agents is also

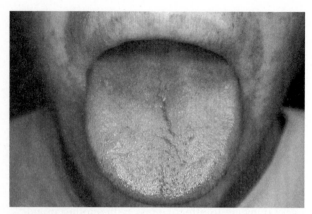

■ FIGURE 10–40   Dorsum of the posterior section of the tongue. (Image courtesy of Instructional Materials for the Dental Team, Lexington, KY.)

recommended to treat and control malodor. This process neutralizes the VSC and influences the gram-negative microflora in the oral cavity. As the most commonly recommended chemotherapeutic agents for neutralizing VSC, chlorhexidine gluconate, chlorine dioxide, zinc, and triclosan have been effective in reducing malodor significantly.[162,231–233] Chlorhexidine and chlorine dioxide also have shown antimicrobial capacity.[162,221] Malodor is primarily associated with the dorso-posterior region of the tongue, which is the common site for production of VSC. Therefore, regular mechanical cleaning of the tongue is a logical measure for the treatment of malodor.[234]

Tongue Cleaners

As previously discussed, the bacteria that collect on the surface of the tongue contribute to oral malodor, compromised wound healing, and oral diseases. Oral malodor can also present a significant social and/or psychologic handicap.[235] Tongue cleaning has been practiced since antiquity.[236] It continues to be an important part of oral hygiene today to control oral malodor and oral diseases.

The large papillary surface area of the tongue dorsum favors the accumulation of oral microorganisms and oral debris. Anatomically, the shorter **fungiform** (mushroom-shaped) papillae and the longer **filiform** (hairlike) papillae create elevations and depressions that can entrap debris and harbor microorganisms, making the tongue an ideal location for bacterial growth. The tongue coating contains nutrients, desquamated epithelial cells, blood cells, and bacteria. One study reported that the bacterial load is about 25 times higher in individuals who have a coated tongue verses those who do not.[226] Bacteria contained in the tongue coating are associated with both dental caries and periodontal diseases.[227, 236]

This tongue coating can contribute to plaque formation in other areas of the mouth.[228] Reduction of the tongue coating by mechanical tongue debridement can reduce plaque accumulation, control oral malodor, and prevent and control oral diseases.[221,237] Smokers or those with coated, deeply fissured tongues, or hairy tongue will find that tongue debridement is especially beneficial in reducing oral bacteria. (Hairy tongue refers to a tongue covered with filiform papillae that are entangled with threads produced by a fungus, *Aspergillus niger* or *Candida albicans*.) The effectiveness of tongue cleaning in reducing dental caries has been established by researchers who have demonstrated significant reduction in *Streptococcus mutans* colonies as a result of regular daily tongue cleaning.[236] Tongue cleaning to control the bacterial load can contribute to the control of periodontal disease.[224] One study found that adding the use of a tongue scraper to toothbrushing controlled morning breath odor more effectively than the use of dental floss combined with toothbrushing.[226] Tongue cleaning, possibly combined with antimicrobial rinsing, has been suggsted to control malodor.[235]

Various designs of tongue cleaners or scrapers are available (Figure 10–41 ■). A soft-bristled toothbrush has also been recommended. Several studies have compared the use of a soft toothbrush with a tongue scraper. Some studies show that the toothbrush is an effective tongue-cleaning device.[119] Other studies show that a tongue cleaner is more effective than a toothbrush.[223] Another study demonstrated that a tongue cleaner that was a combination of a brush and scraper was more effective than a regular scraper or a toothbrush.[238] A Cochrane review reported that small but unreliable evidence supported the efficacy of a tongue scraper over a soft toothbrush for tongue cleaning.[239]

Dental providers should become aware of tongue-cleaning products and methods to be able to recommend the most appropriate one for the individual patient. Patients should be educated about appropriate methods of tongue cleaning to avoid gagging and brushing the tonsil, which could lead to respiratory infection.[234] To clean the tongue effectively and safely with a toothbrush, the patient should protrude the tongue as far as possible to locate the **terminal sulcus.**[234] With the handle held at a right angle to the midline of the tongue, the toothbrush is placed on the terminal sulcus with the bristles directed toward the throat. It is then rolled forward gently with light pressure. The procedure is repeated three to four times without scrubbing the tongue.[234,240]

A variety of special tongue cleaners and scrapers are available, and are made of different materials such as plastics or stainless steel. Patients should be instructed on selection of a tongue cleaner. The same general principles and directions that apply to tongue cleaning with the toothbrush also apply to tongue cleaners (Figure 10–42 ■). Gagging during tongue cleaning can be avoided by use of a

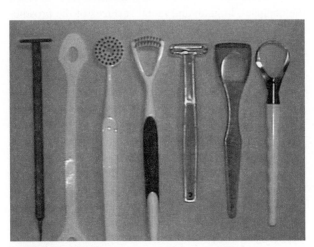

■ **FIGURE 10–41**   Variety of tongue cleaners. Note the third and fourth from the left are a combination brush/cleaner.

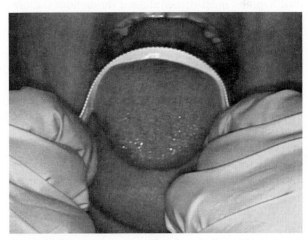

■ **FIGURE 10–42**   Plastic tongue-cleaning device used by pressing it against the dorsum of the tongue in an arc. Serrations on the tongue cleaner provide a scraping action as the cleaner is moved forward on the tongue.

flat tongue cleaner. Damage to the tongue surface is controlled by avoiding sharp metal tongue scrapers, applying gentle pressure, and practicing a sweeping motion instead of scraping.

A research study reported that 60% of participants experienced nausea and another 10% experienced trauma to the tongue mucosa from using a toothbrush to clean the tongue. Participants in this study were more interested in using tongue scrapers than toothbrushes.[223] Microscopic bleeding has also been reported as a result of using a hard toothbrush to clean the tongue.[234] Patient education should include information about the ill effects of the tongue coating, as well as safe and effective ways to clean the tongue. The patient's preferences should be considered as recommendations are made. Rosenberg recommended a positive and suggestive approach by initiating the conversation with "Did you know that people who don't brush their teeth, floss and use tongue cleaners stand the risk of having bad breath?" [222]

PERI-IMPLANT SELF-CARE

The use of dental implants has increased extensively in the past decade. An estimated 300,000 to 400,000 **endosseous implants** (implants placed surgically into the alveolar bone) are performed in the United States annually.[241] Success or failure of an implant depends on many factors, including daily oral hygiene self-care. Because microorganisms from surrounding tissues can be transmitted to the peri-implant area, meticulous daily oral hygiene must be maintained throughout the oral cavity.[7] Especially in patients who are only partially edentulous, there is a potential for cross-contamination from teeth to implants.[242] Accumulation of soft and hard deposits on the abutment, connecting bar, and attached prosthesis can lead to peri-implant mucositis and **peri-implantitis** (inflammation around the area of a dental implant resulting in loss of alveolar bone); these conditions can result in failure of the implant.[243] Research indicates that more plaque deposits accumulate on a titanium implant than on natural teeth. This greater accumulation has contributed to the development of more severe inflammation around implants.[187]

Implant patients need to be educated that maintenance visits are important, and that compliance with good personal self-care is a critical factor in the success of their implants.[49,244,245] These specific self-care recommendations should be based on assessment of the patient's oral health status, ability, motivation, manual dexterity, and mental capacity. Accessibility and ease of cleaning are also affected by the position of the abutment, surrounding anatomy, and design of the final restoration—for example, the length of the abutment, presence of a connecting bar, and amount of space under the prosthesis.[243,246,247]

It is important not only to teach the self-care techniques, but also to communicate the reasons for recommended oral hygiene methods and implements. Patients' compliance with recommendations will depend on their ability to master the techniques, lifestyle issues that affect time availability for a complex self-care regimen, and perception of the value of performing the recommended procedures.[30,40,246] Repeated instructions and continual reinforcement from the oral health professional will enhance compliance.[248]

The objectives of daily oral hygiene around implants are to minimize the subgingival and supragingival microbial accumulation, and to alter the pathogenesis of existing biofilm.[50,246,249] The ultimate goal is to prevent peri-implantitis that can result in failure of the implant. In the process of daily oral hygiene, it is critical to protect the implant surface to minimize surface alterations.[249] Titanium scratches easily, and a scratched surface will trap and hold biofilm that will contribute to peri-implantitis.[50,248] Therefore, implements and products should be selected that will maintain the smooth surface of the titanium. A soft toothbrush, end-tuft brush, gauze, and floss are especially recommended.[248] To prevent scratching, only end-rounded bristles should be recommended for use on implants.

A soft toothbrush can be used effectively to brush the occlusal, lingual, and facial surfaces of the prosthesis. Supplementation of the toothbrush with an end-tuft brush is recommended to accomplish sulcular brushing of the peri-implant area of the abutment. A flat end-tuft brush has been recommended for the facial surface of the abutment, whereas a tapered end-tuft brush with an angled handle has been suggested to more effectively reach the lingual surface of the abutment.[243]

Sonic, rotational, counter-rotational, and oscillating/rotating power toothbrushes have been shown to be more effective than manual toothbrushes to remove plaque and to reduce bleeding and inflammation around implants, and do not damage the titanium surface.[243,250–253] Their use is also safe for the peri-implant area and preferred by patients.[252] Brushing with an anti-calculus dentifrice is recommended, and use of a low-abrasive dentifrice is important to prevent scratching of the titanium.[243]

Daily cleaning of the neck of the abutments and undersurface of the superstructure is critical to prevent peri-implantitis, and will require the use of supplemental interdental aids.[50,248] Interdental aids should be selected according to the features of the implant. Effective interdental self-care for dental implant maintenance may include interdental brushes, different types of floss, dental tape, yarn, floss threaders, toothpicks, a toothpick holder, a rubber-tip stimulator, and application of antimicrobial agents.[249] To prevent scratching of the titanium surface, metal and rough wooden or plastic oral hygiene implements should not be used.[254] The number of recommended aids should be limited to increase compliance with recommendations. Patients are likely to use only two to three aids to supplement toothbrushing, no matter how many are recommended.[30]

Narrow dental floss is recommended for single tooth implants that have a short abutment. Tufted floss is recommended for the underside of a prosthesis that is in close proximity to the soft tissue. With a higher abutment and adequate space under the prosthesis, the abutment circumference and the underside of the prostheses can be cleaned with flossing cords, ribbon floss, other specially designed flosses such as Proxi-Floss and G-Floss, or gauze carried under the surface with a plastic floss threader. The various types of floss can be crisscrossed on the abutment and pulled in a shoeshine method for more effective plaque removal (Figure 10–43A ■). A soft, nylon-coated interproximal brush can also be used (Figure 10–43B ■). Use of metal core interproximal brushes and pipe cleaners is contraindicated (not advisable) because of potential scratching of the titanium.[243,246,254] A rotary brush with a pointed tip, an end-tuft brush (Figure 10–43C ■), a Sulcabrush, and a toothpick with holder have also been recommended. The dental aid should be selected according to the height of the abutment. A brush versus a toothpick will cover a greater surface area of the abutment and is kinder to the peri-implant area.[254]

Adjunctive supragingival and subgingival irrigation with water or antimicrobial agents can be used effectively for self-care of the dental implant.[254] Irrigation with an antimicrobial agent has the advantage of reducing the amount and pathogenesis of plaque around the implant.[187] Daily subgingival irrigation around the abutment with 0.12% chlorhexidine is recommended for this purpose to reduce peri-implant mucositis.[50] The flow rate of an electrical irrigator should be set on the lowest setting and not directed subgingivally to prevent any soft tissue detachment.[243,254]

Although rinsing with an antimicrobial has been shown to reduce plaque formation and increase gingival health around an implant,[255] irrigation with chlorhexidine was shown to be more effective than rinsing. One study demonstrated that subgingival irrigation with 0.06% chlorhexidine had greater reduction of inflammation of the peri-implant area than rinsing with 0.12% chlorhexidine.[250] The AAP suggests the use of topical antimicrobial agents with implant patients.[249] As a measure to prevent staining, chlorhexidine can be applied to specific sites via irrigation devices, cotton tip applicator, single tuft brush, or interproximal brush.[250]

Xerostomia must be managed carefully to enhance implant success. Patients with xerostomia should be monitored with a shorter maintenance interval because of their increased plaque formation. Salivary flow can be stimulated either physiologically or pharmacologically.[256]

In the event that peri-implantitis occurs, it is treated and controlled in the same manner as periodontitis, because they are the same disease.[257] Local delivery of chemotherapeutic agents in the peri-implant area and systemic antibiotics have been used widely to treat peri-implantitis, although a review of their use found variable outcomes after anti-infective treatment of peri-implantitis.[258–260] Only non-acidic agents should be used for rinsing, irrigation, peri-implant anti-infective treatment, and other uses to prevent corrosion and etching of the implant surface.[261,262]

Recommendations for implant self-care must begin with a thorough assessment of the implant patient's needs. Selection of a limited number of aids designed to meet those specific needs, careful instruction, and continual monitoring and reinforcement will contribute to the success of an implant.

SELF-CARE OF DENTURES

Although the incidence of tooth loss is decreasing in our population, the aging trend continues within the population.[33,263] Research indicates that a sizable minority of the population need an increasing number of dentures.[264] Therefore, oral health professionals will be called upon more and more to provide instruction in the care of full and partial dentures.

One-third of the population aged 65 years and older are edentulous, and only about 25% of people older than 60 years wear dentures today.[146,265] Even so, the majority of denture wearers in the United States are older

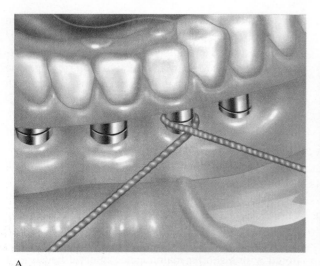

A

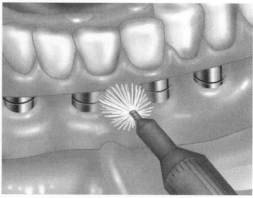

B

C

■ **FIGURE 10–43** Cleaning implants. **A.** Circumferential placement of post-care braided nylon cord criss-crossed to clean all surfaces. **B.** Interproximal brush to clean the proximal surfaces of the implants and the underside of the prosthesis. **C.** Uni-tuft brush to clean the proximal surfaces of the implants and the underside of the prosthesis.

than 65 years.[266] In addition, this population is at higher risk for impairment of salivary flow, which contributes to the formation of plaque and calculus on prosthetic appliances. The materials from which full and partial dentures are constructed, especially methacrylate, provide an irregular surface topography that enhances the attachment of deposits. Deposits that form on dentures include pellicle, biofilm, calculus, oral debris (e.g., desquamated epithelial cells), stain, and food debris. These deposits produce tissue irritation, infection, and malodor.[267–270] Candidal species adhere more easily to methacrylate than to the natural oral surfaces.[268] Failure to adequately clean dentures can result in denture stomatitis and candidiasis, common oral conditions found in denture wearers.[271–273] **Stomatitis** appears as patches of red inflamed areas on the oral mucosa. **Candidiasis** is caused by *Candida* organisms and appears as raised, white patches on the mucosa and tongue. The patches can be easily scraped off to reveal an underlying red, irritated surface.

Patient Education

A summary of procedures for oral self-care of dentures is provided in Table 10–8 ■. It is the responsibility of oral health professionals to provide instruction in the proper care and cleaning of both the dentures and the underlying tissues to improve the successful maintenance of dentures. Denture wearers need to understand the methods, products, and rationale of denture care. As with other oral hygiene instructions, explanation, demonstration, and a return demonstration in which the patient demonstrates the technique just observed will result in improved understanding and compliance.[31] Instruction should be provided verbally and supplemented with written materials for easy reference at a later time.[274] The denture delivery appointment is an excellent time to provide these instructions.[274] The patient's level of manual dexterity should be assessed at this time to provide modifications of cleaning tools and procedures if necessary.

It is also important that denture patients return for annual oral examinations.[275,276] At these regular follow-up appointments, the effectiveness of daily denture care can be monitored, dentures can be professionally cleaned if necessary, instructions can be reinforced, the denture fit can be checked and adjusted as needed, and the oral tissues can be examined.[277] Oral cancer examinations for denture wearers is critical[274] because two-thirds of new cases of oral cancer in the United States are found in persons older than 55 years.[278] Denture wearers must be informed of the importance of this health-protective practice. The Surgeon General's report, *Oral Health in America,* reported that the percentage of seniors that visited the dentist within the previous year in 1993 was 56% for ages 65 to 74 years and 45% for ages 75 years and older.[146] Even more significant, the 1983 *National Health Interview Survey* reported that only 13% of the edentulous population had annual dental visits.[33]

Research has shown that a large percentage of dentures worn by the elderly are not adequately cleaned, and denture wearers are unaware of the inadequacy of their denture hygiene.[279,280] Many do not use proper methods and products to clean their dentures, either because they have not been instructed in denture care or do not follow the advice.[281] In addition, some are not able to practice good denture hygiene and need assistance from their caretakers.[161] Frequently, denture wearers are aware of only the esthetic benefits of maintaining cleanliness. Oral health professionals need to stress the numerous health benefits of denture cleaning. Consistent, effective cleaning

of dentures enhances the sense of oral cleanliness. It also prevents oral malodor, denture stomatitis, and other tissue irritations and infections, and it preserves the esthetic appearance of the denture. Mucosal irritation may impair eating, which can have a negative nutritional impact on a frail, elderly individual.[282–284]

Daily self-care recommendations should also include care of the soft tissues on which a denture rests; these measures include daily removal of the denture overnight or for at least 6 to 8 hours at a time, cleaning and massaging the tissues under the denture daily, and performing regular oral self-examinations to observe and report any irritation or chronic changes in appearance of the tissues.[267,276,285–287] Failure to remove the denture may result in oral malodor, excessive alveolar ridge resorption, candidiasis, denture stomatitis, epulis fissuratum (single or multiple elongated folds of tissue that represent an overgrowth of fibrous connective tissue at the border of an ill-fitting denture), and other oral pathology and infections. A denture should be stored out of the reach of children and pets to keep it safe while it is out of the mouth.[275] It is commonly recommended that dentures be stored in solution while out of the mouth to prevent warping, although Shay has suggested that this inaccurate belief is based on studies with early, antiquated acrylic denture materials.[268]

Massaging the oral mucosa under a denture will stimulate circulation and increase resistance to trauma.[277] These tissues can be cleaned and massaged simultaneously by brushing with a soft end-rounded toothbrush or a power brush twice a day. Massage of the mucosa can also be accomplished by placing the thumb and index finger over the ridge and applying a press-and-release stroke, and by rubbing the palate with the ball of the thumb.[277]

Cleaning the Denture

Commonly practiced cleaning methods include immersion, brushing, or a combination of both. The majority of denture wearers surveyed used either brushing or immersion in a cleanser, although thorough cleaning involves a combination of both immersion and brushing.[271–274]

Brushing of Dentures

Denture materials are easily scratched with abrasive materials; therefore, only compounds designed for use on dentures should be used when brushing them. A denture paste is recommended rather than a toothpaste to protect the acrylic surface from scratching; denture paste is harmless to the denture when used properly.[271,277]

Nonabrasive agents such as hand soap and mild dishwashing liquid are also safe to use.[281] Salt and bicarbonate of soda are mildly abrasive.[277] Abrasive agents such as scouring powders and toothpaste will scratch the acrylic surface, which will dull and remove anatomic and esthetic details from the surface.[275,281]

A specially designed denture brush is recommended rather than a toothbrush to access all surfaces of a denture[274] (Table 10–8 and Figure 10–44 ■). Denture brushes feature stiff bristles. The bristles are all one length on one end, to brush the flat parts of the denture such as the facial, lingual, and palatal surfaces. On the other side, the bristles are set in a pyramid shape, to brush the inner surface of the denture (Figure 10–45 ■). These special brushes have a wide handle for easy gripping. A clasp brush (Figure 10–46 ■) is recommended to reach the inner surfaces of clasps of partial dentures.[277]

A hand or nail brush is adequate to clean a denture if the bristles are long enough to reach into the deeper areas of the inner surface of the denture.[274] A soft toothbrush can also be used if it reaches the curvatures of all surfaces without the need to apply undue pressure in

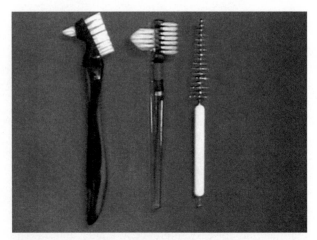

■ **FIGURE 10–44** Sample denture brushes. The brush on the right is a clasp brush.

some areas to clean other areas.[277] If a toothbrush is used, it should not be the same one used to brush any natural teeth still present in the mouth. This precaution is to maintain the condition of the toothbrush for adequate

■ **Table 10–8** Patient Instruction for Daily Denture Care

- Remove dentures after every meal to remove food and debris.
- Always hold the denture over a towel, rubber mat, or a sink filled with several inches of water for protection.
- Grasp denture firmly but gently.
- Rinse and brush dentures with a denture brush.
- If a toothbrush is used on dentures, it should be soft and a different toothbrush from the one used in the mouth.
- Moisten the brush and apply denture paste or mild hand soap (less abrasive).
- Use denture paste rather than toothpaste or any other abrasives.
- Brush every surface, scrubbing gently to avoid damage.
- Pay close attention to deep inner surfaces of the denture.
- Add the use of a clasp brush on partial dentures.
- Rinse the denture thoroughly, and use a brush to remove denture paste that may cling to the irregular denture surface.
- Brush the soft tissues of the mouth with a soft toothbrush before replacing the denture.
- Remove dentures daily either overnight or for at least 6–8 hours at a time.
- Soak dentures in a solution while they are out of the mouth.
- Massage oral tissues daily with a soft toothbrush or the fingers.
- Soak dentures daily in an antimicrobial cleaning solution according to the manufacturer's directions.
- Rinse denture to remove saliva and debris before immersing in cleanser.
- Rinse and brush denture after soaking to remove all traces of chemical solution and softened deposits.
- When dentures are out of the mouth, soak them in cleanser solution or cool water.
- Mix fresh cleanser each time you soak; do not reuse cleanser.
- Keep denture in same safe, handy place to reduce likelihood of misplacement.
- Check a denture for cleanliness by inspecting it visually and running a finger over it to detect slippery plaque.
- If eyeglasses are worn for close work and reading, wear them while cleaning the denture to be able to observe cleanliness of the denture.
- If a denture adhesive is used, clean it out of the denture thoroughly every day.

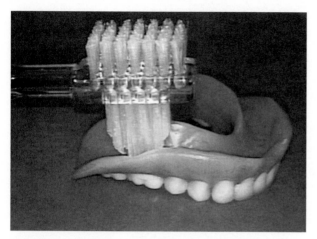

■ **FIGURE 10–45** Pyramid-shaped bristles of a denture brush applied to the inner surface of a denture.

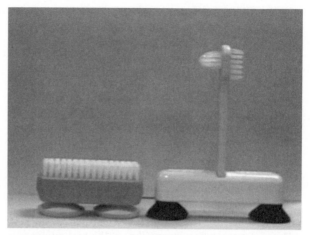

■ **FIGURE 10–47** A nail brush and a denture brush stabilized to the countertop with suction cups for use by a patient who has the use of only one arm or hand.

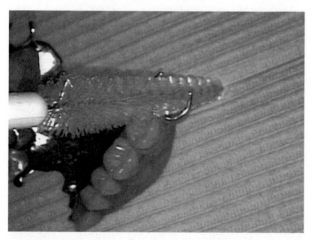

■ **FIGURE 10–46** Clasp brush applied to the inner surface of a partial denture clasp.

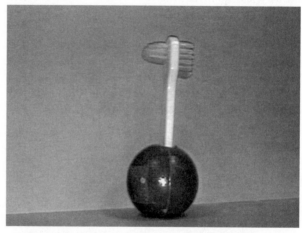

■ **FIGURE 10–48** A denture brush modified for use by an arthritic patient by inserting the handle into a ball.

oral hygiene of the natural teeth.[277] Hard-bristled brushes should not be used on dentures because they will damage the acrylic surface.[267,275]

Although denture brushes are designed with large handles for easy grip, some older denture wearers may require further modifications to their brushes to accommodate arthritis and other disabilities. A denture brush or nail brush can be modified (Figure 10–47 ■) so that it can be attached to the counter top or side of the sink with suction cups, for patients who are limited in the use of one hand or one arm.[288] A denture brush or clasp brush can be inserted into a ball (Figure 10–48 ■), bicycle grip,

or other holder to accommodate the arthritic patient.[289] These and other modified aids are available from suppliers of rehabilitation services or can be created in the dental office or at home.[268,288,289]

The use of a table top ultrasonic cleaner is less common but highly effective to clean and disinfect a denture.[268,290] These small units for individual use at home use a cleaning solution in conjunction with agitation. Only a cleaning solution that is recommended for use with dentures should be used. Use of water that contains ozone with ultrasonication has been found to be as effective as the use of commercial denture cleaners.[291] An ultrasonic cleaner may be especially helpful for individuals with limited dexterity, although they are not designed to replace daily brushing of the denture.[275] Use of an ultrasonic cleaner may be impractical and expensive for use by individual patients at home, but can be useful in long-term facilities.[267] Facility personnel protect owner identification and infection control by placing the denture into the cleaning solution in a sealed plastic bag or secure cup before agitation.[268] A variety of these units are available on the Internet at an affordable cost.

Whichever method is used, the denture should be thoroughly rinsed under running, tepid water before reinsertion into the mouth. This step will remove any cleaning substances to avoid damage to the denture acrylic, inflammatory or allergic reactions of the oral mucosa, or swallowing of traces of caustic agents.[274,277] Both the ADA and Academy of General Dentistry recommend that only cool water be used, because hot water will warp the acrylic denture material.[275,276] Many chemical cleaners leave an unpleasant taste. Soaking overnight in water or briefly in a mouthwash can be recommended to improve the taste of the denture before re-insertion.[281] Overnight soaking in mouthwash is not recommended, because prolonged contact with alcohol or essential oils found in commercial mouthwashes may dry or bleach the denture acrylic.

Immersion Cleaning of Dentures

Immersion of the denture in a cleaning solution is recommended daily to supplement brushing. Use of a combination of immersion and brushing is more effective at removing plaque, debris, and stain than brushing alone.[292] The advantages of immersion are that all areas of the denture are reached by the solution for thorough cleaning, it is easier for denture wearers who have difficulty handling a brush, it offers safe storage, it requires minimum handling of the denture, the risk of dropping the denture during cleaning is reduced, and immersion agents are significantly less abrasive than denture paste.[293] The last three advantages appeal to a caregiver who is cleaning a patient's or loved one's denture.[294] As well as resulting in a cleaner denture, use of commercial immersion solutions will disinfect the denture and control malodor more effectively.[269,281,295]

Selecting an immersion cleaner requires consideration of the type of denture material. The ideal product is easy to use, bactericidal and fungicidal, nontoxic, and harmless to denture materials, and effectively removes deposits.[271] The patient should be instructed on the recommended procedures for use of an immersion cleaner:

- Use a plastic container with a fitted cover.
- Fill the container with enough *warm* water to submerge the denture.
- Soak the denture for the time recommended by the manufacturer.
- Rinse the denture thoroughly after removing it from the container.
- Brush off the loosened deposits while rinsing the denture.
- Empty and clean the container daily.
- Use fresh solution for each soaking.[277]

Several chemicals are used to compound immersion cleaners. Oral health professionals need to be familiar with these cleaning products to guide their patients' selection. No one product is best in all situations. The advantages and disadvantages must be weighed in relation to an individual patient's needs.

Alkaline Peroxide Industry estimates are that 80% of denture wearers use effervescent commercial **alkaline peroxide** denture-cleaning products, which form bubbles when dissolved in water as a result of the release of a gas. These products include compounds for oxidizing (usually an alkaline perborate), effervescing (perborate and/or carbonate), and chelating (ethylenediaminetetraacetic acid; EDTA). When dissolved in water, the compounds decompose and release oxygen bubbles, which mechanically loosen plaque and debris on the denture surface; they also have an antibacterial effect.[271] They are ineffective in removing calculus.[292] The alkaline substances and detergent enhance the mechanical effect of the bubbles. These agents effectively achieve a 99% kill rate of most organisms in the recommended 10- to 20-minute soaking time, and their effects are enhanced by using water at $122°F$.[292] There are no serious disadvantages to the use of these alkaline peroxide cleansers.[271]

Alkaline hypochlorite Alkaline hypochlorite is recommended for 20 minutes of soaking daily, followed immediately by rinsing and soaking the denture in water.[281] This agent has superior action in cleaning dentures, dissolving mucin and plaque matrix, inhibiting calculus formation, and bleaching stains. In addition, alkaline hypochlorite has bactericidal and fungicidal effects.[296] Its tendency to corrode metal-based dentures can be controlled by soaking for periods not to exceed 10 minutes, immediately followed by thorough rinsing and soaking in water.[281] Corrosion occurs not only to exposed metal but possibly also to the metal pins that retain the porcelain denture teeth. The corrosive quality of commercial hypochlorite cleaners has been reduced by the addition of additives.[271]

Acids   Commercial acid cleansers are 3% to 5% solutions of hydrochloric acid alone or in combination with phosphoric acid.[271] They are effective in removing resistant stains and calculus.[271] Because these compounds must be handled with extreme care, they are primarily recommended for use by dental office personnel.[271] They are contraindicated for metal prostheses because of their corrosive nature.[271,281]

Other chemicals   Proteolytic enzymes break down mucin deposits on dentures and thus break up the plaque so that it is easily flushed away.[271] However, they are inferior to alkaline peroxide compounds against *Candida.*[297] Enzyme agents have been added to various commercial immersion cleansers.[277] A new silicone polymer cleanser has been tested with promising results.[268]

Household products   About half of denture wearers clean their dentures with a household product not designed for that purpose.[271] Patients need guidance in how to use these products effectively and safely. The most common household product used to clean dentures is **household bleach** (sodium hypochlorite) diluted 1:10 in tap water. Research has shown that it is an effective antimicrobial for cleaning dentures.[296] It has the disadvantages of corroding and reducing the reflectance of the metal of partial dentures.[298] Also prolonged use can bleach out the pink color of acrylic resin.[299] Addition of 2 teaspoons of Calgon dishwasher detergent has been suggested to control calculus and stain.[268] Daily soaking is recommended for 10 to 15 minutes. Overnight soaking is recommended to help remove calculus and stain from a denture without metal parts that will corrode, but should not be done daily to avoid fading of the acrylic color. [277]

Vinegar is less effective than sodium hypochlorite to kill microorganisms on a denture, but has the advantage of not being as caustic to the oral mucosa if not thoroughly rinsed.[268] Although some denture wearers soak their dentures in an **antimicrobial mouthwash,** effectiveness of these products has not been reported.[268] **Microwave radiation** will kill microorganisms, but remaining non-viable organisms and byproducts can produce a host response. Ultrasonic cleaning or brushing should be done before microwave radiation.[268]

Thorough rinsing and brushing are important after any type of immersion cleaning to remove all cleaning agents. Failure to do this step may result in tissue irritation. Brushing with the tools, products, and procedures already described should be done after immersion cleaning to brush away loosened deposits.[268] During brushing, the denture should be held over a sink filled with water, a rubber mat, or a folded towel to avoid denture fracture if it is dropped. A denture may break if dropped even a few inches.[267,275,288]

Disinfection of the Denture

One of the causes of stomatitis is candidiasis resulting from inadequate denture hygiene.[286] When a patient's denture becomes contaminated with *Candida,* not only is the surface contaminated, but the depths of the porosity within the denture material become contaminated as well. The same types of microorganisms found within the oral mucosa of patients with candidiasis are also impregnated in the denture.[300] Management of this condition is challenging and requires disinfection of the denture at the same time as topical treatment of the mucosa.[286]

Although commercial immersion-type denture cleansers disinfect dentures when they are used on a daily basis, they are not effective in killing *Candida* or *Staphylococcus* when the mucosa and denture are infected.[268,300,301] Soaking dentures in nystatin antifungal suspension has been suggested to manage stomatitis, but research results do not support this approach.[268] An alternative of denture soaks combined with Mycostatin Pastilles (i.e., nystatin lozenges that are allowed to dissolve on the tongue), rather than an oral suspension, were found to be somewhat more effective in decreasing *Candida* and the symptoms of stomatitis.[300]

Soaking the denture for 5 minutes daily in fullstrength household bleach has been recommended for disinfection of a denture that is infected with *Candida.*[277] Soaking must be timed carefully, because of the potential for bleach to fade the color of the acrylic. In addition, it must be followed by thorough rinsing to avoid tissue reaction when the denture is re-inserted into the mouth.[275]

Glass found that soaking a denture for 2 hours in equal parts of automatic dishwasher detergent containing chlorinated bleach, household bleach, and water, followed by a neutralizing counter soak of equal parts of white or apple vinegar and water for 1 hour was effective against *Candida.*[300] This procedure achieved disinfection of the surface and of some depth porosity when used daily. However, it was not effective against other opportunistic or pathogenic microorganisms, which could explain why some patients' symptoms persist even after disinfection of the denture and treatment for candidiasis.

One study demonstrated that ozonated water and ultrasonication reduced the number of *Candida albicans,* although small amounts of the microbe remained after treatment. Treating the microorganism with the appropriate antimicrobial agent, followed by fabrication of a new denture or relining of the existing denture, has resulted in complete recovery in most patients.[286,300]

Denture Liners

Soft temporary denture liners (tissue conditioners) can be damaged by commercial cleaners and brushing.[268] They should be rinsed thoroughly with water after eating and soaked daily in alkaline hypochlorite solution, but not in an effervescent product. A soft cloth or cotton can be used to gently wipe the surface as well. Soft permanent liners (silicone or acrylic resin) should be cleaned by lightly brushing with a soft brush and soap and water, as well as by soaking in a non-effervescent alkaline hypochlorite solution. Other commercial cleaners will damage either type of soft liner and should be avoided.[281]

Denture Adhesives

According to one survey, the use of denture adhesives is not a common practice, but the use of modern adhesives has been suggested for certain patients.[302–304] Compared with older products, adhesives today are improved, providing a stronger, longer hold, and are not harmful to the oral cavity or to the denture.[267,303] Advantages of the use of denture adhesives include increased sense of security and confidence; improved comfort, bite force, retention, and stability of the dentures; and less food-particle collection under the dentures.[274,275,303] Many of these advantages are true even for denture wearers who have good-quality denture support tissues.

Adhesives are especially beneficial to musicians, public speakers, and those who feel the need for the additional sense of security. They are also helpful to those who have very little alveolar ridge left, suffer from xerostomia, have undergone maxillofacial jaw resection, and are neurologically compromised because of stroke, multiple sclerosis, or closed-head injury.[274] Contraindications for the use of denture adhesives include open sores or cuts in the mouth, ill-fitting dentures, dentures that

have not been evaluated recently, poor oral and denture hygiene, and allergic reactions to adhesive products.[274]

Only soluble denture adhesives should be used. Insoluble denture adhesives such as denture liners, pads, and wafers should be avoided. Insoluble adhesives are usually next to the soluble adhesives on the shelf at the store, so patients need to be advised to carefully read labels when selecting an adhesive.[274]

It is fallacy that the correct use of denture adhesives causes tissue irritation, mucosal infection, and bone resorption.[303] Their use can safely enhance denture performance, but they should not be used to compensate for denture deficiencies.[267,274] Studies have demonstrated that denture adhesives can inhibit *Streptococcus mutans* and provide breath protection for up to 6 hours, even after a meal.[305–307]

Patients should be instructed in the appropriate use of denture adhesive.[303] Instructions should include its application to a dry denture, the use of the minimum amount needed, distribution evenly in the inner surface of the denture, re-application when needed, and application only to a thoroughly clean denture.[274] A denture adhesive should be completely cleaned out of the denture with a brush and light pressure during daily denture cleaning.[277] Soaking the denture overnight in water will loosen the adhesive, and allow it to be readily brushed and rinsed off.[274]

A denture adhesive can make it difficult to remove the denture. In this event, the patient should swish vigorously with warm water for a minute or more. Another technique is to alternately puff the cheeks and firmly pull downward with the fingers on the most distofacial flange.[274] It is especially important to stress the need for regular annual examinations to patients who use denture adhesives, because adhesives can modify or eliminate the usual signs of poor fit that require a visit to the dental office.[274]

Xerostomia and the Denture Patient

Greater plaque buildup on the denture will occur more quickly in patients who suffer from xerostomia. Practicing denture hygiene more frequently will compensate for this. An alcohol-free rinse containing aloe or lanolin or water-soluble lubricating jelly can help patients who suffer with dry mouth. The lubricating jelly can be placed in the base of the denture and will release over time. Patients with severe xerostomia caused by a systemic condition may benefit from salivary stimulation by pharmacologic intervention if they can tolerate the side effects.[267]

SUMMARY

In addition to oral conditions, several factors affect the appropriate selection and use of supplemental oral hygiene devices and techniques for the oral health self-care plan. The dexterity, ability, and motivation for performing oral hygiene procedures and the personal preferences for specific devices should be assessed when supplemental oral hygiene aids are recommended. When a device is introduced, it is essential that the proper application in all areas of the mouth be demonstrated, and that the potential for damage with improper use is understood. Instruction should be based on learning theory and health education models, and reinforcement is needed to achieve compliance.

Despite adequate dexterity and ability, attainment of optimal oral health requires motivation and daily compliance in performing oral self-care. To enhance compliance and skill development, the oral health professional should limit the number of recommended oral hygiene devices. Personal preferences for particular oral hygiene aids should also be considered. Although a specific aid may be favored by the oral health professional, it will be ineffective if not used by the patient. If an individual has shown a preference for a specific device, its effective use should be encouraged. For example, if an individual uses a toothpick but presents with inadequate oral hygiene as evidenced by disclosed plaque and/or tissue inflammation, the oral health professional might consider one of the following:

- Instruction to enhance the effectiveness with the toothpick.
- Introduction of a toothpick holder to facilitate access and manipulation of the toothpick.
- Use of the wooden or triangular interdental stick because of its similarity to the toothpick.

A wide variety of interproximal plaque removal devices are available. The oral health professional will need to stay informed of the research describing new devices, as it becomes available. Devices with evidenced-based significance should be considered. Clinical experience and expertise, however, should not be discounted, because they are also important components of evidence-based decision making. It is the obligation of the oral health professional to consistently investigate evidence and apply clinical judgment.

REFERENCES

1. American Academy of Periodontology. (1999). The pathogenesis of periodontal diseases. *J Periodontol,* 70(4):457–70.
2. Fontana, M., & Zero, D. T. (2006). Assessing patients' caries risk. *J Am Dent Assoc,* 137:1231–39.
3. Caton, J., Bouwsma, O., Polson, A., & Espeland, M. (1989). Effects of personal oral hygiene and subgingival scaling on bleeding interdental gingiva. *J Periodontol,* 60(2):84–90.
4. National Institutes of Health Consensus Development Panel. (2001). National Institutes of Health Consensus Development Conference statement. Diagnosis and management of dental caries throughout life, March 26–28, 2001. *J Dent Educ,* 132:1153–61.
5. Albandar, J. M. (2005). Epidemiology and risk factors of periodontal diseases. *Dent Clin North Am,* 49(3):517–32.
6. American Academy of Periodontology. (2001). Treatment of plaque-induced gingivitis, chronic periodontitis, and other clinical conditions. Academy report/position paper. *J Periodontol,* 72(12):1790–800.
7. American Academy of Periodontology (2000). Parameters of care. *J Periodontol,* 71(5 Suppl):847–83.
8. American Academy of Periodontology. (1997). Treatment of gingivitis and periodontitis. *J Periodontol,* 68:1246–53.
9. Dahlen, G., Lindhe, J., Sato, K., Hanamura, H., & Okamoto, H. (1992). The effect of supragingival plaque control on the subgingival microbiota in subjects with periodontal disease. *J Clin Periodontol,* 19:802–809.
10. Loe, H. (2000). Oral hygiene in the prevention of caries and periodontal disease. *Int Dent J,* 50(3):129–39.
11. Axelsson, P., Nystrom, B., & Lindhe, J. (2004). The long-term effect of a plaque control program on tooth mortality, caries and periodontal disease in adults. Results after 30 years of maintenance. *J Clin Periodontol,* 31:749–57.
12. D'Aiuto, F., Parkar, M., & Tonetti, M. S. (2007). Acute effects of periodontal therapy on bio-markers of vascular health. *J Clin Periodontol,* 34:124–29.
13. Jeffcoat, M. K., Geurs, N. C., Reddy, M. S., Cliver, S. P., Goldenberg, R. L., & Hauth, J. C. (2001). Periodontal infection and preterm birth. Results of a prospective study. *J Am Dent Assoc,* 132:875–80.
14. Larkin, M. (2002, July 13). Can flossing teeth foil heart disease? *Lancet,* 360(9327):147.
15. Rosing, C. K., Daudt, F. A. R. L., Festugatto, F. E., & Oppermann, R. V. (2006). Efficacy of interdental plaque control aids in periodontal maintenance patients: A comparative study. *Oral Health Prev Dent,* 4(2):99–103.
16. DeLaRosa, M. R., Guerra, J. Z., Johnston, D. A., & Radike, A. W. (1979). Plaque growth and removal with daily toothbrushing. *J Periodontol,* 50(12):661–64.

17. Lang, N. P., Cumming, B. R., & Loe, H. (1973). Toothbrushing frequency as it relates to plaque development and gingival health. *J Periodontol,* 44(7):396–405.

18. Furuichi, Y., Lindhe, J., Ramberg, P., & Volpe, A. R. (1992). Patterns of de novo plaque formation in the human dentition. *J Clin Periodontol,* 19:423–33.

19. Corbet, E. F., & Davies, W. I. R. (1993). The role of supragingival plaque in the control of progressive periodontal disease. A review. *J Clin Periodontol,* 20:307–13.

20. Wright, G. Z., Banting, D. W., & Feasby, W. H. (1979). The Dorchester dental flossing study: Final report. *Clin Prev Dent,* 1(3):23–26.

21. Mueller-Joseph, L., Homenko, D. F., & Wilkins, E. M. (2005). The professional dental hygienist. In Wilkins, E. M., Ed. *Clinical practice of the dental hygienist* (9th ed.). Philadelphia: Lippincott, Williams, & Wilkins, 3–16.

22. Anusavice, K. (2001). Clinical decision-making for coronal caries management in the permanent dentition. *J Dent Educ,* 65(10):1143–46.

23. Persson, G. R., Mancl, L. A., Martin, J., & Page, R. C. (2003). Assessing periodontal disease risk. A comparison of clinicians' assessment versus a computerized tool. *J Am Dent Assoc,* 134:575–82.

24. Calley, K. H., Rogo, E., Miller, D. L., Hess, G., & Eisenhauer, L. (2000). A proposed client self-care commitment model. *J Dent Hygiene,* 74(1):24–35.

25. Jonsson, B., Lindberg, P., Oscarson, N., & Ohrn, K. (2006). Improved compliance and self-care in patients with periodontitis—a randomized control trial. *International J Dent Hygiene,* 4(2):77–83.

26. Hollister, M. C., & Anema, M. G. (2004). Health behavior models and oral health: A review. *J Dent Hygiene,* 78(3):1–8.

27. Tilliss, T. S. I., Stach, D. J., Cross-Poline, G. N., Annan, S. D., Astroth, D. B., & Wolfe, P. (2003). The transtheoretical model applied to an oral self-care behavioral change: Development and testing of instruments for stages of change and decisional balance. *J Dent Hygiene,* 77(1):16–25.

28. Astroth, D. B., Cross-Poline, G. N., Stach, D. J., Tilliss, T. S. I., Annan, S. D. (2002). The transtheoretical model: An approach to behavioral change. *J Dent Hygiene,* 76(4):286–95.

29. Lees, A., & Rock, W. P. (2000). A comparison between written, verbal, and videotape oral hygiene instruction for patients with fixed appliances. *J Orthodont,* 27(4):323–28.

30. Heasman, P. A., Jacobs, D. J., & Chapple, I. L. (1989). An evaluation of the effectiveness and patient compliance with plaque control methods in the prevention of periodontal disease. *Clin Prev Dent,* 11(2):24–28.

31. Kimbrough, V. J., & Henderson, K. (2006). *Oral health education.* Upper Saddle River, NJ: Pearson Prentice Hall.

32. Cary, J. (2006). Production, products, and your bottom line. *Dent Today,* 25(3):56, 58.

33. Burt, B., A., & Eklund, S. A. (2005). *Dentistry, dental practice, and the community* (6th ed.). St. Louis: Elsevier Saunders.

34. Cobban, S. J., Edgington, E. M., & Compton, S. M. (2007). An argument for dental hygiene to develop as a discipline. *Int J Dent Hygiene,* 5(1):13–21.

35. Pravikoff, D. S. (2004). The evidence-based practice dilemma. *CINAHLnews,* 23(1):6–7.

36. Socher, J. C. (2005). It's a scientific affair: ADA contemplates seal for malodor products, evidence-based dentistry. *CDS Rev,* 98(2):24.

37. Jahn, C. (2004). Evidence for self-care products: Power brushing and interdental aids. *J Pract Hygiene,* 13(1):24–29.

38. Ramberg, P., Lindhe, J., Dahlen, G., & Volpe, A. R. (1994). The influence of gingival inflammation on de novo plaque formation. *J Clin Periodontol,* 21:51–56.

39. Kinane, D. F. (1998). The role of interdental cleaning in effective plaque control: Need for interdental cleaning in primary and secondary prevention. In Lang, N. P., Attstrom, R., & Loe, H., Eds. *European workshop on mechanical plaque control.* Berlin: Quintessence, 156–68.

40. Ower, P. (2003). The role of self-administered plaque control in the management of periodontal diseases: 2. Motivation, techniques and assessment. *Dent Update,* 30(3):110–16.

41. Biesbrock, A., Corby, P. M. A., Bartizek, R., Corby, A. L., Coelho, M., Costa, S., Bretz, W. A. G., & Bretz, W. A. (2006). Assessment of treatment responses to dental flossing in twins. *J Periodontol,* 77(8):1386–91.

42. Terezhalmy, G. T., Bsoul, S. A., Bartizek, R. D., & Biesbrock, A. R. (2005). Plaque removal efficacy of a prototype manual toothbrush versus an ADA reference manual toothbrush with and without dental floss. *J Contemp Dent Prac,* 6(3). Retrieved March 1, 2007 from http://www.thejcdp.com.

43. Bellamy, P., Barlow, A., Puri, G., Wright, K. I. T., Mussatt, A., & Zhou, X. (2004). A new in vivo interdental sampling method comparing a daily flossing regime versus a manual brush control. *J Clin Dent,* 15(3):59–65.

44. Hogan, L M. E., Daly, C. G., & Curtis, B. H. (2007). Comparison of new and 3-month old brush heads in the removal of plaque using a powered toothbrush. *J Clin Periodontol,* 34:130–36.

45. Gorzo, I., Newman, H. N, & Strahan, J. D. (1979). Amalgam restorations, plaque removal and periodontal health. *J Clin Periodontol,* 6(2):98–105.

46. Jansson, L., Ehnevid, H., Lindskog, S., & Blomlof, L. (1994). Proximal restorations and periodontal status. *J Clin Periodontol,* 21(9):577–82.

47. Amundsen, O. C., & Wisth, P. J. (2005). Clinical pearl: LingLock™—the flossable fixed retainer. *J Orthodont,* 32:241–43.

48. Tolboe, H., Isidor, F., Budtz-Jorgensen, E., & Kaaber, S. (1987). Influence of oral hygiene on the mucosal conditions beneath bridge pontics. *Scand J Dent Res,* 95(6):475–82.

49. Sison, S. G. (2003, May/June). Implant maintenance and the dental hygienist. *Access,* Spec Suppl Iss 1:1–12.

50. Meffert, R. M. (1989). Implant therapy. In Nevins, M., Becker, W., & Kornman, K., Proceedings of the world workshop in clinical periodontics. Chicago: American Academy of Periodontology, VIII 1–19.

51. Jackson, M. A., Kellett, M., Worthington, H. V., & Clerehugh, V. (2006). Comparison of interdental cleaning methods: A randomized controlled trial. *J Periodontol,* 77(8):1421–29.

52. Lang, W. P., Ronis, D. L., & Farghaly, M. M. (1995). Preventive behaviors as correlates of periodontal health status. *J Public Health,* 55(1):10–17.

53. Hujoel, P. P., Cunha-Cruz, J., Banting, D. W., & Loesche, W. J. (2006). Dental flossing and interproximal caries: A systematic review. *J Dent Res,* 85(4):298–305.

54. Gisselsson, H., Emilson, C. G., Birkhed, D., & Bjorn, A. L. (2005). Approximal caries increment in two cohorts of schoolchildren after discontinuation of a professional flossing program with chlorhexidine gel. *Caries Res,* 39:350–56.

55. Sarner, B., Lingstrom, P., & Birkhed, D. (2003). Fluoride release from NaF and AmF-impregnated toothpicks and dental flosses in vitro and in vivo. *Acta Odontol Scand,* 61:289–96.

56. Ciancio, S. G., Shibly, O., & Farber, G. A. (1992). Clinical evaluation of the effect of two types of dental floss on plaque and gingival health. *Clin Prev Dent,* 14(3):14–18.

57. Beaumont, R. H. (1990). Patient preference for waxed or unwaxed dental floss. *J Periodontol,* 61(2):123–25.

58. Graves, R. C., Disney, J. A., & Stamm, J. W. (1989). Comparative effectiveness of flossing and brushing in reducing interproximal bleeding. *J Periodontol,* 60(5):243–47.

59. Dorfer, C. E., Wundrich, D., Staehle, H. J., & Pioch, T. (2001). Gliding capacity of different dental flosses. *J Periodontol,* 72(5):672–78.

60. Carr, M. P., Rice, G. L., & Horton, J. E. (2000). Evaluation of floss types for interproximal plaque removal. *Am J Dent,* 13(4):212–14.

61. French, C. I. (1975). The plaque removal ability of waxed and unwaxed dental floss. *Dent Hygiene,* 49(10):449.

62. Lamberts, D. M., Wunderlich, R. C., & Caffesse, R. G. (1982). The effect of waxed and unwaxed dental floss on gingival health. Part I. Plaque removal and gingival response. *J Periodontol,* 53(6):393–96.

63. Perry, D. A., & Pattison, G. (1986). An investigation of wax residue on tooth surfaces after the use of waxed dental floss. *Dent Hygiene,* 60(1):16–19.

64. Ong, G. (1990). The effectiveness of 3 types of dental floss for interdental plaque removal. *J Clin Periodontol,* 17(7):463–66.

65. Halla-Junior, R., & Oppermann, R. V. (2004). Evaluation of dental flossing on a group of second grade students undertaking supervised tooth brushing. *Oral Health Prev Dent,* 2(2):111–18.

66. Crain, N., Klein, B. L., & Mohan, P. (2000). Dental floss ingestion requiring endoscopic retrieval. *Ped Emerg Care,* 16(5):339–40.

67. Gow, A. M., & Kelleher, M. G. D. (2003). Tooth surface floss loss: Unusual interproximal and lingual cervical lesions as a result of bizarre dental flossing. *Dent Update,* 30(6):331–36.

68. Walters, J. D., & Chang, E. I. (2003). Periodontal bone loss associated with an improper flossing technique: A case report. International *J Dent Hygiene,* 1(2), 115–119.

69. Hallmon, W. W., Waldrop, T. C., Houston, G. D., & Hawkins, B. F. (1986). Flossing clefts. Clinical and histologic observations. *J Periodontol,* 57(8):501–504.

70. Kuusela, S., Honkala, E., Kannas, L., Tynjala, J., & Wold, B. (1997). Oral hygiene habits of 11-year-old schoolchildren in 22 European countries and Canada in 1993/1994. *J Dent Res,* 76(9):1602–609.

71. Nield-Gehrig, J. S., & Willmann, D. E. (2003). *Foundations of periodontics for the dental hygienist* (2nd ed.). Philadelphia: Lippincott Williams & Wilkins, 274–81.

72. Melrose, D. (2005). Floss alternatives. *Dimens Dent Hygiene,* 3(10):22, 24, 26. Retrieved March 4, 2007, from http://dimensionsofdentalhygiene.com.

73. Jahn, C. (2000). Review of automated plaque removal products. *J Pract Hygiene,* 9(5):48–52.

74. Lang, W. P. Farghaly, M. M., & Ronis, D. L. (1994). The relation of preventive dental behaviors to periodontal health status. *J Clin Periodontol,* 21:194–98.

75. Rimondini, L., Zolfanelli, B., Bernardi, F., & Bez, C. (2001). Self-preventive oral behavior in an Italian university student population. *J Clin Periodontol,* 28:207–11.

76. Lyle, D. M. (2000). The role of pharmacotherapeutics in the reduction of plaque and gingivitis. *J Pract Hygiene,* 9(6 Supp):46–50.

77. Bergenholtz, A., & Brithon, J. (1980). Plaque removal by dental floss or toothpicks. *J Clin Periodontol,* 7:516–24.

78. Axelsson, P. (1998). Needs-related plaque control measures based on risk prediction. In Lang, N. P., Attstrom, R., & Loe, H., Eds. *Proceedings of the European workshop on mechanical plaque control.* Chicago: Quintessence, 190–247.

79. Jenney, A. W. J., Cherry, C. L., Davis, B., & Wesselingh, S. L. (2001, January 15). Floss and nearly die. *Med J Aust,* 174(2):107–108.

80. Ehrmann, E. H. (2001). Did dental flossing cause endocarditis? Reply. *Aust Dent J,* 46:3.

81. Carroll, G. C., & Sebor, R. J. (1980). Dental flossing and its relationship to transient bacteremia. *J Periodontol,* 51(12):691–92.

82. Dajani, A. S., Taubert, K. A., Wilson, W., Bolger, A. F., Bayer, A., Ferrieri, P., Gewitz, M. H., Shulman, S. T., Nouri, S., Newburger, J. W., Hutto, C., Pallasch, T. J., Gage, T. W., Levison, M. E., Peter, G., & Zuccaro, G. (1997). Prevention of bacterial endocarditis. Recommendations by the American Heart Association. *Circulation,* 96:358–66. Retrieved February 15, 2007 from http://circ.ahajournals.org.

83. Tedesco, L. A., Keffer, M. A., Fleck-Kandath, C. (1991). Self-efficacy, reasoned action, and oral health behavior reports: A social cognitive approach to compliance. *J Behav Med,* 14(4):341–55.

84. Stewart, J. E., & Wolfe, G. R. (1989). The retention of newly-acquired brushing and flossing skills. *J Clin Periodontol,* 16(5):331–32.

85. Ciancio, S. (2003). Improving oral health: Current considerations. *J Clin Periodontol,* 30 (Suppl 5):4–6.

86. Schuz, B., Sniehotta, F. F., Wiedemann, A., & Seeman, R. (2006). Adherence to a daily flossing regimen in university students: Effects of planning when, where, how and what to do in the face of barriers. *J Clin Periodontol,* 33(3):612–19.

87. Mulligan, R., & Wilson, S. (1984). Design characteristics of floss-holding devices for persons with upper extremity disabilities. *Special Care in Dentistry,* 4(4):168–172.

88. Pucher, J., Jayaprakash, P., Aftyka, T., Sigman, L., & Van Swol, R. (1995). Clinical evaluation of a new flossing device. *Quintessence Int,* 26(4):273–78.

89. Kleber, C. J., & Putt, M. S. (1988). Evaluation of a floss-holding device compared to hand-held floss for interproximal plaque, gingivitis, and patient acceptance. *Clin Prev Dent,* 10(4):6–14.

90. Spolsky, V. W., Perry, D. A., Meng, Z., & Kissel, P. (1993). Evaluating the efficacy of a new flossing aid. *J Clin Periodontol,* 20:490–97.

91. Kleber, C. J., & Putt, M. S. (1990). Formation of flossing habit using a floss-holding device. *J Dent Hygiene,* 64(3):140–43.

92. Kinane, D. F., Jenkins, W. M. M., & Paterson, A. J. (1992). Comparative efficacy of the standard flossing procedure and a new floss applicator in reducing interproximal bleeding: A short-term study. *J Periodontol,* 63(9), 757–60.

93. Carter-Hanson, C., Gadbury-Amyot, C., & Killoy, W. (1996). Comparison of the plaque removal efficacy of a new flossing aid (Quik Floss®) to finger flossing. *J Clin Periodontol,* 23:873–78.

94. Honkala, E., Kannas, L., & Rise, J. (1990). Oral health habits of schoolchildren in 11 European countries. *Int Dent J,* 40:211–17.

95. Cronin, M. J., Dembling, W. Z., Cugini, M. A., Thompson, M. C., & Warren, P. R. (2005). A 30-day clinical comparison of a novel interdental cleaning device and dental floss in the reduction of plaque and gingivitis. *J Clin Dent,* 16(2):33–37.

96. Perry, D. A., & Beemsterboer, P. L. (2007). Plaque and disease control for the periodontal patient. In Perry, D. A., & Beemsterboer, P. L., Eds. *Periodontology for the dental hygienist* (3rd ed.). St. Louis: Saunders Elsevier, 235–58.

97. Syme, S. E., & Fried, J. L. (1999). Maintaining the oral health of splinted teeth. *Dent Clin North Am,* 43(1):179–96.

98. Barnes, C. M., Russell, C. M., & Weatherford, T. W. (1999). A comparison of the efficacy of 2 powered toothbrushes in affecting plaque accumulation, gingivitis, and gingival bleeding. *J Periodontol,* 70(8):840–47.

99. Hancock, E. B., & Newell, D. H. (2002). The role of periodontal maintenance in dental practice. *J Indiana Dent Assoc,* 81(2):25–30.

100. Gutkowski, S. (2007). New year new practice. *Prevent Angle,* 6(1), 1–6. Available at newsletter@youngdental.com.

101. Ciancio, S., Shibly, O., Charles, C., & Mather, M. L. (2002). Effect of single versus multiple flossing instruction on gingival health. (Abstract). *J Periodontol,* 73:1245.

102. Schmage, P., Platzer, U., & Nergiz, I. (1999). Comparison between manual and mechanical methods of interproximal hygiene. *Quintessence Int,* 30(8):535–39.

103. Isaacs, R. L., Beiswanger, B. B., Crawford, J. L., Mau, M. S., Proskin, H., & Warren, P. R. (1999). Assessing the efficacy and safety of an electric interdental cleaning device. *J Am Dent Assoc,* 130:104–108.

104. Asadoorian, J. (2006). Flossing: CDHA position paper. Canadian *J Dent Hygiene,* 40(3):1–10.

105. Johansson, L. A., Oster, B., & Hamp, S. E. (1984). Evaluation of cause-related periodontal therapy and compliance with maintenance care recommendations. *J Clin Periodontol,* 11(10):689–99.

106. Jahn, C. A. (2001). Automated oral hygiene self-care devices: Making evidence-based choices to improve client outcomes. *J Dent Hygiene,* 75(2):171–86.

107. Gordon, J. M., Frascella, J. A., & Reardon, R. C. (1996). A clinical study of the safety and efficacy of a novel electric interdental cleaning device. *J Clin Dent,* 7(3):70–73.

108. Cronin, M., Dembling, W., Warren, P., & Braun, A. G. (1997). The safety and efficacy of gingival massage with

an electric interdental cleaning device. *J Clin Dent,* 8(5):130–33.

109. Shibly, O., Ciancio, S. G., Shostad, S., Mather, M., & Boardman, T. J. (2001). Clinical evaluation of an automatic flossing device vs. manual flossing. *J Clin Dent,* 12(3):63–66.

110. Anderson, N. A., Barnes, C. M., Russell, C. M., & Winchester, K. R. (1995). A clinical comparison of the efficacy of an electromechanical flossing device or manual flossing in affecting interproximal gingival bleeding and plaque accumulation. *J Clin Dent,* 6(1):105–107.

111. Hohoff, A., Stamm, T., Kuhne, N., Wiechmann, D., Haufe, S., Lippold, C., Ehmer, U. (2003). Effects of a mechanical interdental cleaning device on oral hygiene in patients with lingual brackets. *Angle Orthodont,* 73(5):579–87.

112. Gutkowski, S. (2006). Power cleaning your teeth. Diabetes self management. Retrieved February 12, 2007 from http://www.diabetesselfmanagment.com.

113. Galvis, D. L. M., & Kreismann, J. (2001). Oral hygiene self-care. In Weinberg, M. A., Westphal, C., Palat, M., & Froum, S. J., Eds. *Comprehensive periodontics for the dental hygienist.* Upper Saddle River, NJ: Prentice Hall, 307–38.

114. Maddox, B. P. (2003). Mechanical plaque control: Interdental care and supplemental aids. In Darby, M. L., & Walsh, M. M., Eds. *Dental hygiene theory and practice* (2nd ed.). St. Louis: Saunders Elsevier, 360–84.

115. Schiff, N., Grosgogeat, B., Lissac, M., & Dalard, F. (2002). Influence of fluoride content and pH on the corrosion resistance of titanium and its alloys. *Biomaterials,* 23:1995–2002.

116. Jahn, C. A., & Wilkins, E. M., (2005). Interdental care. In Wilkins, E. M., Ed. *Clinical practice of the dental hygienist* (9th ed.). Philadelphia: Lippincott Williams & Wilkins, 426–37.

117. Finkelstein, P., Yost, K. G., & Grossman, E. (1990). Mechanical devices versus antimicrobial rinses in plaque and gingivitis reduction. *Clin Prev Dent,* 12(3):8–11.

118. Kiger, R. D, Nyland, K., & Feller, R. P. (1991). A comparison of proximal plaque removal using floss and interdental brushes. *J Clin Periodontol,* 18:681–84.

119. Wolff, D., Joerss, D., & Dorfer, C. E. (2006). In vitro-cleaning efficacy of interdental brushes with different stiffness and different diameter. *Oral Health Prev Dent,* 4(4):279–85.

120. Yost, K. G., Mallatt, M. E., & Liebman, J. (2006). Interproximal gingivitis and plaque reduction by four interdental products. *J Clin Dent,* 17(3):79–83.

121. Bergenholtz, A., & Olsson, A. (1984). Efficacy of plaque-removal using interdental brushes and waxed dental floss. *Scand J Dent Res,* 92(3):198–203.

122. van der Weijden, G. A., Timmerman, M. F., Danser, M. M., Piscaer, M., Jzerman, Y. I., & van der Velden, U.

(2005). Approximal brush head used on a powered toothbrush. *J Clin Peridontol,* 32(3):317–22.

123. Danser, M. M., Timmerman, M. F., Ijzerman, Y., Piscaer, M, van der Velden, U., & van der Weijden, G. A. (2001). Approximal brushhead used on a power toothbrush [Abstract No. 1734]. *J Dent Res,* 80(Spec Iss):743.

124. Jared, H., Zhong, Y., Rowe, M., Ebisutani, K., Tanaka, T., Takase, N. (2005). Clinical trial of a novel interdental brush cleaning system. *J Clin Dent,* 16(2):47–52.

125. Christen, A. G., & Christen, J. A. (2003). A historical glimpse of toothpick use: Etiquette, oral and medical conditions. *J Hist Dent,* 51(2):61–69.

126. Bahn, P. G. (1989). Early teething troubles. *Nature,* 337:693.

127. Ring, M. E. (2001). Further reflections on the toothpick in history and literature. *J Hist Dent,* 49(1):24.

128. Mandel, I. D. (1990). Why pick on teeth? *J Am Dent Assoc,* 121(1):129–32.

129. Bergenholtz, A., Bjornes, A., & Vikstrom, B. (1974). The plaque-removing ability of some common interdental aids. An intraindividual study. *J Clin Periodontol,* 1(3):160–65.

130. Kashani, H., Birkhed, D., & Petersson, L. G. (1998). Fluoride concentration in the approximal area after using toothpicks and other fluoride containing products. *Eur J Oral Sci,* 106:564–70.

131. Sarner, B., Birkhed, D., Huysmans, M. C. D. N. J. M., Ruben, J. L., Fidler, V., & Lingstrom, P. (2005). Effect of fluoridated toothpicks and dental flosses on enamel and dentine on plaque composition in situ. *Caries Res,* 39(1):52–59.

132. Bastos, F. L., Fernandes, P. C., & Attstrom, R. (1992). The effect of 1% chlorhexidine gel delivered with toothpicks on proximal dental plaque. A pilot study. *Braz Dent J,* 3(1):17–23.

133. Kashani, H., Emilson, C. G., Birkhed, D. (1998). Effect of NaF-, SnF$_2$-, and chlorhexidine-impregnated birch toothpicks on mutans streptococci and pH in approximal dental plaque. *Acta Odontol Scand,* 56(4):197–201.

134. Axelsson, P. (1993). New ideas and advancing technology in prevention and nonsurgical treatment of periodontal disease. *Int Dent J,* 43:223–38.

135. Lewis, M. W., Holder-Ballard, C., Selders, R. J., Scarbecz, M., Johnson, H. G., & Turner, E. W. (2004) Comparison of the use of a toothpick holder to dental floss in improvement of gingival health in humans. *J Periodontol,* 75(4):551–56.

136. Beatty, C. F., Fallon, P. A., & Marshall, D. D. (1998). A comparison of the effectiveness of two wooden interdental cleaners. *Contact Int,* 12(2):6–11.

137. Yankell, S. L., & Emling, R. C. (2002). Efficacy and safety of BrushPicks, a new cleaning aid compared to the use of Glide floss. *J Clin Dent,* 13(3):125–29.

138. Tillis, T. S. I., & Keating, J. G. (2004). Oral health self-care supplemental measures to complement toothbrushing. In Harris, N. O., & Garcia-Godoy, F., Eds. *Primary preventive dentistry* (6th ed.). Upper Saddle River, NJ: Pearson Prentice Hall, 145–80.

139. Academy of General Dentistry. (2006). Swallow this: dental tip. (Brochure). Retrieved March 3, 2007, from http://www.agd.org.

140. National Institute of Dental and Craniofacial Research. (2005). Continuing education: Practical oral care series. Retrieved March 4, 2007, from http://www.nidcr.nih.gov.

141. Stefanou, L. B. (2006). You are what you eat—The propensity for tooth wear, caries, and dentin hypersensitivity can be reduced through nutrition and dietary changes. *Dimens Dent Hygiene,* 4(4):20–22. Retrieved February 8, 2007 from dimensionsofdentalhygiene.com.

142. Touger-Decker, R. & van Loveren, C. (2003). Sugars and dental caries. *Am J Clin Nutr,* 78(4):881S–92S.

143. Centers for Disease Control, Task Force on Community Preventive Services. (2001). Promoting oral health: Interventions for preventing caries, oral and pharyngeal cancers, and sports-craniofacial injuries. A report on recommendations of the task force on community preventive services. Retrieved March 3, 2007, from http://www.cdc.gov.

144. Reggiardo, P. A., Feigal, R. J., Casamassimo, P. S., Chan, S. D., Ng, M. W., & Ignelzi, M. A. (2006). Clinical, research, and policy implications of the symposium on the prevention of oral diseases in children and adolescents. *Ped Dent,* 28(2):192–98.

145. Scottish Intercollegiate Guidelines Network. (2000). Preventing dental caries in children at high caries risk. Retrieved March 3, 2007 from http://www.sign.ac.uk/guidelines.

146. United States Department of Health and Human Services. (2000). *Oral health in America: A report of the Surgeon General.* Rockville, MD: U.S. Department of Health and Human Services, National Institutes of Health, National Institute of Dental and Craniofacial Research.

147. Menezes, S. M. S., Cordeiro, L. N., & Viana, G. S. B. (2006). Punica granatum (pomegranate) extract is active against dental plaque. *J Herb Pharmacother,* 6(2):79–92.

148. Elworthy, A., Greenman, J., Doherty, F. M., Newcombe, R. G., & Addy, M. (1996). The substantivity of a number of oral hygiene products determined by the duration of effects on salivary bacteria. *J Periodontol,* 67(6):572–576.

149. Dawes, C., Tsang, R. W. L., & Suelzle, T. (2001). The effects of gum chewing, four oral hygiene procedures, and two saliva collection techniques, on the output of bacteria into human whole saliva. *Arch Oral Biol,* 46(7):625–32.

150. Esposito, E. J., & Gray, W. A. (1975). Effect of water and mouthwashes on pH of oral monkey mucosa. *Pharmacol Therapeut Dent,* 2(1):33–41.

151. Addy, M., Moran, J., & Newcombe, R. G. (2007). Meta-analyses of studies of 0.2% delmopinol mouth rinse as an adjunct to gingival health and plaque control measures. *J Clin Periodontol,* 34:58–65.

152. Bauroth, K., Charles, C. H., Mankodi, S. M., Simmons, K., Zhao, Q., Kumar, L. D. (2003). The efficacy of an essential oil antiseptic mouthrinse vs. dental floss in controlling interproximal gingivitis. *J Am Dent Assoc,* 134(March):359–365.

153. Maruniak, J., Clark, W. B., Walker, C. B., Magnusson, I., Marks, R. G., Taylor, M., & Clouser, B. (1992). The effect of 3 mouthrinses on plaque and gingivitis development. *J Clin Periodontol,* 19:19–23.

154. Fine, D. H., Furgang, D., Sinatra, K., Charles, C., McGuire, A., & Kumar, L. D. (2005). In vivo antimicrobial effectiveness of an essential oil-containing mouth rinse 12 h after a single use and 14 days' use. *J Clin Periodontol,* 32(4):335–40.

155. Grossman, E., Meckel, A. H., Issaacs, R. L., Ferretti, G. A., Sturzenberger, O. P, Bollmer, B. W., Moore, D. J., Lijana, R. C., & Manhart, M. D. (1989). A clinical comparison of antibacterial mouthrinses: Effects of chlorhexidine, phenolics, and Sanguinarine on dental plaque and gingivitis. *J Periodontol,* 60(8):435–40.

156. Santos, A. (2003). Evidence-based control of plaque and gingivitis. *J Clin Periodontol,* 30(Suppl 5):13–16.

157. Sharma, N., Charles, C. H., Lynch, M. C., Qaqish, J., McGuire, J. A., Galustians, J. G., & Kumar, L. D. (2004). Adjunctive benefit of an essential oil-containing mouthrinse in reducing plaque and gingivitis in patients who brush and floss regularly. A six-month study. *J Am Dent Assoc,* 135:496–504.

158. Sharma, C., Charles, C. H., Qaqish, J. G., Galustians, H. J., Zhao, Q., & Kumar, L. D. (2002). Comparative effectiveness of an essential oil mouthrinse and dental floss in controlling interproximal gingivitis and plaque. *Am J Dent,* 15(6):351–55.

159. Zimmer, S., Kolbe, C., Kaiser, G., Krage, T., Ommerborn, M., & Barthel, C. (2006). Clinical efficacy of flossing versus use of antimicrobial rinses. *J Periodontol,* 77(8):1380–85.

160. Wennstrom, J. L. (1998). Rinsing, irrigation and sustained local delivery. In Lang, N. P., Attstrom, R., & Loe, H., Eds. *Proceedings of the European workshop on mechanical plaque control.* Chicago: Quintessence, 131–51.

161. Wilkins, E. M. (2005). *Clinical practice of the dental hygienist* (9th ed.) Philadelphia: Lippincott Williams & Wilkins, 872, 902, 1018.

162. Nachnani, S. (2001). Oral malodor. In Newman, M. G., & van Winkelhoff, A. J., Eds. *Antibiotic and antimicrobial use in dental practice* (2nd ed.). Chicago: Quintessence, 127–41.

163. Slots, J., & Jorgensen, M. G. (2000). Efficient antimicrobial treatment in periodontal maintenance care. *J Am Dent Assoc,* 131:1293–304.

164. Bray, K. K., & Wilder, R. S. (1999, September/October). Full-mouth disinfection: A new approach to non-surgical periodontal therapy. *Access,* 57–61.

165. DeSoetes, M., Mongardi, C., Pauwels, M., Haffajee, A., Socransky, S., vanSteenberghe, D., & Quirynen, M. (2001). One-stage full-mouth disinfection. Long term microbiological results analyzed by checkerboard DNA-DNA hybridization. *J Periodontol,* 72:374–82.

166. Kaplowitz, G. J., & Cortell, M. (2006). Chlorhexidine: A multi-functional antimicrobial drug. Santa Monica, CA: Academy of Dental Therapeutics and Stomatology. Retrieved March 7, 2007, from http://www.ineedce.com.

167. Newbrun, E. (1996). Current treatment modalities of oral problems of patients with Sjögren's syndrome: Caries prevention. *Adv Dent Res,* 10(1):29–34.

168. Featherstone, J. D. B. (2000). The science and practice of caries prevention. *J Am Dent Assoc,* 131(July):887–99.

169. Emilson, C. G. (1994). Potential efficacy of chlorhexidine against mutans streptococci and human dental caries. *J Dent Res,* 73(3):682–91.

170. Whelton, H., & O'Mullane, D. (2001). The use of combinations of caries preventive procedures. *J Dent Educ,* 65(10):1110–13.

171. Dodd, M. J., Larson, P. J., Dibble, S. L., Miaskowski, C., Greenspan, D., MacPhail, L., Hauck, W. W., Paul, S. M., Ignoffo, R., & Shiba, G. (1996). Randomized clinical trial of chlorhexidine versus placebo for prevention of oral mucositis in patients receiving chemotherapy. *Oncol Nurs Forum,* 23(6):921–27.

172. Adamietz, I. A., Rahn, R., Bottcher, H. D., Schafer, V., Reimer, K., & Fleischer, W. (1998). Prophylaxis with povidone-iodine against induction of oral mucositis by radiochemotherapy. *Support Care Cancer,* 6(4):373–77.

173. Potting, C. M. J., Uitterhoeve, R., Scholte Op Reimer, W., & Van Achterberg, T. (2006). The effectiveness of commonly used mouthwashes for the prevention of chemotherapy-induced oral mucositis: A systematic review. *Eur J Cancer Care,* 15(5):431–39.

174. Burkhart, N., Roberts, M., Alexander, M., & Dodds, A. (2005). Communicating effectively with patients suspected of having bulimia nervosa. *J Am Dent Assoc,* 136(3):1–14. Retrieved September 24, 2007 from http://jada.ada.org/cgi/content/full/136/8/1130.

175. American Association of Orthodontists. (2003). The importance of clean teeth: Good oral hygiene during orthodontic treatment. (Brochure). St. Louis: Author. Retrieved March 4, 2007, from http://www.braces.org.

176. Featherstone, J. D. (2004). The continuum of dental caries—evidence for a dynamic disease process. *J Dent Res,* 83(Spec No. C):C39–C42.

177. Wilding, R. J. C. (1999). Evidence based management of dental caries: A review of the repair potential of the pulp-dentine. Retrieved March 3, 2007, from http://www.eclipse.co.uk.

178. Bots, C. P., Brand, H. S., Veerman, E. C., van Amerongen, B. M., & Nieuw Amerongen, A. V. (2004). Preferences and saliva stimulation of eight different chewing gums. *Int Dent J,* 54(3):143–48.

179. Itthagarun, A., & Wei, S. H. (1997). Chewing gum and saliva in oral health. *J Clin Dent,* 8(6):159–62.

180. Milgrom, P., Ly, K. A., Roberts, M. C., Rothen, M., Mueller, G., & Yamaguchi, D. K. (2006). Mutans streptococci dose response to xylitol chewing gum. *J Dent Res,* 85(2):177–81.

181. Featherstone, J. D. (1999). Prevention and reversal of dental caries: Role of low level fluoride. *Commun Dent Oral Epidemiol,* 27:31–40.

182. Greenstein, G. (2000). Nonsurgical periodontal therapy in 2000: A literature review. *J Am Dent Assoc,* 131:1580–92.

183. American Academy of Periodontology. (2005). Position paper: The role of supra- and subgingival irrigation in the treatment of periodontal diseases. *J Periodontol,* 76(11):2015–27.

184. American Dental Association. (2002). Buying oral care products. *J Am Dent Assoc,* 133:1587.

185. Shiloah, J., & Hovious, L. A. (1993). The role of subgingival irrigations in the treatment of periodontitis. *J Periodontol,* 64:835–43.

186. Ernst, C. P., Pittrof, M., Furstenfelder, S., & Willershausen, B. (2004). Does professional preventive care benefit from additional subgingival irrigation? *Clin Oral Invest,* 8, 211–18.

187. Felo, A., Shibly, O., Ciancio, S. G., Lauciello, F. R., & Ho, A. (1997). Effects of subgingival chlorhexidine irrigation on peri-implant maintenance. *Am J Dent,* 10(2):107–10.

188. Jahn, C. A. (2005). Self-care for the orthodontic patient. *J Pract Hygiene,* 14(6):15–18.

189. American Association of Orthodontists. (2006). How do I take care of my braces? (Brochure). Retrieved February 14, 2007, from http://www.braces.org.

190. Etienne, D. (2003). Locally delivered antimicrobials for the treatment of chronic periodontitis. *Oral Dis,* 9 (Suppl 1):45–50.

191. Cobb, C. M., Rodgers, R. L., & Killoy, W. J. (1988). Ultrastructural examination of human periodontal pockets following the use of an oral irrigation device in vivo. *J Periodontol,* 59(3):155–63.

192. Barnes, C. M., Russell, C. M., Reinhardt, R. A., Payne, J. B., & Lyle, D. M. (2005). Comparison of irrigation to floss as an adjunct to tooth brushing: Effect on bleeding, gingivitis, and supragingival plaque. *J Clin Dent,* 16:71–77.

193. Chaves, E. S., Kornman, K. S., Manwell, M. A., Jones, A. A., Newbold, D. A., & Wood, R. C. (1994). Mechanism of irrigation effects on gingivitis. *J Periodontol,* 65:1016–21.

194. Walsh, T. F. (1993). Pulsed oral irrigation in the management of inflammatory periodontal diseases. *Dent Update,* 20(2):65–71.

195. Newman, M. G., Cattabriga, M., Etienne, D., Flemmig, T., Sanz, M., Kornman, K. S., Doherty, F., Moore, D. J., & Ross, C. (1994). Effectiveness of adjunctive irrigation in early periodontitis: Multi-center evaluation. *J Periodontol,* 65(3):224–29.

196. Fine, J. B., Harper, D. S., Gordon, J. M., Hovliaras, C. A., & Charles, C. H. (1994). Short-term microbiological and clinical effects of subgingival irrigation with an antimicrobial mouthrinse. *J Periodontol,* 65(1):30–36.

197. Hoang, T., Jorgensen, M. G., Keim, R. G., Pattison, A. M., & Slots, J. (2003). Povidone-iodine as a periodontal pocket disinfectant. *J Periodont Res,* 38:311–17.

198. Vignarajah, S., Newman, H. N., & Bulman, J. (1989). Pulsated jet subgingival irrigation with a 0.1% chlorhexidine, simplified oral hygiene and chronic periodontitis. *J Clin Periodontol,* 16:365–70.

199. Brownstein, C. N., Briggs, S. D., Schweitzer, K. L., Briner, W. W., & Kornman, K. S. (1990). Irrigation with chlorhexidine to resolve naturally occurring gingivitis. A methodologic study. *J Clin Peridontol,* 17:588–593.

200. Lang, N. P., & Raber, K. (1981). Use of oral irrigators as vehicles for the application of antimicrobial agents in chemical plaque control. *J Clin Periodontol,* 8(3):177–88.

201. Walsh, T. F., Glenwright, H. D., & Hull, P. S. (1992). Clinical effects of pulsed oral irrigation with 0.2% chlorhexidine digluconate in patients with adult periodontitis. *J Clin Periodontol,* 19(4):245–48.

202. Parsons, L. G., Thomas, L. G, Southard, G. L., Woodall, I. R., & Jones, B. J. B. (1987). Effect of sanguinaria extract on established plaque and gingivitis when supragingivally delivered as a manual rinse or under pressure in an oral irrigator. *J Clin Periodontol,* 14(7):381–85.

203. Ehmke, B., Moter, A., Beikler, T., Milian, E., & Flemmig, T. F. (2005). Adjunctive antimicrobial therapy of periodontitis: Long-term effects on disease progression and oral colonization. *J Periodontol,* 76(5):749–59.

204. Pistorius, A., Willershausen, B., Steinmeier, E. M., & Kreislert, M. (2003). Efficacy of subgingival irrigation using herbal extracts on gingival inflammation. *J Periodontol,* 74(5):616–22.

205. Cutler, C. W., Stanford, T. W., Abraham, C., Cederberg, R, A, Boardman, T. J., & Ross, C. (2000). Clinical benefits of oral irrigation for periodontitis are related to reduction of pro-inflammatory cytokine levels and plaque. *J Clin Periodontol,* 27:134–43.

206. Lofthus, J. E., Waki, M. Y, Jolkovsky, D. L., Otomo-Corgel, J., Newman, M. G., Flemmig, T., & Nachnani, S. (1991). Bacteremia following subgingival irrigation and scaling and root planing. *J Periodontol,* 62(10):602–607.

207. Jolkovsky, D. L., Waki, M. Y., Newman, M. G., Otomo-Corgel, J., Madison, M., Flemmig, T. F., Nachnani, S., & Nowzari, H. (1990). Clinical and microbiological effects of subgingival and gingival marginal irrigation with chlorhexidine gluconate. *J Periodontol,* 61(11):663–69.

208. Braun, R. E., & Ciancio, S. G. (1992). Subgingival delivery by an oral irrigation device. *J Periodontol,* 63(5):469–72.

209. Stein, M. (1993). A literature review: Oral irrigation therapy, the adjunctive roles for home and professional use. *Probe,* 27(1):18–25.

210. Parker, D. (2003, October). Oral irrigation. *RDH,* pp. 1–5. Retrieved February 21, 2008 from http://rdhmag.com/articles/article_disply.html?id=190904.

211. Jahn, C. (2002). Automated oral hygiene self-care devices: Making evidence-based choices to improve client outcomes. ADHA CE course retrieved February 21, 2008 from http://www.adha.org/CE_courses/index.html.

212. Watt, D. L., Rosenfelder, C., & Sutton, C. D. (1993). The effect of oral irrigation with a magnetic water treatment device on plaque and calculus. *J Clin Periodontol,* 20(5):314–17.

213. Johnson, K. E., Sanders, J. J., Gellin, R. G., Palesch, Y. Y. (1998). The effectiveness of a magnetized water oral irrigator (Hydro Fioss®) on plaque, calculus and gingival health. *J Clin Periodontol,* 25(4):316–21.

214. Eberhard, J., Damm, S., Freitag, S., Albers, H. K., & Jepsen, S. (2004). Plaque removing capacity of a novel high pressure water irrigator. *Am J Dent,* 17(3):199–202.

215. Frascella, J. A., Fernandez, P., Gilbert, R. D., & Cugini, M. (2000). A randomized, clinical evaluation of the safety and efficacy of a novel oral irrigator. *Am J Dent,* 13(2):55–58.

216. Pallasch, T. J., & Slots, J. (1996). Antibiotic prophylaxis and the medically compromised patient. *Periodontology 2000,* 10:107–38.

217. Berger, S. A., Weitzman, S., Edberg, S. C., Casey, J. I. (1974). Bacteremia after the use of an oral irrigation device. A controlled study in subjects with normal-appearing gingiva: Comparison with use of toothbrush. *Ann Internl Med,* 80(4):510–11.

218. Kleinberg, L., & Westbay, G. (1990). Oral malodor. *Crit Rev Oral Biol Med,* 1(4):247–59.

219. Cicek, Y., Orbak, R., Tezel, A., Orbak, Z., & Erciyas, K. (2003). Effect of tongue brushing on oral malodor in adolescents. *Pediatr Int,* 45(6):719–23.

220. Malcmacher, L. J., & Verburg, J. (2001, June) The hygienist's role in oral malodor treatment. *Dent Today,* 38–41.

221. Bernie, K. M. (2004, April). Advancing the art and science of Dent Hygiene through oral malodor management. *Contemp Oral Hygiene,* 20–26.

222. Rosenberg, M. (2002). Bad breath: A brief update. *Alpha Omegan,* 95(3):10–15.

223. Pedrazzi, V., Sato, S., de Mattos, M. G. C., Lara, E. H. G., Panzeri, H. (2004). Tongue-cleaning methods: A comparative clinical trial employing a toothbrush and a tongue scraper. *J Periodontol,* 75(7):1009–12.

224. Yaegaki, K., & Sanada, K. (1992). Biochemical and clinical factors influencing oral malodor in periodontal patients. *J Periodontol,* 63(9):783–89.

225. Kleinberg, I., & Westbay, G. (1992). Salivary and metabolic factors involved in oral malodor formation. *J Periodontol,* 63(9):768–75.

226. Faveri, M., Hayasibara, M. F., Pupio, G. C., Cury, J. A., Tsuzuki, C. O., & Hayacibara, R. M. (2006). A cross-over study on the effect of various therapeutic approaches to morning breath odour. *J Clin Periodontol,* 33:555–60.

227. Roldan, S., Herrera, D., & Sanz, M. (2003). Biofilms and the tongue: Therapeutical approaches for the control of halitosis. *Clin Oral Invest,* 7:189–97.

228. Richter, J. L. (1996). Diagnosis and treatment of halitosis. *Compendium,* 17(4):370–86.

229. Kostelc, J. G., Preti, G., Zelson, P. R., Brauner, L., Baehni, P. (1984). Oral odors in early experimental gingivitis. *J Periodont Res,* 19:303–12.

230. Zhou, H., McCombs, G. B., Darby, M. L., & Marinak, K. (2004, May 15). Sulphur by-product: The relationship between volatile sulphur compounds and dental plaque-induced gingivitis. *J Contemp Dent Prac,* 5(2). Retrieved March 7, 2007, from http://www.thejcdp.com.

231. Frascella, J., Gilbert, R., Fernandez, P., & Hendler, J. (2000). Efficacy of a chlorine dioxide-containing mouthrinse in oral malodor. *Compend Contin Educ Dent,* 21(3):241–244, 246.

232. Silwood, C. J. L., Grootveld, M. C., & Lynch, E. (2001). A multifactorial investigation of the ability of oral health care products (OHCPs) to alleviate oral malodour. *J Clin Periodontol,* 28:634–41.

233. Loesche, W. J., & Kazor, C. (2002). Microbiology and treatment of halitosis. *Periodontology 2000,* 28:256–79.

234. Yaegaki, K., Coil, J. M., Kamemizu, T., & Miyazaki, H. (2002). Tongue brushing and mouth rinsing as basic treatment measures for halitosis. *Int Dent J,* 52:192–96.

235. Quirynen, M., Zhao, H., & van Steenberghe, D. (2002). Review of the treatment strategies for oral malodour. *Clin Oral Invest,* 6:1–10.

236. White, G. E., & Armaleh, M. T. (2004). Tongue scraping as a means of reducing oral mutans streptococci. *J Clin Ped Dent,* 28(2):163–66.

237. Mcdowell, J. D., & Kassebaum, D. K. (1993). Diagnosing and treating halitosis. *J Am Dent Assoc,* 124:55–64.

238. Seeman, R., Kison, A., Bizhang, M., & Zimmer, S. (2001). Effectiveness of mechanical tongue cleaning on oral levels of volatile sulfur compounds. *J Am Dent Assoc,* 132:1263–67.

239. Outhouse, T. L., Al-Alawi, R., Fedorowicz, Z., & Keenan, J. V. (2006). Tongue scraping for treating halitosis. (Review). *Cochrane Database Syst Rev,* Issue 2, Art. No.: CD005519. DOI:10.1002/14651858.CD005519.pub2.

240. Ray, T. S. (2005). Oral infection control: Toothbrushes and tooth brushing. In Wilkins, E. M., Ed. *Clinical practice of the dental hygienist* (9th ed.). St. Louis: Lippincott Williams & Wilkins, 419–20.

241. American Academy of Periodontology. (2000). Position paper: Dental implants in periodontal therapy. *J Periodontol,* 71(12):1934–42.

242. Beikler, T., & Flemmig, T. F. (2001). Antimicrobials in implant dentistry. In Newman, M. G., & van Winkelhoff, A. J., Eds. *Antibiotic and antimicrobial use in dental practice* (2nd ed.). Chicago: Quintessence, 195–211.

243. Steele, D. L., & Orton, G. S. (1992, June/July). Dental implants: Clinical procedures and homecare considerations. *Pract Hygiene,* 9–12.

244. Koumjian, J. H., Kerner, J., Smith, R. A. (1990). Hygiene maintenance of dental implants. *J Calif Dent Assoc,* 18(9):29–33.

245. Esposito, M., Grusovin, M. G., Coulthard, P., & Worthington, H. V. (2006). Interventions for replacing missing teeth: Treatment of periimplantitis. (Review). *Cochrane Database Syst Rev,* Issue 3, Art. No.: CD004970.DOI:10.1002/14651858.CD004970.pub2.

246. Eskow, R., & Smith, V. (1999). Preventive periimplant protocol. *Compend Contin Educ Dent,* 20(2):137–42.

247. Carlson-Mann, L. D., & Ibbott, C. G. (1991). The maintenance of osseointegrated implants, *J Can Dent Assoc,* 57(8):649–53.

248. McFall, W. T. (1989). Supportive treatment. In Nevins, M., Becker, W., & Kornman, K., Eds. *Proceedings of the world workshop in clinical periodontics.* Chicago: American Academy of Periodontology, IX 1–28.

249. American Academy of Periodontology. (2003). Position paper: Periodontal maintenance. *J Periodontol,* 74:1395–401.

250. Serio, F. G. (1997, December). Tools for the maintenance department. RDH. Retrieved February 21, 2008 from http://www.rdhmag.com/display_article/118024/56/none/none/Feat/Tools-for-the-maintenance-department.

251. Truhlar, R. S., Morris, H. F., & Ochi, S. (2000). The efficacy of a counter-rotational powered toothbrush in the maintenance of endosseous dental implants. *J Am Dent Assoc,* 131(1):101–107.

252. Vandekerckhove, B., Quirynen, M., Warren, P. R., Strate, J., & van Steenberghe, D. (2004). The safety and efficacy of a powered toothbrush on soft tissues in patients with implant-supported fixed prostheses. *Clin Oral Invest,* 8(4):206–10.

253. Wolff, L., Kim, A., Nunn, M., Bakdash, B., & Hinrichs, J. (1998). Effectiveness of a sonic toothbrush in maintenance of dental implants. A prospective study. *J Clin Periodontol,* 25:821–28.

254. Jensen, R. L., & Jensen, J. H. (1991, July/August). Peri-implant maintenance. *Northwest Dent,* 14–23.

255. Ciancio, S. G., Lauciello, F., Shibly, O., Vitello, M., & Mather, M. (1995). The effect of an antiseptic mouthrinse on implant maintenance: Plaque and peri-implant gingival tissues. *J Periodontol,* 66(11):962–65.

256. Beikler, T., & Flemmig, T. F. (2003). Implants in the medically compromised patient. *Crit Rev Oral Biol Med,* 14(4):305–16.

257. Meffert, R. M. (1996). Periodontitis vs. peri-implantitis: The same disease? The same treatment? *Crit Rev Oral Biol Med,* 7(3):278–91.

258. Chen, S., & Darby, I. (2003). Dental implants: Maintenance, care and treatment of peri-implant infection. *Austr Dent J,* 48(4):212–20.

259. Heitz-Mayfield, L. J. A., & Lang, N. P. (2004). Antimicrobial treatment of peri-implant diseases. *Int J Oral Maxillofac Implants,* 19 (Suppl):128–139.

260. Klinge, B., Gustafsson, A., & Berglundh, T. (2002). A systematic review of the effect of anti-infective therapy in the treatment of peri-implantitis. *J Clin Periodontol,* 29 (Suppl 3):213–25.

261. Al-Mayouf, A. M., Al-Swayih, A. A., & Al-Mobarak, N. A. (2004). Effect of potential on the corrosion behavior of a new titanium alloy for dental implant applications in fluoride media. *Mater Corros,* 55(2):88–94.

262. Nakagawa, M., Matsuya, S., Shiraishi, T., & Ohta, M. (1999). Effect of fluoride concentration and pH on corrosion behavior of titanium for dental use. *J Dent Res,* 78(9):1568–72.

263. U.S. Census Bureau. (2004, March 18; modified May 31, 2007). U.S. interim projections by age, sex, race, and Hispanic origin. Retrieved February 21, 2008 from U.S. Census Bureau, Population Division, Population Projections Branch web page at http://www.census.gov/ipc/www/usinterimproj.

264. U.S. Census Bureau. (2004, March 18). U.S. interim projections by age, sex, race, and Hispanic origin. Retrieved March 5, 2007, from http://www.census.gov/pc/www/usinterimproj.

265. Douglass, C. W., & Watson, A. J. (2002). Future needs for fixed and removable partial dentures in the United States. *J Prosthet Dent,* 87(1):9–14.

266. Skarnulis, L. (2007, January 27). 7 Health challenges of aging. Retrieved February 28, 2007, from http://the-headliners.wordpress.com.

267. National Institute of Dental Research. (1987). *Oral health of United States adults: The national survey of oral health in U.S. employed adults and seniors, 1985–1986— National findings* (NIH Publication No. 87-2868). Bethesda, MD: U.S. Department of Health and Human Services, Public Health Service, 3–31.

268. Fehrenbach, M. J. (2004, February). Addressing the needs of denture patients. *RDH,* 1–6. Retrieved February 21, 2008 from http://rdhmag.com/display_article/198336/56/none/none/Feat/Addressing-The-Needs-Of-Denture-Patients.

269. Shay, K. (2000). Denture hygiene: A review and update. *J Contemp Dent Prac,* 1(2):028–041. Retrieved February 28, 2007, from http://www.thejcdp.com.

270. Sazvar, S. M. R., Dashti, M. H., & Afshan, B. K. (2005, March). Effectiveness of a mechanic-chemical method in reducing malodor of dentures. (Abstract). *Oral Dis,* 11(Suppl 1):119.

271. Goldberg, S., Cardash, H., Browning, H., Sahly, H., & Rosenberg, M. (1997). Isolation of Enterobacteriaceae from the mouth and potential association with malodor. *J Dent Res,* 76(11):1770–75.

272. Abelson, D. C. (1985). Denture plaque and denture cleansers: Review of the literature. *Gerodontics,* 1(5):202–206.

273. Gonsalves, W. C., Chi, A. C., & Neville, B. W. (2007, February 15) Common oral lesions: Part I. Superficial mucosal lesions. *Am Fam Physic,* 75(4):501–507.

274. Shulman, J. D., Beach, M. M., & Rivera-Hidalgo, F. (2004). The prevalence of oral mucosal lesions in U.S. adults. *J Am Dent Assoc,* 135(9):1279–86.

275. Shay, K., Grasso, J. E., & Barrack, K. S. (2006, April 17). The complete denture prosthesis: Clinical and laboratory applications—Insertion, patient adaptation, and post-insertion care. (CE Course). Retrieved February 21, 2008 from www.dentalcare.com/soap.conteduc/index.htm.

276. American Dental Association. (2007). Oral health topics A-Z: Dentures: Frequently asked questions. Retrieved February 28, 2007, from http://www.ada.org.

277. Academy of General Dentistry. (2006). What is a denture? (Brochure). Retrieved February 28, 2007 from http://www.agd.org.

278. Ragalis, K. (2005). Care of dental prostheses. In Wilkins, E. M., Ed. *Clinical practice of the dental hygienist* (9th ed.). Philadelphia: Lippincott Williams & Wilkins, 469–84.

279. American Cancer Society. (2006, July 10). What are the key statistics about oral cavity and oropharyngeal cancer? Retrieved March 2, 2007, from http://www.cancer.org.

280. Hoad-Reddick, G., Grant, A. A., & Griffith, C. S. (1990). Investigation into the cleanliness of dentures in an elderly population. *J Prosthet Dent,* 64:48–52.

281. Cosme, D. C., Baldisserotto, S. M., Fernandes, E. D. L., Rivaldo, E. G., Rosing, C. K., & Shinkai, R. S. A. (2006). Functional evaluation of oral rehabilitation with removable partial dentures after five years. *J Appl Oral Sci,* 14(2):1–12. Retrieved February 28, 2007, from http://www.scielo.br/scielo.php.

282. Jagger, D. C., & Harrison, A. (1995). Denture cleaning—the best approach. *Br Dent J,* 178:413–17.

283. de Oliveira, T. R. C., & Frigerio, M. L. M. A. (2004) Association between nutrition and the prosthetic condition in edentulous elderly. *Gerodontology,* 21:205–208.

284. Mobley, C. C. (2005). Nutrition issues for denture patients. *Quintessence Int,* 36(8):627–31.

285. Sahyoun, N. R., & Krall, E. (2003). Low dietary quality among older adults with self-perceived ill-fitting dentures. *J Am Dietet Assoc,* 103(11):1494–99.

286. Akpan, A., & Morgan, R. (2002). Oral candidiasis. *Postgrad Med J,* 78:455–59.

287. Sciubba, J. J. (2005, June 2). Denture stomatitis. E-Medicine from WebMD. Retrieved February 28, 2007, from http://www.emedicine.com.

288. American Cancer Society. (2006a). Oral cancer. (Document No. 300208). Retrieved February 28, 2007, from http://www.cancer.org.

289. Reeson, M. G. (2003). A modified denture cleaning brush for patients with limited manual dexterity. *J Prosthet Dent,* 90(2):205–206.

290. Ragalis, K. (2005). Care of patients with disabilities. In Wilkins, E. M., Ed. *Clinical practice of the dental hygienist* (9th ed.). Philadelphia: Lippincott Williams & Wilkins, 898–99.

291. Gwinnett, A. J., & Caputo, L. (1983). The effectiveness of ultrasonic denture cleaning: A scanning electron microscope study. *J Prosthet Dent,* 50(1):20–25.

292. Arita, M., Nagayoshi, M., Fukuizumi, T., Okinaga, T., Masumi, S., Morikawa, M., Kakinoki, Y., & Nishihara, T. (2005). Microbicidal efficacy of ozonated water against Candida albicans adhering to acrylic dental plates. *Oral Microbiol Immunol,* 20(4):206–10.

293. McCabe, J. F., Murray, I. D, & Kelly, P. J. (1995). The efficacy of denture cleansers. *Eur J Prosthodont Restor Dent,* 3(5):203–207.

294. Harrison, Z., Johnson, A., & Douglas, C. W. I. (2004). An in vitro study into the effect of a limited range of denture cleaners on surface roughness and removal of Candida albicans from conventional heat-cured acrylic resin denture base material. *J Oral Rehab,* 31(5):460–67.

295. Ruiz-Medina, P., Bravo, M., Gil-Montoya, J. A., & Montero, J. (2005). Discrimination of functional capacity for oral hygiene in elderly Spanish people by the Barthel General Index. *Commun Dent Oral Epidemiol,* 33(5):363–69.

296. Dills, S. S., Olshan, A. M., Goldner, S., & Brogdon, C. (1988). Comparison of the antimicrobial capability of an abrasive paste and chemical-soak denture cleaner. *J Prosthet Dent,* 60(4):467–70.

297. Kulac, Y., Arikan, A., Albak, S., Okar, I., & Kazazoglu, E. (1997). Scanning electron microscopic examination of different cleaners: surface contaminant removal from dentures. *J Oral Rehab,* 24(3):209–15.

298. Nakamoto, K., Tamamoto, M., & Hamada, T. (1991). Evaluation of denture cleansers with and without enzymes against Candida albicans. *J Prosthet Dent,* 66(6):792–95.

299. Keyf, F., & Gungor, T. (2003). Comparison of effects of bleach and cleansing tablet on reflectance and surface changes of a dental alloy used for removable partial dentures. *J Biomater Appl,* 18 (July):5–14.

300. Ma, T., Johnson, G. H., & Gordon, G. E. (1999). Effects of chemical disinfectants on surface characteristics and color of three fixed prosthodontic crown materials. *J Prosthet Dent,* 82(5):600–607.

301. Glass, R. T. (1992). The infected toothbrush, the infected denture, and transmission of disease: A review. *Compend Contin Educ Dent,* 13(7):592, 594, 596–98.

302. Tawara, Y., Honma, K., & Naito, Y. (1996). Methicillin-resistant Staphylococcus aureus and Candida albicans on denture surfaces. *Bull Tokyo Dent Coll,* 37(3):119–28.

303. Coates, A. J. (2000). Usage of denture adhesives. *J Dent,* 28(2):137–40.

304. Grasso, J. E. (1996). Denture adhesives: Changing attitudes. *J Am Dent Assoc,* 127(1):90–96.

305. Psillakis, J. (2003). Denture adhesives usage in removable prosthodontics. *Dent Today,* 22(3):90–93.

306. Rajaiah, J., Ramji, N., Barnes, J. E., Kneipp, A. M., Winston, J. L., & Fitzgerald, J. A. (2003). In vitro inhibition of Streptococcus mutans by denture adhesives. Poster presented at American Association of Dental Research. Retrieved March 2, 2007 from http://www.dentalcare.com.

307. Barnes, J. E., Ramji, N., Rajaiah, J., Zhou, X, & Fitzgerald, J. A. (2004). Antimicrobial efficacy of denture adhesives. Poster presented at American Association of Dental Research. Retrieved March 2, 2007, from http://www.dentalcare.com.

308. Myatt, G. J., Hunt, S. A., Barlow, A. P. Winston, J. L., Bordas, A., & Maaytah, M. E. (2002). A clinical study to assess the breath protection efficacy of denture adhesive. *J Contemp Dent Prac,* 3(4). Retrieved February 15, 2007, from http://www.thejcdp.com.

Chapter 11

Community Water Fluoridation

William D. Bailey

OBJECTIVES

After studying this chapter, the student should be able to:

1. Define community water fluoridation.
2. Explain the rationale for using water systems to provide for primary prevention of dental caries.
3. Describe the four historical periods in the evolution and development of community water fluoridation.
4. Describe the caries-preventive benefits of water fluoridation.
5. Define the role of water fluoridation and the impact of multiple sources of fluoride on the decline of dental caries.
6. Describe the effect on caries prevalence when water fluoridation is discontinued in a community.
7. Describe fluorosis classifications and characteristics, by severity, and the need to monitor exposure to fluoride.
8. Describe the economic aspects of water fluoridation.
9. State the optimal fluoride concentration range, in parts per million (ppm F), for maximum caries protection with minimal risk of fluorosis.
10. List the additives used for water fluoridation and briefly describe the technical aspects of fluoridation, including monitoring and surveillance of water fluoridation in the United States.
11. Describe the Safe Drinking Water Act and the Environmental Protection Agency regulatory standards for natural fluoride levels.

KEY TERMS

Community water fluoridation
Fluoridation
Water fluoridation
Clinical discovery phase
Epidemiologic phase
Demonstration phase
Technology transfer phase
Systemic fluoride
Topical fluoride
Exodontia
Dilution
Diffusion
Primary standard
Secondary standard
Idiopathic
Hypofluoridation
Hyperfluoridation
Salt fluoridation
Milk fluoridation

12. Describe the mechanisms by which community water fluoridation may be enacted in the United States.
13. Summarize the readiness assessment factors for initiating a fluoridation campaign.
14. Describe basic principles of risk perception in general terms and as they relate to water fluoridation.
15. Describe strategies and necessary steps to run a successful fluoridation campaign.
16. Summarize the current status of water fluoridation in the United States as it relates to the Healthy People 2010 objective and the percentage of population served.
17. Summarize the current status of fluoridation in other countries and describe alternatives to water fluoridation.

INTRODUCTION

Community water fluoridation, also referred to as **fluoridation,** is defined as the upward adjustment of the natural fluoride level in a community's water supply to a level optimal for dental health. It is a population-based method of primary prevention that uses piped water systems to deliver low doses of fluoride over frequent intervals. By consuming the water, consumers accrue preventive benefits, regardless of age or socioeconomic status. Fluoridation has been cited by the Centers for Disease Control and Prevention (CDC) as one of the top ten public health achievements of the twentieth century. Extensive research spanning more than 60 years has consistently supported the effectiveness, safety, and cost-effectiveness of fluoridation. Fluoridation contributed to a dramatic decline in dental caries from the 1950s to the 1980s, and continues to effectively reduce and prevent tooth decay today when multiple sources of fluoride, such as fluoride toothpaste, are readily available. Continued monitoring of fluoride exposure from all sources, especially from discretionary sources such as fluoride-containing dentifrices, is important to achieve the appropriate balance between maximum caries-preventive benefit and minimal risk of fluorosis. Fluoridation has been shown to be an effective intervention and sound public policy; however, the practice of fluoridating community water supplies has been challenged by vocal opponents since its inception. Fluoridation can be enacted at the state level by legislative action, but more commonly is implemented at the local level through administrative action or a vote of the electorate. Communities often become embroiled in hard-fought, emotional fluoridation referenda that attract significant media attention. Initiation of a fluoridation campaign requires careful planning and coordination, which includes an assessment to determine a community's readiness. Support for fluoridation can be influenced by public opinion; the political climate; the media; voter turnout; knowledge, skills, and political savvy of the campaign committee; external forces; key community leaders; and other factors. Oral health professionals need to remain well informed about issues and events affecting fluoridation by keeping abreast of the scientific literature, as well as relevant state and community policy decisions. Dentists and dental hygienists should to be able to provide accurate information to their patients and address questions about fluoridation benefits or risks. This duty requires not only a grasp of the science, but also an understanding of the forces that affect public attitudes, the policy process, and the strategies employed by the opposition. This chapter defines community water fluoridation, reviews its history, and provides information about effectiveness, cariostatic mechanisms of action, safety, cost-effectiveness, engineering aspects, and strategies used by proponents and opponents of fluoridation. Also included is a section detailing the principles of risk communication, which are important to educational and promotional efforts for fluoridation.

DEFINITION AND BACKGROUND

The American Dental Association (ADA) officially defines **water fluoridation** as the adjustment of the natural fluoride concentration of fluoride-deficient water supplies to the recommended level for optimal dental health.[1] The optimal fluoridation level for any public water system in the United States varies by geographical location according to the temperature and is a value that ranges from 0.7 ppm F to 1.2 ppm F. Parts per million (ppm) and milligrams/liter (mg/l) are essentially equivalent, and the terms are used interchangeably. One part per million is the same concentration as 1 mg/l. Some documents refer to concentrations used in water fluoridation as parts per million; others use milligrams per liter. In this chapter, parts per million will be used.

Fluoride is the reduced form of fluorine, the thirteenth most abundant element on Earth. This naturally occurring substance is found in water, soil, plants, and, even in air. Certain foods, such as tea and fish, contain significant amounts of fluoride.[2] Oceans of the world contain fluoride at concentrations equal to or above levels used for community water fluoridation.[3] Virtually all water sources contain some naturally occurring fluoride, with surface water such as rivers, lakes, and reservoirs normally containing lesser amounts of fluoride than ground water, which is obtained from wells that draw water from beneath the Earth's surface. Because most freshwater sources contain natural levels of fluoride at concentrations below those recommended for optimal dental health, the amount of fluoride is adjusted upward to the optimal level (Figure 11–1 ■).

The Institute of Medicine and the World Health Organization (WHO) identify fluoride as a nutrient important for health.[4,5] Fluoridation can be thought of as a form of nutritional supplementation in which fluoride is added to the drinking water. Nutritional supplementation frequently is used to prevent diseases; examples include the addition of vitamin C to fruit juices to prevent scurvy; vitamin D to milk and breads to prevent rickets; iodine to table salt to prevent goiter; folic acid to grains, cereals, and pastas to prevent birth defects, including spina bifida; and other vitamins and minerals to breakfast cereals to promote normal growth and development. The treatment of water for public consumption is a primary public health activity that has been used by public health agencies to prevent diseases since the 1840s. Water treatment prevents diseases such as amoebic dysentery, cholera, enteropathogenic diarrhea (*Escherichia coli*), giardiasis, hepatitis A, leptospirosis, paratyphoid fever, schistosomiasis, typhoid fever, and many other diseases including dental caries.[6,7]

Fluoridation is an example of an ideal public health intervention in that it (1) benefits people of all ages; (2) is socially equitable and does not exclude any group; (3) imparts continuous protection with no compliance or conscious effort required by consumers, other than drinking optimally fluoridated water; (4) works without requiring individuals to access care or gather in a prescribed location, as with other disease-prevention strategies or programs such as immunizations; (5) does not require the costly services of health professionals; (6) requires no daily-dosage schedules; (7) involves taking no painful inoculations or oral medicines; and (8) is remarkably cost effective.

Every U.S. Surgeon General since 1950 has advocated the adoption of water fluoridation by communities. Dr. Luther Terry, U.S. Surgeon General, 1961 to 1965, described water fluoridation as one of the four great advances in public health, calling it one of the "four horsemen of public health," along with chlorination, pasteurization, and immunization. Dr. C. Everett Koop, U.S. Surgeon General, 1981 to 1989, stated, "Fluoridation is the single most important commitment that a community can make to the oral health of its children and to future generations."[8] In 1992, U.S. Surgeon General Antonia Novello stated that "the optimum standard for the success of any prevention strategy should be measured by its ability to prevent or minimize disease, ease of implementation, high benefit-to-cost ratio, and safety. Community water fluoridation to prevent tooth decay clearly meets this standard."[9] U.S. Surgeon General David Satcher stated, "Community water fluoridation remains one of the great achievements of public health in the twentieth century" and "an inexpensive means of improving oral health that benefits all residents of a community, young and old, rich and poor alike."[10] In the first-ever report on oral health in the United States, released in May 2000, *Oral Health in America: A Report of the Surgeon General,* Dr. Satcher noted that ". . . one of my highest priorities as Surgeon General is reducing the disparities in health that persist among our various populations. Fluoridation holds great potential to contribute toward elimination of these disparities."[11] U.S. Surgeon General Richard Carmona issued a strong endorsement stating, "Policymakers, community leaders, private industry, health professionals, the media, and the public should affirm that oral health is essential to general health and well being and take action to make ourselves, our families, and our communities healthier. I join previous Surgeon Generals in acknowledging the continuing public health role for community water fluoridation in enhancing the oral health of all Americans."[12]

Fluoridation is a population-based method of primary prevention designed to serve as the cornerstone for the prevention of dental caries, one of the most prevalent childhood diseases. More than 16,000 community water systems serving American communities have fluoridated water systems (personal communication, Office

Naturally occurring F in water + Added F = 0.7 ppm to 1.2 ppm F

Optimal Range

■ **FIGURE 11–1** Adjustment of fluoride concentration in water.

of the National Fluoridation Engineer, Centers for Disease Control and Prevention, 2007, October 10). These systems include 43 of the 50 largest American cities.[13] Nearly 70% of the U.S. population on public water supplies consume fluoridated water.[14]

HISTORY OF COMMUNITY WATER FLUORIDATION

The history of community water fluoridation in the United States can be traced back to the first decade of the twentieth century and may be categorized into four separate periods or phases: (1) clinical discovery phase; (2) epidemiologic phase; (3) demonstration phase; and (4) technology transfer phase.[15–18]

The first period, the **clinical discovery phase,** 1901 to 1933, was characterized by the pursuit of knowledge to determine the cause of developmental enamel defects present in people exposed to naturally occurring high levels of fluoride in drinking water in certain western areas of the United States. In 1901, Dr. Frederick McKay, a recent dental school graduate, moved west and set up a dental practice in Colorado Springs, Colorado. He noticed that some of his patients presented with discolored enamel that sometimes exhibited surfaces that were rough, uneven, or even pitted. Local residents called this condition "Colorado Brown Stain." McKay made two important observations about this enamel defect: (1) The stains could not be polished away, meaning that they were intrinsic, or incorporated into the enamel structure; and (2) not everyone's enamel had these characteristics, only a small portion of patients had the condition, and they were limited to a subgroup of patients who had either been born in Colorado Springs or moved there at a very young age. The fact that this uncharacteristic enamel condition was not present among individuals who had not lived in the vicinity as young children led McKay to believe that the etiologic or causal agent was environmental in nature and was incorporated into the enamel structure at the time of tooth formation.

McKay named this condition "mottled enamel" and noted that it appeared to be under-mineralized, or hypomineralized, enamel.[19] McKay sought the consultation of Dr. G. V. Black, one of the time's most well-known and respected researchers, and together they notified the dental profession about this condition by publishing their observations in *Dental Cosmos,* the premier national dental journal of the time[20] (Figure 11–2 ■). Over several decades, McKay examined children in

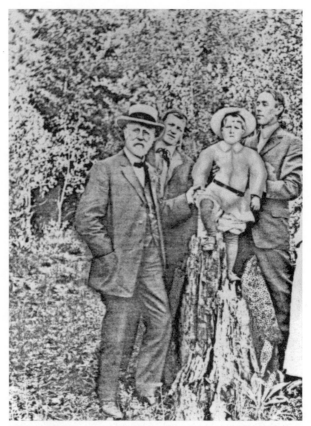

■ **FIGURE 11–2** In 1909, Dr G. V. Black(Lt) visited Dr. F. McKay (Rt) in Colorado Springs to investigate the Colorado brown stain phenomenon.
(Courtesy of the Centers for Disease Control)

various nearby communities and other states to determine the extent of the condition in the population. McKay was able to demonstrate that mottled enamel was confined to specific geographic areas, and he also hypothesized and demonstrated that this condition was directly related to something in the drinking water in these areas.[18,21] In 1927, McKay also published an important corollary finding: People who had enamel fluorosis also experienced less dental decay.[22]

Around the same time period, in the early 1930s, H. V. Churchill, a chemist with the Aluminum Company of America, used a new method of spectrographic analysis to examine the water in the town of Bauxite, Arkansas, a town known to have residents with high levels of mottled enamel. He identified high levels of naturally occurring fluoride in the drinking water supply.[19,23] McKay contacted Churchill and sent him samples of water from Colorado Springs and other areas he had observed to have a high prevalence of mottled enamel. The results showed fluoride concentrations ranging from 2 ppm F to 12 ppm F.[24] McKay had identified his etiologic agent. The high level of fluoride in the water was associated with mottled enamel.

The search for additional information about the role of fluoride in the cause of enamel fluorosis and the prevention of dental caries led to the second period, known as the **epidemiologic phase,** which lasted from 1933 to 1945. Concern about the discovery of fluoride in the water led to the appointment of Dr. H. Trendley Dean, a commissioned officer in the U.S. Public Health Service. Dean was the sole person in what was called the Dental Hygiene Unit, part of the newly established National Institutes of Health (Figure 11–3 ■). The Dental Hygiene Unit evolved over time into the National Institute of Dental Research, which later became the National Institute of Dental and Craniofacial Research.

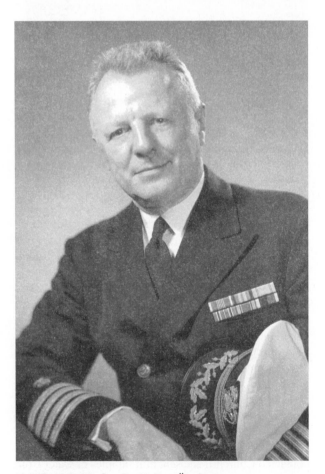

■ **FIGURE 11–3** Dr. H. Trendley Dean.

Dean's job was to map out the prevalence of mottled enamel across the country and to look for a way to reduce or eliminate it. Dean wrote to dental societies across the country asking for their input regarding fluorosis in their locale; in 1933, he published his first map showing the prevalence of mottled enamel in the United States.[25] Although this era predated databases or computers, Dean showed remarkable organizational and epidemiologic prowess in collecting, sorting, and mapping data. By the mid-1930s Dean began using the term *fluorosis* to replace *mottled enamel.* In 1934, Dean developed the Community Fluorosis Index that allowed collection and mapping of severity data in addition to prevalence data.[26] This index assessed not only the location of the condition, but also its severity. Dean later modified the index to classify the full range of enamel conditions, from fine, lacy markings to stained, pitted, damaged enamel. Dean's Fluorosis Index has been the most widely used flurorosis index in the world, and is still used today, especially for surveillance and research activities (Table 11–1 ■).

In addition to studying fluorosis during the epidemiologic phase, researchers began looking at the relationship of fluoride in the water and tooth decay. Dean, with assistance from colleagues at the U.S. Public Health Service's National Institutes of Health, conducted some impressive epidemiologic studies, including the "4 city study" and "Dean's 21-Cities Study." The 4 city study highlighted the difference in dental health and fluorosis among four Illinois cities with differing concentrations of fluoride in the water supply[27] (Table 11–2 ■).

In the 21-city study, Dean examined the data collected by teams of researchers who had examined the teeth of children residing in 21 different communities that had varying levels of naturally occurring fluoride in the drinking water.[28,29] Dean and his team documented the number of carious lesions and fluorosed teeth observed in each of the 21 communities, and compared the findings with the fluoride concentration in the respective water supplies. The findings from Dean's 21-City Study showed that (1) greater concentrations of fluoride in the water correlated with fewer dental caries observed in children, constituting an inverse relationship between the level of natural fluoride in the water and the prevalence of dental caries; and (2) higher levels of fluoride were associated with fluorosis of the teeth, meaning that a direct relationship existed between the level of natural fluoride in the water and the prevalence of enamel fluorosis (Figure 11–4 ■).

■ **Table 11-1** Dean's Fluorosis Index

Diagnosis	Criteria
Normal	Usual translucent semi-vitriform type of structure; smooth, glossy, usually a pale creamy-white color.
Questionable	Slight deviation from normal translucency, ranging from a few white "flecks" to occasional white spots.
Very Mild	Less than 25% of tooth's surface affected. Small, opaque, paper-white areas scattered irregularly over the tooth; tips of cusps often show "snow capping."
Mild	More than 25% but less than 50% of tooth's surface affected. More-extensive, opaque, paper-white areas.
Moderate	All enamel surfaces affected, frequently with brown staining.
Severe	All enamel surfaces affected, with widespread brown staining, and discreet or confluent pitting. Teeth may exhibit a "corroded" appearance.

Dean's results showed that both a reduction of dental caries and an acceptable level of enamel fluorosis could be attained with water containing fluoride levels at approximately 1 ppm of fluoride. At this level, substantial reductions in dental caries of up to 60% were observed, with approximately 10% of the population exhibiting very mild enamel fluorosis. The unattractive form of fluorosis, often called mottling, that was associated with higher levels of fluoride was not observed to occur at the level of 1 ppm F. Consequently, 1 ppm F became the benchmark level used by the U.S. Public Health Service in establishing the optimal range: 0.7 ppm F to 1.2 ppm F. The optimal fluoride level seeks to maximize the benefits of dental caries reduction and minimize the probability of enamel fluorosis (Figure 11–5 ■).

The third period, known as the **demonstration phase,** began in January 1945, and was characterized by a series of community trials in which fluoride levels were adjusted in the public drinking water supply. On January 25, 1945, Grand Rapids, Michigan, became the first city in the world to fluoridate its drinking water as a measure to promote dental health and prevent disease. Grand Rapids was the test, or intervention, city; Muskegon, Michigan, whose water was not fluoridated, was the control city. These cities were the first of four pairs of demonstration cities; the others were (listed by intervention and control) Newburgh and Kingston, New York; Evanston and Oak Park, Illinois; and Brantford and Sarnia, Ontario, Canada. The demonstration cities allowed a comparison of dental and medical observations collected over time from children living in communities with community water fluoridation and those in communities with negligible levels of naturally occurring fluoride. The results were impressive. Sequential cross-sectional surveys, conducted in these communities over 13 to 15 years, showed reductions in dental

■ **Table 11-2** Dean's 4 City Study

City	ppm F in Water	No. of Children[a]	Caries Free (%)	Mean DMFT
Quincy	0.2	291	4.1	6.28
Macomb	0.2	63	14.3	3.68
Monmouth	1.7	99	36.4	2.08
Galesburg	1.8	243	36.2	1.94

DMFT, decayed, missing, filled teeth.
[a] Children ages 12–14 years.
Source: Dean et al, 1939.[27]

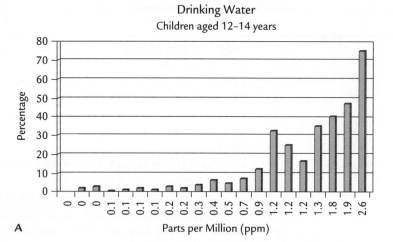

A

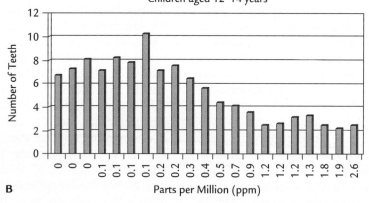

B

■ **FIGURE 11–4** Findings from 21 cities studied by Dean and colleagues in the 1930s showing the prevalence of dental caries and enamel fluorosis.

caries of 50% to 70% among children in the communities with fluoridated water[30] (Table 11–3 ■).

The demonstration phase lasted until about 1954; at that time, the benefits of the optimal adjustment of fluoride levels in drinking water became so apparent that many U.S. cities began fluoridation programs for their citizens. Thus, the demonstration phase overlapped slightly with the fourth period in the history of community water fluoridation, known as the technology transfer phase.

The **technology transfer phase** began about 1950 when planning began in earnest for the implementation of fluoridation in many large U.S. cities. Continuing to this day, the technology transfer phase is characterized by the establishment of a set of national health goals, which includes fluoridation. The year 2010 health objectives for the nation call for the implementation of water fluoridation in all American communities that have communal water sources where implementation is technologically feasible. The target goal for fluoridation is that 75% of the population on community water systems should live in communities with fluoridated water by the year 2010.[31]

Approximately 67% of the U.S. population on community water systems currently enjoy the benefits of water fluoridation (170 million people).[14] This percentage has increased every year since 1945 when fluoridation began

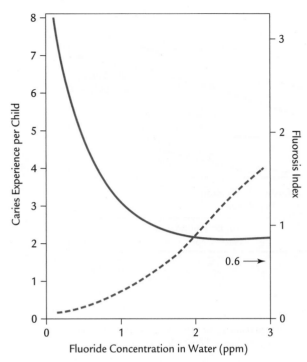

■ **FIGURE 11–5**   Dean's Fluorosis Index/caries/fluorosis curve.

in Grand Rapids, Michigan. Figure 11–6 ■ shows trends in total U.S. population growth, people on public water systems, and people who have optimally fluoridated water.[14] Interestingly, the number of people drinking naturally fluoridated water has not increased, as explained by the fact that most naturally fluoridated waters are groundwater systems serving smaller populations.

In 2002, when the last National Fluoridation Report was published, approximately 170 million Americans were consuming fluoridated water, with an additional 10 million people drinking water with optimal levels of naturally occurring fluoride, equating to 60% of the entire population and 67% of the population served by centralized piped-water systems.[14] State rankings show wide variation in the percentage of the population receiving fluoridation (Table 11–4 ■). Between 1992 and 2002, the population on community water systems served by water fluoridation has grown from 62% to 67%, advancing toward the target of 75%. This datum represented a 38% achievement of the targeted change.[32] Twenty-six states have met or exceeded the Healthy People 2010 goal of 75% of the population being served by community water fluoridation. Of the nation's largest cities, 43 of 50 have adopted fluoridation. Of the seven largest U.S. cities that are not fluoridated—Fresno, Honolulu, Portland, San Diego, San Jose, Tucson, and Wichita—Fresno and Tucson have partially fluoridated water and San Diego has approved fluoridation.[13] The United States has more than 16,000 public water systems with optimal levels of fluoride. Of these water systems, approximately 6,300 have fluoride levels adjusted to optimal levels; more than 3,000 water systems have natural fluoride levels at or above optimal levels; and approximately 6,700 water systems are consecutive with optimal systems (personal communication, Office of the National Fluoridation Engineer, Centers for Disease Control and Prevention, 2007, October 10).

The technology transfer phase has extended fluoridation worldwide, with Singapore implementing fluoridation in 1958, serving 100% of the population.[19] The Republic of Ireland became the first country to actually legislate mandatory nationwide fluoridation in 1960. Israel initiated its mandatory universal fluoridation program in 1981. Countries offering water fluoridation include the United Kingdom, Chile, South Korea, Singapore, Spain, Ireland, the United States, Canada, Brazil,

■ **Table 11–3**   Classic Fluoridation Studies of Paired Cities

	Demonstration Phase	
Fluoridated Cities	*Year of Study*[a]	*Decrease in DMFT of Children Ages 12–14 Years*
Grand Rapids, Michigan	1959	55.5%
Newburgh, New York	1960	70.1%
Evanston, Illinois	1959	48.4%
Brantford, Ontario	1959	56.7%

DMFT, decayed, missing, filled teeth.
[a]Note: All four communities began fluoridating in 1945–1946.
Source: Burt and Eklund, 2005.[23]

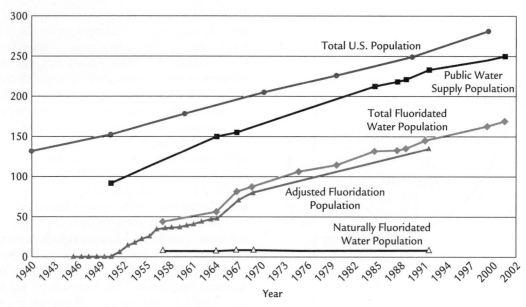

■ **FIGURE 11–6**   Fluoridation growth.
(From Centers for Disease Control and Prevention. *National oral health surveillance statistics/fluoridation status/fluoridation growth.* Retrieved from http://www.cdc.gov/nohss/FSGrowth.htm. Site accessed on 2/12/07.)

Malaysia, Vietnam, Australia, and New Zealand.[13] The WHO issued the following statement in 2005: "Fluoridation of water supplies, where possible, is the most effective public health measure for the prevention of dental decay."[33] Advocated by the WHO, fluoridation benefits over 405 million people in 60 countries worldwide.[13]

Because of its history of effectiveness in reducing the prevalence of dental caries in the United States, water fluoridation was cited as one of the top 10 public health achievements of the twentieth century by the U.S. CDC.[21]

MECHANISMS OF ACTION OF FLUORIDE

Fluoride works in three ways to reduce and prevent tooth decay: (1) systemically, by being ingested and incorporated into the enamel structure during tooth development;[34] (2) topically, by promoting remineralization and inhibiting demineralization of tooth surfaces after eruption;[35,36] and (3) topically, by inhibiting glycolysis in microorganisms, thereby hindering the ability of bacteria to metabolize carbohydrates and produce acid.[37] The greatest effect on reducing and preventing decay is topical;[35] however, both systemic and topical mechanisms are important.

Systemic fluoride is ingested, or taken into the body during consumption of foods or beverages. Systemic fluoride can be incorporated directly into the hydroxyapatite crystalline structure of the developing tooth, with the smaller fluoride ions replacing hydroxyl ions in the crystalline structure of the tooth and producing a less-soluble apatite crystal.[38,39] In the years before water fluoridation was initiated, and for several decades afterwards, the caries-preventive properties of fluoride were attributed almost exclusively to the systemic, or pre-eruptive, effects on the developing teeth. Because it was known that enamel fluorosis could occur only by fluoride being incorporated into the structure of developing teeth, this assumption was reasonable. Today it is accepted that the systemic effect on caries prevention is the lesser effect;[35] however, there is current evidence that systemic exposure to fluoride during tooth formation reduces tooth decay.[40,41]

Topical fluoride concentrates in the plaque and saliva,[35,42] thereby enabling it to come into frequent contact with the surfaces of the teeth. Its effects are posteruptive and can benefit people of nearly all ages by reducing decay on both the coronal and root surfaces.[43,44] The decay process is a continuum that involves both demineralization and remineralizaiton and

■ **Table 11–4**   Percentage of State Populations on Fluoridated Public Water Systems and State Rank, 2002

By State Rank			*Alphabetical by State*		
Location	*Percent*	*State Rank*	*Location*	*Percent*	*State Rank*
United States	65.8		United States	65.8	
District of Columbia	100.0		Alabama	82.0	19
Kentucky	99.6	1	Alaska	57.3	36
Illinois	99.1	2	Arizona	55.4	38
Minnesota	98.4	3	Arkansas	62.1	32
Tennessee	96.0	4	California	27.6	45
North Dakota	95.6	5	Colorado	75.4	24
Indiana	95.5	6	Connecticut	87.6	16
Virginia	93.8	7	District of Columbia	100.0	
Maryland	93.7	8	Delaware	80.9	20
Georgia	93.0	9	Florida	67.4	30
West Virginia	91.5	10	Georgia	93.0	9
South Carolina	91.4	11	Hawaii	8.6	49
Iowa	91.3	12	Idaho	47.5	40
Ohio	90.6	13	Illinois	99.1	2
Wisconsin	89.4	14	Indiana	95.5	6
Rhode Island	89.2	15	Iowa	91.3	12
Connecticut	87.6	16	Kansas	62.1	33
Michigan	86.2	17	Kentucky	99.6	1
North Carolina	84.6	18	Louisiana	45.9	42
Alabama	82.0	19	Maine	74.4	26
Delaware	80.9	20	Maryland	93.7	8
Missouri	80.9	21	Massachusetts	60.7	34
South Dakota	78.0	22	Michigan	86.2	17
New Mexico	76.6	23	Minnesota	98.4	3
Colorado	75.4	24	Mississippi	46.1	41
Oklahoma	74.6	25	Missouri	80.9	21
Maine	74.4	26	Montana	23.8	46
New York	72.9	27	Nebraska	69.5	28
Nebraska	69.5	28	Nevada	69.4	29
Nevada	69.4	29	New Hampshire	42.7	43
Florida	67.4	30	New Jersey	20.8	47
Texas	65.7	31	New Mexico	76.6	23
Arkansas	62.1	32	New York	72.9	27
Kansas	62.1	33	North Carolina	84.6	18
Massachusetts	60.7	34	North Dakota	95.6	5
Washington	58.9	35	Ohio	90.6	13
Alaska	57.3	36	Oklahoma	74.6	25
Vermont	55.7	37	Oregon	19.4	48
Arizona	55.4	38	Pennsylvania	54.0	39
Pennsylvania	54.0	39	Rhode Island	89.2	15
Idaho	47.5	40	South Carolina	91.4	11
Mississippi	46.1	41	South Dakota	78.0	22
Louisiana	45.9	42	Tennessee	96.0	4
New Hampshire	42.7	43	Texas	65.7	31

(*continued*)

■ **Table 11–4**   (*continued*)

By State Rank			Alphabetical by State		
Location	*Percent*	*State Rank*	*Location*	*Percent*	*State Rank*
Wyoming	36.7	44	Utah	2.2	50
California	27.6	45	Vermont	55.7	37
Montana	23.8	46	Virginia	93.8	7
New Jersey	20.8	47	Washington	58.9	35
Oregon	19.4	48	West Virginia	91.5	10
Hawaii	8.6	49	Wisconsin	89.4	14
Utah	2.2	50	Wyoming	36.7	44

Source: Centers for Disease Control and Prevention. (2002). Water fluoridation reporting system (WFRS). Atlanta, GA: Centers for Disease Control and Prevention.

can move in either direction. Just as tooth structure can be lost through demineralization, the enamel can re-form through remineralization. Cycles of demineralization and remineralization continue throughout the lifetime of the tooth (Figure 11–7 ■). Fluoride, especially that held in plaque, is an essential nutrient in the remineralization of teeth.[35]

Cariogenic bacteria residing in dental plaque metabolize sugars and other carbohydrates, producing acid that begins to dissolve, or demineralize, the tooth's enamel crystal surface. Calcium, phosphate, and carbonate are lost from the the enamel and can be captured in the adjacent plaque. The lowered pH caused by the acid also releases fluoride contained in the plaque. Then the fluoride from the plaque and available saliva are taken up by the demineralized enamel along with calcium, phospate, and carbonate; this results in remineralization as the ions re-form into an improved enamel crystal structure that contains more fluoride and less carbonate, and is more resistant to acid (Figure 11–8 ■).[38,39] Fluoride also inhibits the process that bacteria use to metabolize

carbohydrates, thus reducing bacterial acid production and reducing dissolution of tooth enamel.[24,45–50]

One reason why water fluoridation is the most effective method of fluoride delivery is that populations consume small quantities of water throughout the day, not just a couple of times when they brush their teeth or eat. Therefore, on a regular basis, water fluoridation replenishes small quantities of fluoride to the plaque and saliva, which contributes to good oral health.

Systemic fluorides also provide a topical effect because saliva contains some fluoride from ingestion, is continually available at the tooth surface, and becomes concentrated in dental plaque where it inhibits acid-producing cariogenic bacteria from demineralizing tooth enamel.[1,45] Fluoride concentration in the plaque is 50 to 100 times higher than in the whole saliva.[19,51]

In summary, fluoridation has been found to reduce dental decay through three mechanisms: (1) by systemic ingestion of fluoride, which is incorporated into the developing tooth structure and converts hydroxyapatite into fluorapatite, thus reducing the solubility of tooth

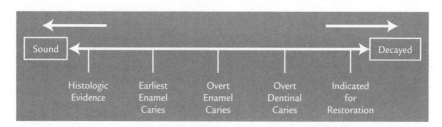

■ **FIGURE 11–7**   Remineralization and demineralization of teeth.

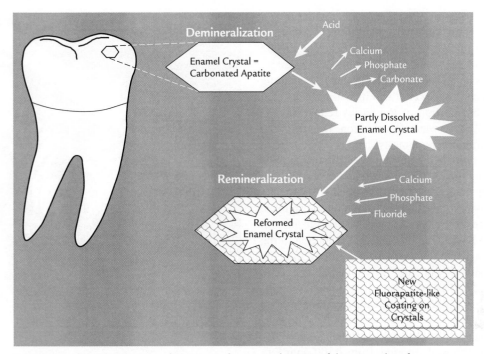

■ FIGURE 11-8 Demineralization and remineralization of the enamel surface.
(From Centers for Disease Control and Prevention, 1999.[89] Adapted from Featherstone, 1999.[35])

enamel in acid and making it more resistant to decay; (2) by topical action of fluoride in the plaque and saliva, which enhances remineralization of tooth enamel that has been demineralized by acids produced by decay-causing bacteria, and (3) by topical interaction with bacteria in the plaque, which reduce the acid production by dental-plaque organisms.

BENEFITS AND EFFECTIVENESS OF FLUORIDATION

Determination of the benefits and effectiveness of community water fluoridation should consider what the oral health of the population was like before fluoridation. It may be difficult to imagine that, during the 1940s in the United States, extractions of first molars in young children were routine; **exodontia** (extraction of teeth) and complete dentures were the norm for older adults; 10% of recruits into World War II were rejected because of poor oral health, which meant those recruits did not have six opposing teeth and 40% needed immediate treatment for relief of pain; and dowries of new brides sometimes included dentures.

Over the past 60+ years, numerous studies have been conducted on the effectiveness of fluoridation and

fluorides in preventing dental caries and decreasing caries rates. When Grand Rapids, Michigan, decided to fluoridate its water supply in 1945, a long-term study of schoolchildren was initiated to determine the effectiveness of fluoridation in decreasing dental caries rates; the study found that, after 11 years of fluoridation, dental caries rates declined by 50% to 63%.[52,53] Corroborative studies in the same era conducted in New York (Newburgh–Kingston) and Illinois (Evanston–Oak Park) reported reductions in caries rates from 57% to 70%.[54,55] Of 73 studies published between 1956 and 1979, the most frequently reported rate of caries reduction was 50% to 60%; it was generally acknowledged that fluoridating a community's water supply would reduce dental decay by half.[19]

Water fluoridation has continued to play a dominant role in the decline in caries, even though the absolute differences in caries prevalence that once were observed between fluoridated and non-fluoridated communities appear to be diminishing.[27] During the early years of fluoridation, the primary source of fluoride was the drinking water, because there were no other discretionary sources of fluoride available, such as fluoride toothpaste, which did not receive the American Dental Association

Seal of Approval until 1964. Consequently, the reductions in dental caries rates attributed to water fluoridation were easily measurable and significant. By 1980, 98% of the available dentifrices contained fluoride.[12,37] As more professional and consumer products containing fluoride came on the market, it was increasingly difficult to measure what portion of the caries reduction was attributable solely to water fluoridation. However, the impact of fluoridation remains evident.

The reduction in the absolute measurable benefits of water fluoridation has been attributed to the dilution and diffusion effects.[19] **Dilution** results from the increased availability of fluoride from multiple sources, diluting the impact of any one source of fluoride, including water.[56–58] Dilution is the apparent reduction in the measurable water fluoridation benefits resulting from the ubiquitous availability of fluoride from other sources in both the fluoridated and the fluoride-deficient comparison community.[15] Today, the most universally available source of fluoride in the United States is a fluoride-containing dentifrice.[17,58] All fluoride-containing dentifrices have very high levels of fluoride, from 1,100 ppm F to 1,500 ppm F, and are a significant potential source of fluoride overexposure and fluorosis. Moreover, they are not meant to be swallowed, especially during the years when the crowns of teeth are forming.[59] The other major modifying factor regarding the effectiveness of fluoridation, the **diffusion** effect, results from the consumption of commercial foods and beverages that were processed in a fluoridated community and transported to fluoride-deficient communities, making fluoride available to consumers in the fluoride-deficient community.[60] Just as ripples in a lake affect water many feet away from the center, foods and beverages produced in fluoridated cities can reach non-fluoridated cities that are hundreds or thousands of miles distant.

Diffusion is described as the extension of benefits of community water fluoridation to residents of fluoride-deficient communities.[19] Diffusion has also been called the "halo effect." The differences in caries-prevalence rates between fluoridated and non-fluoridated communities are diminishing.[6] According to Ripa, the weaker association reported by contemporary studies between exposure to fluoridated drinking water and caries experience, therefore, is not due to a lessening of the effects of waterborne fluoride, but is actually caused by the extension of those effects, through a process of diffusion, of fluoride into fluoride-deficient areas[19] (Figure 11–9 ■). Greater mobility of the population, with increased travel

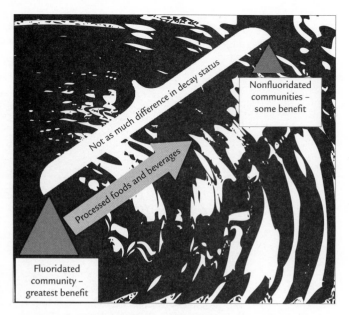

■ **FIGURE 11–9** Diffusion of fluoridation benefits.

to fluoridated communities, impacts the effect of diffusion as well. Also, residents who live in a fluoride-deficient community and work on a military base in the same community may be exposed to fluoridated water, because most military bases have fluoridated water.

In 1986–1987, decades after the initiation of community water fluoridation, an epidemiologic study of more than 39,000 children ages 5 through 17 years was conducted by the National Institute of Dental Research.[56,62] This study determined that younger children who had lived all their lives in optimally fluoridated communities experienced 39% fewer carious lesions and fillings compared with children who had lived in non-fluoridated communities. The impact of water fluoridation and other sources of fluoride on dental caries is apparent from examination of the findings of national surveys assessing the oral health status of school-aged children in the United States, which show a steady decline in rates of caries prevalence and increasing percentages of children who are caries-free (Figure 11–10 ■).

In separate studies, Brunelle and Carlos (1990) and Murray and colleagues (1991) found greater percentages of caries-free children and lower caries-prevalence rates in fluoridated communities where other sources of fluoride were also available.[56,63] After adjusting for other sources of fluoride, they found a 25% difference in dental-caries prevalence. The findings of these two studies

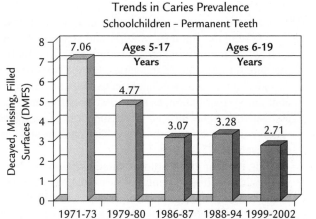

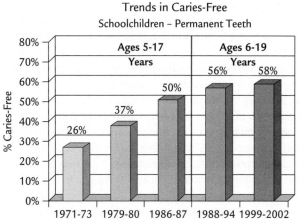

■ **FIGURE 11–10**   Decline in prevalence rates of caries in U.S. schoolchildren. (*Source:* National Survey Findings.)

emphasize that water fluoridation remains an important contributor to caries prevention.[17,56]

Newbrun reported that surveys conducted in the 1980s reported less tooth decay in communities that were fluoridated; fluoridation was credited for preventing 30% to 60% of dental caries in the primary dentition, 20% to 40% in the mixed dentition, and 15% to 35% in the permanent dentition.[64] The decline in percentages of caries reduction has been found in both fluoridated and non-fluoridated communities, with children who had always been exposed to community water fluoridation demonstrating mean scores for decayed, missing, and filled tooth surfaces that ranged from 18% to 40% lower than those who had never lived in fluoridated communities.[64–66] Griffin estimated that fluoridation was responsible for a 27% reduction in tooth decay for adults.[67]

As described above, the decline in dental-caries rates was greatest, up to 65% to 70%, in the earlier years (1940s, 1950s, 1960s) of fluoridation when water was the primary source of fluoride and the availability of other sources of fluoride was limited. The caries-inhibition effectiveness of fluoride in water resulted in a parallel rush to develop other sources of fluorides, resulting in (1) adjunctive systemic fluorides, such as tablets, drops, lozenges, and vitamins with fluoride, meant to be swallowed and dispensed to the public by licensed health professionals; and (2) topical fluorides, which were intended for only topical application and were not meant to be swallowed.[68] Some topical fluorides are used by dental providers in the office, whereas others are used in public health programs and schools. In addition, over-the-counter

products are used by consumers. As more cities adopted fluoridation, and as the ingestion of dietary fluoride supplements increased in fluoride-deficient communities, consumer use of fluoride-containing products such as toothpastes, mouthrinses, and gels also increased. As a result, exposure to fluoride from numerous sources has become more widespread, with benefits accruing at varying levels. At the same time, it is becoming more difficult to accurately determine the level of reduction in caries rates attributed to fluoridated water alone versus other sources. Most researchers now believe that the "dilution" and "diffusion" effects are responsible for the decline in dental caries rates in non-fluoridated, and to a lesser degree, in fluoridated communities.

Although children and adolescents are the major beneficiaries of fluoridation, adults also benefit. The impact of fluoride on the teeth of adults has become more important, because adults are retaining their teeth longer than in previous decades as a result of improved dental health practices, the advent of the dental hygienist, and availability of preventive interventions, especially fluoridation. With aging, teeth remain susceptible to coronal caries,[69] and more of the root surfaces become exposed to the oral environment, resulting in increased susceptibility to root caries.[70] Research indicates that root caries manifests as a significant dental problem as early as ages 35 to 44, doubling in the 45- to 54-year age group, and redoubling in the 55- to 66-year group.[71] Results of a national survey of root caries found that 67% of men and 61% of women between ages 65 and 84+ had root-surface lesions.[72] Studies in adults have consistently reported fewer coronal and root caries in the teeth of adults residing in communities with higher levels of waterborne fluoride.[8] Results of one study of young adults ages 20 to 34 years showed 25% fewer coronal caries (decayed, filled surfaces) in those who resided in fluoridated (adjusted or natural) communities compared with those who had no exposure to fluoridated water.[73] Similar findings were noted in a study of older adults, with mean ages of 40 and 43 years; residents of communities with 1.6 ppm fluoride in the water had 28% fewer coronal caries and 17% fewer root caries than residents of communities with 0.2 ppm fluoride. Newbrun has estimated that the reduction in caries attributable to water fluoridation for adults, aged 20 to 44 years, is between 20% to 30% for coronal caries and 20% to 40% for root caries.[64] A recent examination of studies published during or after 1980 found that any fluoride (self-applied and professionally applied or from fluoridated water) averted 0.29 carious coronal surfaces and 0.22 carious root surfaces in adults.[44] The same study found the prevention fraction attributable to water fluoridation was 27%.[44]

Historically, assessments of effectiveness depended on interpretation of individual studies. In recent years, however, the scientific and health communities have conducted systematic reviews, summarizing the available evidence on a given topic. Systematic reviews use a rule-based process to summarize existing knowledge about the effectiveness of an intervention—in this case, fluoridation. The process of the review is established before the review begins. This rule-based process increases the likelihood that the review captures available knowledge and objectively summarizes methods and results. This objective process seeks to diminish the likelihood of bias that can be introduced by investigators. As such, the systematic review provides the strongest evidence of effectiveness of an intervention.

Several systematic reviews have been conducted on both the safety and effectiveness of fluoridation. The University of York review on fluoridation effectiveness, published in 2000, found that fluoridation of drinking water supplies reduced caries prevalence in variable ranges with a median of 14.6% reduction in rates, as measured by the change in the deft/DMFT indices (decay, extracted, filled in primary teeth and the Decayed, Missing, and Filled in permanent teeth) scores and the proportion of caries-free children.[74] The report also attempted to address the impact of fluoride-containing toothpaste on the effectiveness of fluoridation.[75] The authors of the review acknowledged that the estimates of effectiveness could be biased because of inadequate adjustment for the impact of potential confounding variables.[74] The U.S. Task Force on Community Preventive Services released their systematic findings in 2002 and strongly recommended community water fluoridation as an effective measure for reducing dental caries. On the basis of their included studies, the median effectiveness of starting or continuing fluoridation, as measured by before and after assessments of concurrent comparison groups, was a 29% relative decrease in tooth decay. The median absolute decrease was 1.3 teeth.[76,77]

It is clear from studies cited previously that a worldwide decline in dental-caries rates has occurred, even though certain population groups are still disproportionately affected by dental caries. This decline has been attributed to the widespread use of multiple fluorides from various sources: community water supplies, fluoridated salt, fluoride supplements, fluoride rinses, gels, and varnishes, and dentifrices.

EFFECTS OF DISCONTINUATION OF WATER FLUORIDATION

During the early years of fluoridation, when fluoride in the water supply was the primary source of fluoride, studies showed that dental caries rates increased dramatically when fluoridation was discontinued. In 1960, the city of Antigo, Wisconsin, discontinued fluoridation after having fluoridation for 11 years. Six years later, when Antigo elementary school children were found to have substantial increases in caries rates, ranging from 41% to 70%, fluoridation was reinstated.[78] Similar findings occurred in Scotland upon cessation of fluoridation: In the town of Wick, caries rates increased by 40% in primary teeth and by 27% in permanent teeth. This dramatic increase in dental-caries rates occurred despite ready availability of fluoride toothpaste and a continuing decline in national caries rates in Scotland.[79] Moreover, 5 years after fluoridation was discontinued in the town of Stranraer, caries rates increased to levels approaching those found in the non-fluoridated town of Annan. In Stranraer, restorative dental treatment costs for decay alone rose by 115%.[80]

Similar results can occur if a city changes its water source from one that is optimally fluoridated to one that is fluoride-deficient. The impact would be equivalent to discontinuation of fluoridation, as in the case in Galesburg, Illinois, which in 1959 switched from a water source that was naturally fluoridated to a non-fluoridated source. In 2 years, the caries-prevalence rate increased by 38%.[81] A Public Health Service Report on risks and benefits of fluoride stated that "one way to demonstrate the effectiveness of a therapeutic agent, such as fluoride, is to observe if the benefits are lost when the agent is removed."[82] One of the more notable systematic reviews in recent years was completed in 2002 by the U.S. Task Force on Community Preventive Services, made up of a non-Federal group of health experts. The task force found that communities that stopped community water fluoridation, on average, experienced an 18% increase in dental caries after discontinuation.[77]

Although these studies serve to demonstrate that the discontinuation of community water fluoridation has resulted in the significant loss of the benefits of dental-caries prevention, some more recent studies cannot replicate these results,[83,84] most probably because of the dilution and diffusion effects that introduce fluoride to citizens living in non-fluoridated cities. Still, water fluoridation remains the most efficient way for a community to provide fluoride to its citizens.

The benefits imparted through fluoridation can be lessened by individuals using bottled water as their primary drinking source. Although the fluoride concentrations in bottled water can vary considerably,[85,86] most bottled water contains low fluoride concentrations.[87] Fluoride concentrations are shown on labels only if fluoride is added during the bottling process.[88] The CDC recommended in 2001 that manufacturers include fluoride concentrations on labels.[89] Because fluoridation works by replenishing fluoride concentrations in the plaque and saliva on a frequent basis, substituting optimally fluoridated drinking water for low-fluoride bottled water reduces the overall preventive effect.

ENAMEL FLUOROSIS

Fluoridation has risks as well as benefits. As mentioned earlier in the historical background section, fluoride in water can cause a dental condition known as enamel fluorosis, also referred to as dental fluorosis or fluorosis. Although the mild and very mild forms of fluorosis may be so minimally apparent that individuals may not even realize their teeth are affected,[90] moderate and severe forms of fluorosis result in stained and pitted teeth that are cosmetically objectionable.[91] Regulations, guidelines, and expert panels make this distinction, and normally develop and promote recommendations that protect individuals against the development of moderate and severe fluorosis, but not the lesser types. Although the goal should be to eliminate all moderate and severe

fluorosis, it is improbable to expect elimination of the less-objectionable forms of very mild and mild fluorosis. Decades before community water fluoridation began, investigators such as McKay and Dean found that fluorosis was prevalent in many communities across the country, resulting from natural sources of fluoride.[21,25,26] It should also be noted that, when adjusted fluoridation was initiated in 1945, it was accepted that a portion of the population would develop very mild fluorosis, which was considered an acceptable trade off for the increased caries protection and improved dental health. Fluoridation involves finding the appropriate balance between the benefits of caries prevention and improved oral health, and the potential for cosmetic conditions associated with very mild and mild fluorosis.

Enamel fluorosis results from hypomineralization in enamel surfaces of teeth that have been exposed to fluoride ingested during enamel formation. Enamel fluorosis can present in a number of ways, from barely discernible, white, lacy striae to the most severe form that could be classified as a developmental defect of the enamel.[19,90] The degree of fluorosis depends on the total dose of fluoride from all sources, as well as on the timing and duration of fluoride exposure. Enamel fluorosis occurs in children who consume fluoride when their teeth are developing; fluorosis cannot occur once enamel formation is complete and the teeth have erupted, regardless of intake; therefore, older children and adults are not at risk for enamel fluorosis.[1,92,93] Children ages 8 years or younger are at risk for developing fluorosis, but children ages 6 years and older are considered safe from developing objectionable fluorosis that will show when they speak or smile, because the anterior permanent teeth have formed.[89]

Excessive levels of exposure, those that exceed levels set to protect against moderate and severe fluorosis, can occur in various ways, such as in drinking water that contains higher-than-optimal fluoride levels, as can happen with private wells or community water systems with high levels of naturally occurring fluoride. The Environmental Protection Agency (EPA) considers fluoride content of drinking water higher than 2 ppm F a cosmetic influence and requires public water systems reaching or exceeding this level to issue a public notification. The 1997 Institute of Medicine report established the Tolerable Upper Intake Level of 0.1 mg/kg/day for children younger than 8 years to protect against moderate fluorosis.[4] In 2006 the American Dental Association issued an interim guidance advising, "If liquid concentrate or powdered infant formula is the primary source of nutrition, it can be mixed with water that is fluoride free or contains low levels of fluoride to reduce the risk of fluorosis.[94] The greatest likelihood of exposure to excess fluoride in children results from (1) inadvertent ingestion of toothpaste containing very high concentrations of fluoride; and (2) ingestion of inappropriately prescribed dietary fluoride supplements.[1,95]

Data from the National Health and Nutrition Examination Survey (NHANES) 1999–2002 indicated that approximately 23% of persons ages 6 to 39 years in the United States exhibited fluorosis.[96] This datum represents an increase of 9 percentage points in fluorosis prevalence in the United States since the last national survey (1986–1987 National Survey of Dental Caries in U.S. School Children).[96] In both national surveys, the majority of identified fluorosis cases were classified as being very mild or mild. The minor forms of fluorosis (questionable, very mild, or mild) are not considered to be abnormal, nor are they considered to constitute an adverse health effect. However, both researchers and practitioners should continue to monitor and assess the risk of enamel fluorosis to ensure that the more severe forms of fluorosis do not occur. Although the authors of the NHANES 1999–2002 survey report could not specifically identify the factors responsible for the rise in fluorosis prevalence, they noted that ". . . a potentially important source is toothpaste."[96] In 1936, Dean estimated that approximately 10% of children who drank optimally fluoridated water would develop very mild enamel fluorosis.[97] More recent studies have shown that enamel fluorosis attributed to fluoridation is around 13%.[98] It is probable that about 10% of children will develop a mild form of fluorosis if exposed only to optimally fluoridated drinking water and no other sources of fluoride.[1]

University of Iowa researchers, who have followed a cohort of children from birth through adolescence and documented fluoride intake as reported by parents on questionnaires, have determined that the first 3 years of life are critical to the development of fluorosis.[99] They also found much variation with regard to intake and individual response.[99,100] Even though fluorosis is determined by fluoride exposure, and is related to dose and duration, some children will develop fluorosis and some will not, even when they are exposed to the same level of fluoride. The Iowa researchers have also noted a positive association between fluorosis in the primary and secondary dentition, even when they adjust for fluoride exposure.

The Safe Drinking Water Act, enacted by Congress in 1986, established primary and secondary standards for natural fluoride levels in public drinking water in the United States. The legislation set the **primary standard** (the maximum concentration of fluoride allowed in public drinking water systems) at 4.0 ppm F to protect the public against unwanted health effects such as skeletal fluorosis. A **secondary standard** of 2.0 ppm F was set to protect children from moderate/severe enamel fluorosis. The report *Fluoride in Drinking Water: A Scientific Review of EPA's Standards,*[101] issued by the National Research Council (NRC) in 2006, examined the current EPA water standards. For the first time, the NRC separated severe and moderate enamel fluorosis and considered each separately.[100] In doing so, the committee determined that the current maximum contaminant level goal of 4 ppm F in drinking water was not protective against severe enamel fluorosis. The NRC stated that communities with fluoride concentrations in the public water supply at or near 4 ppm F can expect a 10% frequency of severe enamel fluorosis. For the first time, this expert panel considered severe enamel fluorosis an adverse health effect instead of a cosmetic effect.[65,80,102] Of note, this effect applies to severe enamel fluorosis only, not the other forms of fluorosis. Previous assessments considered all forms of enamel fluorosis to be esthetically displeasing, but not adverse to health, because of the lack of direct evidence that severe enamel fluorosis results in tooth loss, loss of tooth function, or psychologic, behavioral, or social problems. However, in this report the NRC committee noted suggestive but inconclusive evidence that severe enamel fluorosis increased the risk of developing caries.[100] Severe enamel fluorosis results in discrete and confluent pitting and structural damage to the tooth's enamel surface. The committee determined that this damage compromises the function of the tooth surface to protect the dentin and pulp from decay and infection. The report states that the hypothesis of a causal link between severe enamel fluorosis and increased caries risk is plausible and that the evidence for this link is mixed but supportive. In addition, the report acknowledged that restorative dental treatment is often considered for children with the enamel pitting that characterizes this condition.

The NRC report also reported strong evidence of a true population threshold for severe fluorosis at 2 ppm F in the water supply.[101] In other words, severe enamel fluorosis essentially is absent when the water supply contains less than 2 ppm F. Strong evidence exists that lowering the Maximum Contaminant Level Goal for fluoride to a level below 2 ppm F will effectively eliminate severe enamel fluorosis. This observation is supported by an intervention study conducted by Horowitz and others in North Dakota where partial defluoridation of drinking water from 6 ppm F to slightly below 2 ppm F prevented severe fluorosis.[102]

In 1942, H. Trendley Dean developed a system of classification for enamel fluorosis. He established a series of categories that ranged from (1) questionable white flecks or spots or "snow capping"; (2) very mild, small, opaque paper-white areas or streaks known as "veining," covering less than 25% of the tooth surface; (3) mild, opaque white areas covering less than 25% of the tooth surface; (4) moderate marked wear on occlusal/incisal surfaces, which may include brown stains; to (5) severe mottling and brown staining affecting all tooth surfaces.[90]

Dean's Fluorosis Index continues to be widely used today.

Not all enamel opacities or irregularities are caused by fluorosis: Some may be caused by other chemical agents such as strontium and chromium, and pharmaceutical agents such as tetracycline can also change the appearance of the enamel. Other diseases and conditions, such as celiac disease, can result in enamel hypoplasia, which may be mistaken for fluorosis.[104] **Idiopathic** opacities also exist for which the cause is currently unknown.

As previously mentioned, questionable, very mild, and mild stages of fluorosis often result from very young children swallowing too much fluoride-containing toothpaste or from inappropriate supplementation with prescription fluoride products such as (1) physicians or dentists independently prescribing fluoride supplements; or (2) physicians or dentists prescribing fluoride supplements without checking the fluoride content of the child's water supply. In either case, a child gets a "double" dose of fluoride on a daily basis. Monitoring total fluoride intake is complicated, considering the availability of multiple sources of fluoride. Also, fluoride from tablets/drops is ingested and absorbed at one time of day as opposed to fluoride in water in which the ingestion and absorption of low-dose fluoride is distributed throughout the day. These factors have been considered in the establishment of fluoride dosage schedules, which were adjusted downward in the 1990s, particularly for children in the first 6 months of life. The Dietary Fluoride Supplement Schedule approved by the American Dental Association,[105] the American Academy of Pediatrics,[106] and the American Academy of Pediatric Dentistry[107] should be followed when fluoride supplements are prescribed (Table 11–5 ■).

Fluoride ingestion should be reduced during the ages of tooth development, particularly under the age of 2 years. Parents need to assist in attainment of this goal by supervising young children during toothbrushing to

■ **Table 11-5** Dietary Fluoride Supplement Schedule, 1994

Age	Fluoride Ion Level in Drinking Water (ppm)[a]		
	<0.3 ppm F	0.3–0.6 ppm F	>0.6 ppm F
Birth–6 months	None	None	None
6 months–3 years	0.25 mg/day[b]	None	None
3–6 years	0.50 mg/day	0.25 mg/day	None
6–16 years	1.0 mg/day	0.50 mg/day	None

[a] 1.0 part per million (ppm) = 1 milligram/liter (mg/l)
[b] 2.2 mg sodium fluoride contains 1 mg fluoride ion.
Source: Meskin, 1995[105]; American Academy of Pediatrics Committee on Nutrition, 1995[106]; and American Academy of Pediatric Dentistry, 1995[107].

ensure that they use only a small amount of toothpaste (smear or pea-sized) and do not swallow the toothpaste.[89]

REDUCING THE RISK FOR ENAMEL FLUOROSIS

The CDC has developed recommendations to reduce the risk for enamel fluorosis. The CDC report *Recommendations for Using Fluoride to Prevent and Control Dental Caries in the United States* contains the following as well as other recommendations:[89]

- All persons should know whether the fluoride concentration in their primary source of drinking water is below optimal (less than 0.7 ppm F), optimal (0.7–1.2 ppm F), or above optimal (greater than 1.2 ppm F). This knowledge is the basis for all individual and professional decisions regarding use of other fluoride modalities (e.g., fluoride toothpaste for children under 2 years of age, mouthrinses, or supplements).
- Parents of children younger than 6 years should brush the child's teeth (recommended particularly for pre-school children) or supervise the toothbrushing. Because many children at this age have not learned to control the swallowing reflex, parents should encourage the child to spit excess toothpaste into the sink to minimize the amount swallowed.
- Parents and caregivers should consult a dentist or other health care provider before introducing a child younger than 2 years to fluoride toothpaste.
- For children younger than 6 years who use fluoride toothpaste, parents and caregivers should fol-

low the directions on the label and place no more than a pea-sized amount (0.25 grams) of toothpaste on the toothbrush.
- Where community water supply systems and home wells contain a natural fluoride concentration of more than 2 ppm F, children younger than 8 years should have an alternative source of drinking water that preferably contains fluoride at the recommended optimal level.
- Use of other discretionary forms of fluoride, including fluoride mouthrinses and dietary fluoride supplements, should be limited to children who are at a high risk for developing tooth decay. Supplements should be used for only high-risk children living in areas where the drinking water has a low concentration of fluoride. Supplements should be prescribed judiciously and in accordance with the dietary fluoride supplement schedule (Table 11–5).
- Parents of formula-fed infants should weigh the balance between a child's risk for very mild or mild enamel fluorosis and the benefit of fluoride for preventing tooth decay and the need for dental fillings.

Anti-fluoridation groups frequently and inappropriately exhibit photographs of children and/or adults with severe fluorosis in which pitting or mottling of the enamel and brown stains are evident. These groups attribute these manifestations directly to water fluoridation, which is misleading. Fluoridation opponents may also wrongly describe enamel fluorosis as a major risk factor for people of all ages. Severe fluorosis does not occur from fluoridated water alone, and most frequently occurs when there is too much naturally occurring fluoride in water. In making dental-health decisions, patients depend on the dental professional team to assist them in evaluating the risks versus the benefits of a given procedure or public health measure. To do this, dentists and dental hygienists need to stay current with scientific literature and to use this knowledge as a basis for educating themselves and their patients. The risk of developing very mild fluorosis versus the benefit of decreased dental caries and attendant treatment costs should be communicated to patients who express concern.

OPTIMAL FLUORIDE LEVELS

The U.S. Public Health Service established non-regulatory standards for optimal concentrations of fluoride in the drinking water in the United States in 1962. These standards are based on the annual average of maximum daily air temperatures. This methodology is based on the work of Dean, Galagan, and others and is founded on the principle that water consumption is greater in hotter climates and less in colder climates.[25,27,28,108–111] Consequently, the higher the average temperature in a community, the lower the recommended water fluoride level. For every geographic location in the United States, a specific optimal fluoride concentration is recommended for the drinking supply, with optimal levels ranging from 0.7 to 1.2 ppm F (Table 11–6 ■ and Figure 11–11 ■), depending on climate.[112]

Much has changed in the United States since the recommendations for optimal fluoride levels were issued in 1962. Some studies have examined fluid intake and questioned whether temperature influences the amount people drink as it once did, given the widespread use of air conditioning in homes, automobiles, and workplaces.[113,114] Modern consumption patterns of bottled water and other beverages, such as soft drinks and fruit juices, also complicate the matter, because fluoride levels in these beverages vary greatly.[5,115] In addition, optimal fluoride concentrations were recommended at a time before there were other regular sources of fluoride exposure, such as discretionary fluoride toothpaste, mouthrinses, or dietary supplements. Determining daily fluoride intake is influenced by other factors such as consumer use of home distillation and reverse-osmosis water treatment systems, which can remove significant amounts of fluoride from the water supply. The CDC has recommended review of the methodology used to determine optimal levels to see if it is still relevant in this era.[88]

Optimal fluoride concentrations in other countries are not identical to those in the United States; however, most values were originally based on the United States methodology. Some countries (Hong Kong, Singapore) have optimal levels as low as 0.5 ppm F. Several countries, including Canada, Singapore, Vietnam, Ireland, and Hong Kong, have adjusted optimal water fluoride levels downward, citing increased prevalence of fluorosis, to achieve its goal of maximizing the benefits of caries reduction while minimizing the risk of fluorosis in an environment of increased fluoride exposure.[116] Australia conducted a review in 1999 and decided to keep the optimal levels for fluoridation unchanged (0.6 ppm F–1.1 ppm F).[117] These values were affirmed in 2005 with the update of its national guidelines on the use of fluorides.[118] A 1994 WHO report recommended that some regions, especially tropical and subtropical areas, revise the optimal range to establish appropriate higher and lower limits.[5]

■ **Table 11–6**   Recommended Optimal Fluoride Level

Annual Average of Maximum Daily Air Temperature (°F)[a]	Optimal Fluoride Level (ppm F)
40.0–53.7	1.2
53.8–58.3	1.1
58.4–63.8	1.0
63.9–70.6	0.9
70.7–79.2	0.8
79.3–90.5	0.7

[a] Based on average annual temperature over a minimum of 5 years.
Source: Centers for Disease Control. (1991). *Dental disease prevention activity, 1991.* Atlanta, GA: Centers for Disease Control, National Center for Prevention Services.

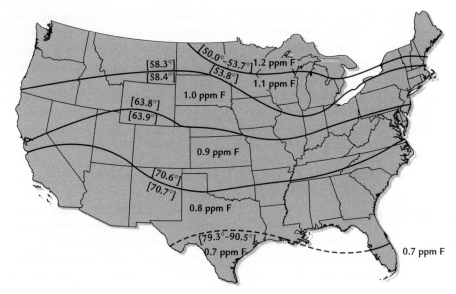

■ **FIGURE 11-11** Optimal fluoride concentrations in the United States.
(From Centers for Disease Control. (1991). *Dental disease prevention activity, 1991.* Atlanta, GA: Centers for Disease Control, National Center for Prevention Services.)

ENGINEERING ASPECTS: CHEMICALS AND TECHNICAL SYSTEMS USED

Three additives are used for water fluoridation in the United States, sodium fluoride (NaF), sodium silicofluoride (NaFS), and hydrofluosilicic acid (H_2SiF_6). States require these additives to meet the standards, testing, and certifications set by the American Water Works Association (AWWA) and the NSF (National Sanitation Foundation) International.[119] The AWWA sets minimum requirements for a product's design, installation, performance, and manufacturing. NSF International sets criteria on the purity of drinking water additives or products, and for protection of the integrity of additives during transport. Fluoridation additives are just one kind of chemical used in the water supply. Water treatment chemicals are used for a number of reasons including disinfection, absorption, algae control, decolorization, oxidation, metal coagulation, water softening, filtration, pH control, iron control, coagulation, corrosion control, chlorination, and fluoridation.[120,121]

Sodium fluoride (granular or powder) and sodium silicofluoride (granular) are used in distribution systems that use "dry" compounds, whereas hydrofluosilicic acid, a liquid, is used in solution or "wet" systems.[122] Sodium fluoride was the first compound used in controlled water fluoridation programs and is still used in

many water systems in smaller communities, usually those serving fewer than 5,000 people.[120] Sodium silicofluoride is substantially less expensive than sodium fluoride and tends to be used in community water systems serving between 5,000 and 50,000 people. Today, the most frequently used compound for water fluoridation in the United States is hydrofluosilicic acid because of its low cost and ease of handling; it is used primarily in larger communities with water distribution systems serving 50,000 or more people and this represents approximately 57% of all fluoridation systems in the United States.[120,123]

Opponents of fluoridation often attempt to distinguish between sodium fluoride and the hexafluorosilicates, sodium silicofluoride and hydrofluosilicic acid, in terms of availability of the fluoride ion. Fluoridation opponents disparage the hexafluorosilicates as "industrial waste dumped into the drinking water" that "contaminates the water with a harmful residue." However, according to EPA scientists, no hexafluorosilicate remains in drinking water at equilibrium, which is readily achieved.[124] This statement has been verified by other research,[125] which implies that there is no difference in the source of fluoride ions from the three chemicals used in fluoridation, as the detractors would have one believe.

Two credible sources for guidelines related to the engineering aspects of water fluoridation, including administration, monitoring, and surveillance; technical requirements; and safety procedures, are the CDC Engineering and Administrative Recommendations for Water Fluoridation[122] and the AWWA Water Fluoridation Principles and Practices.[126]

Determination of the appropriate compound to use in fluoridation depends largely on the type of distribution system used by the individual water plant. The most common methods by which fluoride is added to water supplies in the United States are (1) the volumetric dry-feeder system, which delivers a predetermined quantity of dry fluoride chemical; (2) the acid-feed system, in which a small metering pump is used to add hydrofluosilicic acid to the water supply system; and (3) the saturator-feed system, a system unique to water fluoridation, which uses an up-flow saturator to provide saturated solutions of sodium fluoride in constant strengths of 4%, which are pumped into the water system via a small metering pump.[120,121]

MONITORING AND SURVEILLANCE OF FLUORIDATION

The process of adding fluoride to drinking water supplies to the level recommended to achieve the maximum dental therapeutic benefits is technically simple, uncomplicated, and similar to the processes used when dealing with chlorine and other water treatment chemicals.[120,121] All three types of fluoride additives used in the water fluoridation process are certified as to their purity and safety when used appropriately; fluoride is just one of nearly 50 additional substances approved by the U.S. EPA, and certified as safe for addition to drinking water by the AWWA and NSF International. Contrary to popular perception, fluoride does not affect the taste, odor, color, or turbidity of the water at the levels used for water fluoridation.[120,121]

For fluoridation to be properly implemented, a number of factors should be considered. Of prime importance is the compatibility of the fluoride additive to be used with the existing water treatment and distribution system. Other factors that influence the technical engineering aspects of fluoridation include (1) source of water—underground or surface water; (2) size of the water plant; (3) number and types of point sources of water—one treatment plant or many treatment plants with water coming from wells, reservoirs, rivers, aqueducts, or desalination plants; (4) number of injection points at which fluoride is introduced into the water; (5) fluoride additive costs, including transportation; (6) modification of existing plant versus construction of a new plant;

(7) need for training of water plant operators; and (8) type of monitoring and surveillance system to be used.

Modern water plant design includes engineering controls that ensure excessive amounts of fluoride are prevented from entering the water supply. Properly designed fluoridation systems prevent the addition of excess fluoride to the water system in several ways: (1) Only a limited amount of fluoride is maintained in the day tanks (or hoppers), effectively limiting the bulk amount that could be put into the water system, even in the event of a system failure; (2) positive controls have been installed for feeding fluoride from the hoppers into the dissolving tanks; and (3) metering pumps are electrically connected to the water pump in a manner that ensures failure of one pump stops operation of all pumps—and stops addition of fluoride to the system.[122] Many water plants today use in-line fluoride monitors that give continuous readings of the fluoride concentration in the water supply, providing the ability to assess the fluoride level at any time, not just when the water is tested. In addition to regular testing and documentation of fluoride levels in the water, utilities should have a quality-assurance program in place that includes monthly split sampling.[122] This procedure involves taking two samples of water: One sample is tested at the water plant by normal testing procedures (e.g., ion meter, colorimeter), whereas the other is sent to a reference laboratory, often at the state department of health. The reference laboratory tests the water and compares its results with those from the water plant; if there is a discrepancy, the water plant reviews and adjusts its testing procedures until the results are in agreement. To be certain the results of the reference laboratories are accurate, CDC maintains a national program for proficiency testing, which compares the water plants' results to reference standards with known fluoride concentrations.[127]

Maintaining a constant level of fluoride in the water supply is the responsibility of the water plant operators. Variation in the adjusted water fluoride levels has occurred in water plants where the operators were not properly trained and/or the operator turnover was high.[128] Variability in water fluoride concentration may also occur if a water plant fails to provide adequate and appropriate storage facilities, if there is malfunctioning of feed equipment, or if proper water analysis equipment is lacking, all of which are readily avoidable with proper planning and implementation. Most of the variances in fluoride concentrations that have occurred were due to poor monitoring at water treatment facilities, resulting in fluoride levels below the recommended level (**hypofluoridation**).

For this reason, communities that have implemented fluoridation must continue to monitor the fluoride levels to ensure that the full benefits of fluoridation will accrue in a community. **Hyperfluoridation** occurs when an excess amount of fluoride is added to the drinking water over several days, usually secondary to an overfeed from malfunctioning equipment and/or maintenance errors.[129,130] Over the past 60+ years, seven instances of hyperfluoridation that resulted in outbreaks of acute fluoride poisoning have occurred in the United States, all of which could have easily been prevented.[131] When a community decides to fluoridate its public water supplies, it also must assume the responsibility for monitoring the equipment, training the water plant operators, and implementing performance reviews to ensure that a process is in place to protect the public from an overfeed. The CDC offers national fluoridation training for state fluoridation program managers and has developed a 6-hour training module designed to assist plant operators in sustaining and monitoring their fluoridation systems.[132]

COST OF COMMUNITY WATER FLUORIDATION

Water fluoridation provides significant cost savings for a community and has been described as one of the most cost-effective preventive dental programs available.[19,133] Estimates of the cost of water fluoridation will vary depending on the factors included in the calculations. The size and complexity of the water system, including the number of systems, the number of wells, the use of a dry feeder versus a solution (wet) feeder system, purchase of equipment and installation, purchase of fluoride, labor, and maintenance, as well as the number of service connections and size of the population all factor into the cost of fluoridation.[133–135]

The cost of water fluoridation is usually expressed as the annual cost per person of the population being served.[19] An inverse relationship exists between the cost per person and the size of the population of a community. Consequently, the cost per person is lower in larger communities and higher in smaller communities where the actual cost of fluoridation may approach that of other methods of caries prevention.[134] Fluoridation also eliminates or diminishes additional costs incurred through other forms of fluoride administration, such as costs incurred when accessing professionals to obtain provider-prescribed fluoride products and the lower effectiveness of other forms of fluoride distribution. Fluoridation is the most cost-efficient and cost-effective method of prevention of dental caries for almost all communities.[11]

Another way to look at cost-saving benefits is to determine the dental treatment cost savings of beneficiaries. Employers who pay prepaid dental care fringe benefits for their employees save on costs. Hidden production or service costs caused by dental-related missed workdays by employees are also minimized through fluoridation. Taxpayers who support public programs also benefit from dental treatment cost savings. In fact, skyrocketing dental Medicaid expenditures in California (a state with a low percentage of the population having access to fluoridation) provided the impetus for enactment of a statewide mandatory fluoridation bill in 1995.[136,137] As will be discussed later, studies comparing dental Medicaid expenditures in Louisiana and Texas also demonstrated that treatment costs were significantly higher in non-fluoridated communities than in fluoridated communities.[138,139] Patients can also be expected to benefit from lower health care bills, lower dental care costs, and lower insurance premiums because of lower costs incurred by providers for uncompensated care.

With the availability of baseline levels of dental-caries rates and treatment costs, two different types of analyses can be done to determine (1) the effectiveness of fluoridation as a measure to prevent dental caries (a cost-effectiveness analysis); and (2) associated cost savings (a cost-benefit analysis). It has been postulated that the greater the initial caries prevalence and treatment costs, the greater will be the potential benefits realized by the introduction of fluoridation.[19] The national average for the recurring cost of water fluoridation has been estimated at $0.50 per person per year, whereas the national average cost of one simple restoration is $62.[11] If one were to multiply the approximate average life expectancy of a U.S. resident (75 years) by the annual per capita cost of fluoridation ($0.50), it appears evident that the $37.50 total for a lifetime of protection through fluoridation would more than offset the cost of just one simple restoration for one tooth. In addition, for every carious lesion initially prevented, the need for repeated restorations and treatment of recurrent carious lesions is reduced over a lifetime.[140] Different studies have shown that the replacement rates for amalgam restorations caused by recurrent decay vary between 38% and 50%; the savings to be realized from prevention are substantial.[141,142] The national average benefit-to-cost ratio for fluoridation is 80:1; on average, for every dollar spent on fluoridation, 38 dollars are saved in dental-treatment costs.[135]

Other studies further demonstrate the substantial cost-benefits generated through community water fluoridation. Brown and colleagues, in a comprehensive study for the Texas Department of Health, were able to demonstrate cost savings for the publicly funded Texas Health Steps Program when they compared program costs for clients from fluoridated communities with those from non-fluoridated communities.[137] Similarly, Barsley and colleagues were able to demonstrate that the costs for hospital-based treatment of acute dental conditions to Louisiana's publicly funded Medicaid program were much less for residents of fluoridated communities than for residents of non-fluoridated communities.[138] Finally, Wright and colleagues established conclusively that fluoridation remains an extremely cost-effective public health program in New Zealand in their comprehensive 1999 report for the New Zealand Ministry of Health.[142]

OTHER FLUORIDE VEHICLES

Many countries without centralized water distribution systems have chosen to add fluoride to table salt, a process known as **salt fluoridation,** to provide primary benefits of dental-caries prevention to their populations. Although it is difficult to obtain a verifiable accounting of usage, estimates say as many as 40 to 200 million people in the world use fluoridated salt.[115,143] Using salt as a vehicle of fluoride supplementation is similar to the concept of iodine supplementation and is a relatively inexpensive method of fluoride delivery. Similar to water fluoridation, salt fluoridation results in small amounts of fluoride being released from plasma throughout the day.[145] To achieve dental-caries reductions at levels comparable to water fluoridation, the level of fluoride supplementation of refined salt should be at least 200 mg F/kg as sodium fluoride or potassium fluoride.[146,147] Salt fluoridation requires centralized salt production, as well as monitoring.[116] Because the consumption of high quantities of sodium is a risk factor for hypertension, the use of fluoridated salt is not recommended for those at risk.[116,148] Countries using salt fluoridation include Switzerland, France, Costa Rica, Jamaica, Germany, Mexico, Colombia, Ecuador, Venezuela, and Uraguay. It has also been introduced in a number of other countries.[23] Salt fluoridation is not appropriate for countries where water fluoridation is widely used, because the additional source of fluoride would make management of intake levels difficult.

Milk fluoridation, the addition of 5 mg of fluoride to 1 liter of milk, has been introduced as a vehicle of school-based fluoride delivery in some countries (Bulgaria, Chile, China, the Russian Federation, and the United Kingdom).[5] Additional studies are required to adequately assess milk fluoridation as a viable caries-prevention strategy. According to the WHO report, "The distribution of fluoridated milk can be more complicated than that of fluoride supplements (tablets or drops)."[5] The existence of an established distribution system that includes provisions for pasteurization and refrigeration is a limiting factor in milk-fluoridation programs.

Fluoride mouthrinses were developed in the 1960s as a school-based public health measure designed to provide access to fluoride without requiring a visit to the dentist's office. Studies have reported mixed results on the effectiveness of school-based weekly fluoride rinse programs, which use 0.2% sodium fluoride in preventing coronal caries in school children who are at risk for dental caries. The National Preventive Dentistry Demonstration Project examined preventive efforts from 1976–1981 in ten cities in the United States and reported fluoride mouthrinse programs had little effect in reducing caries, especially among children from fluoridated communities.[149,150] Other studies reported reductions of dental-caries increments ranging from 20% to 35%.[23] Including both weekly and daily mouthrinse programs, the Cochrane Collaboration's systematic review of available evidence found that a 26% reduction in caries (i.e., decayed, missing, filled surfaces) could be expected from supervised school-based mouthrinse programs.[150] Since the establishment of efficacy for fluoride mouthrinses, the level of caries reduction appears to be less than originally observed. In addition, the cost-effectiveness of fluoride mouthrinse programs appears to be diminished because of the declining prevalence of dental caries in general.[11,149]

Implementation of mouthrinse programs requires that enrolled children participate consistently over time to receive maximum benefit. However, many children as they get older (middle/high school years) decline to participate, believing that fluoride rinsing is a program for younger children. Significant coordination and monitoring in the schools, parental consent, tracking of children as they move from elementary school to middle and high school, and commitment on the part of school officials are required for caries-reduction outcomes. According to the CDC, 3.25 million schoolchildren in more than 11,000 sites were participating in fluoride-rinse programs in 1988,[7] but this number has decreased since then.

RISK COMMUNICATION

Fluoridation of community water, while long accepted by qualified scientists and credible professional organizations as a safe, effective, efficient, economic, socially equitable, and environmentally sound public health activity, has endured opposition from groups throughout its 60+-year history. These groups have been effective in creating doubt and raising concern among some members of the public, elected officials, and water plant operators, thus providing convenient excuses to avoid making decisions to fluoridate individual community water systems, while accommodating some in the media who often exploit the issue to portray an apparent rift among experts on both sides of the issue. Most communities successfully work through the controversy, usually as a result of hard work by health professionals and sustained objectivity on the part of community leaders and elected officials. Often misinformation is broadly disseminated, adversely influencing community sentiment such that other measures become necessary to counter the fears generated during the legislative, campaign, or administrative process.

Risk communication is an important tool of health professionals promoting fluoridation in their communities. It serves as a mechanism by which to counter some of the negative community sentiment generated during attempts to fluoridate communities. Sandman has classified this intense negative feeling about what is perceived by some to be a health risk as outrage.[151] According to Sandman, the public defines risk in terms of "levels of outrage." The scientific and health community, who define risk in terms of "hazard," are often too slow to recognize the disparity between actual risk (hazard), as calculated by the scientific community, and perceived risk (outrage), as echoed by the public. Sandman says that the public pays far too little attention to hazard, whereas most experts pay absolutely no attention to outrage. A public whose level of outrage has been heightened by a well-orchestrated anti-fluoridation campaign will be less receptive to educational campaigns by proponents of fluoride until the level of outrage is reduced. Pertinent risk information cannot be communicated when the level of outrage is high, because the intended recipients of the information cannot collate the complex explanations while they are frightened by the fluoridation message and/or angry with the fluoridation messenger.

Scholars of risk perception have defined more than 20 factors that affect the public's level of outrage. A few factors are presented as follows:[152]

- *Voluntariness:* A voluntary risk is much more acceptable to people than a risk they perceive as coerced, because a voluntary risk generates little or no outrage. Voluntariness helps explain why anti-fluoridation propagandists will offer organized, voluntary fluoride-supplement programs as an acceptable (to them) alternative to "coerced" community water fluoridation.
- *Control:* When disease prevention and exposure mitigation are in the hands of individuals (fluoride supplements), the risk (but not the hazard) is perceived by them to be much lower than when the same programs are controlled by a government agency (municipal water system and health department).
- *Fairness:* People who feel that they are enduring greater risks than their neighbors, especially if they feel that they are without access to greater benefits, are naturally outraged, more so if the rationale for increasing their risk appears to have been decided through the political process rather than through science. Even though fluoridation benefits people of all ages, older Americans often assume that it benefits only children and frequently complain that they are being put at risk without accruing any benefits themselves.
- *Process:* Sometimes the process by which fluoridation is approved becomes the principle focus of the public's outrage, particularly when the agency or group promoting fluoridation portrays itself as arrogant rather than concerned, dishonest rather than trustworthy, and manipulative rather than collaborative.
- *Morality:* American society has evolved in its thinking about pollution to feel that it is not just harmful, but that it is morally evil. Fluoridation opponents often attempt to portray fluoridation as a form of pollution and claim that fluoride chemicals are products marketed by the chemical industry as beneficial (fluoridation) to avoid paying the costs to dispose of these chemicals. When fluoridation proponents start talking about cost-risk trade offs in this kind of political climate, they often appear to be callously advocating a morally relevant risk.
- *Familiarity:* Exotic, high-technology facilities and processes (computer-monitored water treatment plants that add fluoride and other chemicals) provoke more outrage than do familiar risks (fluoride-containing toothpaste as part of home dental care).

- *Memorability:* A memorable accident—especially one involving chemicals or radiation, such as Love Canal (New York), Bhopal (India), Times Beach (Missouri), Three-Mile Island (Pennsylvania), or Chernobyl (Ukraine), makes the potential risk easier to imagine and, therefore, perceived to be more risky. A strategy used by fluoridation opponents is to attempt to engender fear among the public by emphasizing the statistically minute potential of over-fluoridation, or hyperfluoridation, as if it were a likely catastrophic event.
- *Dread:* Illnesses such cancer, AIDS, Alzheimer's disease, or end-stage renal disease are more dreaded than dental caries. Fluoridation opponents help incite fear among the public by falsely claiming that fluoridation causes these dreaded diseases or makes them incurable, while at the same time attempting to minimize fluoridation's strong preventive effect on dental caries.
- *Diffusion in time and space:* Hazard-A (rampant dental caries) ultimately could result in the deaths of 50 or more anonymous people a year across the country, whereas Hazard-B (a poorly monitored and poorly operated fluoridation system) resulted in one very well publicized death recently, despite 56 years of safe, effective fluoridation efforts that daily benefited tens of millions of people.

Myths and Actions Related to Risk Communication

Some of those involved in community organization for promotion of fluoridation fail to properly consider the role of outrage in the community decision-making process. They assume that the public will trust them and that by merely presenting the scientific data, the public will be "won over." By ignoring the role of outrage, they miss the opportunity to succeed through use of a collaborative effort in community education and community decision making. Chess and others have categorized a number of myths and actions related to risk communication,[153] ten of which follow:

- *Myth 1:* Because the fluoridation referendum is so close, we do not have enough time and resources to have a risk communication program.

  —Action 1: Train fluoridation proponents to communicate more effectively. Plan projects to allow time to involve the public in priority setting and decision making.

- *Myth 2:* Telling the public about a potential risk related to fluoridation is more likely to unduly alarm people than keeping quiet.

  —Action 2: Fluoridation proponents can decrease the potential for alarm by giving the public a chance to express their concerns and by appropriately responding to those concerns.

- *Myth 3:* Communication is less important than education. If people knew the true risks related to fluoridation, they would accept them.

  —Action 3: Pay as much attention to your process for dealing with people and their fears of fluoridation as you do to explaining the scientific data.

- *Myth 4:* We should not go to the public until we can provide answers or solutions to all their perceived fears about fluoridation.

  —Action 4: Provide information about fluoridation and discuss concerns about risk-management options. Involve the community in the development of strategies in which they have a stake.

- *Myth 5:* The issues and scientific data regarding fluoridation are too difficult for the public to understand.

  —Action 5: Separate public disagreement with your fluoridation promotion practices from misunderstanding of the highly technical issues related to fluoridation.

- *Myth 6:* One of the easiest myths for dental professionals to embrace is that technical decisions should be left in the hands of technical people.

  —Action 6: Provide the public with information about fluoridation. Listen to community concerns about fluoridation. Involve people with diverse backgrounds on the fluoridation committee so that much thought and discussion go into developing fluoridation policies and strategies.

- *Myth 7:* I am just a dentist/dental hygienist; risk communication is not my job.

  —Action 7: As a public servant, whether the fluoridation promoter works for a health department or has a private dental/dental hygiene practice, you have a responsibility to the public. Learn to integrate risk communication into your efforts and help others from the fluoridation committee do the same.

- *Myth 8:* If we give them an inch, they will take a mile.

  —Action 8: If you listen to people when they are asking for inches, they are less likely to demand miles. Avoid the battleground that could result from attempts to stifle discussion about all aspects of fluoridation. Do not attempt to stifle discussion of issues about which fluoridation proponents are uncomfortable. Involve the public early and often.

- *Myth 9:* If we listen to the public complain about risks from fluoridation, we will devote scarce resources to issues that are not really a great threat to the public's health.

  —Action 9: Listen carefully and early to avoid controversy and the potential for disproportionate attention to lesser issues.

- *Myth 10:* Activist anti-fluoride groups are responsible for stirring up unwarranted concerns.

  —Action 10: Anti-fluoride activists help to focus public anger. Work hard to gain the public's trust early so that you can work with responsible public groups to promote the adoption of responsible public policy regarding fluoridation.

Covello and Allen have developed a list of Ten Deadly Sins of Communication, which are fairly self-explanatory: (1) appearing unprepared; (2) handling questions improperly; (3) apologizing for yourself or your organization; (4) not knowing knowable information; (5) unprofessional use of audiovisual aids; (6) seeming to be off schedule; (7) not involving participants; (8) not establishing rapport; (9) appearing disorganized; and (10) providing the wrong content.[154,155]

It remains obvious that the mere dissemination of information to the public, without any attempts to communicate the complexities and uncertainties of risk, does not necessarily ensure that the public will understand or accept community water fluoridation. Well-managed risk-communication efforts will help ensure that the public is provided with messages that are constructively formulated, transmitted, and received, and that the efforts are more likely to result in positive thoughts and an acceptance of fluoridation. In the words of Baruch Fischhoff, "If we have not gotten our message across, then we ought to assume that the fault is not with our receivers."[156]

PRINCIPLES OF RISK COMMUNICATION

The principles of risk communication, if practiced universally, can go a long way toward increasing the speed with which the public accepts community water fluoridation as a local policy option. Covello and Allen have developed Seven Cardinal Principles of Risk Communication, all designed to help fluoridation promoters accomplish their goals.[155]

1. **Accept and involve the public as a partner.** Your goal is to produce a public that is informed about the advantages of fluoridation, not to defuse public concerns or replace actions.
2. **Plan carefully and evaluate your efforts.** - Different goals, audiences, and media require different approaches and different actions.
3. **Listen to the public's specific concerns.** People often care more about trust, credibility, competence, fairness, and empathy than about statistics and details.
4. **Be honest, frank, and open.** Trust and credibility are difficult to obtain and, once lost, are almost impossible to regain.
5. **Work with other credible sources.** Conflicts and disagreements among organizations make communication with the public much more difficult.
6. **Meet the needs of the media.** The media are usually more interested in controversy than risk, simplicity than complexity, and danger than safety. Help them understand the differences.
7. **Speak clearly and with compassion.** Never let your efforts prevent your acknowledging the tragedy of an illness, injury, or death, or even their potential. Acknowledge and empathize with people's fears. People can understand risk information, but they may still not agree with you. Some people will never be satisfied with your answers.

SUMMARY

Community water fluoridation is the prime example of community-based prevention in which the benefits accrue to all individuals consuming drinking water that is optimally fluoridated without regard to socioeconomic status. Fluoridation remains a safe, effective health measure to prevent dental caries. It also fulfills all of the requirements of an excellent public policy.

REFERENCES

1. American Dental Association Council on Access, Prevention and Interprofessional Relations. (2005). *Fluoridation facts 2005.* Chicago: American Dental Association.

2. U.S. Department of Agriculture. (2004). *USDA national fluoride database of selected foods and beverages.* Retrieved on 03/03/08 from http://www.ars.usda.gov/Services/docs.htm?docid=6312.

3. Whitford, G. M. (1989). The metabolism and toxicology of fluoride. *Monogr Oral Sci,* 13:1–160.

4. Institute of Medicine, Food and Nutrition Board. (1997). *Dietary reference intakes: Calcium, phosphorus, magnesium, vitamin D, and fluoride.* Washington, DC: National Academy Press, 288–313.

5. World Health Organization. (1994). Fluorides and oral health. (Technical Report Series 846). Geneva: World Health Organization.

6. Easley, M. (2000). Opposition to community water fluoridation and connections to the "alternative medicine" movement. *Sci Rev Altern Med,* 5 (1):24–31.

7. Easley, M. W. (1995). Celebrating 50 years of fluoridation: A public health success story. *Br Dent J,* 21:72–75.

8. U.S. Department of Health and Human Services. (1983, February 8). *Surgeon General statement on community water fluoridation* (Dr. C. Everett Koop). Washington, DC: U.S. Department of Health and Human Services, Public Health Service.

9. U.S. Department of Health and Human Services. (1995, December 14). *Surgeon General statement on community water fluoridation* (Dr. Antonio Novello). Washington, DC: U.S. Department of Health and Human Services, Public Health Service.

10. U.S. Department of Health and Human Services. (2000, March 25). *First-ever Surgeon General's report on oral health finds profound disparities in nation's population.* Bethseda, MD: U.S. Department of Health and Human Services, National Institute of Dental and Craniofacial Research, National Institutes of Health.

11. U.S. Department of Health and Human Services. (2000). *Oral health in America: A report of the Surgeon General* (NIH Publicaton No. 00-4713). Rockville, MD: U.S. Department of Health and Human Services, National Institute of Dental and Craniofacial Research, National Institutes of Health.

12. U.S. Department of Health and Human Services. (2004, July 28). *Surgeon General statement on community water fluoridation* (Dr. R. Carmona). Washington, DC: U.S. Department of Health and Human Services, Public Health Service.

13. The British Fluoridation Society. (2004). *One in a million—The facts about water fluoridation.* Manchester, England: the UK Public Health Association, the British Dental Association, the Faculty of the Public Health of the Royal College of Physicians. Retrieved on 06/06/07 from http://www.bfsweb.org/onemillion/onemillion.htm.

14. Centers for Disease Control and Prevention. *Oral health resources; water supply statistics 2002; status of water fluoridation in the United States.* Retrieved on 06/12/08 from http://www.cdc.gov/nohss/FSSupplyStats.htm.

15. Ripa, L. W. (1999). Water fluoridation. In Harris, N.O., & Garcia-Godoy, F., Eds. *Primary preventive dentistry* (5th ed.). Stamford, CT: Appleton and Lange, 658.

16. McClure, F. J. (1970). *Water fluoridation. The search and the victory.* Washington, DC: U.S. Government Printing Office.

17. Murray, J. J., Rugg-Gunn, A. J., & Jenkins, G. N. (1991). *Fluorides in caries prevention* (3rd ed.). Oxford: Butterworth-Heinemann, Ltd.

18. Leske, G. S. (1983). Water fluoridation. In Mellberg, J. R., & Ripa, L. W., Eds. *Fluoride in preventive dentistry.* Chicago: Quintessence Publishing, 290.

19. Harris, N. O., & Garcia-Godoy, F., Eds. (1999). *Primary preventive dentistry* (5th ed.). Stamford, CT: Appleton and Lange, 658.

20. Black, G. V., & McKay, F. S. (1916). Mottled teeth—An endemic developmental imperfection of the teeth heretofore unknown in the literature of dentistry. *Dent Cosmos,* 58:129–56.

21. McKay, F. S. (1933). Mottled enamel: The prevention of its further production through a change of water supply at Oakley, Idaho. *J Am Dent Assoc,* 20:1137–49.

22. McKay, F. S. (1928). The relation of mottled enamel to caries. *J Am Dent Assoc,* 15:1429–37.

23. Burt, B. A., & Eklund, S. A. (2005). *Dentistry, dental practice, and the community* (6th ed.). St. Louis: Elsevier Saunders.

24. Centers for Disease Control & Prevention. (1999). Achievements in public health, 1900–1999: Fluoridation of drinking water to prevent dental caries. *MMWR Morb Mortal Wkly Rep,* 48:933–40. Retrieved from http://www.cdc.gov/mmwr/preview/mmwrhtml/mm4841a1.htm.

25. Dean, H. T. (1993). Distribution of mottled enamel in the United States. *Public Health Rep,* 48:703–34.

26. Dean, H. T., Dixon, R. M., & Cohen, C. (1935). Mottled enamel in Texas. *Public Health Rep,* 50:424–42.

27. Dean, H. T., Jay P., Arnold, Jr., F. A., McClure, F. J., & Elvove, E. (1939). Domestic water and dental caries, including certain epidemiological aspects of oral *L. acidophilus. Public Health Rep,* 54:862–88.

28. Dean, H. T., Jay, P., Arnold, Jr., F. A., & Elvove, E. (1941). Domestic water and dental caries. II. A study of 2,832 white children aged 12–14 years, of eight suburban Chicago communities, including *L. acidophilus* studies of 1,761 children. *Public Health Rep,* 56:761–92.

29. Dean, H. T., Arnold, Jr., F. A., & Elvove, E. (1942). Domestic water and dental caries. V. Additional studies of the relation of fluoride domestic waters to dental caries experience in 4,425 white children aged 12–14 years of 13 cities in 4 states. *Public Health Rep,* 157:1155–79.

30. Ast, D. B., & Fitzgerald, B. (1962). Effectiveness of water fluoridation. *J Am Dent Assoc,* 65:581–87.

31. U.S. Department of Health and Human Services. (1998, September 15). *Healthy people 2010 objectives: Draft for public comment.* (Oral Health Section). Washington, DC: U.S. Government Printing Office.

32. Department of Health and Human Services. *Healthy people—progress toward healthy people 2010 targets.* Retrieved on 03/12/08 from http://www.healthypeople .gov/data/midcourse/pdf/fa21.pdf.

33. World Health Organization. (2005). *Statement on water fluoridation.* Geneva: World Health Organization.

34. Groeneveld, A., Van Eck, A. A., & Backer Dirks, O. (1990). Fluoride in caries prevention: Is the effect pre- or post-eruptive? *J Dent Res,* 69.

35. Featherstone, J. D. (1999). Prevention and reversal of dental caries: Role of low level fluoride. *Community Dent Oral Epidemiol,* 27:31–40.

36. Rolla, G., & Edstrand, J. (1996). Fluoride in oral fluids and dental plaque. In Fejerskov, O., Ekstrand, J., & Burt, B. A, Eds. *Fluoride in dentistry* (2nd ed.). Copenhagen: Munksgaard, 215–19.

37. Hamilton, I. R. (1990). Biochemical effects of fluoride on oral bacteria. *J Dent Res,* 69 Spec Iss):660–67.

38. Chow, L. C. (1990). Tooth-bound fluoride and dental caries. *J Dent Res,* 69 (Spec Iss):595–600.

39. Kidd, E. A., Thylstrup, A., Fejerskov, O., & Bruun, C. (1980). Influence of fluoride in surface enamel and degree of dental fluorosis on caries development in vitro. *Caries Res,* 14:196–202.

40. Singh, K. A., Spencer, A. J., & Brennan, D. S. (2007). Effects of water fluoride exposure at crown completion and maturation on caries of permanent first molars. *Caries Res,* 41:34–42.

41. Singh, K. A., Spencer, A. J., & Armfield, B. A. (2003). Relative effects of pre- and post-eruption water fluoride on caries experience of permanent first molars. *J Public Health Dent,* 63:11–19.

42. Koulourides, T. (1990). Summary of session II: Fluoride and the caries process. *J Dent Res,* 69 (Spec Iss):558.

43. Newbrun, E. (1989). Effectiveness of water fluoridation. *J Public Health Dent,* 49 (Spec Iss):279–89.

44. Griffin, S. O., Regnier, E., Griffin, P. M., & Huntley, V. (2007). Effectiveness of fluoride in preventing decay in adults. *J Dent Res,* 86:410–15.

45. Lambrou, D., Larsen, M., Fejerskov, O., & Tachos, B. (1981). The effect of fluoride in saliva on remineralization of dental enamel in humans. *Caries Res,* 15:341–45.

46. Backer-Dirks, O., Kunzel, W., & Carlos, J. P. (1978). Caries-preventive water fluoridation. In Ericcson, Y., Ed. Progress in caries prevention. *Caries Res,* 12 (Suppl 1):7–14.

47. Silverstone, L. M. (1983, May). Remineralization and enamel caries: New concepts. *Dent Update,* 10(4):261–73.

48. Featherstone, J. D. (1987). The mechanism of dental decay. *Nutr Today,* 22 (3):10–16.

49. Fejerskov, O., Thylstrup, A., & Larsen, M. J. (1981). Rational use of fluorides in caries prevention. *Acta Odontol Scan,* 39:241–49.

50. Silverstone, L. M., Wefel, J. S., Zimmerman, B. F., Clarkson, B. H., & Featherstone, M. J. (1981). Remineralization of natural and artificial lesions in human dental enamel in vitro. *Caries Res,* 15:138–57.

51. Bowen, W. H., & Geddes, D. A. M. (1990). Summary of Session III: Fluoride in saliva and dental plaque. *J Dent Res,* 69 (Spec Iss):637.

52. Arnold, Jr., F. A., Likins, R. C., Russell, A. L., & Scott, D. B. (1962). Fifteenth year of the Grand Rapids fluoridation study. *J Am Dent Assoc,* 65:780–85.

53. Arnold, Jr., F. A., Dean, H. T., & Knutson, J. W. (1953). Effect of fluoridated public water supplies on dental caries incidence. Results of the seventh year of study at Grand Rapids and Muskegon, Mich. *Public Health Rep,* 68:141–48.

54. Ast, D. B., Finn, S. B., & McCaffrey, I. (1950). The Newburgh-Kingston Caries Fluorine Study. I. Dental findings after three years of water fluoridation. *Am J Public Health,* 40:716–24.

55. Blaney, J. R., & Tucker, W. H. (1948). The Evanston Dental Caries Study. II. Purpose and mechanism of the study. *J Dent Res,* 27:279–86.

56. Brunelle, J. A., & Carlos, J. P. (1990). Recent trends in dental caries in U.S. children and the effect of water fluoridation. *J Dent Res,* 69 (Spec Iss):723–27.

57. Rozier, R. G. (1995). The effectiveness of community water fluoridation: Beyond dummy variables for fluoride exposure. *J Public Health Dent,* 55:195.

58. Horowitz, H. S. (1996). The effectiveness of community water fluoridation in the United States. *J Public Health Dent,* 56 (5 Spec No.):253–58.

59. Stookey, G. K. (1994). Review of fluorosis risk of self-applied topical fluorides: Dentifrices, mouthrinses and gels. *Community Dent Oral Epidemiol,* 22:181–86.

60. Griffin, S. O., Gooch, B. E., Lockwood, S. A., & Tomar, S. L. (2001). Quantifying the diffused benefit from water fluoridation in the United States. *Community Dent Oral Epidemiol,* 29:120–29.

61. Slade, G. D., Davies, M. J., Spencer, A. J., & Stewart, J. F. (1995). Associations between exposure to fluoridated drinking water and dental caries experience among children in two Australian states. *J Public Health Dent,* 55:218–28.

62. Newbrun, E. (1992). Current regulations and recommendations concerning water fluoridation, fluoride supplements, and topical fluoride agents. *J Dent Res,* 67:1255–65.

63. Murray, J. J., Breckon, J. A., Reynolds, P. J., Tabari, E. D., & Nunn, J. H. (1991). The effect of residence and social class on dental caries experience in 15–16-year-old children living in three towns (natural fluoride, adjusted fluoride and low fluoride) in the north east of England. *Br Dent J,* (171)10:319–22.

64. Newbrun, E. (1989). Effectiveness of water fluoridation. *J Public Health Dent,* 49 (Spec Iss):279–89.

65. Kaminsky, L. S., Mahoney, M. C., Leach, J., Melius, J., & Miller, M. J. (1990). Fluoride: Benefits and risks of exposure. *Crit Rev Oral Biol Med,* 1:261–81.

66. Barnard, P. D., & Sivaneswaran, S. (1990). Oral health of Tamworth schoolchildren 24 years after fluoridation. *J Dent Res,* 69 (Div Abstr):934. Abstract 9.

67. Griffen, S. O., Regnier, E., Griffin, P. M., Huntley, V. N. (2007). Effectiveness of fluoride in preventing caries in adults. *J Dent Res,* 86(5):410–14.

68. Burt, B. A. (1985). Fluoride: How much of a good thing? *J Public Health Dent,* 5:37–38.

69. Griffin, S. O., Griffin, P. M., Swann, J. L., & Zlobin, N. (2005). New coronal caries in older adults: Implications for prevention. *J Dent Res,* 84:715–20.

70. Griffin, S. O., Griffin, P. M., Swann, J. L., & Zlobin, N. (2004). Estimating rates of new root caries in older adults. *J Dent Res,* 83:634–38.

71. Stamm, J. W., Banting, D. W., & Imrey, P. B. (1990). Adult root caries survey of two similar communities with contrasting natural water fluoride levels. *J Am Dent Assoc,* 120:143–49.

72. U.S. Department of Health and Human Services. (1987). *Oral health of United States adults. The national survey of oral health in U.S. employed adults and seniors: 1985–1986. National findings* (NIH Publication No. 87-2868). Bethesda, MD: U.S. Department of Health and Human Services, National Institutes of Health.

73. Grembowski, D., Fiset, L., & Spadafora, A. (1992). How fluoridation affects adult dental caries. *J Am Dent Assoc,* 123:49–54.

74. McDonagh, M., Whiting, P., Bradley, M., Cooper, J., Sutton, A., Chestnutt, I., Misso, K., Wilson, P., Treasure, E., & Kleijnen, J. (2000). A systematic review of public water fluoridation. University of York, NHS Centre for Reviews and Dissemination, York, England.

75. Morris, J., & White, D. (2000, December). The York Review of Water Fluoridation—Key points for the busy practitioner. *Dent Update,* 474–75.

76. Centers for Disease Control and Prevention. (2001). Promoting oral health: Interventions for preventing dental caries, oral and pharyngeal cancers, and sports-related craniofacial injuries: A report on the recommendations of the Task Force on Community Preventive Services. *MMWR Morb Mortal Wkly Rep,* 50 (RR-14):1–42.

77. Truman, B. I., Gooch, B. F., Sulemana, I., Gift, H. C., Horowitz, A. M., Evans, Jr., C. A., Griffin, S. O., & Carande-Kulis, V. G. (2002). The task force on community preventive services. Reviews of evidence on interventions to prevent dental caries, oral and pharangeal cancers, and sports-related craniofacial injuries. *Am J Prev Med,* 23 (1S):21–54.

78. Lemke, C. W., Doherty, J. M., & Arra, M. C. (1970). Controlled fluoridation: The dental effects of discontinuation in Antigo, Wisconsin. *J Am Dent Assoc,* 80:782–86.

79. Stephen, K. W., McCall, D. R., & Tullis, J. I. (1987). Caries prevalence in Northern Scotland before and 5 years after water defluoridation. *Brit Dent J,* 163:324–26.

80. Attwood, D., & Blinkhorn, A. S. (1991). Dental health in schoolchildren 5 years after water fluoridation ceased in south-west Scotland. *Int Dent J,* 41:43–48.

81. Way, R. M. (1964). The effect on dental caries of a change from a naturally fluoridated to a fluoride-free communal water. *J Dent Child,* 31:151–57.

82. U.S. Department of Health and Human Services. (1991). *Public Health Service committee to coordinate environmental health and related programs. Review of fluoride: Benefits and risk.* Washington, DC: U.S. Department of Health and Human Services, Public Health Service.

83. Maupome, G., Clark, D. C., Levy, S. M., & Berkowitz, J. (2001). Patterns of dental caries following the cessation of water fluoridation. *Community Dent Oral Epidemiol,* 29:37–47.

84. Burt, B. A., Keels, M. A., & Heller, K. E. (2000). The effects of a break in water fluoridation on the development of dental caries and fluorosis. *J Dent Res,* 79:761–69.

85. Flaitz, C. M., Hill, E. M., & Hicks, M. J. (1989). A survey of bottled water usage by pediatric dental patients: Implications for dental health. *Quintessence Int,* 20:847–52.

86. Bartels, D., Haney, K., & Khajotia, S. S. (2000). Fluoride concentrations in bottled water. *J Okla Dent Assoc.* 2000 Summer; 91(1):18–22.

87. Tate, W. H., & Chen, J. T. (1994). Fluoride concentrations in bottled and filtered waters. *Gen Dent,* 42:362–66.

88. Food and Drug Administration. 1995. Beverages: Bottled Water; Final Rule. Federal Register, 21 CFR Part 103 et al. 60, 57075–57130.

89. Centers for Disease Control and Prevention. (2001). Recommendations for using fluoride to prevent and control dental caries in the United States. *MMWR Morb Mortal Wkly Rep,* 50 (RR-14):1–42.

90. Dean, H. T. (1942). The investigation of physiological effects by the epidemiological method. In Mouton, F. R., Ed. *Fluorine and dental health.* Washington, DC: American Association for the Advancement of Science, 19:23–31.

91. Fejerskov, O., Manji, F., & Baelum, V. (1990). The nature and mechanisms of dental fluorosis in man. *J Dent Res,* 69 (Spec Iss):692–700.

92. Whitford, G. M. (1996). *The metabolism and toxicity of fluoride* (2nd rev. ed.). (Monographs in Oral Science). Basel, Switzerland: Karger, 16.

93. Horowitz, H. S. (1986). Indexes for measuring dental fluorosis. *J Public Health Dent,* 46:179–83.

94. American Dental Association. (2006, November). ADA offers interim guidance on infant formula and fluoride. Retrieved on 03/12/08 from http://www.ada.org/prof/resources/positions/statements/fluoride_infants.asp.

95. Pendrys, D. G. (2000). Risk of enamel fluorosis in non-fluoridated and optimally fluoridated populations: Considerations for the dental professional. *J Am Dent Assoc,* 131:746–55.

96. Beltran-Aguilar, E. D., Barker, L. K., Canto, M. T., Dye, B. A., Gooch, B. F., Griffin, S. O., Hyman, J., Jaramillo, F., Kingman, A., Nowjack-Raymer, R., Selwitz, R., & Wu, T. (2005). Surveillance for dental caries, dental sealants, tooth retention, edentulism, and enamel fluorosis. *MMWR CDC Suveill Summ,* 54 (3):1–44.

97. Dean, H. T. (1936). Chronic endemic dental fluorosis. *J Am Med Assoc,* 107:1269–73.

98. Lewis, D. W., & Banting, D. W. (1994). Water Fluoridation: Current effectiveness and dental fluorosis. *Community Dent Oral Epidemiol,* 22:153–58.

99. Hong, L., Levy, S. M., Broffitt, B., Warren, J. J., Kanellis, M. J., Wefel, J. S., & Dawson, D. V. (2006). Timing of fluoride intake in relation to development of fluorosis on maxillary central incisors. *Community Dent Oral Epidemiol,* 34:299–305.

100. Levy, S. M., Warren, J. J., Davis, C. S., Kirchner, H. L., Kanellis, M. J., & Wefel, J. S. (2001). Patterns of fluoride intake from birth to 36 months. *J Public Health Dent,* 61:70–77.

101. National Academy of Sciences, National Research Council. (2006). *Fluoride in drinking water: A scientific review of EPA's standards.* Washington, DC: National Academies Press.

102. Clark, D. C., Hann, H. J., Williamson, M. F., & Berkowitz, J. (1993). Aesthetic concerns of children and parents in relation to different classifications of the Tooth Surface Index of Fluorosis. *Community Dent Oral Epidemiol,* 21:360–64.

103. Horowitz, H. S., Heifetz, S. B., & Driscoll, W. S. (1972). Partial defluoridation of a community water supply and dental fluorosis. *Health Serv Rep,* 87:451–55.

104. National Institutes of Health. Consensus Development Conference Statement, NIH Consensus Development Conference on Celiac Disease. June 28–30, 2004. Retrieved on 3/12/08 from http://consensus.nih.gov/2004/2004CeliacDisease118html.htm.

105. Meskin, L. H., Ed. (1995). Caries diagnosis and risk assessment: A review of preventive strategies and management. *J Am Dent Assoc,* 126 (Suppl):1S–24S.

106. American Academy of Pediatrics Committee on Nutrition. (1995). Fluoride supplementation for children: Interim policy recommendations. *Pediatrics,* 95:777.

107. American Academy of Pediatric Dentistry. (1995). Special issue: Reference manual 1994–95. *Pediatr Dent,* 16 (Spec Iss):1–96.

108. Galagan, D. J. (1953). Climate and controlled fluoridation. *J Am Dent Assoc,* 47:159–70.

109. Galagan, D. J., & Vermillion, J. R. (1957). Determining optimum fluoride concentrations. *Public Health Rep,* 72:491–93.

110. Galagan, D. J., Vermillion, J. R., Nevitt, G. A., Stadt, Z.M., & Dart, R.E. (1957). Climate and fluid intake. *Public Health Rep,* 72:484–90.

111. U.S. Public Health Service. (1962). *Public Health Service drinking water standards 1962* (PHS Publication No. 956). Washington, DC: Government Printing Office.

112. Heller, K. E., Sohn, W., Burt, B. A., & Eklund, S. A. (1999). Water consumption in the United States in 1994–96 and implications for water fluoridation policy. *J Public Health Dent,* 59:3–11.

113. Sohn, W., Heller, K. E., & Burt, B. A. (2001). Fluid consumption related to climate among children in the United States. *J Public Health Dent,* 61:99–106.

114. Levy, S. M., Kiritsy, M. C., & Warren, J. J. (1995). Sources of fluoride intake in children. *J Public Health Dent,* 55:39–52.

115. Kiritsy, M. C., Levy, S. M., Warren, J. J., Guha-Chowdhury, N., Heilman, J. R., & Marshall, T. (1996). Assessing fluoride concentrations of juices and juice-flavored drinks. *J Am Dent Assoc,* 127:895–902.

116. Review of water fluoridation and fluoride intake from discretionary fluoride supplements. Review for the National Health and Medical Research Council by the Royal Melbourne Institute of Technology – Key Centre for Applied and Nutritional Toxicology in conjunction with the Monash University Medical School's Centre for Epidemiology and Preventive Medicine. Melbourne, Australia. 15 April 1999.

117. Australian Research Centre for Population Oral Health, Dental School, The University of Adelaide, South Australia. (2006). The use of fluorides in Australia: Guidelines. *Australian Dent J,* 51:195–99.

118. Centers for Disease Control and Prevention. (2007, September 17). *Water fluoridation additives.* Retrieved from http://cdc.gov/fluoridation/fact_sheets/engineering/wfadditives.htm.

119. Reeves, T. G. (1996). Technical aspects of water fluoridation in the United States and an overview of fluoridation engineering world-wide. *Community Dent Health,* 13 (Suppl 2):21–26.

120. U.S. Department of Health and Human Services. (1986). *Water fluoridation. A manual for engineers and technicians 1986.* Bethesda, MD: U.S. Department of Health and Human Services. U.S. Public Health Service, Centers for Disease Control.

121. Centers for Disease Control and Prevention. (1995). Engineering and administrative recommendations for water fluoridation, 1995. *MMWR Morb Mortal Wkly Rep,* 44 (No. RR-13):1–40.

122. Hinman, A. R., Sterritt, G. R., & Reeves, T. G. (1996). The U.S. experience with fluoridation. *Community Dent Health,* 13 (Suppl 2):5–9.

123. Urbansky, E. T., & Schock, M. R. (2000). Can fluoridation affect lead (II) in potable water? Hexafluorosilicate and fluoride equilibria in aqueous. *Intern J Environ Studies,* 57:597–637.

124. Finney, W. F., Wilson, E., Callendar, A., Morris, M. D., & Beck, L. W. (2006, April 15). Reexamination of hexafluorosilicate hydrolysis by 19F NMR and pH measurements. *Environ Sci Technol,* 40:2572–77.

125. American Water Works Association. (2004). *Water fluoridation principles and practices. Manual of Water Supply Practices - M4.* Fifth Ed., USA.

126. Centers for Disease Control and Prevention. (2007, September 27). *Fluoride proficiency testing program.* Retrieved December 11, 2007, from http://cdc.gov/fluoridation/engineering.htm#4.

127. Lalumandier, J. A., & Jones, J. L. (1999). Fluoride concentrations in drinking water. *J Am Water Works Assoc,* 91:42–51.

128. Leland, D. E., Powell, K. E., & Anderson, R. S. (1980). A fluoride overfeed incident at Harbor Springs, Michigan. *J Am Water Works Assoc,* 72:238–43.

129. Petersen, L. R., Denis, D., Brown, D., Hadler, J. L., & Helgerson, S. D. (1998). Community health effects of a municipal water supply hyperfluoridation accident. *Am J Public Health,* 78:711–13.

130. Gessner, B. D., Beller, M., Middaugh, J. P., & Whitford, G. M. (1994). Acute fluoride poisoning from a public water system. *N Engl J Med,* 330:95–99.

131. Centers for Disease Control and Prevention. (2007, September 27). *Oral health resources: Community water fluoridation.* Retrieved December 11, 2007, from http://www.cdc.gov/fluoridation/engineering.htm.

132. White, B. A., Antezak-Bouckoms, A. A., & Weinstein, M. C. (1989). Issues in the economic evaluation of community water fluoridation. *J Dent Educ,* 53:646–57.

133. Ringelberg, M. L., Allen, S. J., & Jackson Brown, L. (1992). Cost of fluoridation: 44 Florida communities. *J Public Health Dent,* 52:75–80

134. Griffin, S. O., Jones, K., & Tomar, S. L. (2001). An economic evaluation of community water fluoridation. *J Public Health Dent,* 61:78–86.

135. Neenan, M. E. (1996). Obstacles to extending fluoridation in the United States. *Community Dent Health,* 13 (Suppl 2):10–20.

136. Speier and Brown, Assembly Members, and Maddy, California Legislature, 1995–96, Regular Session Senator, Assembly Bill No. 733, February 22, 1995.

137. Brown, J. P. (2000, May). *Water fluoridation costs in Texas: Texas Health Steps (EPSDT-Medicaid).*

138. Centers for Disease Control and Prevention. (1999). Water fluoridation and the costs of medicaid treatment for dental decay, Louisiana, 1995–1996. *MMWR Morb Mortal Wkly Rep,* 48:753–57.

139. Mjor, I. A. (1989). Amalgam and composite resin restorations: Longevity and reasons for replacement. In Anusavice, K. J., Ed. *Quality evaluations of dental restorations.* Chicago: Quintessence Publishing, 61–72.

140. MacInnis, W. A., Ismail, A., Brogan, H., & Kavanagh, M. (1990). Placement and replacement of restorations in a military population. *J Dent Res,* 69 (Spec Iss):179. Abstract 564.

141. Qvist, J., Qvist, V., & Mjor, I. A. (1990). Placement and longevity of amalgam restorations in Denmark. *J Dent Res,* 69 (Spec Iss):236. Abstract 1018.

142. Wright, J., Bates, M., Cutress, T., & Lee, M. (1999). The cost-effectiveness of fluoridating water supplies in New Zealand: A report for the New Zealand Ministry of Health. Porirua, New Zealand: Institute of Environmental Science and Research, 1–31.

143. World Health Organization. (2003). *World oral health report 2003.* Geneva: World Health Organization.

144. Bergmann, K. E., & Bergmann, R. L. (1995). Salt fluoridation and general health. *Adv Dent Res,* 9:138–43.

145. Mejia, R., Espinal, F., Velez, H., & Aguirre, M. (1976). Estudio sobre la fluoruracion de la sal. VIII Resultados obtenidos de 1964 a 1972. *Boll Of Sanit Panam,* 80:67–80.

146. Kunzel, W. (1993). Systemic use of fluoride—Other methods: salt, sugar, milk, etc. *Caries Res,* 27 (Suppl 1):16–22.

147. Intersalt Cooperative Research Group. (1988). Intersalt: An international study of electrolyte excretion and blood pressure. Results for 24 hour urinary and potassium excretion. *Br Med J,* 297:319–28.

148. Klein, S. P., Bohannan, H. M., Bell, R. M., Disney, J. A., Foch C. B., & Graves, R. C. (1985). The cost and effectiveness of school-based preventive dental care. *Am J Public Health,* 75:382–91.

149. Disney, J. A., Graves, R. C., Stamm, J. W., Bohannan, H. M., & Abernathy, J. R. (1989). Comparative effects of a 4-year fluoride mouthrinse program on high and low caries forming grade 1 children. *Community Dent Oral Epidemiol,* 17:139–43.

150. Marinho, V. C., Higgins, J. P., Logan, S., & Sheiham, A. The Cochrane Collaboration. (2005). Fluoride mouthrinses

for preventing dental caries in children and adolescents. (Review). *Cochrane Database Syst Rev,* 2003;(3): CD002284. Review.

151. Sandman, P. M. (1990, April). Hazard vs Outrage: Public Perception of Fluoridation Risks. *Journal of Public Health Dentistry,* 50 (4):285–287.

152. Hance, B., Chess, C., & Sandman, P. (1990). Industry risk communication manual. Boca Raton, FL: CRC Press/Lewis Publishers.

153. Chess, C., Hance, B., & Sandman, P. (1988). *Improving dialogue with communities: A risk communication manual for government.* Trenton, NJ: Division of Science and Research, New Jersey Department of Environmental Protection.

154. Covello, V. (1989). Issues and problems in using risk comparisons for communicating right-to-know information on chemical risks. *Environ Sci Technol,* 23:1444–49.

155. Covello, V., & Allen, F. (1988). *Seven Cardinal Rules of Risk Communication.* Washington, DC: U.S. Environmental Protection Agency, Office of Policy Analysis.

156. Fischoff, B., Lichtenstein, S., Slovic, P., & Keeney, D. (1981). *Acceptable risk.* Cambridge: Cambridge University Press.

Chapter 12

Topical Fluoride Therapy

Patricia R. Campbell

OBJECTIVES

After studying this chapter, the student should be able to:

1. List the fluoride compounds used to control caries and indicate their relative effectiveness.
2. Describe the possible chemical reactions associated with the topical application of sodium fluoride, stannous fluoride, and acidulated phosphate fluoride.
3. Identify what percentages of sodium fluoride and stannous fluoride are available for office and home use.
4. Describe how topical fluoride is applied to the teeth.
5. Explain why the early dentifrices did not produce the expected caries decrements.
6. State the expected decreases in caries formation following use of dentifrices and mouthrinses containing fluoride.
7. Describe fluoridated varnishes and fluoride-releasing dental restorative materials, and the potential of these materials to inhibit demineralization and enhance remineralization.

KEY TERMS

Topical fluoride therapy
Enamel maturation
Sodium fluoride (NaF)
Stannous fluoride
APF, acidulated phosphate fluoride
Cariostatic
Sodium monofluorophosphate
Thixotropic
Pedodontists
Multiple fluoride therapy

INTRODUCTION

When public water supplies are available, community water fluoridation clearly represents the most effective, efficient, and economical of all known measures for the prevention of dental caries, although similar results have been observed with fluoridated salt in many countries. Unfortunately, fluoridated water is available to only about two-thirds of the population. Thus, it is obvious that additional measures are needed for the dental profession to provide greater protection against caries to as many segments of the population as possible.

The term **topical fluoride therapy** refers to the use of systems containing relatively large concentrations of fluoride that are applied locally, or topically, to erupted tooth surfaces to prevent the formation of dental caries. This term encompasses the use of fluoride rinses, dentifrices, pastes, gels, foams, and varnishes, which are applied in various manners.

MECHANISM OF ACTION OF TOPICAL FLUORIDE TREATMENTS

Studies of the use of professional topical fluoride applications for the control of dental caries began in the early 1940s. Since that time, it has been generally accepted that the fluoride content of enamel is inversely related to the prevalence of dental caries.

Using in vivo enamel-sampling techniques and improved analytic methods, investigators have been better able to quantitate this relationship. For example, Keene and coworkers explored this relationship in young naval recruits 17 to 22 years of age; their observations are summarized in (Table 12–1 ■).[1] These data suggest that the presence of elevated levels of fluoride in surface enamel is associated with a minimal caries experience.

A much more extensive investigation of this relationship was reported by DePaola and coworkers.[2] These investigators similarly examined 1,447 subjects, 12 to 16 years of age, who were lifetime residents of selected fluoridated and non-fluoridated communities; again the inverse relationship between enamel fluoride content and caries prevalence was apparent.

At the time of tooth eruption, the enamel is not yet completely calcified and undergoes a post-eruptive period, approximately 2 years in length, during which enamel calcification continues. Throughout this stage, called the period of **enamel maturation,** fluoride and other elements continue to accumulate in the more superficial portions of enamel. This fluoride is derived from the saliva as well as from the exposure of the teeth to fluoride-containing water and food.[3] Following the period of enamel maturation, relatively little additional fluoride is incorporated from such sources into the enamel surface.[4] Thus, most of the fluoride that is incorporated into the developing enamel occurs during the pre-eruptive period of enamel formation and the post-eruptive period of enamel maturation.

The continued deposition of fluoride into enamel during the later stages of enamel formation, and especially during the period of enamel maturation, results in a concentration gradient of fluoride in enamel. Invariably the highest concentration of fluoride occurs at the very outermost portion of the enamel surface, with the fluoride content decreasing as one progresses inward toward the dentin.[5,6] This decrease in fluoride concentration is extremely rapid in the outermost 5 to 10 microns of enamel, and is much less pronounced thereafter. This characteristic fluoride concentration gradient has been observed in un-erupted and erupted teeth, and in both the permanent and deciduous dentition, regardless of the amount of previous exposure to fluoride.

■ **Table 12–1** Relationship Between Surface Enamel Fluoride Content and Caries Prevalence in Young Adults

Number of Subjects	Caries Prevalence (DMFT)	Enamel Fluoride Content (ppm)
47	0	3459
31	5–11	2229
29	12–26	1944

DMFT, decayed, missing, or filled teeth.
Values calculated from data presented by Keene et al, 1973.[1]

The presence of elevated concentrations of fluoride in surface enamel serves to make the tooth surface more resistant to the development of dental caries. Fluoride ions, when substituted into the hydroxyapatite crystal, fit more perfectly into the crystal than do hydroxyl ions. This fact, coupled with the greater bonding potential of fluoride, serves to make the apatite crystals more compact and stable. Such crystals are thereby more resistant to the acid dissolution that occurs during caries initiation.[7,8] This effect is even more apparent as the pH of the enamel environment decreases because of the momentary loss of minute quantities of fluoride from the dissolving enamel and its nearly simultaneous re-precipitation as a fluorhydroxyapatite.[9–11]

Most of the initial studies concerning topical fluoride applications were conducted with **sodium fluoride (NaF).** It was recognized at that time that prolonged exposure of the teeth to low concentrations of fluoride in the dental office was not practical. To overcome this problem, researchers explored two approaches: increasing the fluoride concentration and decreasing the pH of the application solution.

Although the ability of NaF to increase the resistance of enamel to acid dissolution had been reported on several occasions, it had also been reported that lowering the pH of the NaF solution greatly increased protection against enamel decalcification. Five clinical caries studies were conducted to evaluate the effectiveness of acidulated NaF topical solutions. The fluoride solutions were acidulated (made acidic) by various methods (e.g., acetic acid, acid phthalate) and used under varying conditions, but in no instance was a statistically significant caries-preventive effect observed. Thus, the use of acidulated NaF systems was abandoned, at least temporarily.

On the other hand, the observed results of increasing concentrations of fluoride were very encouraging, particularly when multiple applications were used. Although it was initially proposed that the effectiveness of topically applied NaF was due to the formation of a fluorhydroxyapatite, subsequent investigations indicated that the primary reaction product involved the transformation of surface hydroxyapatite to calcium fluoride.[12–19]

$$Ca_{10}(PO_4)_6(OH)_2 + 2OF^- \longleftrightarrow$$
hydroxyapatite

$$10CaF_2 + 6HPO_4^\equiv + 2(OH)^-$$
calcium fluoride

The preceding reaction involves the breakdown of the apatite crystal into its components, followed by the reaction of fluoride and calcium ions to form calcium fluoride, with a net loss of phosphate ions from treated enamel. Newer fluoride systems incorporate a means of preventing such phosphate loss. The early investigators of the reaction between soluble fluoride and enamel observed that the nature of the reaction products was markedly influenced by a number of factors, including fluoride concentration, the pH of the solution, and the length of exposure.

For example, the use of acidic fluoride solutions greatly favored the formation of calcium fluoride.[14] Neutral NaF solutions with fluoride concentrations of 100 ppm or less resulted primarily in the formation of fluorapatite, whereas higher fluoride concentrations resulted in the formation of calcium fluoride.[18] Because topical applications of NaF involve the use of 2.0% solutions (slightly over 9,000 ppm), the use of these solutions essentially involves the formation of calcium fluoride.[17]

The second fluoride compound developed for topical use in the dental office during the 1950s was **stannous fluoride** (SnF_2).[19–21] Compared with that of NaF, the reaction of SnF_2 with enamel is unique in that both the cation (stannous) and the anion (fluoride) react chemically with enamel components. This reaction is commonly depicted as follows:

$$Ca_{10}(PO_4)_6(OH)_2 + 19nF_2 \longrightarrow$$
hydroxyapatite   stannous fluoride

$$10CaF_2 + 6Sn_3F_3PO_4 + SnO \cdot H_2O$$
calcium   stannous   hydrated
fluoride   fluorophosphate   tin oxide

As indicated by the equation, formation of stannous fluorophosphate prevents, at least temporarily, the phosphate loss typical of NaF applications. Incidentally, the exact nature of the tin-containing reaction products varies depending on reaction conditions, including pH, concentration, and length of exposure (or reaction time).[22,23]

A third topical fluoride system for professional use was developed during the 1960s and is widely known as **APF, acidulated phosphate fluoride.** This system was developed by Brudevold and coworkers in an effort to achieve greater amounts of fluorhydroxyapatite and lesser amounts of calcium fluoride formation.[24,25] These investigators reviewed the various chemical reactions of fluoride with hydroxyapatite and concluded that (1) if the pH of the fluoride system was made acidic to enhance the rate of reaction of fluoride with hydroxyapatite and (2) if phosphoric acid was used as the acidulant to increase the concentration of phosphate present at the reaction site, it should be possible to obtain greater amounts of fluoride deposited in surface enamel as fluorhydroxyapatite, with minimal formation of calcium fluoride and minimal loss of enamel phosphate. On the basis of this chemical reasoning, APF systems were developed and shown to be effective for caries prevention.

Subsequent independent studies of the reactions of APF with enamel indicated, however, that the original chemical objectives were only partially achieved. The major reaction product of APF with enamel is also calcium fluoride, although a greater amount of fluorhydroxyapatite is formed than with the previous topical fluoride systems.[15,26,27] The chemical reaction of APF with enamel may be written as follows:

$$\underset{\text{hydroxyapatite}}{Ca_{10}(PO_4)_6(OH)_2} + \underset{\text{stannous fluoride}}{F^-} \longrightarrow$$

$$\underset{\substack{\text{calcium} \\ \text{fluoride}}}{CaF_2} + \underset{\text{fluorhydroxyapatite}}{Ca_{10}(PO_4)_6(OH)_{2x}F_x}$$

It is obvious from the preceding discussion that the primary chemical reaction product with all three types of topical fluoride systems (i.e., NaF, SnF_2, and APF) is the formation of calcium fluoride on the enamel surface.

The initial deposition of calcium fluoride on the treated tooth surfaces is by no means permanent; a relatively rapid loss of fluoride occurs within the first 24 hours, with some continued loss occurring during the following 15 days.[28–32] The rate of loss varies between patients and is influenced by the nature of the fluoride treatment.[33,34]

Nevertheless, it is known that each individual, professionally applied fluoride treatment results in an increase in the permanently bound fluoride content of the outermost layers of the enamel, with a subsequent decrease in the susceptibility of the enamel for caries initiation and progression.

Numerous investigations of professional fluoride applications have focused on the role that calcium fluoride deposits on the enamel surface play in providing the observed **cariostatic** benefits, that is, benefits from preventing formation of dental caries. It is known that the most desirable form of fluoride in enamel for caries prevention is fluorhydroxyapatite, and that the most efficient means of forming this reaction product occurs with prolonged exposure of the enamel to low concentrations of fluoride. It is also known that calcium fluoride may serve as a fluoride source for enamel remineralization, and that calcium fluoride dissolves much more slowly in the oral environment than in an aqueous solution because of the presence of a phosphate or protein-rich coating of the globular deposits of calcium fluoride on the enamel surface.[35–38] As a result of this continued research, a growing body of convincing evidence suggests that the deposits of calcium fluoride serve as an important fluoride reservoir, and that these phosphate-coated globules are dissolved in the presence of plaque acids, providing an available source of both fluoride and phosphate to facilitate the remineralization of decalcified areas.[39]

Regardless of the mechanism of action of professionally applied topical fluoride treatments, the results of clinical trials clearly indicate that the benefits are related to the number of treatments. (Table 12–2 ■) summarizes a clinical study in which schoolchildren were given a dental prophylaxis and a topical application of 8% SnF_2 at 6-month intervals throughout a 3-year period.[40] Dental

■ **Table 12–2** Clinical Reductions in Incremental Caries as a Function of the Number of Topical Fluoride Applications

		Caries Reduction (%)	
Study Period (Years)	*Total Number of Topical Applications*	*DMFT*	*DMFS*
1	2	2.8	12.6
2	4	29.2	34.1
3	6	47.4	51.5

DMFT, decayed, missing, or filled teeth; DMFS, decayed, missing, or filled surfaces.
Values calculated from data presented by Beiswanger et al, 1980.[40]

caries examinations were performed initially and each year thereafter. It is apparent from these data that the caries-preventive benefits increased in relation to the number of treatments. Similar observations have been noted with the other two fluoride systems used for professional applications. The original NaF topical application procedure developed by Knutson specified a series of four treatments during a 2-week period.[41] Mellberg and coworkers have also indicated the need for repeated topical applications of APF to obtain maximal benefits.[42,43] Thus, it is apparent that maximal patient benefits can be obtained with only repeated topical applications regardless of the nature of the fluoride system used.

It was noted earlier that the reaction of SnF_2 with enamel resulted in the formation of tin-containing compounds. Although much less is known about the precise nature and ultimate fate of these compounds, it appears that they contribute significantly to the cariostatic activity of SnF_2. The tin reaction products formed on sound enamel surfaces appear to be leached from the enamel in a manner similar to that for calcium fluoride.[44] The greatest accumulation of stannous complexes occurs in circumscribed areas of enamel defects; typically such areas are hypomineralized and are frequently the result of decalcification associated with the initiation of the caries process. Extremely high concentrations of tin, about 20,000 ppm, have been reported in these locations.[45] Clinically, these areas, which have been described as frank carious areas, become pigmented (presumably because of the presence of the tin complexes) and appear to be more calcified following the application of SnF_2. This pigmentation has thus been suggested as indicative of the arrest of carious lesions and is typically retained for 6 to 12 months or longer, implying that these stannous reaction products are of considerably greater significance than those formed on sound enamel.

At reduced concentrations of 0.10% to 0.15% fluoride, all of the foregoing fluoride compounds have also been approved for use in dentifrices and gels intended for personal use, and NaF at a concentration of 0.05% has also been approved for use in mouthrinses sold over the counter. In general, it is recognized that the mechanism of action of these fluoride compounds is similar at all the concentrations used for both professional and self-care products.

One additional fluoride compound, **sodium monofluorophosphate,** has been approved for use in dentifrices; this compound has the empirical formula Na_2PO_3F and is commonly known as MFP. Although

evaluated in one study as an agent for topical fluoride application in the dental office, its use in this manner has received little consideration. Although the mechanism of action of MFP is thought to involve a chemical reaction with surface enamel, the precise nature of this reaction is poorly understood. Some investigators have suggested that the fluorophosphate moiety (component) PO_3F^5 may undergo an exchange reaction with phosphate ions in the apatite structure, but the presence of PO_3F^5 in enamel has never been demonstrated; such a reaction mechanism appears unlikely. Others have suggested that the PO_3F^5 complex is enzymatically dissociated by phosphatases present in saliva and dental plaque into PO_3^2 and F^2, with the ionic fluoride reacting with hydroxyapatite in a manner similar to that described earlier. That treatment of enamel with MFP results in less fluoride deposition and less protection against enamel decalcification than observed with simple inorganic fluoride compounds such as NaF, while still imparting nearly comparable cariostatic activity, indicates a more complex mechanism of action.

For the most part, the foregoing discussion of the chemical reactions of concentrated fluoride solutions with enamel suggests that the reactions occur on the outer enamel surface and serve to make that surface more resistant to demineralization. It is apparent that this process is particularly predominant in newly erupted teeth that are undergoing continued enamel maturation and calcification, for the first 2 years following eruption into the oral cavity. In such instances, some of the applied fluoride readily penetrates the relatively permeable enamel surface to depths of 20 to 30 mm and readily reacts with the calcifying apatite to form a fluorhydroxyapatite. Furthermore, the dissolution of the calcium fluoride deposited on the enamel surface provides additional fluoride ions, which become incorporated in maturing enamel.

It has become increasingly apparent that application of fluoride to sound, fully matured enamel results in very little fluoride deposition that lasts more than 24 hours. This situation apparently occurs regardless of the nature of the fluoride compound, the concentration of fluoride, or the manner of application. Thus, there appears to be no preventive benefits from the application of fluoride to maturated, sound enamel.

The caries process begins with a demineralization of the apatite adjacent to the crystal sheaths. Demineralization permits the diffusion of weak acids into the subsurface enamel, and because the subsurface enamel has a lower fluoride content and is less resistant to acid demineralization, it is preferentially dissolved, forming an incipient, subsurface lesion. As this process continues, it becomes clinically apparent as a so-called "white spot" that, in reality, is a rather extensive subsurface lesion covered by a relatively intact enamel surface. Thus, enamel surfaces that clinically appear to be sound or free of demineralization frequently have areas that have been slightly decalcified with minute subsurface lesions that are not yet detectable clinically.[46] This situation is particularly likely to exist in patients with clinical evidence of caries activity on other teeth.

It now appears that the predominant mechanism of action of fluoride involves its ability to facilitate the remineralization of these demineralized areas. Topically applied fluoride clearly diffuses into these demineralized areas, and reacts with calcium and phosphate to form fluorhydroxyapatite in the remineralization process. It is also noteworthy that such remineralized enamel is more resistant to subsequent demineralization than was the original enamel. This process has been shown to occur with all forms and concentrations of fluoride, including concentrations as low as 1 ppm such as is found in optimally fluoridated drinking water. Studies have clearly shown that the amount of fluoride deposition in subsurface lesions after a topical fluoride application is much greater than that occurring after the use of lesser concentrations of fluoride provided by fluoride rinses or dentifrices. As a result, topical fluoride applications appear to be an effective means of inducing the remineralization of incipient lesions.

EFFECTS OF FLUORIDE ON PLAQUE AND BACTERIAL METABOLISM

Thus far, the assumption has been that the cariostatic effects of fluoride are mediated through a chemical reaction between this ion and the outermost portion of the enamel surface. Overwhelmingly, data support this view. A growing body of information suggests, however, that the caries-preventive action of fluoride may also include an inhibitory effect on the oral flora involved in the initiation of caries. The ability of fluoride to inhibit glycolysis (breaking down of glucose) by interfering with the enzyme enolase has long been known; concentrations of fluoride as low as 50 ppm have been shown to interfere with bacterial metabolism. Moreover, fluoride may accumulate in dental plaque in concentrations above 100 ppm. Although the fluoride normally present in plaque is largely bound and thus unavailable for antibacterial

action, it dissociates to ionic fluoride when the pH of plaque decreases (i.e., when acids are formed). Thus, when the carious process starts and acids are formed, plaque fluoride in ionic form may serve to interfere with further acid production by plaque microorganisms. In addition, it may react with the underlying layer of dissolving enamel, promoting its remineralization as fluorhydroxyapatite. The end result of this process is a physiologic restoration of the initial lesion by remineralization of enamel and the formation of a more resistant enamel surface. The ability of fluoride to promote the re-precipitation of calcium phosphate solutions in apatitic forms has been repeatedly demonstrated.

In addition to these possible effects of fluoride, several investigators have reported that the presence of tin, especially as provided by SnF_2, is associated with significant antibacterial activity, which has been reported to decrease both the amount of dental plaque and gingivitis in both animals and adult humans.[47,48] Existing evidence suggests that these antibacterial effects of fluoride and tin may also contribute to the observed cariostatic activity of topically applied fluorides.

TOPICAL FLUORIDE APPLICATIONS

The use of concentrated fluoride solutions applied topically to the dentition for the prevention of dental caries has been studied extensively during the past 50 years, although few studies have been conducted since the 1970s. This procedure results in a significant increase in the resistance of the exposed tooth surfaces to the development of dental caries and, as a result, has become a standard procedure in most dental offices.

At present, three different fluoride systems have been adequately evaluated and approved for use in this manner in the United States. These three systems are 2% sodium fluoride (NaF), 8% stannous fluoride (SnF_2), and acidulated phosphate fluoride (APF) systems containing 1.23% fluoride.

Available Forms

When topical fluoride applications became available to the profession, the fluoride compounds, NaF and SnF_2, were obtained in powder or crystalline form, and aqueous solutions were prepared immediately prior to use. Subsequently, it was realized that NaF solutions were stable if stored in plastic containers, and this compound became available in liquid, gel, and powder form. Several factors resulted in a trend toward the use of ready-to-use, stable, flavored preparations in gel and foam form: Continued research of different types of agents; professional recognition of disadvantages of existing forms with regard to patient acceptance and stability; and the need to use professional time more efficiently. The "one-minute foams" are also popular, but research supports use of only the 4-minute foams.

Sodium Fluoride

This material is available as a powder, gel, foam, liquid, and varnish. The compound is recommended for use in a 2% concentration, which may be prepared by dissolving 0.2 g of powder in 10 ml of distilled water. The prepared solution or gel has a basic pH and is stable if stored in plastic containers. Ready-to-use 2% solutions and gels of NaF are commercially available. Because of the relative absence of taste considerations with this compound, these solutions generally contain little flavoring or sweetening agents.

Stannous Fluoride$_2$

This compound is available in powder form, either in bulk containers or preweighed capsules. The recommended and approved concentration is 8%, which is obtained by dissolving 0.8 g of the powder in 10 ml of distilled water. Stannous fluoride solutions are quite acidic, with a pH of about 2.4 to 2.8. Aqueous solutions of SnF_2 are not stable because of the formation of stannous hydroxide and, subsequently, stannic oxide, which is visible as a white precipitate. As a result, solutions of this compound must be prepared immediately prior to use. As will be noted later, SnF_2 solutions have a bitter, metallic taste. A stable, flavored solution can be prepared with glycerine and sorbitol to retard hydrolysis of the agent and with any of a variety of compatible flavoring agents, thus eliminating the need to prepare this solution from the powder and improving patient acceptance.

Acidulated Phosphate Fluoride

This treatment system is available as a solution, foam, or gel; all forms are stable and ready to use.[49,50] All contain 1.23% fluoride, generally obtained by the use of 2.0% NaF and 0.34% hydrofluoric acid. Phosphate is usually provided as orthophosphoric acid in a concentration of 0.98%. The pH of true APF systems should be about 3.5. Gel preparations feature a greater variation in composition, particularly with regard to the source and concentration of phosphate. In addition, the gel preparations generally contain thickening (binders), flavoring, and coloring agents.

Another form of APF for topical applications, namely thixotropic gels, is also available. The term **thixotropic** denotes a solution that sets in a gel-like state but is not a true gel. With application of pressure, thixotropic gels behave like solutions; it has been suggested that these preparations are more easily forced into the interproximal spaces than conventional gels. The active fluoride system in thixotropic gels is identical to conventional APF solutions. Although the initial thixotropic gels exhibited somewhat poorer biologic activity in in vitro studies, subsequent formulations were at least equivalent to conventional APF systems. Even though few clinical efficacy studies have been reported, the collective data were considered adequate evidence of activity.[51]

A foam form of APF is also available. Laboratory studies indicate that the amount of fluoride uptake in enamel after applications using the foam is comparable to that observed with conventional APF gels and solutions. The primary advantage of foam preparations is that appreciably less material is used for a treatment; therefore, lesser amounts are likely to be inadvertently swallowed by young children during professional application.[50] Equally important, foam applications are better tolerated by patients owing to the pleasant taste.

Application Procedures

In essence, three procedures are available for administering topical fluoride treatments. One procedure, in brief, involves the isolation of teeth and continuously painting the liquid solution onto the tooth surfaces. The second, and more popular, procedure involves the use of fluoride foams or gels applied with a disposable tray. Most recently, fluoride varnish has been used for young children and individuals with developmental disabilities; it is easily painted on the tooth surfaces without the need for isolation.

In the past, it was assumed that it was necessary to administer a thorough dental prophylaxis prior to the topical application of fluoride. This hypothesis was supported by the results of an early study that suggested topically applied NaF was more effective if a prophylaxis preceded the treatment.[52] The results of four clinical trials have indicated that a prophylaxis immediately prior to the topical application of fluoride is not necessary.[53–56] In these studies, the children were given topical applications of APF in the conventional manner, except that three different procedures were used to clean the teeth immediately prior to each treatment: a dental prophylaxis, toothbrushing and flossing, or no cleaning procedure. The results indicated that the cariostatic activity of the APF treatment was not influenced by the different pre-application procedures. Thus, the administration of a dental prophylaxis prior to the topical application of fluoride must be considered optional; it should be performed if there is a general need for a prophylaxis, but it need not be performed as a prerequisite for topical fluoride applications.

It should be stressed that various precautions should be taken routinely to minimize the amount of fluoride that is inadvertently swallowed by the patient during the application procedure. A number of reports have shown that 10 to 30 mg of fluoride may be inadvertently swallowed during the application procedure, and it has been suggested that the ingestion of these quantities of fluoride by young children may contribute to the development of dental fluorosis in teeth that are un-erupted and in the developmental stage.[57–63] Precautions that should be undertaken include (1) using only the required amount of the fluoride solution or gel to perform the treatment adequately; (2) positioning the patient in an upright position; (3) using efficient saliva aspiration, or suctioning, apparatus; and (4) requiring the patient to expectorate thoroughly on completion of the fluoride application. The use of these procedures has been shown to reduce the amount of inadvertently swallowed fluoride to less than 2 mg, which may be expected to be of little consequence.[64]

After the topical application is completed, the patient is advised not to rinse, drink, or eat for 30 minutes. The necessity of the latter procedure has not been substantiated; the fact that it has been followed in most of the prior clinical studies serves as the primary basis for this recommendation. This recommendation is supported, however, by a 1986 study that measured the amount of fluoride deposition in incipient lesions (subsurface enamel demineralization) in patients who either were, or were not, permitted to rinse, eat, or drink during this 30-minute posttreatment period.[65] It was found that significantly greater fluoride deposition occurred when the patients were not permitted to rinse, eat, or drink following the fluoride treatment.

Whichever fluoride system is used for topical fluoride applications, the teeth should be exposed to the fluoride for 4 minutes for maximal cariostatic benefits.[66–69] This treatment time has consistently been recommended for both NaF and APF. Some confusion has arisen, however, with regard to SnF_2, because shorter application periods of 15 to 30 seconds with SnF_2 have been reported

to result in significant cariostatic benefits. Nevertheless, the collective results of these and subsequent clinical investigations indicate that maximum caries protection is achieved only with the use of the longer exposure period. Thus, although reduced exposure periods of 30 to 60 seconds might be appropriate as a fluoride maintenance or preventive measure in patients with very little caries activity, the use of the longer, 4-minute application should be required for patients with existing or potential caries activity. The 1-minute time period advertised by some companies on available fluorides are not adequate for most patients, because more time is needed for the product to be maximally effective.

Application of Fluoride Gels and Foams

The commonly used, and convenient, technique for providing treatments with fluoride gels and foams involves the use of a soft, styrofoam tray. These trays can be bent to insert in the mouth and are soft enough to produce no discomfort when they reach the soft tissues. These trays, as well as some of the previous types of trays, allow simultaneous treatment of both arches.

As with the use of topical fluoride solutions, the treatment may be preceded by a prophylaxis if indicated by existing oral conditions. With the tray application technique, the armamentarium (equipment and pharmaceutical agents) consists simply of a suitable tray and the fluoride gel or foam.

Many different types of trays are available; selection of a tray adequate for the individual patient is an important part of the technique.[70] Most manufacturers offer sizes to fit patients of different ages. An adequate tray should cover all the patient's dentition; it should also have enough depth to reach beyond the cementoenamel junction and to contact the alveolar mucosa to prevent saliva from diluting the fluoride gel or foam.

If a prophylaxis is given, the patient is permitted to rinse, and the teeth of the arch to be treated are dried with compressed air. A ribbon of gel or foam is placed in the trough portion of the tray and the tray seated over the entire arch. The method used must ensure that the gel/foam reaches all of the teeth and flows interproximally. If, for instance, a soft pliable tray is used, the tray is pressed or molded against the tooth surfaces, and the patient may also be instructed to bite gently against the tray. Some of the early trays contained a sponge-like material that "squeezed" the gel against the teeth when the patient was asked to bite lightly or to simulate a chewing motion after the trays were inserted. It is recommended that the trays be kept in place for a 4-minute treatment period for optimal fluoride uptake, although some systems recommend a 1-minute application time. As noted previously, the patient is advised not to eat, drink, or rinse for 30 minutes following the treatment.[65] Figure 12–1 ■ illustrates the tray technique of fluoride gel application.

Application of Fluoride Varnish

Teeth should be relatively dry before applying fluoride varnish. The paint brush that comes with the product is used to paint the varnish on all selected tooth surfaces. Patients should be instructed that some varnishes leave a temporary, yellow stain that may last for 24 hours. In addition, patients should not eat abrasive food or brush their teeth until the next morning for optimum effectiveness. Fluoride varnish has shown promising results in preventing early childhood caries in young children, and in treating exposed root surfaces in adults.

Application Frequency

As previously mentioned, although a single, topical application is accepted as not being able to impart maximal caries protection, considerable confusion has arisen regarding the preferred frequency for administering topical fluoride treatments. Much of this confusion is caused by the absence of controlled, clinical evaluations of this variable, particularly with the most commonly used agent APF.

The original Knutson technique for the topical application of NaF consisted of a series of four applications provided at approximately 1-week intervals, with only the first application preceded by a prophylaxis.[41] It was further suggested that this series of applications be administered at ages 3, 7, 10, and 13 years, with these ages selected, or varied, in accordance with the eruption pattern of the teeth.[71] The objective of the timing was to provide protective benefits to the permanent teeth during the period of changing dentition. Because this treatment sequence did not coincide with the common patient-recall pattern in the dental office, Galagan and Knutson explored the possible use of longer intervals of 3 or 6 months between the individual applications in each treatment series.[72] The results of their work indicated that although significant benefits were obtained with single applications provided at 3- or 6-month intervals, maximal benefits were obtained only with a series of treatments. Nevertheless, the administration of single applications of NaF at 3- to 6-month

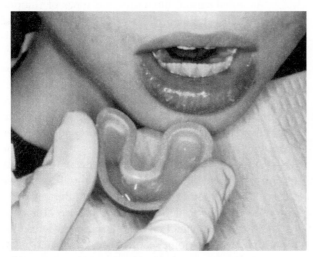
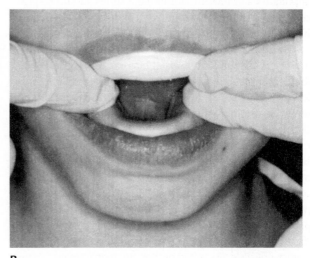

A B

■ **FIGURE 12–1** Fluoride trays. Appropriate-sized soft styrofoam trays are used to avoid pinching the soft tissues. A ribbon of gel is dispensed into the trough of the tray. Enough gel should be used to cover all tooth surfaces, but care should be used to avoid an excess that will flow into the mouth. (Experience will teach the operator how much gel to use.) The patient is shown with the loaded mandibular tray **A.** which is ready for insertion. **B.** The maxillary tray is inserted after the mandibular is in place. The patient is then asked to bite together so as to be more comfortable and, at the same time, to force the gel against the teeth. The use of thixotropic gels facilitates the wetting of all tooth surfaces. The trays should be maintained in place for 4 minutes.

intervals became a common practice, because these intervals were more convenient to the dentist's normal recall system.

When SnF$_2$ and APF were subsequently developed and evaluated, apparently little, if any, attempt was made to determine the optimal treatment frequency. Instead, the treatments were administered as single applications provided at 6- or 12-month intervals, which were convenient to the normal office schedules. Because these treatment intervals resulted in significant cariostatic benefits, the procedure that was ultimately approved and recommended involved this application frequency.

In view of this background, it seems that the frequency of topical applications should be dictated by the conditions and needs presented by each patient and not by the convenience of the dental office. This conclusion is supported by the data cited earlier, which reveal that a series of applications is required to impart maximal caries resistance to the tooth surface. Current studies support this recommendation.[73–75]

Thus, it is recommended that new patients, regardless of age, with active caries be given an initial series of four topical fluoride applications within a period of 2 to 4 weeks. If desired, the initial application may be preceded by a thorough prophylaxis and the remaining three applications of the initial treatment series should be preceded by toothbrushing to remove plaque and oral debris. It should be obvious that this series of treatments may be very conveniently combined with plaque control, dietary counseling, and initial restorative programs that the dental provider has devised for these patients. Following this initial series of treatments, the patient should be given single, topical applications at intervals of 3, 6, or 12 months, depending on the patient's caries status. Patients with little evidence of existing or anticipated caries should be given single applications every 12 months as a preventive measure.

Special effort should be made by the dental provider to schedule topical fluoride applications so as to provide treatment to newly erupted teeth within 12 months after eruption, and preferably as close to eruption as possible. As noted earlier, an approximate 2-year enamel maturation period occurs immediately following tooth eruption. The preventive benefits of fluoride are invariably much greater on newly erupted teeth than on previously erupted teeth.[76–79] This finding is apparent regardless of the fluoride system used and is presumably due to the greater reactivity, permeability, and ease of formation of fluorhydroxyapatite in enamel still undergoing calcification (or maturation).

Although it is important to expose newly erupted teeth to topical fluoride, it may be more appropriate to use a fluoride varnish for newly erupted primary teeth. Children at this young age may swallow too much of a topical fluoride gel or foam and may have pre-cooperative behavior (i.e., show lack of intellectual ability to cooperate), making it difficult to use typical topical fluoride gels or foams.

EFFICACY OF TOPICAL FLUORIDE THERAPY

Clinical studies demonstrate that topical fluoride therapy contributes significantly to the partial control of dental caries. Unfortunately, the practitioner is frequently concerned, and sometimes confused, about which procedure or agent should be used in a given situation to provide a maximal degree of dental caries protection for the patient. Such concern and confusion are understandable when it is realized that dental caries investigators themselves frequently do not agree on these matters.

The results of the numerous clinical investigations of various topical fluoride agents and treatment procedures have been the subject of several reviews.[79–93] Therefore no attempt is made to repeat these reviews here.

As noted earlier, three different types of fluoride systems (NaF, SnF$_2$, and APF) have been evaluated and approved as safe and effective for topical fluoride applications by the Food and Drug Administration (FDA).[94] To determine which of these systems may be the most effective, one would have to compare the results of independent clinical studies in which all three systems have been tested when used in the recommended manner. Unfortunately, such data are not available, and alternative procedures must be sought.

Different approaches have been taken to estimate the magnitude of the cariostatic benefits that may be expected from topical applications of the different approved fluoride systems. One approach is simply to list all of the pertinent clinical trials and then determine the arithmetic mean of the reported caries reduction. This approach has been used by several investigators, who observed the results for children residing in a non-fluoridated community.[84–86] Another approach is to use an empirically based procedure with existing clinical data to predict the efficacy of different systems[95] (Table 12–3 ■). Whatever the approach, study designs varied in a number of ways, such as the number and frequency of topical applications and the study duration. These variations serve to confound estimates of cariostatic efficacy. Nevertheless, it

■ **Table 12–3** Comparative Effectiveness of Different Topical Fluoride Systems (Average Percentage Reduction in Caries Incidence)

Fluoride System (%)	Form Used	Ripa[84] 1981	Mellberg & Ripa[85] 1983	Stookey[83] 1987	Clark et al.[95] 1985
Stannous fluoride (2.0)	Solution	29	29	27	NA
Stannous fluoride (8.0)	Solution	32	32	36	NA
Acidulated phosphate fluoride (1.2)	Solution	28	28	36	38
Acidulated phosphate fluoride (1.2)	Gel	19	19	25	26

is apparent from Table 12–3 that all three types of topical fluoride systems result in appreciable cariostatic benefits of comparable magnitude, with percentage reductions ranging from 27% to 36%. Furthermore, the data suggest that fluoride applied in gel form may be slightly less effective than solutions.

Considerably less information is available to document the efficacy of topical fluoride applications in adults. A total of 14 clinical trials were conducted in adults during the period 1944–1974, but the studies used a wide variety of experimental conditions, including the type of topical fluoride system, frequency of applications, and duration of the test period.[96–109] Although most of the methods resulted in a significant cariostatic benefit, the magnitude of this effect varied considerably, as might be expected. Furthermore, none of these studies used the application frequency suggested earlier for children.

It is generally recognized by dental scientists that the dental caries process is fundamentally the same in both children and adults, although the rate of progression in young and middle-aged adults is frequently much slower because of a variety of factors, including more efficient oral hygiene and fewer between-meal snacks. Conversely, in older adults, the rate of progression may increase because of medications that reduce salivary flow. A common assumption is that topical fluoride applications are effective for prevention of coronal caries regardless of the age of the patient. Root caries will be discussed later. Once again the frequency of application should be dictated by the needs of the patient; in the presence of frank or incipient caries activity, an initial series of applications should be given followed by maintenance applications at 3, 6, or 12 months, depending on patient needs (i.e., evidence and extent of caries activity). Similarly, the choice of the fluoride system may be at the discretion of the dentist, because there appears to be little, if any, difference in their efficacy.

On occasion it has been suggested that present topical fluoride treatment systems involve the use of excessive concentrations of fluoride. For example, some have suggested that the use of 0.4% rather than 8% SnF_2 is adequate to obtain maximal benefits from topical applications of this compound. The basis for such suggestions invariably rests with the results of in vitro studies, quite commonly enamel-solubility studies, in which maximal effects are achieved with lesser concentrations of fluoride. Unfortunately, in vitro data do not necessarily predict clinical effects, and the results of a clinical investigation clearly contradict these suggestions.[110] As shown in (Table 12–4 ■), the use of lower concentrations of SnF_2 resulted in smaller caries-preventive benefits in children. Thus, until considerably more clinical data to the contrary become available, there is no legitimate basis for using concentrations of fluoride for topical applications other than those that have been adequately evaluated clinically and approved by review groups.

The relative superiority of APF gel or solution systems is a frequent topic for research. Five clinical trials directly investigated this question, and the results are summarized in (Table 12–5 ■). Four of these studies involved single annual applications; another one involved semiannual treatments.[51,78,111–113] These data suggest that the two forms are quite comparable, particularly when applied semiannually. In practice, the gels are greatly preferred because of their ease of application and reduced chair time when trays are used.

ROOT-SURFACE CARIES

As noted elsewhere, the increased retention of the teeth during adulthood because of various caries-preventive measures, and the increase in life expectancy in many countries, has resulted in an increased prevalence of root-surface caries in adults. According to the 1985–1986 United States

■ **Table 12-4** Clinical Effectiveness of Varying Concentrations of Topically Applied Stannous Fluoride

Stannous Fluoride Concentration (%)	Number of Subjects	Caries Reduction (%)	
		DMFT	DMFS
8	135	54.7	57.2
4	140	44.1	43.5
0.4	138	29.0	27.4

DMFT, decayed, missing, or filled teeth; DMFS, decayed, missing, or filled surfaces.
Source: Mercer and Muhler, 1972.[110]

Public Health Service (USPHS) survey of adults, about one-half of U.S. adults are afflicted with root-surface caries by age 50, with an average prevalence of about three lesions by age 70.[114] Interestingly, a study conducted at the University of Iowa has indicated that adults over age 65 can expect an incidence of about 0.9 newly decayed, missing, or filled (DMF) coronal surfaces per year as well as about 0.6 new DMF root surfaces per year.[115] A more recent study reported similar results on the incidence of coronal and root caries in elderly Iowans between 1987 and 1998.[116] Thus, this form of caries has received increased attention from dental scientists, with investigations covering both its cause and measures for prevention.[117]

Quite clearly, fluoride is very effective for the prevention of root-surface caries as evidenced by a limited number of clinical trials and numerous in vitro as well as in situ studies. For example, the results of several epidemiologic studies and reports have demonstrated that the presence of fluoridated drinking water throughout the lifetime of an individual prevents the development of root-surface caries.[118–122] The magnitude of this effect is consistently greater than 50%. Furthermore, it has been observed that the use of an NaF dentifrice results in a significant decrease in root-surface caries of more than 65%.[124]

Much less information is available, however, to document the effect of topical fluoride applications on the prevention of root caries and particularly the relative efficacy of different fluoride systems. Nyvad and Fejerskov reported the arrestment of root-surface caries following the topical application of 2% NaF and the daily use of a fluoride dentifrice.[125] Wallace and coworkers reported a 70% reduction in the incidence of root-surface caries following semiannual applications of an APF gel during a 4-year study period.[126] To obtain some perspective on the potential efficacy of different topical fluoride systems, an established animal root caries model was used.[127,128] The results of this investigation are summarized in (Table 12–6 ■). From these data, it is apparent that all three approved topical fluoride systems decreased the formation of root caries by 63% to 76% in this preclinical model. In the absence of the results of similar clinical

■ **Table 12-5** Comparative Effectiveness of Topically Applied APF Gels and Solutions

Clinical Trial	Reduction in Caries Incidence	
	APF Solution (%)	APF Gel (%)
Ingraham and Williams[111]	11	41
Cons et al.[112]	0	22
Horowitz and Doyle[113]	28	24
Szwejda[78]	28	4
Cobb et al.[51]	34	35

APF, acidulated phosphate fluoride.

■ **Table 12–6**   Effect of Professional Topical Fluoride Systems on Root Caries in Hamsters

Topical Fluoride System	Root Caries Score	Percent Reduction
Control (Water)	8.2	NA
Stannous fluoride (0.4%) + acidulated phosphate fluoride (0.3%)	4.9	40.2
Acidulated phosphate fluoride (1.2%)	3.0	63.4
Sodium fluoride (2.0%)	2.3	72.0
Stannous fluoride (8.0%)	2.0	75.6

Source: Stookey, G. K. et al., 1989.[129]

data and with the recognition that the application of 8% SnF_2 imparts a brown pigmentation to exposed dentin, it seems appropriate to recommend the topical use of 2% NaF for the prevention of root caries and dentin hypersensitivity.

RECOMMENDATIONS: TOPICAL FLUORIDE TREATMENTS

On the basis of the foregoing discussion, it is apparent that, although periodic topical applications of any of the three approved agents provide protection against dental caries, maximal patient benefits may be expected only through the use of selected procedures previously mentioned.

FLUORIDE VARNISHES

Fluoride-containing varnishes are available in the United States and are being recommended to provide topical fluoride treatments, particularly for very young children. Most varnishes contain 5.0% NaF (2.26% fluoride); a typical application requires only 0.3 to 0.5 ml of the varnish, which contains 3 to 6 mg of fluoride. The application procedure involves cleaning the tooth surfaces by toothbrushing and painting the varnish on the teeth. The varnish is retained for 24 to 48 hours, during which time fluoride is released for reaction with the underlying enamel.[129–132] It is recommended that the applications be repeated at 4- to 6-month intervals.

The efficacy of fluoride varnishes for caries prevention has been repeatedly demonstrated in Europe, where they have been in common use for many years; the results of these studies have been summarized in recent reviews.[91,133,134] These studies have consistently demonstrated a significant reduction in the incidence

of dental caries and also have indicated that the magnitude of the benefit is related to the frequency of application, particularly in children at high risk for caries. Promising research has been conducted in the United States, specifically aimed at using fluoride varnishes as a preventive agent for children at high risk for early childhood caries.[135]

Little information is available to compare the effectiveness of fluoride varnishes with professionally applied topical fluoride solutions or gels. The results of a clinical study conducted on children in India, comparing the efficacy of a fluoride varnish with topical applications of an APF gel, indicated that the fluoride varnish was more effective, although both treatments resulted in a significant reduction in caries.[136] Seppa and coworkers reported the results of a clinical trial comparing semiannual applications of the NaF varnish with similar applications of an APF gel in 12- and 13-year-old children with a history of caries, and observed no significant differences between the two treatment regimens.[137] In the absence of additional clinical data, these two treatment procedures appear to be at least equivalent.

INITIATION OF THERAPY

Practitioners frequently wonder when they should recommend and initiate a topical fluoride application program. All too frequently the tendency is to defer such treatments until the child is 8 to 10 years of age, when a majority of the permanent dentition has already erupted.

As discussed earlier, it is well established that the enamel surface of a newly erupted tooth is not completely calcified; therefore, the period when the tooth is most susceptible to carious attack is the first few months after eruption. Furthermore, it has been shown that topical fluoride treatments are effective for both the deciduous and permanent dentitions. Thus, it follows that topical fluoride therapy should be initiated when the child is about 2 years of age, when most of the deciduous dentition should have erupted. The treatment regimen should be maintained at least on a semiannual basis throughout the period of increased caries susceptibility, which persists for about 2 years after eruption of the permanent second molars (i.e., until the child is about 15 years of age).

It should be added that the susceptibility of dentition to dental caries does not end at 15 years of age. It is probable, however, that the gradual decrease in caries susceptibility with increasing age will permit a less-frequent topical application program to maintain cariostasis in many patients; annual fluoride treatments may suffice.

DISADVANTAGES OF FLUORIDE TREATMENTS

Some clinical situations may alter the selection of the treatment agent. For example, the use of SnF_2 may be contraindicated for esthetic reasons in specific instances. The reaction of tin ions with enamel, particularly carious enamel, results in the formation of tin phosphates, some of which are brown in color. Thus, the use of this agent produces a temporary brownish pigmentation of carious tooth structure. This stain may exaggerate existing esthetic problems when the patient has carious lesions in the anterior teeth that will not be restored. Stannous fluoride, however, has not been found to discolor composite restorative materials.

Another problem frequently raised, particularly by **pedodontists** (pediatric dentists), concerns the strong, unpleasant, metallic taste of SnF_2. Although experienced practitioners can handle this problem, there is no question that flavored APF preparations are much better accepted by children. Until the taste problem of SnF_2 is solved, most pedodontists agree that the agent of choice for children is APF.

Acidulated phosphate fluoride systems have the disadvantage of possibly etching ceramic or porcelain surfaces. As a result, porcelain veneer facings and similar restorations should be protected with cocoa butter, vaseline, or isolated prior to applying APF. Alternatively, NaF may be used instead of APF.

Without doubt, the tendency in many dental offices is to use a specific topical fluoride system and treatment regimen for every patient. It should be emphasized, however, that the specific needs of the patient should be determined initially and a specific treatment program developed to fulfill those needs.[138] For example, the use of a series of four or more topical fluoride applications within a 4-week period followed by repeated single applications at 3- to 6-month intervals should be considered for a patient with a severe caries problem. Likewise, a reduced topical application time of 30 seconds, as opposed to 4 minutes, may be adequate to maintain a patient with little or no current caries activity. In other words, the practitioner should be familiar with the indications and contraindications for using various approaches, and should select the treatment system and conditions that best meet the needs of the patient.

FLUORIDE-CONTAINING PROPHYLACTIC PASTES

Fluoride-containing prophylactic pastes have been available and widely used in dental offices for many years to clean and polish accessible tooth surfaces and restorations. Abrasives are needed to clean and polish teeth efficiently. Because the abrasives are harder than enamel, inevitably a small amount of the enamel surface will be removed by abrasion during the prophylaxis. The actual amount of enamel removed during a prophylaxis is very small and has been shown to involve the loss of surface enamel to a depth of about 0.1 to 1.0 microns during a 10-second polishing.[139,140] Because it has been noted that the greatest concentrations of fluoride in enamel occur in the outermost surface layers, it follows that the loss of even this small amount of surface enamel during a prophylaxis results in the exposed enamel surface having a lower concentration of fluoride than was present prior to the prophylaxis.[141,142]

When fluoride-containing prophylactic pastes first became available in the 1950s, it was thought that the use of the preparations to perform a routine dental prophylaxis would result in a significant reduction in the subsequent development of dental caries. Consequently, a number of clinical trials were conducted to determine the magnitude of this benefit. The results of these investigations, considered collectively, indicated that the use of these pastes resulted in a very modest increase in the resistance of the tooth surfaces to the development of dental caries, but the magnitude of this effect was not statistically significant. As a result, fluoride-containing prophylactic pastes have never been accepted as therapeutic agents by the FDA. However, the pastes are commonly recommended for use during a prophylaxis to at least replace the fluoride lost from the enamel surface by abrasion during the procedure. In summary, the following recommendations are proposed:

- When a simple prophylaxis is administered, which will not be followed by a topical fluoride application, fluoride-containing prophylactic pastes should be used to replenish the fluoride lost during the procedure.
- When a topical fluoride application is given to a caries-susceptible patient and a prophylaxis is deemed to be necessary, it is advisable to administer the preceding prophylaxis with a fluoride-containing paste. Although no definitive proof of the additive benefits of both procedures exists as yet, an increased benefit has been shown in some studies. Even when doubt exists, it is preferable to give the patient the possible benefit of any increased protection.

MULTIPLE FLUORIDE THERAPY

From the prior discussions of various measures to apply fluoride to erupted teeth, it is apparent that no single fluoride treatment provides total protection against dental caries. Recognition of this fact led early investigators to evaluate the use of combinations of fluoride measures.

Multiple fluoride therapy is a term that has been used to describe these fluoride combination programs. As originally developed, this program included the application of fluoride in the dental office in the form of both a fluoride-containing prophylactic paste and a topically applied fluoride solution, along with self-care using an approved fluoride dentifrice. In addition, some form of systemic fluoride ingestion, preferably communal-water fluoridation, was included.

The only published reports of clinical investigations that attempted to assess the total effect of this type of multiple fluoride therapy on dental caries involved the use of SnF_2 topical systems.[143-148] In each of these studies, the topical fluoride treatments were administered semiannually; the results are summarized in (Table 12–7 ■). The results of these investigations indicate that the combination of topical fluoride applications and self-care using a fluoride dentifrice resulted in about 59% fewer carious lesions.

The fact that the magnitude of this benefit is somewhat less than that of the components evaluated individually indicates that the caries-protective effects of the individual components (i.e., prophylactic paste, topical solution, and dentifrice) are only partially additive. Nevertheless, it is important to note that the combination of SnF_2 treatments not only reduced the incidence of caries by more than 50% in both children and young adults, but it did so in both the presence and absence of communal fluoridation. If one accepts a 50% caries reduction attributable to water fluoridation and another 50% reduction of the remaining caries from the use of multiple fluoride treatments, it is apparent that the use of multiple fluoride therapy, including communal fluoridation, results in an overall reduction in caries of about 75%.

Clinical investigators have explored combinations of fluoride treatments using agents other than SnF_2 with variable success. For example, Beiswanger and coworkers reported that additive benefits were observed with topical applications of APF and self-care using an SnF_2 dentifrice.[149] Neither Downer and associates nor Mainwaring and Naylor were able to demonstrate additive

■ **Table 12-7** Results of Clinical Studies Using Multiple Fluoride Therapy Involving Stannous Fluoride–Containing Prophylactic Paste, Topical Fluoride, and Dentifrice

Clinical Investigation	Study Population	Fluoride in Water	Study Duration	Caries Reduction (%)
Gish and Muhler[145]	Children	Yes	3 years	55
Bixler and Muhler[144]	Children	No	3 years	58
Muhler et al.[146]	Adults	Yes	30 months	64
Scola and Ostrom[148]	Adults	No	2 years	58[a]
Scola[149]	Adults	No	2 years	56[a]
Obersztyn et al.[147]	Adults	No	1 year	60

[a]Average reduction for multiple similar groups.

benefits from the combined use of an MFP dentifrice and topical application of APF.[150,151]

The available data relating to multiple fluoride therapy thus suggest additive benefits from the use of either SnF_2 or APF in the dental office and self-care using dentifrices containing fluoride.[152] This finding does not necessarily mean that other combinations of fluoride treatments may not provide additive benefits, but merely that they have not yet been evaluated. In the meantime, the dental practitioner is strongly advised to use combinations of fluoride treatments to provide maximal caries protection for patients.

FLUORIDE RINSES

In 1960, reports began to appear indicating that the regular use of neutral NaF solutions decreased the incidence of caries. In an attempt to identify topical fluoride measures especially appropriate for use in dental public health programs, this approach was studied extensively during the subsequent 15 years. Whereas these studies used a wide variety of experimental conditions, a number of investigations involved either the daily use of solutions containing 200 to 225 ppm or the weekly use of solutions containing about 900 ppm fluoride. The majority of these studies were conducted in schools with supervised use of the rinse throughout the school year.

The results of these investigations have been summarized on several occasions and will not be repeated here.[94,152–156] In general, both types of fluoride rinses resulted in significant caries reduction of about 30% to 35%. On the basis of these findings, the simplicity of administration, and the lack of need for professional dental supervision, weekly fluoride-rinse programs in schools became increasingly popular. A "Guide to the Use of Fluoride" was published in the September 1986 issue of the *Journal of the American Dental Association.* The composition and recommended use of approved products are shown in (Table 12–8 ■).

Nearly all of the early investigations using fluoride rinses involved children residing in areas in which the drinking water was deficient in fluoride. As a result, the approvals given to fluoride rinses were related to their use in non-fluoridated communities. Reports indicated, however, significant benefits from fluoride rinses used in the presence of an optimal concentration of fluoride in the drinking water.[76,157,158] Results from three additional reports concerning the use of fluoride rinses in children residing in fluoridated communities indicate that cariostatic benefits provided by fluoride rinses are additive to those derived from communal fluoridation.[159–161] In view of these collective observations, there appears to be no reason to restrict the use of fluoride rinses to non-fluoridated communities.

The approval of fluoride rinses by the FDA for use in public health programs opened the door for self-care with these products as a component of multiple fluoride preventive programs. Although the approved preparations were intended to be available strictly by prescription, a 0.05% neutral NaF rinse (Fluorigard) was subsequently introduced for over-the-counter (OTC) sale. Ultimately, approval was given to OTC fluoride rinses for oral self-care, although some restrictions were required. These restrictions included the distribution of quantities containing no more than 300 mg fluoride in a single container, a label cautioning users to avoid swallowing the product, and an indication that the preparations should not be used by children younger than 6 years of age. At present there are several fluoride rinses distributed in this manner; these products contain about 225 ppm fluoride and are intended for daily use.

■ **Table 12–8** Composition and Usage of Approved Fluoride Rinses

Source of Fluoride	Fluoride Content		Recommended Usage
	Percent	*ppm*	
Sodium fluoride	0.20	900	Weekly
Sodium fluoride	0.02	100	Twice daily
Sodium fluoride	0.05	225	Daily
Acidulated phosphate fluoride	0.02	200	Daily
Stannous fluoride	0.10	243	Daily

The question of additivity of the effects of fluoride rinses to those obtained using fluoride with other vehicles has received contradictory answers. Ashley and associates found a modest additivity of benefits from the supervised daily rinsing in school with an APF rinse coupled with supervised brushing in school plus normal self-care using an MFP dentifrice.[162] A similar observation was reported by Triol and coworkers.[163] On the other hand, Blinkhorn and coworkers failed to observe any indication of additive caries protection between the similar supervised daily use of a neutral 0.05% NaF and self-care using the same dentifrice.[164] Likewise, Ringelberg and associates failed to find additivity between a daily NaF rinse and self-care using an SnF_2 dentifrice.[165] Similarly, Horowitz and coworkers, in a study involving the supervised weekly use of an NaF rinse and daily fluoride tablets plus self-care with approved fluoride dentifrices, observed a caries reduction comparable in magnitude to that reported earlier by these investigators with fluoride tablets or rinses used individually.[166]

Additive effects can also be inferred from the numerous school fluoride-rinse studies in which caries reductions from 30% to 35% were observed. Because the majority of these children in both the control and experimental groups used fluoride-containing dentifrices, it follows that the benefits observed in those studies were above those provided by the fluoride dentifrices. The same conclusion can be reached from the data reported by Birkeland and coworkers in Norway, a country where over 90% of the children use fluoride dentifrices.[153] After 10 years of a mouthrinsing program, these authors found a caries reduction of over 50% and reduction in the need for restoration of more than 70%.

It can thus be concluded that fluoride rinses have a place as a component of a preventive program along with, but not as substitutes for, other modalities of fluoride use. Fluoride rinses are used mainly for patients with a high risk of contracting caries. Although existing evidence may lead some to doubt whether additional benefits for the patients accrue from the use of rinses, it is preferable in these instances to give the patients the benefit of the doubt. Examples of patients for whom fluoride rinses should be recommended include:

- Patients who, because of the use of medication, surgery, radiotherapy, and so on, have reduced salivation and increased caries formation.
- Patients who have orthodontic appliances or removable prostheses, which act as traps for plaque accumulation.

- Patients who are unable to achieve acceptable oral hygiene.
- Patients who have extensive dental restorations and multiple restorative margins, which represent sites of high caries risk.
- Patients who need fluoride in their self-care regimen but cannot tolerate a custom-fitted tray.
- Patients who have gingival recession and susceptibility to root caries.
- Patients who have rampant caries, at least as long as the high caries activity persists.

As a general rule, daily rinses should be recommended rather than a weekly regimen; not only does the daily procedure appear to be slightly more effective, but, as a practical consideration, it is easier for patients to remember and comply with a daily procedure. In all these instances, it is important to remember that the rinses should not be used in place of any of the other modalities of fluoride use, but as part of a comprehensive, preventive program that should also comprise plaque control, regular professional dental hygiene appointments, frequent fluoride topical applications, self-care using a fluoride dentifrice, diet control, and testing to determine if and when the oral environment is no longer conducive to caries. For children living in non-fluoridated areas, the prescription fluoride supplements or rinses for self-care may also be considered.

FLUORIDE GELS FOR ORAL SELF-CARE

A number of fluoride gels have become available as additional measures that may be used to help achieve caries control. These products contain 0.4% SnF_2 (1,000 ppm fluoride) or 1.0% NaF (5,000 ppm) and are formulated in a nonaqueous gel base that does not contain an abrasive system. Their recommended method of use involves toothbrushing with a gel (similar to using a dentifrice), allowing the gel to remain in the oral cavity for 1 minute, and then expectorating thoroughly.

Even though no controlled clinical trials have been conducted on the products used in this manner, a number of them have been approved by the ADA's Council on Dental Therapeutics as an additional caries-preventive measure for use in patients with rampant caries. The basis for the approval of these products has been the numerous prior clinical caries studies using dentifrices that contain the same amount of SnF_2, coupled with analytic data demonstrating the stability of these preparations.

From a practical point of view, the recommended use of fluoride gels is generally similar to that cited earlier for fluoride rinses. In other words, they may be considered as an alternative to the use of fluoride rinses, and an adjunct to the use of professional, topical fluoride applications and fluoride dentifrices as a collective means of achieving caries control in patients who are especially prone to caries formation. Like fluoride rinses, the use of these gels is generally restricted to the period required to achieve caries control. Compared with fluoride rinses, however, fluoride gels appear to have an advantage in terms of patient compliance. Because these preparations are only distributed to patients by their dentists, it is commonly thought that patients are more likely to use them in compliance with the recommendations of their dentist.

It should be stressed that fluoride gels should not be used in place of fluoride dentifrices. Because the gels contain no abrasive system to control the deposition of pellicle, their use in place of a dentifrice results in the accumulation of stained pellicle in the majority of patients within a few weeks. Nevertheless, the proper use of these preparations in combination with professional topical fluoride applications and self-care with fluoride dentifrices may be expected to help achieve caries control in caries-active patients.

FLUORIDE-RELEASING DENTAL MATERIALS

Fluoride-releasing dental restorative materials may provide an additional benefit in preventive dentistry. Although not currently available in the United States, a fluoride-releasing amalgam has demonstrated recurrent caries inhibition at enamel and dentin restoration margins.[167] Likewise, both chemical-cured and light-cured glass ionomer cements have demonstrated caries inhibition at these restoration margins.[168–171] Fluoride-releasing resin composites and sealants have also consistently demonstrated recurrent caries inhibition at enamel margins, yet there are conflicting results whether caries inhibition occurs at dentin margins.[168,169,171–173] Preliminary studies indicate that glass ionomer cement and fluoride-releasing resin composite have synergistic effects with fluoride rinses and fluoridated dentifrices, in the remineralization of incipient enamel caries.[174–177] The materials may act as a fluoride delivery system. Upon exposure to additional external fluoride, the material surface undergoes an increase in fluoride. This fluoride is subsequently released, and has demonstrated inhibition of demineralization and even the occurrence of remineralization at the adjacent tooth structure. Further clinical research to evaluate these fluoride-releasing restorative materials may provide more information for clinical recommendations.

TOXICOLOGY OF FLUORIDE

The handling of fluorides is carefully regulated in industry by occupational safety health legislation and in the marketplace by the FDA. Commercial dental fluoride products and professional practices can be toxic and even lethal when used inappropriately. The lethal dose for an adult is somewhere between 2.5 and 10 g, with the average lethal dose being 4 to 5 g. The use of the term *average lethal dose* is a very imprecise designation that makes it difficult to predict the outcome of an accidental swallowing of an excess of fluoride. To correct this problem, investigators have recommended a probable toxic dose (PTD) standard based on body weight as a more practical approach to making treatment decisions. With it, the urgency for first aid and more definitive emergency treatment can be determined rapidly. The PTD approach, first reported by Bayless and Tinanoff,[178] bases the level and urgency of treatment on the number of multiples of 5 mg/kg of fluoride ingested (Table 12–9 ■).

If the amount ingested is less than 5 mg/kg, the office use of available calcium, aluminum, or magnesium products as first-aid antidotes should suffice. If the amount is over 5 mg/kg, first-aid measures should be expeditiously applied, followed by hospital observation for possible further care. Finally, if the amount of fluoride ingested approaches or exceeds 15 mg/kg, the immediate first-aid treatment should be followed by a most urgent action to move the patient swiftly into a hospital emergency room where cardiac monitoring, electrolyte evaluation, and shock support are available. Ingestion of 15 mg/kg fluoride can be lethal.

Fluoride Toxicity

Excessive intake of fluoride results in four general reactions: (1) When a concentrated fluoride salt contacts moist skin or mucous membrane, hydrofluoric acid forms, causing a chemical burn; (2) fluoride, a general protoplasmic poison, acts to inhibit enzyme systems; (3) it binds calcium needed for nerve action; and (4) hyperkalemia (exessive amount of phosphate in the blood stream) occurs, contributing to cardiotoxicity (damage to the heart muscle).

■ **Table 12–9** Emergency Treatment for Fluoride Overdose

Milligrams Fluoride Ion per Kilogram Body Weight[a]	*Treatment*
Less than 5 mg/kg	1. Give calcium (milk) orally to relieve gastrointestinal symptoms. Observe for a few hours. 2. Induced vomiting not necessary.
More than 5 mg/kg	1. Empty stomach by inducing vomiting with emetic. For patients with depressed gag reflex caused by age (<6 months old), Down syndrome, or severe mental retardation, induced vomiting is contraindicated, and endotracheal intubation[b] should be performed before gastric lavage. 2. Give orally soluble calcium in any form (e.g., milk, 5% calcium gluconate, or calcium lactate solution). 3. Admit to hospital, and observe for a few hours.
More than 15 mg/kg	1. Admit to hospital immediately. 2. Induce vomiting. 3. Begin cardiac monitoring and be prepared for cardiac arrhythmias. Observe for peaking T waves and prolonged QT intervals. 4. Slowly administer intravenously 10 ml of 10% calcium gluconate solution. Additional doses may be given if clinical signs of tetany or QT interval prolongation develops. Electrolytes, especially calcium and potassium, should be monitored and corrected as necessary. 5. Adequate urine output should be maintained using diuretics if necessary. 6. Use general supportive measures for shock.

[a] Average weight per age: 1–2 years = 10 kg; 2–4 years = 15 kg; 4–6 years = 20 kg; 6–8 years = 23 kg.
[b] Insertion of an endotracheal tube through the mouth into the trachea to aspirate fluoride secretions.
Source: Bayless & Tinanoff, 1985.[179]

When dry fluoride powder contacts the mucous membrane or the moist skin, a reddened lesion occurs, and later the area becomes swollen and pale; still later, ulceration and necrosis may occur. In past years, skin burns of this type were common for many water engineers who emptied drums of fluoride agents into the hoppers feeding water supplies. Federal and state occupational safety acts have greatly reduced this danger.

Following excessive ingestion of fluoride, nausea and vomiting can occur. The vomiting is usually caused by the formation of hydrofluoric acid in the acid environment of the stomach, causing damage to the lining cells of the stomach wall. Local or general signs of muscle tetany (intermittent, prolonged spasms) ensue from a drop in blood calcium (hypocalcemia). This effect can be accompanied by abdominal cramping and pain. Finally, as the hypocalcemia and hyperkalemia intensify, the severity of the condition becomes ominous with the onset of the three C's that can indicate death—coma, convulsions, and cardiac arrhythmias (irregular heartbeat). Generally, death from ingestion of excessive fluoride occurs within 4 hours; if the individual survives for 4 hours, the prognosis is guarded to good.

Emergency Treatment

Four actions are especially significant in treating fluoride poisoning: (1) immediate treatment, (2) induced vomiting, (3) protection of the stomach by binding fluoride with orally administered calcium or aluminum preparations, and (4) maintenance of blood calcium levels with intravenous calcium. Urgent and decisive treatment is mandatory once the PTD of 15 mg/kg has been approached or exceeded. The speed of initiating proper treatment can be critical to a person's chance for survival.[79] The blood level of fluoride reaches its maximum from 0.5 to 1 hour after the fluoride is ingested. By that time it can be too late.

If an excessive amount of NaF is ingested, first-aid treatment can be initiated. Milk, or better yet, milk and eggs should be given, for two reasons: (1) as demulcents, they help protect the mucous membrane of the upper gastrointestinal tract from chemical burns; and (2) they provide the calcium that acts as a binder for the fluoride. Lime water (calcium hydroxide) or Maalox (an aluminum preparation) can be ingested to accomplish the same purpose. Plenty of fluid, preferably milk, should be ingested to help dilute the fluoride compound in the stomach. Vomiting is beneficial and often occurs spontaneously. When vomiting does occur, the majority of the ingested fluoride is often expelled. Preferably, the patient should be taken directly to the emergency room of a hospital. Otherwise, the closest emergency medical service unit or physician capable of dealing with fluoride toxicity is an alternative. Once in a well-equipped medical facility, several options are possible, such as gastric lavage (use of a fluid to wash fluoride out of the stomach), blood dialysis (diffusion of blood across a semipermeable membrane to remove the fluoride), or oral intravenous delivery of calcium gluconate to maintain blood calcium levels. Every effort should be made to rid the body rapidly of the fluoride or to negate its toxicity before refractory (resistant to treatment) hyperkalemia and cardiac fibrillation (rapid, irregular contraction of muscle fibers in the heart) become a greater problem than the fluoride intoxication.[180]

Chronic Fluoride Exposure

At high levels of industrial fluoride exposure, as experienced by cryolite and bauxite workers prior to the era of occupational safety regulations, the combined intake of fluoride through inhalation, ingestion, and water consumption often resulted in a daily dose of over 20 mg. This exceedingly high level of continual intake for 10 to 20 years resulted in a severe skeletal fluorosis characterized by osteosclerosis (abnormal increase in thickness and density of bone), calcification of the tendons, and the appearance of multiple exostoses (bony growths that arise from the bone's surface). This same crippling bone fluorosis can also occur from long-term consumption of naturally fluoridated waters found in some parts of the

world, which contain 14 ppm or more of fluoride. Other factors that increase the severity of bone fluorosis are high temperatures with a concomitant increase in drinking episodes, an elevated intake of fluoride in food, nutritional diseases, and low-calcium diets. No cases of skeletal fluorosis had been reported in the United States where water-fluoridation concentrations at that time were under 3.9 ppm.[181]

Despite all precautions, there is a potential for signs and symptoms of fluoride toxicity in dental office and patient use of topical fluoride. The most probable cause is in children in the 15- to 30-month age bracket having an excess of dentifrice placed on the toothbrush and then swallowing the fluoride-laden saliva. In most cases, this results in a very mild, often unnoticeable change in the enamel of erupting teeth around 6 years of age. A more serious toxicity can arise in the dental office from the mishandling and ingestion of fluoride salts used for professional purposes. To be prepared for such an unlikely emergency, the professional staff should be trained to institute emergency procedures if necessary.

Home Security of Fluoride Products

The lack of secure home storage of OTC and prescription fluoride products poses hazards to consumers. As presently packaged, the fluoride content of OTC fluoride products can exceed the PTD for children.[182] That the danger at home is real is attested by two deaths of children after swallowing fluoride tablets: one in Austria, and the other in Australia.[183] In 1 year (1986–1987), 13 cases of fluoride poisoning were reported to the North Carolina Poison Center. It was noted by the poison center that no health care providers who contacted the center were familiar with the treatment of the gastrointestinal symptoms induced by fluoride poisoning.[184] Clearly, parents need to be educated about the hazards of fluoride-containing dental products. Dentifrices, mouthrinses, and fluoride supplements need to be securely stored. Also, health professionals need to be educated about the emergency treatment protocol for excessive intake of fluoride.

The American Association of Poison Control Centers reported the occurrence in 2004 of 24,180 exposures involving toothpaste with fluoride. Of these, only 440 cases were actually treated in the emergency department.[186] Children younger than 6 years of age accounted for 21,890 of these exposures. No deaths from fluoride exposure were reported in 2004; however, there was one death from ingestion of fluoride toothpaste in 2002.[185]

SUMMARY

A number of different aspects of topical fluoride therapy have been reviewed in the foregoing material. Without doubt, the use of topical fluoride therapy contributes significantly to the control of dental caries; however, one cannot expect to control dental caries completely through the use of fluorides alone. Furthermore, because no single fluoride treatment procedure provides the maximal degree of caries protection possible with fluoride, the use of multiple fluoride therapy is advocated. In particular, the dentist should identify the needs of each patient and institute a multiple fluoride treatment program designed specifically to fulfill those needs.

REFERENCES

1. Keene, H. J., Mellberg, J. R., & Nicholson, C. R. (1973). History of fluoride, dental fluorosis, and concentrations of fluoride in surface layer of enamel of caries-free naval recruits. *J Public Health Dent,* 33:142–48.

2. DePaola, P. F., Brudevold, F., Aasenden, R., Moreno, E. C., Englander, H., Bakhos, Y., Bookstein, F., and Warram, B. (1975). A pilot study of the relationship between caries experience and surface enamel fluoride in man. *Arch Oral Biol,* 20:859–64.

3. Eakle, W. S., Featherstone, J. D., Weintraub, J. A. Shain, S. G., & Gansky, S. A. (2004). Salivary fluoride levels following application of fluoride varnish or fluoride rinse. *Community Dent Oral Epidemiol,* 32:462–69.

4. Weatherall, J. A., Hallsworth, A. S., & Robinson, C. (1973). The effect of tooth wear on the distribution of fluoride in the enamel surface of human teeth. *Arch Oral Biol,* 18:1175–89.

5. Aasenden, R., Moreno, E. C., & Brudevold, F. (1973). Fluoride levels in the surface enamel of different types of human teeth. *Arch Oral Biol,* 18:1403–10.

6. Brudevold, F. (1975). Fluoride therapy. In Bernier, J. L., & Muhler, J. C., Eds. *Improving dental practice through preventive measures* (3rd ed.). St. Louis: C. V. Mosby.

7. Isaac, S., Brudevold, F., Smith, F. A., & Gardner, D. E. (1958). Solubility rate and natural fluoride content of surface and subsurface enamel. *J Dent Res,* 37:254–63.

8. Thylstrup, A. (1979). A scanning electron microscopical study of normal and fluorotic enamel demineralized by EDTA. *Acta Odont Scand,* 37:127–35.

9. Recommendations for using fluoride to prevent and control dental caries in the United States. (2000). Centers for Disease Control and Prevention. *MMWR Recomm Rep,* 50(RR-14):1–42.

10. Diefenderfer, K. E. (2003). Maximizing fluoride's potential. *Dimens Dent Hygiene,* Nov/Dec:26–28.

11. Brudevold, F., & McCann, H. G. (1968). Enamel solubility tests and their significance in regard to dental caries. *Ann N Y Acad Sci,* 153:20.

12. Bibby, B. G. (1944). Use of fluorine in the prevention of dental caries. I. Rationale and approach. *J Am Dent Assoc,* 31:228–36.

13. Phillips, R. W., & Muhler, J. C. (1947). Solubility of enamel as affected by fluorides of varying pH. *J Dent Res,* 26:109–17.

14. Fischer, R. B., & Muhler, J. C. (1952). The effect of sodium fluoride upon the surface structure of powdered dental enamel. *J Dent Res,* 31:751–55.

15. Frazier, P. D., & Engen, D. W. (1966). X-ray diffraction study of the reaction of acidulated fluoride with powdered enamel. *J Dent Res,* 45:1144–48.

16. Gerould, C. H. (1945). Electron microscope study of the mechanisms of fluoride deposition in teeth. *J Dent Res,* 24:223–33.

17. Joost-Larsen, M., & Fejerskov, O. (1978). Structural studies on calcium fluoride formation and uptake of fluoride in surface enamel in vitro. *Scand J Dent Res,* 86:337–45.

18. McCann, H. G., & Bullock, F. A. (1955). Reactions of fluoride ion with powdered enamel and dentin. *J Dent Res,* 34:59–67.

19. Scott, D. B., Picard, R. G., & Wyckoff, W. G. (1950). Studies of the action of sodium fluoride on human enamel by electron microscopy and electron diffraction. *Public Health Rep,* 65:43–56.

20. Muhler, J. C., & Van Huysen, G. (1947). Solubility of enamel protected by sodium fluoride and other compounds. *J Dent Res,* 26:119–27.

21. Muhler, J. C., Boyd, T. M., & Van Huysen, G. (1950). Effects of fluorides and other compounds on the solubility of enamel, dentin, and tricalcium phosphate in dilute acids. *J Dent Res,* 29:182–93.

22. Jordan, T. H., Wei, S. H. Y., Bromberger, S. H., & King, J. C. (1971). $Sn_3F_3PO_4$: The products of the reaction between stannous fluoride and hydroxyapatite. *Arch Oral Biol,* 16:241–46.

23. Wei, S. H. Y., & Forbes, W. C. (1974). Electron microprobe investigations of stannous fluoride reactions with enamel surfaces. *J Dent Res,* 53:51–56.

24. Brudevold, F., Savory, A., Gardner, D. E., Spinelli, M., & Speirs, R. (1963). A study of acidulated fluoride solutions. *Arch Oral Biol,* 8:167–77.

25. Wellock, W. D., & Brudevold, F. (1963). A study of acidulated fluoride solutions. II. The caries inhibition effect of single annual topical applications of an acidic fluoride and phosphate solution, a two year experience. *Arch Oral Biol,* 8:179–82.

26. DeShazer, D. O., & Swartz, C. J. (1967). The formation of calcium fluoride on the surface of fluorhydroxyapatite after treatment with acidic fluoride-phosphate solution. *Arch Oral Biol,* 12:1071–75.

27. Wei, S. H. Y., & Forbes, W. C. (1968). X-ray diffraction and analysis of the reactions between intact and powdered enamel and several fluoride solutions. *J Dent Res,* 47:471–77.

28. Mellberg, J. R., Laakso, P. V., & Nicholson, C. R. (1966). The acquisition and loss of fluoride by topically fluoridated human tooth enamel. *Arch Oral Biol,* 11:1213–20.

29. Bruun, C. (1973). Uptake and retention of fluoride by intact enamel in vivo after application of neutral sodium fluoride. *Scand J Dent Res,* 81:92–100.

30. Lovelock, D. J. (1973). The loss of topically applied fluoride from the surface of human enamel in vitro using 18F. *Arch Oral Biol,* 18:27–29.

31. Mellberg, J. R. (1973). Topical fluoride controversy symposium. Enamel fluoride uptake from topical fluoride agents and its relationship to caries inhibition. *J Am Soc Prev Dent,* 3:53–54.

32. Rinderer, L., Schait, A., & Muhlemann, H. R. (1965). Loss of fluoride from dental enamel after topical fluoridation. Preliminary report. *Helv Odont Acta,* 9:148–50.

33. Ahrens, G. (1976). Effect of fluoride tablets on uptake and loss of fluoride in superficial enamel in vivo. *Caries Res,* 10:85–95.

34. Wei, S. H. Y., & Schulz, E. M., Jr. (1975). In vivo microsampling of enamel fluoride concentrations after topical treatments. *Caries Res,* 9:50–58.

35. Kanauya, Y., Spooner, P., Fox, J. L., Higuchi, W. I., & Muhammad, N. A. (1983). Mechanistic studies on the bioavailability of calcium fluoride for re-mineralization of dental enamel. *Int J Pharmacol,* 16:171–79.

36. Chandler, S., Chiao, C. C., & Fuerstenau, D. W. (1982). Transformation of calcium fluoride for caries prevention. *J Dent Res,* 61:403–407.

37. Featherstone, J. D. B. (1999). Prevention and reversal of dental caries: Role of low level fluoride. *Community Dent Oral Epidemiol,* 27:31–40.

38. Rolla, G. (1988). On the role of calcium fluoride in the cariostatic mechanism of fluoride. *Acta Odontol Scand,* 46:341–45.

39. ten Cate, J. M. (1997). Review on fluoride, with special emphasis on calcium fluoride mechanisms in caries prevention. *Eur J Oral Sci,* 105:461–65.

40. Beiswanger, B. B., Mercer, V. H., Billings, R. J., & Stookey, G. K. (1980). A clinical caries evaluation of a stannous fluoride prophylactic paste and topical solution. *J Dent Res,* 59:1386–91.

41. Knutson, J. W. (1948). Sodium fluoride solution: Technique for applications to the teeth. *J Am Dent Assoc,* 36:37–39.

42. Mellberg, J. R. (1977). Enamel fluoride and its anticaries effects. *J Prev Dent,* 4:8–20.

43. Mellberg, J. R., Nicholson, C. R., Miller, B. G., & Englander, H. R. (1970). Acquisition of fluoride in vivo by enamel from repeated topical sodium fluoride applications in a fluoridated area: Final report. *J Dent Res,* 49:1473–77.

44. Puttnam, N. A., & Bradshaw, F. (1964). X-ray fluorescence studies on the effect of stannous fluoride on human teeth. *Adv Fluorine Res Dent Caries Prev (ORCA),* 3:145–50.

45. Hoermann, K. C., Klima, J. E., Birks, L. S., Nagel, D. J., Ludwick, W. E., Lyon H. W. (1966). Tin and fluoride uptake in human enamel in situ: Electron probe and chemical microanalysis. *J Am Dent Assoc,* 73:1301–305.

46. Ferreira, M. S., Latorre, Mdo. R., Rodrigues, C. S. & Lima, K. C. (2005). Effect of regular fluoride gel application on incipient carious lesions. *Oral Health Prev Dent,* 3:141–49.

47. McDonald, J. L., Schemehorn, B. R., & Stookey, G. K. (1978). Influence of fluoride upon plaque and gingivitis in the beagle dog. *J Dent Res,* 57:899–902.

48. Beiswanger, B. B., McClanahan, S. F., Bartizek, R. D., Lanzalaco, A. C., Bacca, L. A., & White, D. J. (1997). The comparative efficacy of stabilized stannous fluoride dentifrice, peroxide/baking soda dentifrice and essential oil mouthrinse for the prevention of gingivitis. *J Clin Dent,* 8:46–53.

49. Garcia-Godoy, F., Hicks, J., & Flaitz, C. (2002). APF foam application: Caries initiation and progression in vitro. *J Dent Res,* 81(Spec Iss):Abstract 3541.

50. Pimlott, J. F. L. (1999). Professionally applied topical fluorides: Providing optimal patient care using an evidence-based approach. *Probe Sci J,* 33:175–79.

51. Cobb, H. B., Rozier, R. G., & Bawden, J. W. (1980). A clinical study of the caries preventive effects of an APF solution and an APF thixotropic gel. *Pediatr Dent,* 2:263–66.

52. Knutson, J. W., Armstrong, W. D., & Feldman, F. M. (1947). Effect of topically applied sodium fluoride on dental caries experience. IV. Report of findings with two, four, and six applications. *Public Health Rep,* 62:425–30.

53. Houpt, M., Koenigsberg, S., & Shey, Z. (1983). The effect of prior toothcleaning on the efficacy of topical fluoride treatment. Two-year results. *Clin Prev Dent,* 5(4):8–10.

54. Katz, R. V., Meskin, L. H., Jensen, M. E., & Keller, D. (1984). Topical fluoride and prophylaxis: A 30-month clinical trial. *J Dent Res,* 63: Abstract 771.

55. Ripa, L. W., Leske, G. S., Sposato, A., & Varma, A. (1983). Effect of prior toothcleaning on biannual professional APF topical fluoride gel-tray treatments. Results after two years. *Clin Prev Dent,* 5(4):3–7.

56. Bijella, M. F., Bijella, V. T., Lopes, E. S., & Bostos, J. R. (1985). Comparison of dental prophylaxis and toothbrushing prior to topical APF applications. *Community Dent Oral Epidemiol,* 13:208–11.

57. Ekstrand, J., & Koch, G. (1980). Systemic fluoride absorption following fluoride gel application. *J Dent Res,* 59:1067.

58. Ekstrand, J., Koch, G., Lindgren, L. E., & Petersson, L. G. (1981). Pharmacokinetics of fluoride gels in children and adults. *Caries Res,* 15:213–20.

59. LeCompte, E. J., & Whitford, G. M. (1982). Pharmacokinetics of fluoride from APF gel and fluoride tablets in children. *J Dent Res,* 61:469–72.

60. LeCompte, E. J., & Doyle, T. E. (1982). Oral fluoride retention following various topical application techniques in children. *J Dent Res,* 61:1397–1400.

61. LeCompte, E. J., & Rubenstein, L. K. (1984). Oral fluoride rentention with thixotropic and APF gels and foam-lined and unlined trays. *J Dent Res,* 63:69–70.

62. McCall, D. R., Watkins, T. R., Stephan, K. W., Collins, W. J., & Smalls, M. J. (1983). Fluoride ingestion following APF gel application. *Br Dent J,* 155:333–36.

63. Pourbaix, S., & Desager, J. P. (1983). Fluoride absorption: A comparative study of 1% and 2% fluoride gels. *J Biol Buccale,* 11:103–108.

64. LeCompte, E. J., & Doyle, T. E. (1985). Effects of suctioning devices on oral fluoride retention. *J Am Dent Assoc,* 110:357–60.

65. Stookey, G. K., Schemehorn, B. R., Drook, C. A., & Cheetham, B. L. (1986). The effect of rinsing with water immediately after a professional fluoride gel application on fluoride uptake in demineralized enamel: An in vivo study. *Pediatr Dent,* 8(3):153–57.

66. Marinho, V. C., Higgins, J. P., Logan, S., & Sheiham, A. (2002). Fluoride gels for preventing dental caries in children and adolescents. *Cochrane Database Syst Rev,* Issue 2. Art. No.: CD002280.

67. Jiang, H., Bian, Z., Tai, B. J., Du, M. A., & Peng, B. (2005). The effect of a bi-annual professional application of APF foam on dental caries increment in primary teeth: 24 month clinical trial. *J Dent Res,* 84:265–68.

68. Jiang, H., Tai, B., Du, M., & Peng, B. (2005). Effect of professional application of APF foam on caries reduction in permanent first molars in 6–7 year old children: 24 month clinical trial. *J Dent,* 33:469–73.

69. American Dental Association Council on Scientific Affairs. (2006). Professionally applied topical fluoride, evidence-based clinical recommendations. *J Am Dent Assoc,* 137:1151–59.

70. Lavigne, S. (2000). Not all trays are created equal: An analysis of fluoride tray fit. *Probe Scientific J,* 6:217–24.

71. Averill, H. M., Averill, J. E., & Ritz, A. G. (1967). A two-year comparison of three topical fluoride agents. *J Am Dent Assoc,* 74:996–1001.

72. Galagan, D. F., & Knutson, J. W. (1948). Effect of topically applied sodium fluoride on dental caries experience. VI. Experiments with sodium fluoride and calcium chloride. Widely spaced applications. Use of different solution concentrations. *Public Health Rep,* 63:1215–21.

73. Scheifele, E., Studen-Pavlovich, D., & Markovic, N. (2002). Practitioner's guide to fluoride. *Dent Clin North Am,* 46:831–46.

74. Featherstone, J. D. B. (2001). Elements of a successful adult caries preventive program. *Compend Cont Educ Oral Hygiene,* 8:3–9.

75. Berger, E. K. (2006). Review of professional and take-home fluorides. *Contemp Oral Hyg,* 6:8–9.

76. Horowitz, H. S., & Heifetz, S. B. (1969). Evaluation of topical fluoride applications of stannous fluoride to teeth of children born and reared in a fluoridated community: Final report. *J Dent Child,* 36:355–61.

77. Muhler, J. C. (1960). The anticariogenic effectiveness of a single application of stannous fluoride in children residing in an optimal communal fluoride area. II. Results at the end of 30 months. *J Am Dent Assoc,* 61:431–38.

78. Szwejda, L. F. (1972). Fluorides in community programs: A study of four years of various fluorides applied topically to the teeth of children in fluoridated communities. *J Public Health Dent,* 32:25–33.

79. Brudevold, F., & Nanjoks, R. (1978). Caries preventive fluoride treatment of the individual. *Caries Res,* 12 (Suppl 1):52–64.

80. Forrester, D. J. (1971). A review of currently available topical fluoride agents. *J Dent Child,* 38:52–58.

81. Horowitz, H. S., & Heifetz, S. B. (1970). The current status of topical fluorides in preventive dentistry. *J Am Dent Assoc,* 81:166–77.

82. Forrester, D. J., & Shulz, E. M., Eds. (1974). *International workshop of fluorides and dental caries reductions.* Baltimore: University of Maryland.

83. Stookey, G. K. (1970). Fluoride therapy. In Bernier, J. L., & Muhler, J. C., Eds. *Improving dental practice through preventive measures* (2nd ed.). St. Louis: Mosby, 92–156.

84. Ripa, L. W. (1981). Professionally (operator) applied topical fluoride therapy: A critique. *Int Dent J,* 31:105–20.

85. Mellberg, J. R., & Ripa, L. W. (1983). Professionally applied topical fluoride. In *Fluoride in preventive dentistry. Theory and clinical applications.* Chicago: Quintessence, 181–214.

86. Katz, S., McDonald, J. L., & Stookey, G. K. (1979). *Preventive dentistry in action* (3rd ed.). Upper Montclair, NJ: DCP Publishing Company.

87. Ripa, L. W. (1989). Review of the anticaries effectiveness of professionally applied and self-applied topical fluoride gels. *J Public Health Dent,* 49:297–309.

88. Ripa, L. W. (1990). An evaluation of the use of professional (operator-applied) topical fluorides. *J Dent Res,* 69:786–96.

89. Wei, S. H. Y., & Yiu, C. K. Y. (1993). Evaluation of the use of topical fluoride gel. *Caries Res,* 27 (Suppl 1):29–34.

90. Johnston, D. W. (1994). Current status of professionally applied topical fluorides. *Community Dent Oral Epidemiol,* 22:159–63.

91. Horowitz, H. S., & Ismail, A. I. (1966). Topical fluorides in caries prevention. In Fejerskov, O., Ekstrand, J., & Burt, B. A., Eds. *Fluoride in dentistry* (2nd ed.). Copenhagen: Munksgaard, 311–27.

92. Featherstone, J. D. (2006). Delivery challenges for fluoride, chlorhexidine and xylitol. *BMC Oral Health,* 6 (Suppl 1):S8.

93. Adair, S. M. (2006). Evidence-based use of fluoride in contemporary pediatric dental practice. *Pediatr Dent,* 28:133–42.

94. Fine, S. D. (1974). Topical fluoride preparations for reducing incidence of dental caries. Notice of status. *Fed Reg,* 39:17245.

95. Clark, D. C., Hanley, J. A., Stamm, J. W., Weinstein, D. L. (1985). An empirically based system to estimate the effectiveness of caries-preventive agents. A comparison of the effectiveness estimates of APF gels and solutions, and fluoride varnishes. *Caries Res,* 19:83–95.

96. Arnold, F. A., Jr., Dean, H. T., & Singleton, D. C., Jr. (1944). The effect on caries incidence of a single topical application of a fluoride solution to the teeth of young adult males of a military population. *J Dent Res,* 23:155–62.

97. Frank, R. (1950). Research and clinical evaluation of local applications of sodium fluoride. *Schweiz Mschr Zahnh,* 60:283–87.

98. Driak, F. (1951). Kariesprophlaxe mit besonderer Berücksichtigung der Impragnierungsmethoden. *Oester Ztschr Stomat,* 48:153–68.

99. Klinkenberg, E., & Bibby, B. G. (1950). Effect of topical applications of fluorides on dental caries in young adults. *J Dent Res,* 29:4–8.

100. Rickles, N. H., & Becks, H. (1951). The effects of an acid and a neutral solution of sodium fluoride on the incidence of dental caries in young adults. *J Dent Res,* 30:757–65.

101. Kutler, B., & Ireland, R. L. (1953). The effect of sodium fluoride application on dental caries experience in adults. *J Dent Res,* 32:458–62.

102. Carter, W. J., Jay, P., Shklair, I. L., & Daniel, L. H. The effect of topical fluoride on dental caries experience in adult females of a military population. *J Dent Res,* 34:73–76.

103. Muhler, J. C. (1957). Effect on gingiva and occurrence of pigmentation on teeth following the topical application of stannous fluoride or stannous chlorofluoride. *J Periodont,* 28:281–86.

104. Muhler, J. C. (1958). The effect of a single topical application of stannous fluoride on the incidence of dental caries in adults. *J Dent Res,* 37:415–16.

105. Protheroe, D. H. (1961). A study to determine the effect of topical application of stannous fluoride on dental caries in young adults. *Roy Can Dent Corps Q,* 3:18–23.

106. Harris, N. O., Hester, W. R., Muhler, J. C., & Allen, J. F. (1964). *Stannous fluoride topically applied in aqueous solution in caries prevention in a military population* (SAM-TDR-64-26). Brooks Air Force Base, TX: United States Air Force School of Aerospace Medicine.

107. Obersztyn, A., Kolwinski, K., Trykowski, J., & Starosciak, S. (1979). Effects of stannous fluoride and amine fluorides on caries incidence and enamel solubility in adults. *Aust Dent J,* 24:395–97.

108. Viegas, Y. (1970). The caries inhibiting effect of a single topical application of an acidic phosphate solution in young adults. A one year experience. *Rev Saude Publica,* 4:55–60.

109. Curson, I. (1973). The effect on caries increments in dental students of topically applied acidulated phosphate fluoride (APF). *J Dent,* 1:216–18.

110. Mercer, V. H., & Muhler, J. C. (1972). Comparison of single topical application of sodium fluoride and stannous fluoride. *J Dent Res,* 51:1325–30.

111. Ingraham, R. Q., & Williams, J. E. (1970). An evaluation of the utility of application and cariostatic effectiveness of phosphate-fluorides in solution and gel states. *J Tenn Dent Assoc,* 50:5–12.

112. Cons, N. C., Janerich, D. T., & Senning, R. S. (1970). Albany topical fluoride study. *J Am Dent Assoc,* 80:777–81.

113. Horowitz, H. S., & Doyle, J. (1971). The effect on dental caries of topically applied acidulated phosphate-fluoride: Results after three years. *J Am Dent Assoc,* 82:359–65.

114. U.S. Public Health Service. (1987, August). *Oral health of United States adults. The national survey of oral health in U.S. employed adults and seniors: 1985–1986. National findings* (NIH Publication No. 87–2868). Bethesda, MD: National Institutes of Health.

115. Hand, J. S., Hunt, R. S., & Beck, J. D. (1988). Incidence of coronal and root surface caries in an older adult population. *J Pub Health Dent,* 48:14–19.

116. Hamasha, A. A., Warren, J. J., Hand, J. S., & Levy, S. M. (2005). Coronal and root caries in the older Iowans: 9-11 year incidence. *Spec Care Dent,* 25:106–10.

117. National Institutes of Health. (2001). *Diagnosis and management of dental caries throughout life. NIH consensus statement 2001 March 26–28,* 18(1):1–24. Retrieved August 4, 2006, from http://consensus.nih.gov/2001/2001DentalCaries115html.htm.

118. Burt, B. A., Ismail, A. I., & Eklund, S. A. (1986). Root caries in an optimally fluoridated and a high-fluoride community. *J Dent Res,* 65:1154–58.

119. Brustman, B. A. (1986). Impact of exposure to fluoride-adequate water on root surface caries in elderly. *Gerodontics,* 2:203–207.

120. Hunt, R. J., Eldredge, J. B., & Beck, J. D. (1989). Effect of residence in a fluoridated community on the incidence of coronal and root caries in an older adult population. *J Pub Health Dent,* 49:138–41.

121. Stamm, J. W., Banting, D. W., & Imrey, P. B. (1990). Adult root caries survey of two similar communities with

contrasting natural water fluoride levels. *J Am Dent Assoc,* 120:143–49.

122. Jones, S., Burt, B. A., Petersen, P. E., & Lennon, M. A. (2005). The effective use of fluorides in public health. *Bull World Health Org,* 83:670–76.

123. Petersen, P. K. The World Oral Health Report 2003. (2003). Continuous improvement of oral health in the 21st century—The approach of the WHO Global Oral Health Programme. Geneva: World Health Organization.

124. Jensen, M. E., & Kohout, F. J. (1988). The effect of a fluoridated dentifrice on root and coronal caries in an older adult population. *J Am Dent Assoc,* 117:829–32.

125. Nyvad, B., & Fejerskov, O. (1986). Active root surface caries converted into inactive caries as a response to oral hygiene. *Scand J Dent Res,* 94:281–84.

126. Wallace, M. C., Retief, D. H., & Bradley, E. L. (1993). The 48-month increment of root caries in an urban population of older adults participating in a preventive dental program. *J Pub Health Dent,* 53:133–37.

127. Stookey, G. K. (1990). Critical evaluation of the composition and use of topical fluorides. *J Dent Res,* 69:805–12.

128. Stookey, G. K., Rodlun, C. A., Warrick, J. M., & Miller, C. H. (1989). Professional topical fluoride systems vs root caries in hamsters. *J Dent Res,* 68:372. Abstract 1521.

129. Hong, L., Watkins, C. A., Ettinger, R. L., & Wefel, J. S. (2005). Effect of topical fluoride and fluoride varnish on in vitro root surface lesions. *Am J. Dent,* 18:182–87.

130. Berger, E. K. (2006). Fluoride varnish treatment for reducing caries: A brief review of the literature. *Contemp Oral Hyg,* 6:8, 9.

131. Beltran-Aguilar, E. D., Goldstein, J. W., & Lockwood, S. A. (2000). Fluoride varnishes—A review of their clinical use, cariostatic mechanism, efficacy and safety. *J Am Dent Assoc,* 131:589–596.

132. Semler, S. (2006). Evidence-based solutions to clinical challenges: Prevention-based dentistry—Fluoride varnish. *Journal of Practical Hygiene,* 15:23, 25.

133. Petersson, L. G. (1993). Fluoride mouthrinses and fluoride varnishes. *Caries Res,* 27 (Suppl 1):35–42.

134. Petersson, L. G., Arthursson, L., Ostberg, C., Jonsson, G., & Gleerup, A. (1991). Carries-inhibiting effects of different modes of Duraphat varnish reapplication: A 3-year radiographic study. *Caries Res,* 25:70–73.

135. Weinstein, P., Domoto, P., Koday, M., & Leroux, B. (1994). Results of a promising trial to prevent baby bottle tooth decay: A fluoride varnish study. *J Dent Child,* 61:338–41.

136. Shobha, T., Nandlal, B., Prabhakar, A. R., & Sudha, P. (1987). Fluoride varnish versus acidulated phosphate fluoride for school children in Manipal. *J Ind Dent Assoc,* 59:157–60.

137. Seppa, L., Leppanen, T., & Hausen, H. (1995). Fluoride varnish versus acidulated phosphate fluoride gel: A 3-year clinical trial. *Caries Res,* 29:327–30.

138. Fontana, M., & Zero, D. T. (2006). Assessing patients' caries risk. *J Am Dent Assoc,* 137:1231–39.

139. Biller, I. R., Hunter, E. L., Featherstone, M. J., & Silverstone, L. M. (1980). Enamel loss during a prophylaxis polish in vitro. *J Int Assoc Dent Child,* 11:7–12.

140. Stookey, G. K. (1978). In vitro estimates of enamel and dentin abrasion associated with a prophylaxis. *J Dent Res,* 57:36.

141. Vrbic, V., Brudevold, F., & McCann, H. G. (1967). Acquisition of fluoride by enamel from fluoride pumice pastes. *Helv Odont Acta,* 11:21–26.

142. Vrbic, V., & Brudevold, F. (1970). Fluoride uptake from treatment with different fluoride prophylaxis pastes and from the use of pastes containing a soluble aluminum salt followed by topical application. *Caries Res,* 4:158–67.

143. Bixler, D., & Muhler, J. C. (1966). Effect on dental caries in children in a nonfluoride area of combined use of three agents containing stannous fluoride: A prophylactic paste, a solution, and a dentifrice. II. Results at the end of 24 and 36 months. *J Am Dent Assoc,* 72:392–96.

144. Gish, C. W., & Muhler, J. C. (1965). Effect on dental caries in children in a natural fluoride area of combined use of three agents containing stannous fluoride: A prophylactic paste, a solution, and a dentifrice. *J Am Dent Assoc,* 70:914–20.

145. Muhler, J. C., Spear, L. B., Jr., Bixler, D., & Stookey, G. K. (1967). The arrestment of incipient dental caries in adults after the use of three different forms of SnF$_2$ therapy: Results after 30 months. *J Am Dent Assoc,* 75:1402–406.

146. Obersztyn, A., Piotrowski, Z., Kowinski, K., & Ekler, B. (1973). Stannous fluoride in the prophylaxis of caries in adults. *Czas Stomat,* 26:1181–87.

147. Scola, F. P., & Ostrom, C. A. (1968). Clinical evaluation of stannous fluoride when used as a constituent of a compatible prophylactic paste, as a topical solution, and in a dentifrice in naval personnel. II. Report of findings after two years. *J Am Dent Assoc,* 77:594–97.

148. Scola, F. P. (1970). Self-preparation stannous fluoride prophylactic technique in preventive dentistry: Report after two years. *J Am Dent Assoc,* 81:1369–72.

149. Beiswanger, B. B., Billings, R. J., Sturzenberger, O. P., & Bollmer, B. W. (1978). Effect of an SnF$_2$Ca$_2$P$_2$O$_7$ dentifrice and APF topical applications. *J Dent Child,* 45:137–41.

150. Downer, M. C., Holloway, P. J., & Davies, T. G. H. (1976). Clinical testing of a topical fluoride caries prevention program. *Br Dent J,* 141:242–47.

151. Mainwaring, P. J., & Naylor, N. M. (1978). A three-year clinical study to determine the separate and combined caries-inhibitory effects of sodium monofluorophosphate toothpaste and an acidulated phosphate fluoride gel. *Caries Res,* 12:202–12.

152. Marinho, V. C., Higgins, J. P., Sheiham, A., & Logan, S. (2004). Combinations of topical fluoride (toothpastes,

mouthrinses, gels, varnishes) versus single topical fluoride for preventing dental caries in children and adolescents. *Evid Based Dent,* 5:38.

153. Birkeland, J. M., Broch, L., & Jorkjend, J. (1977). Benefits and prognoses following 10 years of a fluoride mouthrinsing program. *Scand J Dent Res,* 85:31–37.

154. Birkeland, J. M., & Torell, P. (1978). Caries-preventive fluoride mouthrinses. *Caries Res,* 12 (Suppl 1):38–51.

155. Reports on Councils and Bureaus, Council on Dental Therapeutics, American Dental Association. (1975). Council classifies fluoride mouthrinses. *J Am Dent Assoc,* 91:1250–52.

156. Torell, P., & Ericsson, Y. (1974). The potential benefits to be derived from fluoride mouth-rinses. In Forrester, D. J., & Schulz, E. M., Jr., Eds. *International workshop on fluorides and dental caries reductions.* Baltimore: University of Maryland, 113–76.

157. Heifetz, S. B., Franchi, G. J., Mosley, G. W., MacDougall, O., & Brunelle, J. (1979). Combined anticariogenic effect of fluoride gel-trays and fluoride mouthrinsing in an optimally fluoridated community. *J Clinic Prevent Dent,* 6:21–23.

158. Radike, A. W., Gish, C. W., Peterson, J. K., King, J. D., & Zegreto, V. A. (1973). Clinical evaluation of stannous fluoride as an anticaries mouthrinse. *J Am Dent Assoc,* 86:404–408.

159. Driscoll, W. S., Swango, P. A., Horowitz, A. M., & Kingman, A. (1981). Caries-preventive effects of daily and weekly fluoride mouthrinsing in an optimally fluoridated community: Findings after 18 months. *Pediatr Dent,* 3:316–20.

160. Jones, J. C., Murphy, R. F., & Edd, P. A. (1979). Using health education in a fluoride mouthrinse program: The public health hygienist's role. *Dent Hyg,* 53:469–73.

161. Kawall, K., Lewis, D. W., & Hargreaves, J. A. (1981). The effect of a fluoride mouthrinse in an optimally fluoridated community—Final two year results. *J Dent Res,* 60 (Spec Iss A):471. Abstract 646.

162. Ashley, F. P., Mainwaring, P. F., Emslie, R. D., & Naylor, M. N. (1977). Clinical testing of a mouthrinse and a dentifrice containing fluoride. A two-year supervised study in school children. *Br Dent J,* 143:333–38.

163. Triol, C. W., Franz, S. M., Volpe, A. R., Frankl, N., Alman, J. E., & Allard, R. L. (1980). Anticaries effect of a sodium fluoride rinse and an MFP dentifrice in a nonfluoridated water area. A thirty-month study. *Clin Prev Dent,* 2:13–15.

164. Blinkhorn, A. S., Holloway, P. J., & Davies, T. G. H. (1977). The combined effect of a fluoride mouthrinse and dentifrice in the control of dental caries. *J Dent Res,* 56 (Spec Iss D):D111.

165. Ringelberg, M. L., Webster, D. B., Dixon, D. O., & Lezotte, D. C. (1979). The caries-preventive effect of amine fluorides and inorganic fluorides in a mouthrinse or dentifrice after 30 months of use. *J Am Dent Assoc,* 98:202–208.

166. Horowitz, H. S., Heifetz, S. B., Meyers, R. J., Driscoll, W. S., & Korts, D. C. (1979). Evaluation of a combination of self-administered fluoride procedures for the control of dental caries in a nonfluoride area: Findings after four years. *J Am Dent Assoc,* 98:219–23.

167. Skartveit, L., Wefel, J. S., & Ekstrand, J. (1991). Effect of fluoride amalgams on artificial recurrent enamel and root caries. *Scand J Dent Res,* 99:287–94.

168. Donly, K. J. (1995). Enamel and dentin demineralization inhibition of fluoride-releasing materials. *Am J Dent,* 7:275–78.

169. Erickson, R. L., & Glasspoole, E. A. (1995). Model investigations of caries inhibition by fluoride-releasing dental materials. *Adv Dent Res,* 9:315–23.

170. ten Cate, J. M., & van Duinen, R. N. B. (1995). Hypermineralization of dentinal lesions adjacent to glass-ionomer cement restorations. *J Dent Res,* 74:1266–71.

171. Donly, K. J., Segura, A., Kanellis, M., & Erickson, R. L. (1999). Clinical performance and caries inhibition of resin-modified glass ionomer cement and amalgam restorations. *J Am Dent Assoc,* 130:1459–66.

172. Rawls, H. R. (1991). Preventive dental materials: Sustained delivery of fluoride and other therapeutic agents. *Adv Dent Res,* 5:50–56.

173. Vatanatham, K., Trairatvorakul, C., & Tantbironjn, D. (2006). Effect of fluoride- and nonfluoride-containing resin sealants on mineral loss of incipient artificial carious lesion. *J Clin Pediatr Dent,* 30:320–24.

174. Jones, D. W., Jackson, G., Suttow, E. J., Hall, A. C., & Johnson, J. (1988). Fluoride release and fluoride uptake by glass ionomer materials. *J Dent Res,* 67(A):197. Abstract 672.

175. Marinelli, C. B., Donly, K. J., Wefel, J. S., Jakobsen, J. R., & Denehy, G. E. (1997). An in vitro comparison of three fluoride regimens on enamel remineralization. *Caries Res,* 31:418–22.

176. Bynum, A. M., & Donly, K. J. (1999). Enamel demineralization on teeth adjacent to fluoride releasing materials without dentifrice exposure. *ASDC J Dent Child,* 66:89–92.

177. Donly, K. J., Segura, A., Wefel, J. S., & Hogan, M. M. (1999). Evaluating the effects of fluoride-releasing dental materials on adjacent interproximal caries. *J Am Dent Assoc,* 130:817–25.

178. Bayless, J. M., & Tinanoff, N. (1985). Diagnosis and treatment of acute fluoride toxicity. *J Am Dent Assoc,* 110:209–11.

179. Heifetz, S. B., & Horowitz, H. S. (1986). The amounts of fluoride in current fluoride therapies; safety considerations for children. *J Dent Child,* 77:876–82.

180. Melvor, M. E. (1987). Delayed fatal hyperkalemia in a patient with acute fluoride intoxication. *Ann Emerg Med,* 16:1165–67.

181. Department of Health and Human Services. (1991). U.S. Public Health Service. *Report of the ad hoc subcommittee to coordinate environmental health and related programs. Review of fluoride benefits and risks.* Washington, DC: U.S. Department of Health and Human Services.

182. Whitford, G. M. (1987). Fluoride in dental products: Safety considerations. *J Dent Res,* 66:1056–60.

183. Newbrun, E. (1992). Current regulations and recommendations concerning water fluoridation, fluoride supplements, and topical fluoride agents. *J Dent Res,* 67:1255–65.

184. Keels, M. A., Osterhout, S., & Vann, W. F., Jr. (1988). Incidence and nature of accidental fluoride ingestions. *J Dent Res,* 67 (Spec Iss):335. Abstract 1778.

185. Nochimson, G. Toxicity, fluoride. Retrieved February 29, 2008, from http://www.emedicine.com/emerg/topic181.htm.

Chapter 13

Dental Sealants

Denise Muesch Helm

OBJECTIVES

After studying this chapter, the student should be able to:

1. Describe how sealants prevent dental caries.
2. Describe the history of sealant development.
3. List the criteria for selecting teeth for sealant placement.
4. Describe the essentials in attaining maximum retention of sealants.
5. Describe the placement of a sealant.
6. Compare the advantages and disadvantages of light-cured and self-cured sealants.
7. List reasons given for the underuse of sealants by practitioners, and analyze the validity of the reasons.

KEY TERMS

Dental sealant
Enameloplasty
Prophylactic odontotomy
Filled sealants
Unfilled sealants
Polymerization
Photocure
Photoactivation
Light activation
Cold cure
Autopolymerization
Chemical activation
Chemical-cured Sealants
Alternative restorative technique (ART)
Tags
Fossa
Etchants
Articulating paper

INTRODUCTION

Fluorides are highly effective in reducing the number of carious lesions that occur on the smooth surfaces of enamel and cementum. Unfortunately, fluorides are not equally effective in protecting the occlusal pits and fissures, where the majority of carious lesions occur.[1] The placement of sealants is a highly effective means of preventing carious lesions in the pits and fissures in both primary and permanent teeth.[2–4] A Cochrane systematic review examined the effectiveness of second-generation resins compared with no treatment; the resin-based sealants were highly effective in preventing caries in permanent first molars in individuals under 20 years of age, and in children 5 to 10 years of age.[5] Another systematic review examined the efficacy of professional measures for caries prevention in high-risk individuals; sealants presented an 88% reduction in caries in that population.[6] Sealants present great preventive value when placed correctly and monitored regularly. A sealant is indicated if an occlusal fissure, fossa, or incisal lingual pit is present. When in doubt, seal and monitor is the preferred course of action.

A liquid resin, more commonly called a **dental sealant,** is placed over the occlusal surface of the tooth where it penetrates the deep fissures to fill areas that cannot be cleaned with the toothbrush (Figure 13–1 ■). The resin then solidifies and, subsequently, the hardened sealant presents a barrier between the tooth and the hostile oral environment. Concurrently, there is a significant reduction of *Streptococcus mutans* on the treated tooth surface.[7] Pits and fissures serve as reservoirs for mutans streptococci; therefore, sealing the niche reduces their oral count.

HISTORICAL PERSPECTIVE

Historically, several agents have been tried to protect deep pits and fissures on occlusal surfaces. In 1895, Wilson reported the placement of dental cement in pits and fissures to prevent caries.[1] In 1929, Bödecker suggested that deep fissures could be broadened with a large round bur to make the occlusal areas more self-cleansing, a procedure that is called **enameloplasty.**[8,9] Two major disadvantages, however, accompany enameloplasty. First, it requires a dentist, which immediately limits its use. Second, in modifying a deep fissure by this method, it is often necessary to remove more sound tooth structure than would be required to insert a small restoration.

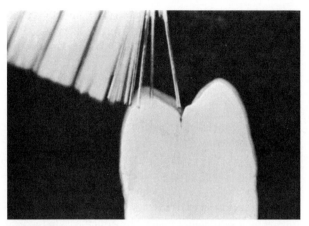

■ **FIGURE 13–1**   One reason that 50% of the carious lesions occur on the occlusal surface is that the toothbrush bristle has a greater diameter than the width of the fissure. (Courtesy of Dr. J. McCune, Johnson & Johnson.)

In 1923 and again in 1936, Hyatt advocated the early insertion of small restorations in deep pits and fissures before carious lesions had the opportunity to develop.[10] He termed this procedure **prophylactic odontotomy.** Again, this operation is more of a treatment procedure than a preventive approach, because it removes sound tooth structure.

Several materials have been unsuccessfully used in an attempt to either seal or make the fissures more resistant to caries. These attempts have included the use of topically applied zinc chloride, potassium ferrocyanide, and ammoniacal silver nitrate; copper amalgam has also been packed into the fissures.[11–13]

A final course of action to manage a deep pit and fissure is one that is often used: Do nothing; wait and watch. This option avoids the need to cut good tooth structure until a definite carious lesion is identified. It also results in many teeth being lost when individuals do not return for periodic examinations. This approach, although used, is a violation of the ethical principle of beneficence (providing a benefit) and patient autonomy.

SEALANT USE IN DENTAL CARE

In the late 1960s and early 1970s, another option became available, the use of pit-and-fissure sealants.[14] Buonocore first described placing sealants using a method to bond polymethylmethacrylate (PMMA) to human enamel conditioned with phosphoric acid.[14] Practical use of this concept, however, was not realized until the development of bisphenol A–glycidyl methylacrylate (Bis-GMA), urethane dimethacrylate (UDMA), and triethylene glycol dimethacrylate (TEGDMA) resins, which possessed better physical properties than PMMA. The first successful use of resin sealants was reported by Buonocore in the 1960s.[14]

Bisphenol A–glycidyl methylacrylate is now the sealant of choice. It is a mixture of Bis-GMA and methyl methacrylate. Nuva-Seal, the first successful commercial sealant, was placed on the market in 1972. Since then, more effective sealants have become available. The first sealant clinical trials used cyanoacrylate-based materials, which were later replaced by dimethacrylate-based products. The primary difference between sealants is the method of polymerization; these methods are discussed in the following section.

Some sealants contain fillers, which makes it desirable to classify the commercial products into filled and unfilled sealants. The **filled sealants** contain microscopic glass beads, quartz particles, and other fillers used in composite resins. The fillers are coated with products such as silane to facilitate their combination with the Bis-GMA resin. The fillers make the sealant more resistant to abrasion and wear. Because filled sealants are more resistant to abrasion, the occlusion should be checked, and the sealant height may need to be adjusted after placement. In contrast, **unfilled sealants** wear quicker but usually do not need occlusal adjustment.

POLYMERIZATION OF SEALANTS

The common sealant is a liquid resin called a monomer (a molecule that can be bound to similar molecules to form a polymer, which contains two or more monomers). When the catalyst acts on the monomer, repeating chemical bonds begin to form, increasing in number and complexity as the hardening process, **polymerization,** proceeds (Figure 13–2 ■). Finally, the resultant hard product is known as a polymer.

Two methods have been used to catalyze polymerization. The first method is light curing with the use of a visible blue light; synonyms for this method are **photocure, photoactivation,** and **light activation.** Some light-cured sealants contain a catalyst, such as camphoroquinone, which is placed in the monomer at the time of manufacture. The catalyst is sensitive to visible blue-light frequencies. When the monomer is exposed to the visible blue light, polymerization is initiated. The second method is self-curing, in which a monomer and a catalyst are

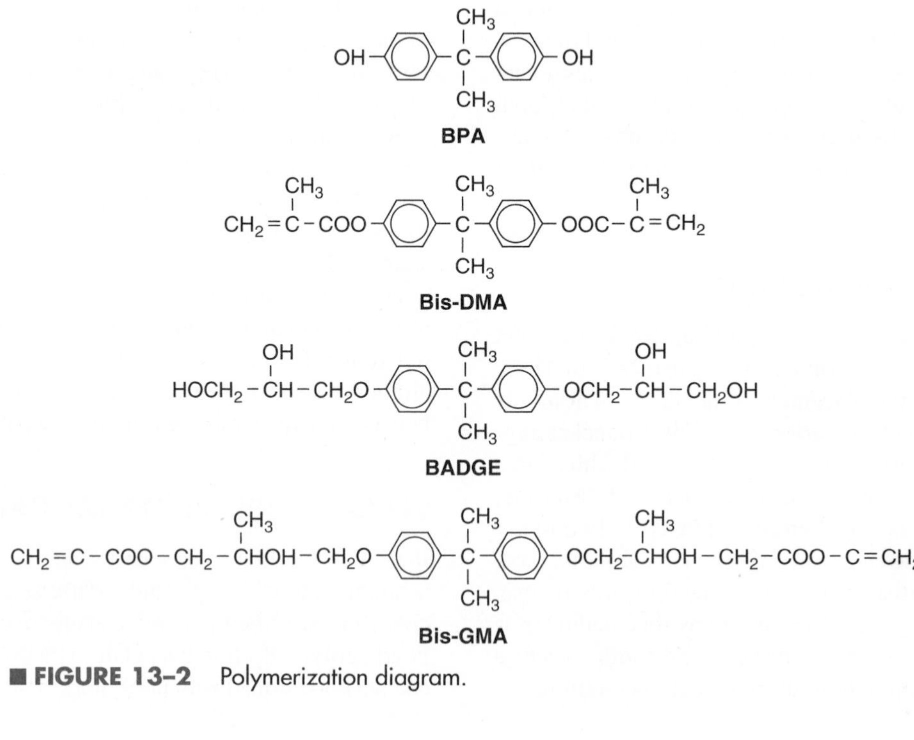

■ **FIGURE 13–2** Polymerization diagram.

mixed together to induce polymerization without the use of a light source; synonyms for this process are **cold cure, autopolymerization,** and **chemical activation.**

In first-generation sealants, polymerization was initiated by ultraviolet light; these sealants were replaced by other light-cured sealants that instead required visible blue light. Second-generation sealants were autopolymerized, and third-generation sealants used visible blue light. Fourth- and fifth-generation sealants added a step in which dental-bonding agents were used as a primer before the sealants were placed. Sixth-generation sealants use a self-etching process. Less frequently, glass ionomer cement is used as a dental sealant.

Light-Cured Sealants

The main advantage of the light-cured sealant is that the operator can initiate polymerization at any suitable time. Polymerization time is shorter with the light-cured products than with the self-curing sealants. The light-cured process does require purchase of a light source, but this light is also used for polymerization of composite restorations, and is available in all dental offices. Light-cured sealants have become the product of choice in most offices. Light-cured sealants should be stored away from bright office lighting, which can sometimes initiate polymerization. The light-cured sealants have a higher compressive strength and a smoother surface, probably because air is introduced into the self-cure resins during mixing.

The light-emitting device consists of a high-intensity white light, a blue filter to produce the desired blue color, usually between 400 to 500 nm, and a light-conducting rod. Some other systems consist of a blue light produced by light-emitting diodes (LED) (Figure 13–3 ■). Most systems have timers for automatically switching off the lights after a predetermined time interval. In use, the end of the rod is held only a few millimeters above the sealant during the first 10 seconds, after which time the rod can be rested on the hardened surface of the partially polymerized sealant. The time required for polymerization is set by the manufacturer and is usually around 20 to 30 seconds. The depth of cure is influenced by the intensity of the light, which can differ greatly with different products and length of exposure. Often it is desirable to set the automatic light timer for longer than the manufacturer's instructions. Even after cessation of light exposure, a final, slow polymerization can continue over a 24-hour period.[15]

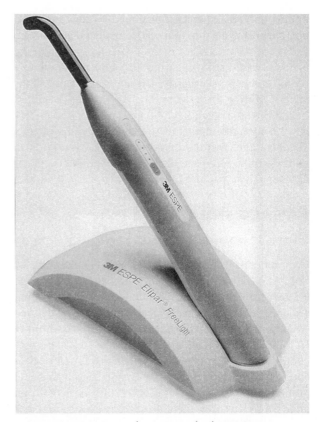

■ **FIGURE 13–3**   Light-emitting diode (LED) curing unit for direct, intraoral exposure.

Long-term exposure to the intense light may cause damage to the eyes. Staring at the lighted operating field is uncomfortable and does produce afterimages. This problem is circumvented by the use of a round, 4-inch, dark-yellow disk, which fits over the light housing. The disk filters out the intense blue light in the 400- to 500-nm range and is sufficiently dark to subdue other light frequencies.

Self-Cured Sealants

Autopolymerizing sealants, sometimes referred to as **chemical-cured sealants,** incorporate a catalyst with the monomer; in addition, another bottle contains an initiator, usually benzoyl peroxide. When the monomer and the initiator are mixed, polymerization begins.

The self-curing resins do not require an expensive light source. However, a great disadvantage is that once mixing has started, if some minor problem is experienced in the operating field, the operator must either continue mixing or stop and make a new mix. For the autopolymerizing resin, the time allowed for sealant manipulation and placement must not be exceeded, even though the material might still appear liquid. Once the hardening begins, it occurs very rapidly, and any manipulation of the material during this critical time jeopardizes retention. In addition, the operating field must remain completely dry for a longer amount of time, which is obviously a disadvantage. Despite these differences, retention in both the light-cured and the self-cured products appear to be equal.[16,17]

TYPES OF SEALANTS

Glass Ionomer Cement Sealants

Glass ionomer cements have been used as dental sealants. Studies have indicated that they do not have the same effective retention rates as those of conventional sealants.[18] Glass ionomer cement is most frequently used when providing the **alternative restorative technique (ART).** This technique is defined as the treatment procedure for caries prevention that involves removal of soft/demineralized tooth tissue using a hand instrument alone, followed by restoration of the tooth with an adhesive restorative material, such as a glass ionomer cement.[19] This technique is especially valuable in areas of the country where there are shortages of dentists and where dental hygienists have been trained to place sealants. In fact, ART is used extensively throughout the world as a method to alleviate pain and infection.[20]

Sealants with Bonding Agents

Recently, bonding agents or primers have been added to dental sealant systems. A clincial study conducted over 5 years reported a 50% reduction in occlusal sealant failure and a 66% reduction in buccal–lingual sealant failure when bonding agents were used.[21] The use of a bonding agent also increases the time and cost for sealant materials.

Self-Etching Light-Cured Sealants

A new sealant has been introduced that has revolutionized sealant placement. This sealant material contains a self-etching additive, which allows placement of the sealant material after a tooth surface is cleaned by oil-free pumice and dried. After waiting 15 seconds for the etching to occur, the light is placed on the sealant for 20 seconds. This procedure is much faster than previous methods, and these sealants also include fluoride.

Fluoride-Releasing Sealants

The addition of fluoride to sealants was considered about 20 years ago, and was based on the finding that the incidence and severity of secondary caries were reduced around fluoride-releasing materials such as the silicate cements used for anterior restorations. Use of a fluoridated resin-based sealant was thought to possibly provide an additional anti-cariogenic effect if the fluoride released from its matrix was incorporated into the adjacent enamel, because fluoride uptake would increase the enamel's resistance to the caries effect.[22]

Fluoride is added to sealants by two methods. The first method involves adding a soluble fluoride to the unpolymerized resin. The second method involves adding an organic fluoride compound that will bind chemically to the resin to form an ion exchange resin. Fluoride-releasing sealants have shown antibacterial properties as well as a greater artificial caries resistance compared with a non-fluoridated sealant.[23–27] Fluoridated sealants have also demonstrated a caries-inhibiting effect, with a significant reduction in lesion depth in adjacent surface enamel and a reduction in the frequency of wall lesions.[27] Moreover, the fluoridated sealant's laboratory bond strength to enamel is similar to that of non-fluoridated sealants.[28]

However, recent reviews revealed that, compared with resin-based sealants, fluoride-containing sealants have a poor retention rate after 48 months; they also have not proven to act as a fluoride reservoir with long-term release of fluoride into the oral environment.[17,27,29]

Colored versus Clear Sealants

Both clear and colored sealants are available. Colored sealants vary from translucent (clear) to white, yellow, and pink. Some manufacturers sell both clear and colored sealants in either the light-curing or autopolymerizing form. The selection of a colored versus a clear sealant is a matter of individual preference. The colored products permit a more precise placement of the sealant, with the visual assurance that the periphery extends halfway up the inclined planes. Retention can be more accurately monitored by both the patient and the operator placing the sealant. A clear sealant, however, may be considered more esthetically acceptable.

Some clinicians prefer the clear sealants, because they are more discrete than white sealants. Others prefer the white sealants, because they are easier to monitor at recall appointments. On the other hand, some clinicians seem to prefer the clear sealants, because it is possible to see under the sealant to detect if a carious lesion is active or advancing. However, no clinical study has comprehensively compared these issues. Some pit-and-fissure sealants actually change color as they become light-polymerized. Color change has not been fully investigated and seems to have only a relative advantage to the dental provider applying the sealant.

SEALANT RETENTION

Resin sealants are retained better on recently erupted teeth than on teeth with a more mature surface. Moreover, they are retained better on first molars than on second molars, and are better retained on mandibular than on maxillary teeth. This latter finding is possibly caused by the mandibular teeth being more accessible and easier to see; also, gravity aids the flow of the sealant into the fissures. Sealants appear to be equally retained on occlusal surfaces in primary and permanent teeth.[3] One-year retention rates on primary teeth sealed with a flowable resin material were significantly higher than non-flowable materials.[30]

Sealed teeth from which the dental sealants were later lost still had fewer lesions than control teeth.[31] This finding is possibly due to the presence of tags that are retained in the enamel after the bulk of the sealant has been sheared from the tooth surface. When the resin sealant flows over the prepared surface, it penetrates the finger-like depressions created by the etching solution. These projections of resin into the etched areas are called **tags** (Figure 13–4 ■). The tags are essential for retention. Scanning electron microscope examination of

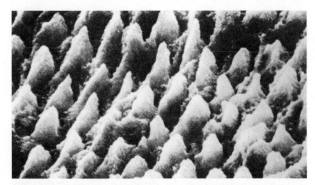

■ **FIGURE 13–4**   Tags, 30 micron. Sealant was flowed over etched surface and allowed to polymerize. The tooth surface subsequently dissolved away in acid, leaving tags. (Courtesy of Silverstone, L. M., Dogon, IL. *The acid etch technique.* St. Paul, MN: North Central Publishing, 1975.)

sealants that were not retained has demonstrated large areas devoid of tags or incomplete tags, usually caused by saliva contamination during the sealing process. If a sealant is forcefully separated from the tooth by masticatory pressures, many of these tags are retained in the etched depressions.

The number of retained sealants decreases at a curvilinear rate. Over the first 3 months, the rapid loss of sealants is probably caused by faulty technique in placement. The fallout rate then begins to plateau, with the ensuing sealant losses probably caused by abnormal masticatory stresses. After a year or so, the sealants become very difficult to see or to discern tactilely, especially if they are abraded to the point that they fill only the fissures. In research studies, this lack of visibility often leads to underestimating the effectiveness of the sealants that remain but cannot be identified. Because the most rapid falloff of sealants occurs in the early stages, an initial 3-month recall after placement to determine if sealants have been lost should be routine, although the recall is not generally done. If sealants are lost, the teeth should be resealed. Teeth successfully sealed for 6 to 7 years are likely to remain sealed.[32]

Long-term studies reported that, at the 20-year follow-up examination of the first molars, 65% showed complete retention of sealants and 27% partial retention without caries. At a 15-year follow-up of the same sealants, the second molars demonstrated corresponding retention rates of 65% and 30%, respectively.[33,34] Mertz-Fairhurst cited studies in which 90% to 100% of the original sealants were retained over a 1-year period[32] (Figure 13–5 ■). More recent studies report 82% of the sealants placed are retained for 5 years.[35] When resealing is accomplished as needed at recall appointments, a higher and more continuous level of protection is achieved. Pit-and-fissure sealants applied during childhood have a long-lasting, caries-preventive effect.[33,34]

CRITERIA FOR SELECTING TEETH FOR SEALANT PLACEMENT

A sealant is indicated if:

- The **fossa** (shallow depression) selected for sealant placement is well isolated from another fossa with a restoration.
- The area selected is confined to a fully erupted fossa, even though the distal fossa is impossible to seal because of inadequate eruption.

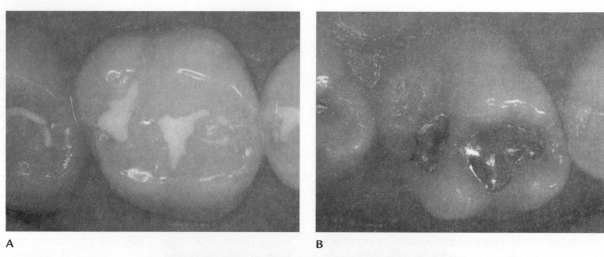

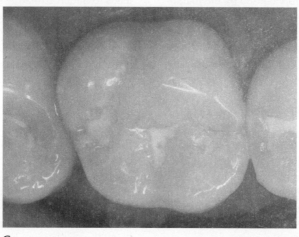

■ **FIGURE 13–5** **A.** 5-year sealant: Five years after placement of a white pit-and-fissure sealant in the matched pair to the control subject. Sealant and control subjects were matched on age, gender, caries history, and other factors. **B.** 5-year control: This matched pair to the sealed patient did not receive sealant. The first permanent molar has already been restored with two amalgam restorations in the previous 5-year period. **C.** 15-year sealant: 15 years after the single application of a white pit-and-fissure sealant. This is the same tooth as in **A.,** but 10 years later. As can be seen, the sealant has served its purpose even though there has been some loss in the peripheral fissures. (Courtesy of Dr. Richard J. Simonsen, DDS.)

- The selected tooth has an intact occlusal surface when the contralateral tooth surface (surface of tooth in opposite arch) is carious or restored; teeth on opposite sides of the arches usually are equally prone to caries.
- An incipient lesion exists in the pit-and-fissure area.
- Sealant material can be flowed over a conservative class I composite or amalgam to improve the marginal integrity, and into the remaining pits and fissures to further prevent recurrent decay.

All teeth meeting the previous criteria should be sealed and re-sealed as needed. Sealants should be placed on the teeth of adults if there is evidence of existing or impending caries susceptibility, as would occur following excessive intake of sugar, methamphetamine use, or xerostomia induced by drugs or radiation therapy. Sealants should also be used in communities where fluoride levels in the water supply is optimized, as well as in non-fluoridated communities.[35] The following cases are two good illustrations of this philosophy. After a 3-year study, Ripa and colleagues concluded that the time the teeth had been in the mouth (some for 7 to 10 years) had no effect on the vulnerability of occlusal surfaces to caries attack.[36] Also, the incidence of occlusal caries in young Air Force recruits, who were usually in their late teens or early twenties, is relatively high.[37]

When priorities must be based on economic factors, such as in many public health programs, ages 3 and 4 years (preschool) are the most important times for sealing the eligible deciduous teeth; ages 6 to 7 years (second grade) for the first permanent molars; and ages 11 to 13 years (sixth grade) for the second permanent molars and premolars.[38] Currently, 77% of the 12- to 17-year-old children in the United States have dental caries in their permanent teeth.[39] Combining sealant placement and regular fluoride exposure would save many school days, and school dental health clinics or mobile dental health programs would achieve better dental health.[40] If limited resources is a primary factor in treatment planning, the disease susceptibility of the tooth should be considered when selecting teeth for sealants, as opposed to the age of the individual.

A sealant is contraindicated if:

- Patient behavior does not permit use of adequate dry-field techniques throughout the procedure.
- An open, frank, carious lesion exists on the same tooth.
- Caries exist on other surfaces of the same tooth in which restoration will disrupt an intact sealant.
- A large occlusal restoration is already present.

SEALANT PLACEMENT

For sealant retention, the surface of the tooth must (1) have a maximum surface area, (2) have deep, irregular pits and fissures, (3) be clean, and (4) for most sealant materials, be absolutely dry at the time of sealant placement and uncontaminated with saliva residue. These are the four commandments for successful sealant placement, and they cannot be violated.

Increasing the Surface Area

Sealants do not bond directly to the teeth. Instead, they are retained mainly by adhesive forces. Increasing the surface area, which in turn increases the adhesive potential, requires the use of tooth conditioners (also called **etchants**), which are composed of a 30% to 50% concentration of phosphoric acid; the etchants are placed on the occlusal surface prior to placement of the sealant.[41] The etchant may be in liquid or gel form. Both forms are equal in abetting retention.[42] Once a tooth is etched, it appears chalky white as shown in Figure 13–6 ■. If any etched areas on the tooth surface are not covered by the sealant or if the sealant is not retained, the normal appearance of the enamel returns within 1 hour to a few weeks owing to remineralization of the enamel by salivary constituents.[43]

The etchant should be carefully applied to avoid contact with the soft tissues. If not confined to the occlusal surface, the acid may produce a mild inflammatory response. It also produces a sharp acid taste that is often objectionable.

Pit-and-Fissure Depth

Deep, irregular pits and fissures offer a much more favorable surface contour for sealant retention compared with broad, shallow fossae (Figure 13–7 ■). The deeper fissures protect the resin sealant from the shear forces occurring as a result of masticatory movements. Of parallel importance is the possibility of caries development increasing as the fissure depth and slope of the inclined planes increase.[44] Thus, as the potential for caries increases, so does the potential for sealant retention.

Surface Cleanliness

The need and methods for cleaning the tooth surface prior to sealant placement are controversial. Methods used to clean the tooth surface include, air polishing, use of hydrogen peroxide, polishing with pumice, brushing with a nonfluoridated toothpaste, and use of laser.[45–48] Comparison

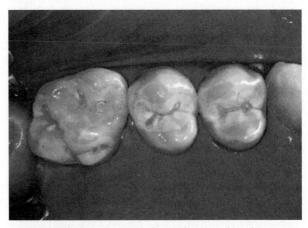

■ **FIGURE 13–6**   Tooth after etchant is placed.

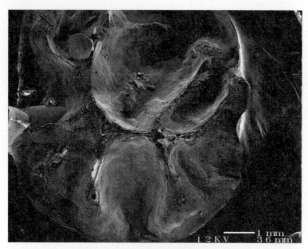

■ **FIGURE 13–7** An electron-scanning microscope view of the deep pits and fissures of the occlusal surface of a molar. (Courtesy of Dr. A. J. Gwinnett, State University of New York, Stony Brook.)

of acid etching with laser alone did not demonstrate any significant difference of sealant retention or microleakage. In light of the expense of laser equipment, using a laser prior to sealant placement provides no advantage.[17] Furthermore, cleaning teeth with the newer prophylaxis pastes with or without fluoride (NuPro, Topex) was not shown to affect the bond strength of sealants.[49] Interestingly, in the most cited studies on sealant longevity, Simonsen accomplished the most effective sealant longevity without use of a prior prophylaxis.[33] However, cleaning the tooth surface with oil-free pumice is recommended for sixth-generation sealant material. Whatever the cleaning preferences, either by acid etching or other methods, all heavy stains, deposits, debris, and plaque should be removed from the occlusal surface before applying the sealant material.

It was once thought that the use of fluoride prior to sealant placement would decrease sealant retention. The literature indicates that this concern is not true and that, if the tooth is treated with fluoride and the sealant is not retained, the tooth will still benefit from the prior fluoride placement.[50,51]

Preparing the Tooth for Sealant Application

The preliminary steps for the light-activated and the autopolymerized resins are similar up to the time of application of the resin to the teeth. After the selected teeth are isolated, they are thoroughly dried. If a liquid etchant is being used, it is dabbed on the tooth with a small resin sponge or cotton pledget held with cotton pliers. A gel etchant would be placed directly on the tooth by the supplied syringe/canula delivery system. Following the manufacturer's direction for etch time is important; typically 20 to 30 seconds of enamel-etching time is recommended. The etched tooth is then rinsed and dried (Figure 13–8 ■).

The dried tooth surface should have a white, dull, frosty, or chalky appearance, because the etching removes approximately 5 to 10 micron of the original surface, although at times inter-rod penetrations of up to 100 micron may occur.[52,53] The etching does not always involve the inter-rod areas; sometimes the central portion of the rod is etched, and the periphery is unaffected. The pattern on any one tooth is unpredictable.[54] In any event, the surface area is greatly increased by the acid etch.

Drying the Tooth Surface

The teeth must be dry at the time of sealant placement because sealants are hydrophobic. The presence of saliva on the tooth is even more detrimental than water, because its organic components interpose a barrier between the tooth and the sealant. Whenever the teeth are dried with an air syringe, the air stream should be checked to ensure that it is not moisture-laden. Otherwise, if sufficient moisture is sprayed on the tooth, adhesion of the sealant to the enamel will be prevented. A check for moisture can be accomplished by directing the air stream onto a cool mouth mirror; any fogging indicates the presence of moisture. The omission of this simple step possibly accounts for the inter-operator variability in the retention of fissure sealants.

A dry field can be maintained in several ways including use of cotton rolls, and/or the placement of bibulous (absorbent) pads over the opening of the parotid duct. The most successful sealant studies have used cotton rolls for isolation.[33] In one study comparing the retention rate of a rubber dam versus cotton rolls, the sealant retention was approximately equal.[55] Other studies have shown excellent sealant retention after 3 years and after 10 to 20 years.[33,34,56] Another promising dry-field–isolating device for single-operator use, especially when used with cotton rolls, is ejector moisture-control systems, which suction and eject saliva from the mouth.

The use of two operators, such as a dental hygienist or a dentist and a dental assistant, is preferred, because it increases the likelihood that a dry field can be maintained.

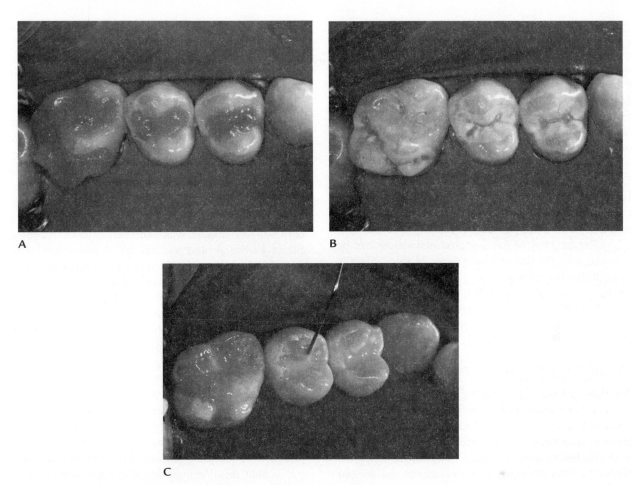

■ **FIGURE 13–8**   Sealant placement. **A.** Gel etchant is applied to teeth, including the lingual cusp on the first molar. **B.** Etched surface has a "frosty" appearance. **C.** Application of resin-based sealant. (Courtesy of Dr. Chris Bryant.)

In the event that it becomes necessary to replace a wet cotton roll, it is essential that no saliva contacts the etched tooth surface. If saliva contact is suspected, it is necessary to repeat all procedures up to the time the dry field was compromised, including repeated etching to remove any residual saliva.

Sealant Application

With either the light-cured or autopolymerized sealants, the material should be placed first in the fissures of maximum depth. At times penetration of the fissure is negated by the presence of debris, air entrapment, narrow orifices, and excessive viscosity of the sealant.[57] The sealant should not only fill the fissures, but some bulk over the fissure should be present. After the fissures are adequately covered, the material is then brought to a knife edge approximately halfway up the inclined plane.

Following polymerization, the sealants should be examined carefully before the dry field is discontinued. If any voids are evident, additional sealant can be added without the need for any additional etching. The hardened sealant leaves an oil residue on the surface. This residue is unreacted monomer that can be either wiped off with a gauze sponge or left on the surface. If a sealant requires repair at any time after the dry field is discontinued, it is prudent to repeat the initial etching and drying procedures. Because all commercial sealants, light-cured and self-cured, are of the same Bis-GMA chemical family, they easily bond to one another.[58]

Occlusal and Interproximal Discrepancies

At times, excess sealant may inadvertently flow into a fossa or into the adjoining interproximal spaces. To remedy the first problem, the occlusion should be checked visually or, if indicated, with **articulating paper,** which has a pigment coating on one or both sides to mark teeth where their occlusal surfaces contact the paper. The marked surfaces indicate the contact points of the teeth. Usually any minor discrepancies in occlusion are rapidly removed by normal chewing action. A large, no. 8, round cutting bur may be used to rapidly create a broad resin fossa, if the premature contact is unacceptable.

The integrity of the interproximal spaces can be checked with the use of dental floss. If any sealant is present, the use of scalers may be required to accomplish removal. If the sealant still cannot be removed, the area should be re-etched to remove the sealant. These corrective actions are rarely needed once proficiency of placement is attained.

Evaluating Retention of Sealants

The finished sealant should be checked for retention without using undue force. If the sealant does not adhere, the placement procedures should be repeated, with only about 15 seconds of etching needed to remove the residual saliva before again flushing, drying, and applying the sealant. If two attempts are unsuccessful, the sealant application should be postponed until remineralization occurs and the patient can comply with the procedure.

PLACEMENT OF SEALANTS OVER CARIOUS LESIONS

Sealing over a carious lesion is important because of the professional concern about the possibility of caries progression under the sealant sites. Teeth that were examined in vivo and later subjected to histologic examination after extraction for orthodontic reasons were often found to have areas of incipient or overt caries under many fissures, which cannot be detected by the explorer. In one study, sealants were purposely placed over small, overt lesions; when compared with control teeth, many of the sealed carious teeth were diagnosed as sound 3 and 5 years later.[59] Handelman has indicated that sealants can be considered a viable modality for arrest of pit-and-fissure caries.[60] The number of bacteria recovered from the area decreased rapidly when the lesion was sealed.[24,59–61] This

decrease in bacterial population is probably due to the integrity of the seal between the resin and the etched tooth surface, which does not permit the movement of fluids or tracer isotopes between the sealant and the tooth.[62,63]

Sealants have been placed over more extensive lesions in which carious dentin is involved.[64] Even with these larger lesions, there is a decrease in the bacterial population and arrest of the carious process as a function of time. Clinically detectable lesions in the dentin were covered for 5 years with Nuva-Seal. After that time the bacterial cultures were essentially negative, and an apparent 83% reversal from a caries-active to a caries-inactive state was achieved.[61] More recently, Mertz-Fairhurst and colleagues demonstrated that sealed lesions became inactive bacteriologically, with arrested carious lesions.[65] This ability to arrest incipient and early lesions is highlighted by the statement in the 1979 publication of the ADA's Council on Dental Therapeutics: "Studies indicate that there is an apparent reduction in microorganisms in infected dentin covered with sealant. These studies appear to substantiate that there is no hazard in sealing carious lesions." The statements end with the cautionary note: "However, additional long-term studies are required before this procedure can be evaluated as an alternative to traditional restorative procedures."[66] Sealants that have been placed over incipient lesions should be monitored at subsequent recall/annual dental examination. In addition, there have been reports of sealants being used to achieve penetration of incipient smooth-surface lesions ("white spots") of facial surfaces.

Many times dental providers perform enameloplasty using a bur or air abrasion to remove demineralized areas and then place a dental sealant. In fact, enameloplasty has no significant differences compared with etching before sealants. Enameloplasty also requires a dentist, which increases the cost of placing sealants.

DENTAL PROVIDERS

The cost of sealant placement increases directly with the level of professional education of the operator. In view of the cost-effectiveness, dental hygienists and dental assistants should be considered the logical providers to place sealants. In most states, dental hygienists are now allowed to place sealants without the presence of a dentist; however, in many states the dentist is required to examine the tooth to make the decision regarding sealant placement. This requirement hinders the ability of the dental hygienist to assess and place the sealant concurrently, increasing the number of dental providers required for placement. Basically, it increases the time spent in providing sealants and increases the cost of placing the sealants by increasing the number of dental providers required for the procedure.

ECONOMICS

Bear in mind that not every tooth receiving a sealant would necessarily become carious, but the cost of preventing a single carious lesion is greater than the cost of a single sealant application. For instance, calculations revealed that five sealants would need to be placed on sound teeth to prevent one lesion over a 5-year period, that is, an estimated one tooth for every three sealant applications are prevented from becoming carious.[67] Sealants would be most cost-effective if they could be placed in only those pits and fissures that are destined to become carious. Unfortunately, we do not have a caries predictor test of such exactitude, but the use of visual examination plus an economic, portable electronic device that objectively measures conductance (or resistance) would greatly aid in evaluating occlusal risk. Without such a device, it is necessary to rely on professional judgment, which is based on the severity of indicators for caries activity: number of demineralized fissures, level of plaque index, number of incipient and overt lesions, and microbiologic test indications.

In an office setting, it is estimated to cost 1.6 times more to treat a tooth than to seal it. A panel of seven experts found that placing sealants, especially on teeth with high caries risk, was a cost-effective measure with positive outcomes.[68] The Task Force on Community Preventive Services, an independent, non-federal group formed to evaluate oral health interventions, was charged with determining interventions that promote and improve oral health. The Task Force examined the cost of six public health programs for placing pit-and-fissure sealants, revealing a mean cost of $39.10 per person.[69]

DISPARITIES IN DENTAL SEALANT USE

Significant disparities in the number of placed sealants exist. Disparities are found mostly among young children, but are also linked to race/ethnicity, income levels, and education.[70] One study reported that white children and children from high income backgrounds were 60% more likely to have sealants than other racial/ethnic minorities or those from lower incomes. Adults and the elderly generally have lower sealant use, even though many of them suffer from xerostomia, which would make them ideal candidates for sealant use.

Barriers that affect the delivery of sealants include (1) legal restrictions on dental hygienists and dental assistants placing sealants without the approval and/or presence of a dentist; (2) lack of consumer knowledge of the effectiveness of sealants and a resultant lack of demand for the product; (3) a shortage of dentists willing to accept patients on Medicaid; and (4) dental providers' concern over the falsely perceived detrimental effect of sealing over a carious lesion.[71]

The safety of dental sealant placement has been demonstrated by many studies showing that, even when placed over incipient and minimally overt caries sites, progression did not occur as long as the sealant remained intact.[72] In addition, several clinical studies have pointed out that sealants could be applied by dental hygienists and dental assistants, thus providing a more economical workforce for private practice and public health programs.

Dental and public health organizations support the use of dental sealants. The economics and education of the profession and the public are the prime requisites for expanded acceptance of sealants.[71]

SUMMARY

The majority of all carious lesions that occur in the mouth occur on the occlusal surfaces. Which teeth will become carious cannot be predicted; however, if the surface is sealed with a pit-and-fissure sealant, no caries will develop as long as the sealant remains in place. Recent studies indicate an approximate 90% retention rate of sealants 1 year after placement. Even when sealants are eventually lost, most studies indicate that the caries incidence for these teeth is less than that of control surfaces that had never been sealed. Research data also indicate that many incipient and small overt lesions are arrested when sealed. Not one report has shown that caries developed in pits or fissures under an intact sealant.

Sealants are easy to apply, but their application is an extremely sensitive technique. The surfaces that are to receive the sealant must be completely isolated from the saliva during the entire procedure, and etching, flushing, and drying procedures must be timed to ensure adequate preparation of the surface for the sealant. Sealants are comparable to amalgam restorations for longevity, but do not require the cutting of tooth structure. Sealants cost less to place than amalgams. Despite their advantages, the use of sealants has not been embraced by all dental providers, even though sealants are endorsed by the American Dental Association, American Dental Hygienist' Association, and the U.S. Public Health Service. Even when small overt pit-and-fissure lesions exist, they can be dealt with conservatively by using ART. What now appears to be required is that the dental and dental hygiene schools teach sealants as an effective intervention, that the dental professional use them, that the dental hygienist and dental assistant be permitted to apply them, and that the public demand them.

REFERENCES

1. Wilson, I. P. (1985). Preventive dentistry. *Dent Diagn,* 1:70–72.
2. Hotuman, E., Rolling, I., & Poulsen, S. (1998). Fissure sealants in a group of 3–4-year-old children. *Int J Paediatr Dent,* 8:159–60.
3. Garcia-Godoy, F., & Donly, K. J. (2002). Dentin/enamel adhesives in pediatric dentistry. *Pediatr Dent,* 24:462–64.
4. Bletram-Aguilar, E. D., Barker, L. K., Canto, M. T., Dye, B. A., Gooch, B. F., Hyman, J., Jaramillo, F., Kingman, A., Nowjack-Raymer, R., Selwitz, R. H., & Wu, T. (2005). Surveillance for dental caries, dental sealants, tooth retention, edentulism, and enamel fluorosis—US, 1988–1994 and 1999–2002. *Morb Mortality Wkly Rep MMWR,* 54(03):1–44.
5. Ahovuo-Saloranta, A., Hiiri, A., Nordblad, A., Worthington, H., & Makela, M. (2004). Pit and fissure sealants for preventing dental decay in the permanent teeth of children and adolescents. *Cochrane Database Syst Rev,* Issue 3. Art. No.: CD001830.
6. Bader, J. D., Shugars, D. A., & Bonito, A. J. (2001). A systematic review of selected caries prevention and management methods. *Community Dent Oral Epidemiol,* 29:399–411.
7. Mass, E., Eli, I., Lev-Dor-Samovici, B., & Weiss, E. I. (1999). Continuous effect of pit and fissure sealing on *S. mutans* presence in situ. *Pediatr Dent,* 21:164–68.
8. Bödecker, C. F. (1929). The eradication of enamel fissures. *Dent Items Int,* 51:859–66.
9. Sturdevant, C. M., Barton, R. E., Sockwell, C. L., & Strickland, W. D. (1985). *The art and science of operative dentistry.* St. Louis: C. V. Mosby.
10. Hyatt, T. P. (1936). Prophylactic odontotomy: The ideal procedure in dentistry for children. *Dent Cosmos,* 78:353–370.
11. Ast, D. B., Bushel, A., & Chase, C. C. (1950). A clinical study of caries prophylaxis and zinc chloride and potassium ferrocyanide. *J Am Dent Assoc,* 41:437–42.
12. Klein, H., & Knutson, J. W. (1942). Studies on dental caries. XIII. Effect of ammoniacal silver nitrate on caries in the first permanent molar. *Am Dent Assoc,* 29:1420–26.
13. Miller, J. (1951). Clinical investigations in preventive dentistry. *Br Dent J,* 91:92–95.
14. Buonocore, M. G. (1971). Caries prevention in pits and fissures sealed with an adhesive resin polymerized by ultraviolet light: A two-year study of a single adhesive application. *J Am Dent Assoc,* 82:1090–93.
15. Leung, R. L., Adishian, S. R., & Fan, P. L. (1985). Postirradiation comparison of photoactivated composite resins. *J Prosthet Dent,* 54:645–49.
16. Houpt, M., Fuks, A., Shapira, J., Chosack, A., & Eidelman, E. (1987). Autopolymerized versus light-polymerized fissure sealant. *J Am Dent Assoc,* 115:55–56.
17. Muller-Bolla, M., Lupi-Pegurier, L., Tardieu, C., Velly, A. M., & Antomarchi, C. (2006). Retention of resin-based pit and fissure sealants: A systematic review. *Community Dent Oral Epidemiol,* 34:321–36.
18. Poulsen, S., Laurberg, L., Vaeth, M., Jensen, U., & Haubek, D. (2006). A field trial of resin-based and glass-ionomer fissure sealants: Clinical and radiographic assessment of caries. *Comm Dent Oral Epid,* 34:36–40.
19. American Academy of Pediatric Dentistry. (2004). *Policy on alternative restorative treatment.* Chicago: (ART) American Academy of Pediatric Dentistry.
20. Retrieved from http://www.who.org. The work of WHO in the Eastern Mediterranean Region. Annual Report of the Regional Director. 1 January– 31 December 1998 Chapter 4. Retrieved 4/29/08 from http://www.enro.who.int/Ra/AnnualReports/1998/ExecutiveSummary.htm.
21. Feigal, R. J., Musherure, P., Gillespie, B., Levy-Polack, M., Quelhas, I., & Hebling, J. I. (2000). Improved sealant retention with bonding agents: A clinical study of two-bottle and single-bottle systems. *J Dent Res,* 79:1850–56.
22. Forsten, L. (1977). Fluoride release from a glass ionomer cement. *Scand J Dent Res,* 85:503–504.
23. Kozai, K., Suzuki, J., Okada, M., Nagasaka, N. (2000). In vitro study of antibacterial and antiadhesive activities of fluoride-containing light-cured fissure sealants and a glass ionomer liner/base against oral bacteria. *ASDC J Dent Child,* 67:117–22.
24. Carlsson, A., Petersson, M., & Twetman, S. (1997). 2-year clinical performance of a fluoride-containing fissure sealant in young schoolchildren at caries risk. *Am J Dent,* 10:115–19.
25. Loyola-Rodriguez, J. P., & Garcia-Godoy, F. (1996). Antibacterial activity of fluoride release sealants on mutans streptococci. *J Clin Pediatr Dent,* 20:109–11.

26. Jensen, M. E., Wefel, J. S., Triolo, P. T., & Hammesfahr, P. D. (1990). Effects of a fluoride-releasing fissure sealant on artificial enamel caries. *Am J Dent* 3:75–78.

27. Hicks, M. J., Flaitz, C. M., & Garcia-Godoy, F. (2000). Fluoride-releasing sealant and caries-like enamel lesion formation in vitro. *J Clin Pediatr Dent,* 24:215–19.

28. Marcushamer, M., Neuman, E., & Garcia-Godoy, F. (1997). Fluoridated and nonfluoridated unfilled sealants show similar shear strength. *Pediatr Dent,* 19:289–90.

29. Garcia-Godoy, F., Abarzua, I., De Goes, M. F., & Chan, D. C. (1997). Fluoride release from fissure sealants. *J Clin Pediatr Dent,* 22:45–49.

30. Corona, S. A., Borsatto, M. C., Garcia, L., Ramos, R. P., & Palma-Dibb, R. G. (2005). Randomized, controlled trial comparing the retention of a flowable restorative system with a conventional resin sealant: One-year follow up. *Int J Paediatr Dent,* 15:44–50.

31. Hinding, J. (1974). Extended cariostasis following loss of pit and fissure sealant from human teeth. *ASDC J Dent Child,* 41:201–203.

32. Mertz-Fairhurst, E. J. (1984). Current status of sealant retention and caries prevention. *J Dent Educ,* 48:18–26.

33. Simonsen, R. J. (1987). Retention and effectiveness of a single application of white sealant after 10 years. *J Am Dent Assoc,* 115:31–36.

34. Wendt, L. K., Koch, G., & Birkhed, D. (2001). On the retention and effectiveness of fissure sealant in permanent molars after 15–20 years: A cohort study. *Community Dent Oral Epidemiol,* 29:302–307.

35. Bohannan, H. M. (1983). Caries distribution and the case for sealants. *J Public Health Dent,* 43:200–204.

36. Ripa, L. W., Leske, G. S., & Varma, A. O. (1988). Longitudinal study of the caries susceptibility of occlusal and proximal surfaces of first permanent molars. *J Public Health Dent,* 48:8–13.

37. Foreman, F. J. (1994). Sealant prevalence and indication in a young military population. *J Am Dent Assoc,* 125:182–84, 186.

38. Simonsen, R. J. (1984). Pit and fissure sealant in individual patient care programs. *J Dent Educ,* 48:42–44.

39. National Institutes of Health. (2001). *Diagnosis and management of dental caries throughout life. NIH consensus statement 2001 March 26–28;* 18(1):1–24. Retrieved December 4, 2007, from http://consensus.nih.gov/2001/2001DentalCaries115html.htm.

40. U.S. Department of Health and Human Service. (2002, November). Oral health (section 21). In *Healthy People 2010, Vol. 2* (2nd ed.). Washington, DC: U.S. Government Printing Office.

41. Gwinnett, A. J., & Buonocore, M. G. (1965). Adhesives and caries prevention; a preliminary report. *Br Dent J,* 119:77–80.

42. Garcia-Godoy, F., & Gwinnett, A. J. (1987). Penetration of acid solution and gel in occlusal fissures. *J Am Dent Assoc,* 114:809–10.

43. Arana, E. M. (1974). Clinical observations of enamel after acid-etch procedure. *J Am Dent Assoc,* 89:1102–106.

44. König, K. G. (1963). Dental morphology in relation to caries resistance with special reference to fissures as susceptible areas. *J Dent Res,* 2:461–76.

45. Garcia-Godoy, F., & de Araujo, F. B. (1994). Enhancement of fissure sealant penetration and adaptation: The enameloplasty technique. *J Clin Pediatr Dent,* 19:13–18.

46. Kanellis, M. J., Warren, J. J., & Levy, S. M. (2000). A comparison of sealant placement techniques and 12-month retention rates. *J Public Health Dent,* 60:53–56.

47. Chan, D. C., Summitt, J. B., Garcia-Godoy, F., Hilton, T. J., & Chung, K. H. (1999). Evaluation of different methods for cleaning and preparing occlusal fissures. *Oper Dent,* 24:331–36.

48. Sol, E., Espasa, E., Boj, J. R., & Canalda, C. (2000). Effect of different prophylaxis methods on sealant adhesion. *J Clin Pediatr Dent,* 24:211–14.

49. Bogert, T. R., & Garcia-Godoy, F. (1992). Effect of prophylaxis agents on the shear bond strength of a fissure sealant. *Pediatr Dent,* 14:50–51.

50. Warren D. P., Infante, N. B., Rice, H. C., Turner, S. D., & Chan, J. T. (2001). Effect of topical fluoride on retention of pit and fissure sealant. *J Dent Hyg,* 75:21–24.

51. El-Housseiny, A. A., & Sharaf, A. A. (2005). Evaluation of fissure sealant applied to topical fluoride treated teeth. *J Clin Pediatr Dent,* 29:215–19.

52. Pahlavan, A., Dennison, J. B., & Charbeneau, G. T. (1976). Penetration of restorative resins into acid-etched human enamel. *J Am Dent Assoc,* 93:1170–76.

53. Silverstone, L. M. (1974). Fissure sealants. Laboratory studies. *Caries Res,* 8:2–26.

54. Bozalis, W. G., & Marshall, G. W. (1977). Acid etching patterns of primary enamel. *J Dent Res,* 56:185.

55. Straffon, L. H., Dennison, J. B., & More, F. G. (1985). Three-year evaluation of sealant: Effect of isolation on efficacy. *J Am Dent Assoc,* 110:714–17.

56. Wood, A. J., Saravia, M. E., & Farrington, F. H. (1989). Cotton roll isolation versus Vac-Ejector isolation. *ASDC J Dent Child,* 56:438–41.

57. Silverstone, L. M. (1983). Fissure sealants: The enamel-resin interface. *J Public Health Dent,* 43:205–15.

58. Myers, C. L., Rossi, F., & Cartz, L. (1974). Adhesive taglike extensions into acid-etched tooth enamel. *J Dent Res,* 53:435–41.

59. Mertz-Fairhurst, E. J., Williams, J. E., Pierce, K. L., Smith, C. D., Schuster, G. S., Mackert, J. R., Jr., Sherrer, J. D., Wenner, K. K., Richards, E. E., & Davis, Q. B. (1991). Sealed restorations: 4-year results. *Am J Dent,* 4:43–49.

60. Handelman, S. L., Washburn, F., & Wopperer, P. (1976). Two-year report of sealant effect on bacteria in dental caries. *J Am Dent Assoc,* 93:967–70.

61. Going, R. E., Loesche, W. J., Grainger, D. A., & Syed, S. A. (1978). The viability of microorganisms in carious lesions five years after covering with a fissure sealant. *J Am Dent Assoc,* 97:455–62.

62. Theilade, E., Fejerskov, O., Migasena, K., & Prachyabrued, W. (1977). Effect of fissure sealing on the microflora in occlusal fissures of human teeth. *Arch Oral Biol,* 22:251–59.

63. Jensen, O. E., & Handelman, S. L. (1978). In vitro assessment of marginal leakage of six enamel sealants. *J Prosthet Dent,* 39:304–306.

64. Handelman, S. L. (1982). Effect of sealant placement on occlusal caries progression. *Clin Prev Dent,* 4:11–16.

65. Mertz-Fairhurst, E. J., Schuster, G. S., & Fairhurst, C. W. (1986). Arresting caries by sealants: Results of a clinical study. *J Am Dent Assoc,* 112:194–97.

66. American Dental Association. (1982). *Accepted dental therapeutics* (39th ed.). Chicago: American Dental Association.

67. Rock, W. P., & Anderson, R. J. (1982). A review of published fissure sealant trials using multiple regression analysis. *J Dent,* 10:39–43.

68. Quinonez, R. B., Downs, S. M., Shugars, D., Christensen, J., & Vann, W. F., Jr. (2005). Assessing cost-effectiveness of sealant placement in children. *J Public Health Dent,* 65:82–89.

69. Truman, B. I., Gooch, B. F., Sulemana, I., Gift, H. C., Horowitz, A. M., Evans, C. A., Griffin, S. O., & Carande-Kulis, V. G. (2002). Task Force on Community Preventive Services (2002). Reviews of evidence on interventions to prevent dental caries, oral and pharyngeal cancers, and sports-related craniofacial injuries. *Am J Prev Med,* 23:21–54.

70. U.S. Department of Health and Human Services. (2000). *Oral health in America: A report of the Surgeon General: Executive summary.* Rockville, MD: U.S. Department of Health and Human Services, National Institute of Dental and Craniofacial Research, National Institutes of Health.

71. Cohen, L., LaBelle, A., & Romberg, E. (1988). The use of pit and fissure sealants in private practice: A national survey. *J Public Health Dent,* 48:26–35.

72. Handelman, S. L. (1991). Therapeutic use of sealants for incipient or early carious lesions in children and young adults. *Proc Finn Dent Soc,* 87:463–75.

Chapter 14

Nutrition, Diet, and Associated Oral Conditions

Carole A. Palmer

Linda D. Boyd

OBJECTIVES

After studying this chapter, the student should be able to:

1. Describe the rationale for the Dietary Reference Intakes, MyPyramid, Dietary Guidelines for Americans, and food labels.
2. Describe the potential oral effects of poor nutrition during organogenesis.
3. Evaluate the effect of dietary patterns and food composition on cariogenic potential.
4. Describe the effects of food on saliva's buffering capacity.
5. Describe the role of nutrition in oral diseases.
6. Explain nutritional factors that place groups with certain medically compromising conditions or special needs at higher risk for oral disease.

KEY TERMS

Nutritional risk
Dietary guidance
U.S. Preventive services task force guidelines
Food and nutrition board (FNB)
Recommended dietary allowances (RDAs)
Dietary reference intakes (DRIs)
Tolerable upper intake Level [UL]
Dietary guidelines for americans
2005 Dietary guidelines for americans
Body mass index (BMI)
MyPyramid
Food guide pyramid
Nutrition facts
National labeling and education act of 1990
Daily values
Significant scientific agreement (SSA)
Qualified health claims
Optimal nutrition
Malnutrition
Calcium
Vitamin D and phosphorus
Hypomineralization
Iron deficiency anemia

(continued)

KEY TERMS (CONTINUED)

Zinc deficiency
Vitamin A deficiency
Vitamin C deficiency
B-Complex vitamins
Dental demineralization
Physical form
Retentiveness
Sequence
Protective

Cariogenic potential indices
Diet evaluation
Patient counseling
Early Childhood Caries (ECC)
Baby bottle tooth decay
Severe Early Childhood Caries (S-ECC)
Anorexia nervosa
Bulimia nervosa
Binge-Eating Disorder (BED)
Poorly controlled diabetes

INTRODUCTION

Oral health, diet, and nutritional status are closely linked (Figure 14–1 ■). Nutrition is essential for the growth, development, and maintenance of oral structures and tissues. During periods of rapid cellular growth, nutrient deficiencies can have an irreversible effect on the developing oral tissues. Before tooth eruption, nutritional status can influence tooth enamel maturation and chemical composition as well as tooth morphology and size.[1] Early malnutrition increases a child's susceptibility to dental caries in the deciduous teeth.[2] Throughout life, nutritional deficiencies or toxicities can affect host resistance, healing, oral function, and oral-tissue integrity. For example, immune response to local irritants and healing of periodontal tissues may be impaired when nutritional status is compromised. Because the oral epithelium has more rapid cell turnover than most other tissues in the body, clinical signs of malnutrition often manifest first in the oral cavity.

After tooth eruption, diet affects the dentition topically rather than systemically. Dietary factors and eating patterns can initiate, exacerbate, or minimize dental decay. Fermentable carbohydrates are essential for the implantation, colonization, and metabolism of bacteria in dental plaque. Factors such as eating frequency and carbohydrate retentiveness on the dentition influence the progression of carious lesions, whereas foods containing calcium and phosphorus, such as cheese, enhance remineralization. Frequent intake of acidic foods or beverages can cause enamel erosion. Conversely, impaired dental function may lead to poor nutritional health. Older adults with loose or missing teeth, or ill-fitting dentures often reduce their intake of foods that require chewing, such as fresh fruits, vegetables, meats, and breads.[3] When the variety of foods in a diet is reduced, there is greater risk of nutrient inadequacies. The patient who undergoes oral or periodontal surgery may require dietary guidance to prevent deleterious changes in the diet. Patients with diabetes mellitus, oral cancer, or depressed immune function may suffer from oral conditions that compromise nutritional status. The dental clinician needs to

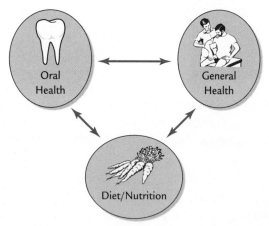

■ **FIGURE 14–1** Relationships between nutrition and health.

understand how diet and nutrition can affect oral health, and how oral conditions can affect food choices and ultimately nutritional status. This chapter provides an overview of the relationships between diet, nutrition, and dental practice, and offers appropriate suggestions for patient guidance.

DIET ASSESSMENT AND COUNSELING IN DENTAL CARE

The modern dental practitioner is concerned not only with educating patients for the prevention of caries and periodontal disease, but also plays an important role in screening patients for other health risks. Just as a medical history and blood pressure evaluation are used to screen for underlying medical conditions, a dietary assessment and screening can help pinpoint potential nutritional problems that may affect, or be affected by, dental care. Because of the large number of patients seen regularly in a dental practice, the dentist and dental hygienist are in an excellent position to recognize areas of **nutritional risk.** The role of the dental provider should be to screen patients for nutritional risk, provide **dietary guidance** related to oral health, and refer patients to nutrition professionals for treatment of other nutrition-related systemic conditions.[3]

Patients should be carefully screened and/or assessed to determine the level of prevention and nutrition guidance needed as outlined in the following **U.S. Preventive Services Task Force guidelines.**[4]

Primary Prevention

This strategy targets a subset of the total population deemed to be at risk for caries for a variety of reasons.[4] Examples include:

- Adolescents at risk of caries because of high intake of soft drinks and snack foods.
- Caries-prevention counseling for patients with xerostomia or cariogenic diet patterns.
- Proactive diet suggestions for new denture wearers or those having jaw fixation.
- Diet advice before radiation or chemotherapy.

Using current diet patterns as a basis for discussion, patients should be taught the role of diet in caries, what are cariogenic and noncariogenic eating patterns, and how to adapt the current diet to lower cariogenic risk.

Secondary Prevention

This strategy targets individuals showing early danger signs of caries, such as extensive cervical demineralization.[4] Examples include:

- Adolescents with cervical decalcification after removal of orthodontic appliances.
- Adults with decalcification due to gastroesophageal reflux disease.

These individuals need the immediate aforementioned interventions as well as more-detailed guidance on how to reduce cariogenicity of their current diet. This guidance would involve determining the factors influencing current habits, and working with the patient to develop appropriate and acceptable strategies for improvement.

Tertiary Prevention

This strategy provides supportive and rehabilitative services to maximize the quality of life.[4] Examples include:

- Adults with a history of caries and many restorations.
- An elderly person with new prosthetic devices.

This level of prevention may require ongoing dietary counseling to promote long-term change to prevent recurrence of caries. In addition, it may require dietary counseling to identify methods of preparing foods to facilitate consumption of a healthy diet when chewing may be compromised by tooth loss or new dentures.

THE BASIS FOR A HEALTHY DIET
Dietary Reference Intakes

Daily food intake must meet metabolic requirements for energy (calories), and provide the essential nutrients that the body cannot synthesize in sufficient quantities to meet physiologic needs. Since the 1940s, the **Food and Nutrition Board (FNB)** of the National Academy of Sciences has published the **Recommended Dietary Allowances (RDAs),** which were recommendations for daily nutrient intake that would support growth and maintenance of body tissues, and prevent deficiency diseases.[5] Beginning in 1997, the FNB began to make major changes to the format and purpose of the nutrition recommendations. The **Dietary Reference Intakes (DRIs)** expand and replace the RDAs[6] by addressing the prevention of chronic degenerative diseases and the risk of excess intake of nutrients.[6]

The DRIs are quantitative estimates of nutrient values to be used for planning and assessing diets for healthy people.[6] These reference values vary by gender and life stage group. DRIs consist not only of RDAs but also the three other types of reference values shown in (Table 14–1 ■). The most recently released RDAs also report the upper limit of nutrient intake considered safe (i.e., **Tolerable Upper Intake Level [UL]**). This reference value was needed because increased intake of nutrients, primarily as dietary supplements, can have harmful effects.

A comprehensive nutritional assessment of an individual's status requires a combination of clinical, biochemical, and anthropometric data.[5,6] For example, if an individual reports an intake of a nutrient below the RDA, more information would be necessary to assess the patient for a nutrient deficiency. Nutrient intakes generally average out over time, so it is unusual for healthy people eating a varied diet to exhibit nutrient deficiencies.

Dietary Guidelines for Americans

The **Dietary Guidelines for Americans** were first published in 1980 and are revised every 5 years.[7] The guidelines are designed to complement the DRIs by making recommendations for a pattern of eating to promote health. The **2005 Dietary Guidelines for Americans** were redesigned and include nine interrelated focus areas.[7] Each of the focus areas has several associated key recommendations.[7] The key recommendations consist of both general recommendations and recommendations for special population groups, such as pregnant women and the elderly. The focus areas and general recommendations can be found in (Table 14–2 ■).[7] In comparison with previous editions, these new guidelines place more emphasis on consuming a nutrient-dense diet that does not exceed energy needs, having regular physical activity, and maintaining a healthy weight. The focus on preventing obesity results from the increased risk obesity presents for many chronic and degenerative diseases, such as heart disease, stroke, diabetes, arthritis, high blood pressure, and some kinds of cancer. The recommendations emphasize balance, moderation, and variety in food choices; they also promote increased use of whole grains, fruits, and vegetables, and decreased use of saturated fat, added sugars, cholesterol, and salt. In addition, the guidelines address food safety in an effort to combat food-borne illness, an important public health concern.[7] For the first time these guidelines recommend good oral hygiene and a reduction in cariogenic foods to reduce dental caries.

The 2005 Dietary Guidelines for Americans focus on a healthy weight according to the **body mass index (BMI)** and waist circumference. The BMI is a medical standard for defining obesity that not only is highly correlated with independent measures of body fat, but is also used to determine if a person is at increased health risk because of excess weight[8] (Table 14–3 ■). A healthy BMI of 19 to 24.9 is associated with the lowest statistical health risk.[9] Persons with BMI above 25 are considered obese, and the recommendation is to lose 1 to 2 BMI units (10 to 15 pounds) to reduce their risk for chronic

---

■ **Table 14–1** Types of Daily Reference Intakes (DRI)

Estimated Average Requirement (EAR)
The daily nutrient intake value estimated to meet the needs of half (50%) of all healthy people in a life stage and gender group.

Recommended Dietary Allowance (RDA)
The average daily nutrient value considered adequate to meet the nutrient needs of nearly all (97%–98%) healthy people in a life stage and gender group.

Adequate Intake (AI)
An intake value assumed to be adequate for healthy people in each life stage and gender group when there is not enough data to determine an RDA.

Tolerable Upper Intake Level (UL)
The highest level of daily nutrient intake likely not to pose adverse health risks for almost all individuals in a life stage and gender group. The risk of adverse effects increases with intakes above the UL.

Source: Food and Nutrition Board, 1989.[6]

■ **Table 14–2**   2005 Dietary Guidelines for Americans

Adequate Nutrients within Calorie Needs
- Consume a variety of nutrient-dense foods and beverages in the basic food groups while choosing foods that limit the intake of saturated and trans fats, cholesterol, added sugars, salt, and alcohol.
- Meet recommended intakes within energy needs by adopting a balanced eating pattern.

Weight Management
- To maintain body weight in a healthy range, balance calories from foods and beverages with calories expended.
- To prevent gradual weight gain over time, make small decreases in food and beverage calories and increase physical activity.

Physical Activity
- Engage in regular physical activity and reduce sedentary activities to promote health, psychological well-being, and a healthy body weight.
- Achieve physical fitness by including cardiovascular conditioning, stretching exercises for flexibility, and resistance exercises or calisthenics for muscle strength and endurance.

Food Groups to Encourage
- Consume a sufficient amount of fruits and vegetables while staying within energy needs.
- Choose a variety of fruits and vegetables each day.
- Consume 3 or more ounce equivalents of whole-grain products per day.
- Consume 3 cups per day of fat-free or low-fat milk or equivalent milk products.

Fats
- Consume less than 10% of calories from saturated fatty acids and less than 300 mg/day of cholesterol.
- Keep total fat intake between 20% and 35% of calories, with most fats coming from sources of polyunsaturated and monounsaturated fatty acids.
- When selecting and preparing meat, poultry, dry beans, and milk or milk products, make choices that are lean, low-fat, or fat-free.
- Limit intake of fats and oils high in saturated and/or trans fatty acids, and choose products low in such fats and oils.

Carbohydrates
- Choose fiber-rich fruits, vegetables, and whole grains often.
- Choose and prepare foods and beverages with little added sugars or caloric sweeteners.
- Reduce the incidence of dental caries by practicing good oral hygiene and consuming sugar- and starch-containing foods and beverages less frequently.

Sodium and Potassium
- Consume less than 2,300 mg (approximately 1 teaspoon of salt) of sodium per day.
- Choose and prepare foods with little salt.

Alcoholic Beverages
- Those who choose to drink alcoholic beverages should do so sensibly and in moderation—defined as the consumption of up to one drink per day for women and up to two drinks per day for men.
- Alcoholic beverages should not be consumed by some individuals, including those who cannot restrict their alcohol intake, women of childbearing age who may become pregnant, pregnant and lactating women, children and adolescents, individuals taking medications that can interact with alcohol, and those with specific medical conditions.
- Alcoholic beverages should be avoided by individuals engaging in activities that require attention, skill, or coordination, such as driving or operating machinery.

Food Safety
- To avoid microbial foodborne illness:
  - Clean hands, food contact surfaces, and fruits and vegetables. Meat and poultry should not be washed or rinsed.
  - Separate raw, cooked, and ready-to-eat foods while shopping, preparing, or storing foods.
  - Cook foods to a safe temperature to kill microorganisms.
  - Chill (refrigerate) perishable food promptly and defrost foods properly.
  - Avoid raw (unpasteurized) milk or any products made from unpasteurized milk, raw or partially cooked eggs or foods containing raw eggs, raw or undercooked meat and poultry, unpasteurized juices, and raw sprouts.

Source: Food and Nutrition Board, 2006.[6]

■ Table 14-3 Body Mass Index (BMI)

To use the table, find the appropriate height in the left-hand column labeled "Height." Move across to a given weight. The number at the top of the column is the BMI at that height and weight. Pounds have been rounded off.

BMI	19	20	21	22	23	24	25	26	27	28	29	30	31	32	33	34	35
Height (inches)									**Body Weight (pounds)**								
58	91	96	100	105	110	115	119	124	129	134	138	143	148	153	158	162	167
59	94	99	104	109	114	119	124	128	133	138	143	148	153	158	163	168	173
60	97	102	107	112	118	123	128	133	138	143	148	153	158	163	168	174	179
61	100	106	111	116	122	127	132	137	143	148	153	158	164	169	174	180	185
62	104	109	115	120	126	131	136	142	147	153	158	164	169	175	180	186	191
63	107	113	118	124	130	135	141	146	152	158	163	169	175	180	186	191	197
64	110	116	122	128	134	140	145	151	157	163	169	174	180	186	192	197	204
65	114	120	126	132	138	144	150	156	162	168	174	180	186	192	198	204	210
66	118	124	130	136	142	148	155	161	167	173	179	186	192	198	204	210	216
67	121	127	134	140	146	153	159	166	172	178	185	191	198	204	211	217	223
68	125	131	138	144	151	158	164	171	177	184	190	197	203	210	216	223	230
69	128	135	142	149	155	162	169	176	182	189	196	203	209	216	223	230	236
70	132	139	146	153	160	167	174	181	188	195	202	209	216	222	229	236	243
71	136	143	150	157	165	172	179	186	193	200	208	215	222	229	236	243	250
72	140	147	154	162	169	177	184	191	199	206	213	221	228	235	242	250	258
73	144	151	159	166	174	182	189	197	204	212	219	227	235	242	250	257	265
74	148	155	163	171	179	186	194	202	210	218	225	233	241	249	256	264	272
75	152	160	168	176	184	192	200	208	216	224	232	240	248	256	264	272	279
76	156	164	172	180	189	197	205	213	221	230	238	246	254	263	271	279	287

Source: www.cdc.gov/nccdphp/dnpa/bmi/adult_BMI/about_adult_BMI.htm

disease.[9] The waist circumference serves as an approximation of abdominal fat and may be predictive of an increased health risk when the BMI is in the normal range. High-risk waist circumferences are greater than 40 inches for men and 35 inches for women.[10]

MyPyramid

MyPyramid is based on the dietary guidelines and the DRIs. It translates this information into a diet that meets individual nutrition needs and urges moderation of dietary components that are commonly consumed in excess.[11] MyPyramid remains a pyramid symbol with the six food categories depicted as vertical bands rather than the horizontal bands that were used in the previous **Food Guide Pyramid.** The major addition to the new pyramid is the symbol depicting a person climbing the

side of the pyramid to indicate the need for being physically active every day (Figure 14–2 ■). As in previous nutrition guidelines, foods are grouped according to similar nutrient composition. The food groups are represented by different colors to indicate variety. The food categories are whole grains, vegetables, fruits, oils, milk, and meats and beans. Variety is essential to ensure adequate nutrition, because each group provides some, but not all, essential nutrients. The width of the food group bands is meant to indicate proportionality, which refers to how much food a person should choose from each food group. It is recommended that people eat more of some foods (fruits, vegetables, whole grains, and fat-free or low-fat milk products) and less of other foods (saturated and trans fats, added sugars, cholesterol, salt, and alcohol).[11] Rather than providing specific numbers of servings, MyPyramid directs people to

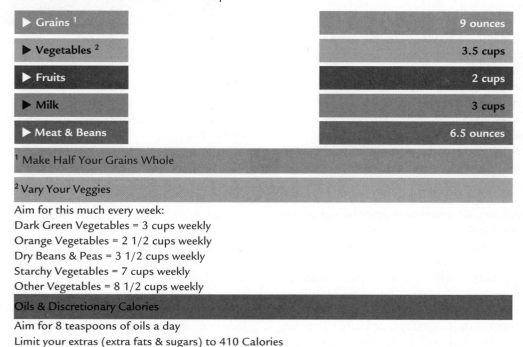

Based on the information you provided and the average needs for your age, gender and physical activity [Age: 45, Sex: male, Physical Activity: 30 to 60 Minutes] your results indicate that you should eat these amounts from the following food groups daily.

Your results are based on a 2600 calorie pattern*.

▶ Grains [1]	9 ounces
▶ Vegetables [2]	3.5 cups
▶ Fruits	2 cups
▶ Milk	3 cups
▶ Meat & Beans	6.5 ounces

[1] Make Half Your Grains Whole

[2] Vary Your Veggies

Aim for this much every week:
Dark Green Vegetables = 3 cups weekly
Orange Vegetables = 2 1/2 cups weekly
Dry Beans & Peas = 3 1/2 cups weekly
Starchy Vegetables = 7 cups weekly
Other Vegetables = 8 1/2 cups weekly

Oils & Discretionary Calories

Aim for 8 teaspoons of oils a day
Limit your extras (extra fats & sugars) to 410 Calories

*This calorie level is only an estimate of your needs. Monitor your body weight to see if you need to adjust your calorie intake.

■ **FIGURE 14–2** MyPyramid: A Guide to Daily Food Choices is a guide for healthy eating.
(From U.S. Department of Agriculture, 2005.[13])

the MyPyramid.gov Web site for personalized recommendations. (Figure 14–2) The narrowing of the band as it approaches the peak of the pyramid is meant to symbolize moderation. The narrowest part of each band indicates foods that should be minimized because they contain more added sugars and fat. The slogan "Steps to a Healthier You" encourages gradual improvement in diet and lifestyle each day (Table 14–4 ■, Figure 14–3 ■).[11]

Food Labels

The **Nutrition Facts** panel found on most processed food packages helps the consumer select foods that meet the dietary guidelines (Figure 14–4 ■). The **National Labeling and Education Act of 1990** requires that comprehensive nutrition information must appear on the labels of most processed foods, processed meats, and poultry products. In addition, nutrition information at point of purchase is voluntary for fresh fruits, vegetables, and raw fish. In accordance with the most recent mandatory food labeling regulations published by the Food and Drug Administration (FDA) January 1, 2006,[12] the nutrition panel on processed foods must include the following:

- A standardized serving size (designed to make nutritional comparisons of similar products easier, and reflecting the serving sizes that people actually eat).
- The number of servings per container.
- The amounts of total calories and calories from fat per serving.
- The number of grams per serving of total fat, saturated fat, trans fat, cholesterol, sodium, total carbohydrates, dietary fiber, sugars, and protein.

In addition, the nutritional contribution of one serving of the product must be stated as a percentage of the **Daily Values.** These values are based on the RDA for protein, vitamins, and minerals, and on standards designed especially for food labels for nutrients not covered in the RDA such as fat, cholesterol, total carbohydrates, dietary fiber, and sodium. The calculations to determine the percentages of Daily Values are based on a 2,000-calorie diet. Depending on a person's age, gender, and activity level, a person may need more or less than 100% of a Daily Value. The Daily Value

■ **Table 14–4** Tips to Get Started

- Make half your grains whole.
- Vary your veggies.
- Focus on fruit.
- Get your calcium-rich foods.
- Go lean with protein.
- Find your balance between food and physical activity.

Source: U.S. Department of Health and Human Services, October 2000.[10]

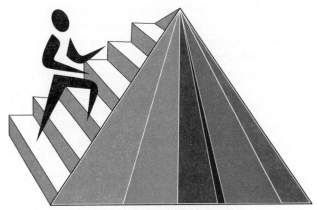

■ **FIGURE 14–3** Sample MyPyramid Recommendations
(From U.S. Department of Agriculture, 2005.[13])

also helps consumers see how a food fits into an overall daily diet.

Other information, such as the amounts of polyunsaturated or monounsaturated fats or other vitamins and minerals, is optional. In addition, descriptors such as "free," "low," "high," "light," "lean," or "reduced" may be used on the label as long as a standard portion meets defined criteria. For example, to be labeled "low-calorie" a serving must have no more than 40 calories. To be labeled "low-fat," no more than 3 grams of fat per serving is allowed.

A health claim, by definition, demonstrates scientific evidence about a substance that may include a food, food component, or dietary ingredient and a disease or health-related condition. There are currently two categories of health claims: health claims with **significant scientific agreement (SSA)** and **qualified health**

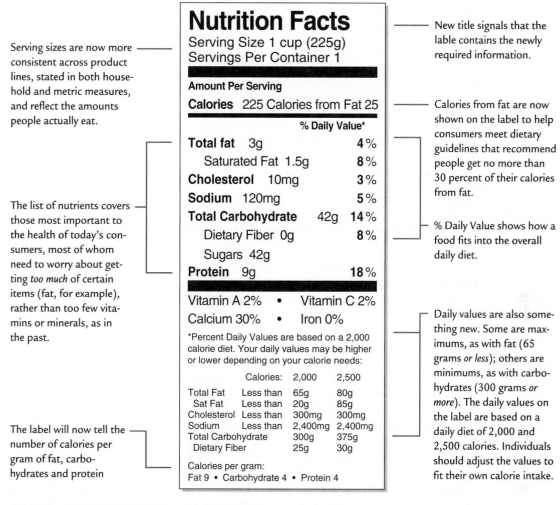

Serving sizes are now more consistent across product lines, stated in both household and metric measures, and reflect the amounts people actually eat.

The list of nutrients covers those most important to the health of today's consumers, most of whom need to worry about getting *too much* of certain items (fat, for example), rather than too few vitamins or minerals, as in the past.

The label will now tell the number of calories per gram of fat, carbohydrates and protein

Nutrition Facts
Serving Size 1 cup (225g)
Servings Per Container 1

Amount Per Serving

Calories   225 Calories from Fat 25

                                    % Daily Value*

Total fat   3g   **4**%
     Saturated Fat 1.5g   **8**%
Cholesterol   10mg   **3**%
Sodium   120mg   **5**%
Total Carbohydrate   42g   **14**%
     Dietary Fiber 0g   **8**%
     Sugars 42g
Protein   9g   **18**%

Vitamin A 2%   •   Vitamin C 2%
Calcium 30%   •   Iron 0%

*Percent Daily Values are based on a 2,000 calorie diet. Your daily values may be higher or lower depending on your calorie needs:

		Calories:	2,000	2,500
Total Fat	Less than		65g	80g
Sat Fat	Less than		20g	85g
Cholesterol	Less than		300mg	300mg
Sodium	Less than		2,400mg	2,400mg
Total Carbohydrate			300g	375g
Dietary Fiber			25g	30g

Calories per gram:
Fat 9 • Carbohydrate 4 • Protein 4

New title signals that the lable contains the newly required information.

Calories from fat are now shown on the label to help consumers meet dietary guidelines that recommend people get no more than 30 percent of their calories from fat.

% Daily Value shows how a food fits into the overall daily diet.

Daily values are also something new. Some are maximums, as with fat (65 grams *or less*); others are minimums, as with carbohydrates (300 grams *or more*). The daily values on the label are based on a daily diet of 2,000 and 2,500 calories. Individuals should adjust the values to fit their own calorie intake.

*This label is only a sample. Exact specifications are in the final rules.
Source: Food and Drug Administration 1992.

■ **FIGURE 14–4**   Food label.

claims. Significant scientific agreements are supported by significant scientific evidence with widespread agreement between different studies and researchers.[13] These claims undergo rigorous review and are approved by the FDA. The qualified health claims also rely on scientific evidence, but the evidence does not have to be as strong as that required for SSAs. Qualified health claims differ from SSAs in that they must be accompanied by a disclaimer.[13] Current health claims with SSA that are allowed to be placed on food labels are shown in (Table 14–5 ■).[13] As of October 14, 2006, a health claim for the use of fluoridated water to reduce the risk of dental caries was approved.

NUTRITIONAL FACTORS AFFECTING THE ORAL CAVITY

Nutrition plays an important role in the initial growth and development of oral tissues and in their continuous integrity through the lifespan. **Optimal nutrition** during periods of hard and soft tissue development allow these tissues to reach their optimal potential for growth and

■ **Table 14–5** Health Claims Allowed on Food Labels

1. Calcium and osteoporosis
2. Dietary lipids (fat) and cancer
3. Dietary saturated fat, cholesterol and coronary heart disease (CHD)
4. Dietary non-cariogenic carbohydrate sweeteners and dental caries
5. Fiber-containing grain products, fruits, and vegetables and cancer
6. Folic acid and neural tube defects
7. Fruits and vegetables and cancer
8. Fruits, vegetables, and grain products that contain fiber, particularly soluble fiber, and the risk for CHD
9. Sodium and hypertension
10. Soluble fiber from certain foods and risk of heart disease
11. Soy protein and CHD
12. Sterols and plant stanol esters and risk of CHD
13. Fluoridated water and reduced risk of dental caries

Source: Food and Drug Administration.[13]

resistance to disease. **Malnutrition,** either over- or under-nutrition, during critical periods of organogenesis can have irreversible effects on developing tissues. Examples of this effect can be seen in the tetracycline staining of teeth, dental fluorosis, enamel defects in children born prematurely, and the fever-induced enamel hypoplasia seen in the primary teeth.[14,15] In the dentition, malnutrition is less well documented in humans than in animals, but it appears that, during the "critical periods," malnutrition can result in dentition with increased caries susceptibility.[16] Malnutrition after initial organ and tissue development is usually reversible, but can still compromise tissue regeneration and healing and increase susceptibility to oral diseases. Nutrients for which deficiencies or excesses have been directly associated with oral conditions are calories; protein; calcium; phosphorus; vitamins C, A, and D; iodine; and fluoride. A summary of the oral symptoms of nutrient deficiencies can be found in (Table 14–6 ■).

Protein/Calorie Malnutrition

Protein, the most abundant organic compound in the body, is required for the synthesis of virtually all body tissues and structures. Proteins account for the structure of DNA, the tensile strength of collagen, and the viscosity of saliva. Thus, aberrations in protein nutrition can have far-reaching oral and systemic effects.

The normal turnover of epithelial tissue in the oral cavity requires a continual supply of nutrients. For example, every 3 to 6 days, the basal epithelium of the gingiva undergoes renewal.[17] Thus, any severe deficiency of protein/calorie intake will result in a decrease in mitotic activity in the crevicular epithelium, as well as elsewhere throughout the body.[18] In a comparison of periodontal involvement in patients with severe malnutrition, kwashiorkor, with that of healthy controls in South India, fewer caries and more periodontal diseases were found among the undernourished group.[19] Because the oral hygiene indices of both groups were similar, it was assumed that the difference was due to nutritional factors. It should be noted that any malnutrition of the severity of kwashiorkor represents a multi-nutrient deficiency. Impaired protein synthesis has been found if protein malnutrition occurs during the developmental stage in animals.[20] In animal models, short-term (4 days) fasting resulted in a 40% reduction in collagen production.[21] In the same study, a 10% decrease in collagen synthesis was noted with a reduced dietary intake meeting 20% of requirements.[21] These findings suggest that even short-term states of undernutrition may impact collagen synthesis.

In chronically malnourished children, several studies have shown delays in tooth eruption patterns and increased tooth enamel solubility, leading to increased caries susceptibility.[22–28]

The linear hypoplasia reported in the enamel of primary teeth of children in underprivileged populations is thought to contribute to their high prevalence of dental caries. This type of hypoplasia appears to be related to the severity of the malnutrition.[29]

With the exception of the cleansing and diluting effects of saliva, oral defense mechanisms depend on an adequate supply of proteins. The glycoproteins that result in aggregation of bacteria arise from the salivary

■ **Table 14–6** Oral Symptoms of Nutrient Deficiencies

Nutrient	Oral Symptom of Deficiency	Dietary Considerations
Riboflavin (vitamin B_2) or iron	Cheilosis or angular stomatitis	• Rule out other etiology • Palliative treatment • Refer to MD/RD for treatment with diet modifications and/or supplements
Riboflavin (vitamin B_2) or iron	Glossitis (magenta tongue)	• Rule out other etiology • Palliative treatment • Refer to MD/RD for treatment with diet modifications and/or supplements
Niacin (vitamin B_3) or vitamin B_{12}	Bright red, sore tongue	• Rule out other etiology • Palliative treatment • Refer to MD/RD for diet modifications: avoiding spicy or acidic foods, eating foods at room temperature, eating nutrient and energy-dense foods that are soft and moist
Riboflavin	Hyperemia and edema of the pharyngeal and oral mucous membranes	• Rule out other etiology • Refer to MD/RD for treatment with diet modifications and/or supplements
Folate	Atrophic glossitis	• Rule out other etiology • Refer to MD/RD for treatment with diet modifications and/or supplements
Biotin	Red, scaly, skin rash, frequently around the eyes, nose, and mouth (rare)	• Rule out other etiology • Refer to MD/RD for treatment with diet modifications and/or supplements
Vitamin C	Inflamed, bleeding gingiva and impaired wound healing (symptoms of scurvy, which is rare in the United States)	• Rule out other etiology • Treat with diet modifications and/or supplements
Vitamin A	Changes in taste	• Rule out other etiology • Refer to MD/RD for treatment with diet modifications to include nutrient and energy-dense foods and/or supplements • Avoid foods that may cause aversion
Iron	Esophageal webs that may result in dysphagia	• Rule out other etiology • Palliative treatment • Refer to MD/RD for treatment with diet modifications to include iron-rich foods and/or supplements

MD, physician; RD, registered dietitian.
Source: Food and Nutrition Board, 2006;[8] deMenzes et al., 1984.[44]

glands. Lysozyme, salivary peroxidase, and lactoferrin are also glycoproteins. Secretory immunoglobulin A (sIgA) arises mainly from the labial and buccal glands.[30] The cell types involved in cellular immunity, polymorphonuclear lymphocytes and macrophages as well as the enzymes used in phagocytosis, also require protein for their production.[31]

Probably one of the most deleterious effects of protein/calorie deficiency is the *depletion of the cellular and immuno-cellular defenses* of both the oral and the connective sides of the barrier epithelial cells lining the gingival crevice. In general, the severity of the impaired immunologic response parallels the severity of the protein or calorie deficiency.[31] Chronic undernutrition may also compromise cytokine response and affect immune cell function. In other words, undernutrition may impact immune response tissue regeneration, and response to insult or infection.[32]

Minerals

Calcium, in association with **vitamin D and phosphorus,** is essential for proper development and maintenance of mineralized tissues, especially teeth and alveolar bone. A deficiency of these nutrients during critical phases of tooth development in children results in **hypomineralization** of developing teeth and possible delayed eruption patterns.[33] The rate of enamel hypoplasia in primary teeth in children born prematurely is more than threefold that of children born at term.[33] In addition, the rate of enamel hypoplasia in permanent teeth in these children is more than twofold that of controls.[33] Preterm infants miss the intrauterine period when 80% of the body calcium, phosphorus, and magnesium are accumulated. As a result, these infants have much higher requirements for calcium and phosphorus.[34,35] In addition, very low birthweight infants have immature kidneys and may not metabolize adequate levels of vitamin D, further impairing tooth development.[35]

Iron is of interest because iron deficiency is the most common nutrient deficiency in the United States. **Iron deficiency anemia** manifests in the oral cavity as pallor of oral tissues, especially the tongue. The tongue may appear shiny, with blunted filiform papillae. The effects of iron deficiency on mineralized tissues are less clear. In rats, even a marginal deficiency of iron in the diet predisposes the rats to caries.[36] Conversely, supplementing a caries-promoting diet with iron produced a major reduction in caries, with the greatest effect shown in the neonatal period.[36] In addition, iron serves as a cofactor with ascorbic acid in collagen synthesis, as does copper.[37]

Zinc regulates function in inflammation by inhibiting the release of lysosomal enzymes and histamines. A **zinc deficiency** can inhibit collagen formation and reduce cell-mediated immunity.[38–40] Zinc deficiency can also result in delayed wound healing, defective keratinization of epithelial cells, epithelial thickening, atrophic oral mucosa, and xerostomia. In addition, zinc is essential for

taste and odor sensitivity. Declines in taste experienced by many elders may be a result of zinc deficiency. The effect of zinc in modifying periodontal defense mechanisms has been shown in rabbits, but has yet to be clearly delineated in humans.[40,41]

Vitamins

Vitamin A is essential for the development and continued integrity of all body organs and tissues, including the epithelial mucosa of the oral cavity. In **vitamin A deficiency,** cell differentiation is impaired. The result is defective tissue formation and impaired healing. Vitamin A deficiency also results in impairment of both specific and nonspecific immuno-protective mechanisms. Deficiency can affect tissue response to bacterial infection, mucosal immunity, parasitic and viral infection, activity of natural killer cells, and phagocytosis.[41] Vitamin A toxicity can show similar effects, with impaired healing response being the most direct affect in the oral cavity.[39] Other effects include proliferation of oral epithelium, reduction of the keratin layer, thickening of the basal membrane, and increase in the granular layer.

In a case report, a patient who took 200,000 IU of vitamin A daily for over 6 months presented with painful gingival lesions, along with nausea, vomiting, xerostomia, and headaches. Clinical examination revealed gingival erosions, ulcerations, bleeding, swelling, loss of keratinization, color changes, and desquamation of the lips.[42] All pathologic manifestations disappeared within 2 months of the elimination of the vitamin A supplements without a change in oral hygiene habits.

In addition to the effects of high levels of vitamin A intake on soft tissue, a review of twenty studies demonstrates that high doses of vitamin A may result in an increased risk for hip fracture.[43] Whether this effect may impact alveolar bone health is unclear, but it is an area requiring further research.

Vitamin C, ascorbic acid, is essential to oral health. Synthesis of hydroxyproline, an essential component of collagen, requires ascorbic acid. Defects in collagen synthesis are responsible for the many manifestations of **vitamin C deficiency** called scurvy. Signs of scurvy in the oral cavity include spontaneous bleeding, infusions of blood into interdental papillae, loosening and exfoliation of teeth, detachment of oral epithelial tissue, and impaired wound healing (Figure 14–5 ■).

The effects of vitamin C deficiency are best studied in animal models in which all factors can be controlled.[44]

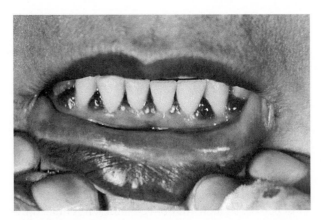

■ FIGURE 14–5 Scurvy.

Acute scurvy was produced by placing monkeys on a vitamin C deficient diet for 12 weeks. The hydroxyproline content of the gingiva started to decline in the first four weeks and occurred at a faster rate than in skin. By the end of the eighth week, the synthesis of hydroxyproline was totally impaired. The results were extensive gingival pocket formation and tooth mobility due to degradation of the collagen making up periodontal ligament fibers.

Although frank scurvy is rare, even marginal deficiencies may result in alterations in collagen synthesis (Figure 14–5). Thus deficient or marginal ascorbic acid intakes may be a conditioning factor in the development of gingivitis and one of the early manifestations of vitamin C deficiency.[45] The most recent epidemiologic data from the Third National Health and Nutrition Examination Survey (NHANES III) suggest that the odds of having periodontal disease are 1.2 times greater in those with low dietary vitamin C intakes.[46] In the same study, smokers and former smokers with low vitamin C intake are at 1.6 times greater risk of having periodontal disease.[46] In a recent clinical study, patients with periodontitis were found to have lower plasma vitamin C levels than healthy controls. After grapefruit consumption by patients with periodontitis, plasma vitamin C levels rose and bleeding scores improved.[47] Research findings suggest that people with marginal vitamin C deficiency supplemented with ascorbic acid have a statistically significant increase in hydroxyproline in periodontal tissues.[48]

Ascorbic acid is essential to immune-related functions, such as resistance to oral infection, via its role in leukocyte formation and subsequent phagocytosis. In addition, vitamin C protects the integrity of cells from damage during the oxidative stress that occurs during the inflammatory response. Therefore, during infections and stress, vitamin C levels in the plasma and leukocytes decline rapidly.[49]

Conversely, chronic vitamin C excess may precipitate a scurvy-like condition (rebound scurvy) upon cessation of the vitamin. Because the impact of deficient levels of vitamin C is first observed in gingival tissues, dentists and dental hygienists in clinical practice may be the first to diagnose the phenomenon.[50]

The **B-complex vitamins** primarily function as coenzymes in energy metabolism. B-complex vitamins are found widely in foods, and are usually found together. With the exception of B_{12} in the elderly and folic acid in pregnant women, deficiencies of single B vitamins are uncommon (except in alcoholics). The Dietary Guidelines for Americans 2005 provides specific recommendations for people older than 50 years to consume vitamin B_{12} in its crystalline form (i.e., fortified foods or supplements) because of a reduced ability to absorb naturally occurring vitamin B_{12}.[7] Oral signs and symptoms of B-complex vitamin deficiencies include cracks in the corners of the mouth referred to as cheilosis, and inflammation, burning, redness, pain and swelling of the tongue.[51]

DIET AND ENAMEL DEMINERALIZATION

Dental demineralization can result from excessive toothbrushing, regurgitation of stomach acid, as in the eating disorder bulimia, or from excessive consumption of acid-containing foods or beverages. The demineralizing effect of acid from the diet is magnified in the presence of xerostomia, because saliva helps to neutralize acids and remove them from the oral cavity.

Dietary sources of acid may include citrus fruits and juices, acidogenic sports drinks, snacks containing citrus acid, carbonated beverages, chewable vitamin C tablets, or excessive regurgitation of gastric contents into the mouth.[52–56] Recently, attention has been focused on the constant use of carbonated beverages, both regular and diet. Both contain acids and are possible contributors to an increase in enamel demineralization, leading to dental caries in young people.[57] It is important to differentiate this type of erosion or demineralization from the caries process in which acid produced from plaque bacteria causes the enamel demineralization.

DIET AND DENTAL CARIES
Role of Carbohydrates

Dental caries is a diet-related, infectious, and transmissible disease that is strongly affected by diet. *Streptococcus mutans* are the predominant oral bacteria that initiate the caries process. Development of clinical caries is contingent upon the interaction of three local factors in the mouth: *a susceptible tooth, cariogenic bacteria, and fermentable carbohydrate.* Newly erupted teeth with a thin enamel layer, like those found in many children born prematurely, are very susceptible to caries. Tooth morphology, especially the presence of deep pits and fissures, influences the likelihood that mutans streptococci will attach to and colonize the tooth's surface. Plaque bacteria ferment starches and sugars, producing organic acids. These acids demineralize dental enamel.[58]

Other dietary factors counteract the damaging effects of carbohydrates. The presence of protective minerals and ions, such as fluoride, calcium, and phosphorus in plaque and saliva, promote remineralization of incipient lesions. In addition to transporting minerals, saliva contains buffering agents, bicarbonate and phosphates, which neutralize organic acids. Thus, the amount and composition of saliva affect the caries process. Other host factors that influence caries risk include genetic predisposition, immune status, malnutrition during tooth formation, education level, and income status.

In the most recent national health and nutrition examination survey (NHANES III, phase I) 94% of adults showed evidence of coronal caries and 22.5% of adults had root caries.[59] In the same survey, 25% of the children and teens aged 5 to 17 years had 80% of the dental caries detected in the permanent teeth.[60] For these caries-prone children and adults, nutrition counseling about the damaging effects of fermentable carbohydrates on teeth is essential.

Through epidemiologic and clinical studies, the causal relationship between sugar consumption and dental caries has been established. Animal studies suggest that an increase in the concentration of sucrose in the diet reduces dental plaque formation and increases the incidence of dental caries.[61,62] People with very low sugar intakes have low caries scores. People in nations that have high sugar intakes have high rates of caries.[63] Sucrose plays a more dominant role than other sugars in the development of smooth-surface caries, because not only can it be fermented by oral bacteria but, unlike the other simple sugars, it is a substrate for mutans streptococcus synthesis of intracellular and extracellular polysaccharides.[64] Extra-cellular dextran, a storage form of sugar, allows for continued acid formation even when eating and drinking are not occurring. One of these extracellular polysaccharides is called glucan; it enables the *Streptococcus mutans* to adhere to the smooth enamel surfaces and contributes to the structural integrity of plaque biofilm.[64] It also appears that the plaque biofilm formed in relation to sucrose intake contains low concentrations of calcium, phosphorus, and fluoride, which are critical elements in the demineralization and remineralization of the tooth surface, and may further increase sucrose's cariogenic potential.[64]

Although the consumption of sugars is high among most persons in industrialized countries, it is more difficult to demonstrate a correlation between caries prevalence and the amount of sugar consumed in these countries than in developing countries where sugar intake is lower. Three recent clinical trials of UK, United States, and Canadian schoolchildren examined the relationship between sugar intake and dental caries. In England, 405 children with a mean age of 11.6 years were followed for 2 years. Total sugar intake of 118 grams per day, or 21% of total calorie intake, had the highest significant correlation with caries rates.[65] Intake of sugary foods before bedtime was highly correlated with caries incidence. In the United States, 499 children, aged 11 to 15 years and living in non-fluoridated rural Michigan communities, were followed for 3 years. The average increase in decayed, missing, and filled surfaces over the 3 years was 3.1 in girls and 2.7 for boys.[66] The daily average sugar intake was 142 grams, which represented 26.5% of their total energy intake.[66] Children who obtained a higher percentage of their total calories from sugars had more proximal surface caries. The average number of eating occasions and the number of sugary between-meal snacks consumed were not related to caries increment in these studies.[66]

Fifty percent of 232 11-year-old children in a Canadian study had inadequate diets. Children with superior diets tended to develop fewer caries; however, the association was not statistically significant.[67] Differences in eating patterns and intake of caries-promoting foods among the children in these studies may have been too small to result in significant differences in caries experience.

Caries has declined in Western countries in recent years. Factors thought to contribute to this decline include fluoride intake from water, the use of fluoridated dentifrices, improved plaque control, the use of dental sealants, and more frequent visits to a dental provider.[68]

The use of sugar alcohols and alternative sweeteners in foods has played a role in reducing caries. Perhaps one of the most promising sugar substitutes to be studied is xylitol, a sugar alcohol that has been demonstrated to be non-cariogenic as well as a promotor of remineralization.[69] Xylitol's ability to inhibit metabolic acid production by mutans streptococci results in minimal depression of plaque pH. Maintenance of the plaque pH close to the saliva pH also fosters remineralization of teeth.[70] In addition, the substitution of xylitol for fermentable sugars in the diet results in a less-cariogenic bacterial flora. The importance of other non-fermentable sweeteners in caries control is detailed in Chapter 15.

Simple sugars are not the only carbohydrate that influences the development of a carious lesion. Highly refined, cooked starch–sugar combinations such as doughnuts, cookies, potato chips, and some ready-to-eat breakfast cereals produce a prolonged acidogenic response when retained in interproximal spaces.[71] When starches are cooked, they are partially degraded, which allows the salivary alpha-amylase to convert starch particles retained on the tongue, oral mucosa, and teeth to maltose. Making maltose available to plaque bacteria extends the length of time that plaque pH will remain low and permit enamel demineralization to occur. Thus, retentive high-starch foods may be more acidogenic than high-sugar, low-starch foods that are rapidly eliminated from the mouth.[72]

Effects of Eating Patterns and Physical Form of Foods

Other dietary factors that may hinder or enhance caries development include the frequency of eating, the **physical form** of the carbohydrate (liquid versus solid), **retentiveness** of a food on the tooth surface, the **sequence** in which foods are consumed (e.g., cheese eaten before a sweet food limits the pH drop), and the presence of minerals in a food.

Frequent between-meal snacking on sugar or processed starch-containing foods increases plaque formation and extends the length of time that bacterial acid production can occur. When total daily sugar intake was held constant, increasing the frequency of sugar intake for groups of rats resulted in increased number of *Streptococcus mutans* in plaque and the amount of caries experienced.[73] The positive relationship between frequency of sugar intake and caries in humans was first demonstrated in the Vipeholm study.[74] Subjects who consumed candies between meals developed more caries than those who were fed equal amounts of sugars with meals. Frequent snacking between meals keeps the plaque pH

low and extends the time for enamel and dentin demineralization to occur.

Bacterial fermentation can continue as long as carbohydrate adheres to the enamel and exposed dentinal tooth surfaces. Even though starchy foods vary in their cariogenic potential, the highly refined starchy foods, such as soft bread and potato chips, which are retained on tooth surfaces for prolonged periods of time, result in a lowered pH that may last up to 60 minutes.[72,75] High-sucrose confectionery foods deliver high levels of sugar to the oral bacteria immediately after the foods are consumed, whereas high-starch foods deliver progressively increasing concentrations of sugars over a considerably longer period of time.

The sequence in which foods are eaten affects how much the plaque pH falls and how long it remains depressed. Sugared coffee consumed at the end of a meal will cause the plaque pH to remain low for a longer time than when an unsweetened food is eaten following intake of sugared coffee.[76] If peanuts are eaten before or after sugar-containing foods, the plaque pH is less depressed.[77]

Caries-Protective Foods and Nutrients

Some components of foods are **protective** against dental caries. Protein, fat, phosphorus, and calcium inhibit caries in rats.[78,79] Aged natural cheeses have been shown to be cariostatic.[80] When cheese is eaten after a sucrose rinse, the plaque pH remains higher than when no cheese follows a sucrose rinse. In addition, enamel demineralization, measured using the intraoral cariogenicity test, is reduced. The protective effect of cheeses is attributed to their texture, which stimulates salivary flow, and their protein, calcium, and phosphate content, which neutralizes plaque acids. Many dairy products are now fortified with probiotic *Lactobacillus rhamnosus GG,* which has been shown to have an inhibitory affect on a wide range of bacteria including *Streptococcus* species.[81] Studies have demonstrated a 37% to 56% reduction in caries risk with short- and long-term exposure, respectively, to these probiotic dairy products.[81,82] Fluoride found in drinking water, foods, and dentifrices increase a tooth's resistance to demineralization and enhance remineralization of carious lesions.

Lipids seem to accelerate oral clearance of food particles. Some fatty acids, linoleic and oleic, in low concentration, inhibit growth of mutans streptococcus. Lectins, proteins found in plants, appear to interfere with microbial colonization and may affect salivary function.[83]

Measuring the Cariogenic Potential of Foods

Because it is unethical to conduct human experiments to measure the true cariogenic potential of foods, other indirect tests have been developed. These tests enable researchers to classify foods into at least three categories: protective, low, and high cariogenic potential. Currently the cariogenic potential or the ability to induce caries in humans may be assessed indirectly by measuring the ability of a test food to cause caries formation in animals, acid production in dental plaque, or demineralization of enamel.[1]

Animal studies have been conducted using a programmed feeding machine. In one study, 20 common snack foods were presented to rats at specified intervals during the day.[84] After sulcal and smooth-surface caries were scored in the animals, **cariogenic potential indices** (CPIs) were computed for each food. The sucrose group had a CPI value of 1 (Table 14–7 ■). A food with a CPI of 0.4 had low cariogenic potential. Those snack foods with high cariogenic potential had 1% or more hydrolyzable starch in combination with sucrose or other sugars.

Acid production in the mouth during bacterial fermentation of a food is predictive of the contribution of that food to the caries process. Measurement of plaque acidogenicity can be measured by determining the pH of a plaque sample taken from the mouth or in situ.[1] Foods that cause the plaque pH to fall below the critical demineralization level (pH 5.5–5.0) are considered acidogenic. Measurement of oral plaque pH requires placement of a wire-telemetric appliance containing a pH microelectrode in the space where a tooth is missing in the mouth. As the test food is chewed, the pH under undisturbed plaque at the site of the indwelling electrode is continually transmitted to an external receiver. The rate of the fall and rise of the pH at an interproximal site can be recorded continuously by plaque telemetry. Foods found to have low acidogenic potential using this method include aged cheeses, some vegetables, meats, fish, and nuts.[85] To assess the ability of a food to demineralize dental enamel, investigators developed an intraoral cariogenicity. Bovine or human

■ **Table 14–7**   Cariogenic Potential of Foods in Animal Models[79]

Foods	Caries Potential Index	
	Buccal	*Sulcal*
Raisins	1.3	0.95
Bananas	1.2	1.17
French fried (chips)	1.2	0.98
Granola (a breakfast cereal)	1.1	0.64
Sucrose	**1.0**	**1.0**
Bread	0.82	0.90
Grahams (digestive biscuits)	0.66	0.79
Cupcakes	0.62	1.73
Chocolate	0.59	0.81
Cornstarch	0.47	0.76
Sponge cake	0.44	0.95
Rye crackers	0.36	0.86
Saltines (savory crackers)	0.36	0.69
Peanuts	0.30	0.43
Pretzels	0.21	0.77
Jello (fruit jelly)	0.11	0.43
Yogurt	0.11	0.65
Corn chips	0.10	0.54

Source: Adapted from Mundorff SA, Featherstone JDB, Eisenberg AD, et al. Cariogenicity of foods: Rat study. *J Dent Res.* 64:(special issue) 1985; 294. Abstract 1071.

dental enamel slabs are imbedded in a prosthesis and placed in the mouth where a tooth is missing. After ingesting a test food, changes in surface micro-hardness or enamel porosity are determined.[86] Because each test measures a different aspect of cariogenicity, foods will be ranked differently. It is recommended that two testing methods be used to determine food acidogenicity and cariogenicity potential.[87,88] (Table 14–8 ■) shows the acidogenic potential of foods. (Table 14–9 ■) provides diet suggestions for caries prevention.

NUTRITION AND PERIODONTAL DISEASES

Like caries, periodontal disease is an infectious disease, is multifactorial in etiology, and occurs when virulence of the bacterial challenge is greater than the host defense and repair capability. The course of periodontal disease involves periods of progression and remission. Unlike the direct causative relationship between carbohydrates and caries, nutritional factors seem to play a much more subtle role in periodontal status. Nutritional factors can alter host susceptibility to periodontal disease and/or modulate its progress.[89] The nutritional factors related to preventing infection and enhancing wound healing in general applies to the prevention and management of periodontal disease as well.[90] If both the challenge to, and the defense and repair capabilities of, the periodontal tissues are in balance, nutrition could be the deciding factor in whether health or disease results. Even when the periodontium is healthy, there is continual need for nutrients to maintain the tissues. Once inflammation is established, the need for nutrients increases. There is a close relationship between malnutrition and infection, with infection aggravating malnutrition and malnutrition abetting infection. Host defense in the gingival crevice and connective tissue requires an adequate intake of all nutrients to ensure adequate production and function of defense and supporting cells.[91–94] With the increased needs of cellular immunity and the additional demands by the tissue cells attempting to maintain and repair damaged areas, a greater supply of all nutrients is needed. This phenomenon has led to evidence showing that nutrient requirements may be higher at local sites of increased stress than in the rest of the body. Such localized challenges may result in end-organ nutrient deficiencies.[95,96] Epidemiologic research also indicates that increasing intake of whole grains may reduce the risk for periodontitis.[97]

■ **Table 14–8** Acidogenic Potential of Foods

Non- to Low-Acidogenic		Acidogenic
Raw vegetables, for example:	Lower	Cooked vegetables
Broccoli		Fresh fruits, especially bananas
Cauliflower		Fruit juices, fruit drinks
Cucumbers		Sweetened beverages
Lettuce		Nondairy creamers
Dill pickles		Sweetened canned or cooked fruits
Carrots		Ice cream, sherbet, pudding, gelatin, flavored
Peppers		yogurts
Meat, fish, poultry		Potato chips, pretzels
Beans, peas		Dried fruits, fruit rolls
Nuts, natural peanut butter		Marshmallows
Milk, cheeses		Starches: bread, rice, pasta, sweetened cereals
Popcorn		Cookies, cakes, pies, pastry
Fats, oils, butter, margarine		Crackers
Nonsugar sweeteners		Candy, especially slowly dissolving breath mints, cough drops
	Higher	

■ **Table 14–9** Diet Suggestions for Caries Prevention

Food Group	*Suggestions*
General	• Limit number of meals/snacks. • Avoid sticky or retentive foods.
Grains/cereals (3–8 ounce equivalents/day[a])	• Have whole grains. • Have popcorn for snacks. • Avoid crackers, donuts, potato chips between meals.
Fruits (1–2 cups/day)	• All fruits are fine: fresh, frozen, canned, juices. • Have fruits for dessert/snacks. • Avoid dried fruits or fruit roll-ups. • Do not sip slowly or often on fruit juices. • Avoid fruit drinks.
Vegetables (1–3 cups/day)	• All vegetables are fine: fresh, frozen, canned, juices, potatoes. • Limit sweetened salad dressings. • Have raw vegetables for snacks.
Protein (2–6 ounces/day)	• All proteins are fine: meat, fish, poultry, eggs, beans (lentils, etc.), tofu, nuts. • Have nuts for snacks.
Dairy[b] (2–3 cups/day)	• Have milk in coffee, soup. • Have cheese in sandwiches, casseroles, etc. • Have cheese for snacks.
Oils and sweets	• Avoid slowly dissolving candies. • Have sweets as dessert with a meal, not between meals. • Avoid constant sipping on sweet beverages (soda, sports drinks).
Other	• Have flavored club soda or diet soda. • Use sugar-free gum, preferably one containing xylitol. • Have water between meals and with snacks.

[a] 1 ounce equivalent = one slice of bread, 1 cup of cereal, or 1/2 cup cooked rice, pasta, or cereal.
[b] Aim for fat-free or low-fat products unless increased calories are indicated.

■ **Table 14–10** Dietary Suggestions for Patients with Periodontal Disease

• Eat a *nutritionally adequate diet* following the food pyramid guidelines.
• Increase the use of saliva-stimulating fibrous foods.
• Take multivitamin/mineral supplements in doses *no higher* than 1–2 times RDA levels.
• *Avoid fad diets:* they could be deficient in nutrients.
• Avoid *single-vitamin* supplements.
• *Avoid potentially detrimental megadoses* of vitamins and minerals (10 times RDA or higher).

RDA, Recommended Dietary Allowance.

Whenever routine scaling, prophylaxis, and oral plaque-control procedures fail to reverse gingivitis and before any treatment for periodontitis is attempted, a session involving thorough **diet evaluation** and **patient counseling** is indicated. The patient should be informed about the importance of systemic nutrition in the defense and repair of oral tissues. Recommendations should be made to help ensure optimal nutrition to help prevent and manage periodontal disease. These recommendation are listed in (Table 14–10 ■).

LIFESTYLE DIET AND ORAL HEALTH ISSUES

Early Childhood Caries

Early Childhood Caries (ECC), which used to be referred to as "**baby bottle tooth decay**" or "nursing caries" is defined as one or more decayed, missing (due to caries), or filled tooth surfaces in any primary tooth in a pre-school age child between birth and 71 months of age. **Severe Early Childhood Caries (S-ECC)** refers to a more severe pattern of progressive or rampant caries in pre-school children. Inappropriate feeding practices may result in progressive dental caries on the buccal and lingual surfaces of newly erupted primary maxillary anterior teeth of infants and toddlers. The overall prevalence of ECC in the NHANES, 1999–2002 is estimated to be 27.9%.[98] This value is an increase from 24.2% prevalence in the NHANES, 1988–1994.[97] However, a much higher prevalence has been seen among Alaskan and Oklahoma Native American children (53%), Navajo (72%), and Cherokee (55%) children attending Head Start programs.[99,100]

Primary risk factors for ECC include putting a child to sleep at naptime or bedtime with a bottle containing a liquid other than plain water, allowing an infant to breast-feed at will during the night, and extended use of the nursing bottle or sippy cup beyond 1 year of age. Results of the 1991 National Health Interview Survey show that 16.7% or 3.5 million children between 6 months and 5 years of age are put to sleep with a liquid in the bottle other than plain water.[101] Inappropriate feeding practices were reported more often by parents with less than a high school education, low annual family income, young maternal age, single-parent homes, Hispanic backgrounds, and those parents whose children had not been to a dentist in the past year.[102] Other risk factors for ECC include childhood illness and the use of liquid prescription medications with high-sucrose content, such as amoxicillin, for extended lengths of time.[102]

Children who develop maxillary anterior caries are at increased risk of developing posterior caries in the future.[103] To prevent early childhood caries, dentists, dental hygienists, pediatricians, and other health care professionals should ask parents about their infant-feeding practices. Those parents who report inappropriate feeding practices should receive counseling. Programs serving low-income families, such as the Special Supplemental Food Program for Women, Infants, and Children (WIC), can play a major role in providing education to parents at higher risk for using inappropriate feeding practices. (Table 14–11 ■) provides dietary recommendations to reduce the risk of EEC.

Eating Disorders

Eating disorders are often first diagnosed in the dental office because of the pain and discomfort caused by dental complications.[104] There are a number of types of eating disorders, but the primary types include anorexia nervosa, bulimia nervosa, and binge-eating disorder. The prevalence of anorexia nervosa and bulimia nervosa is estimated to be between 0.5% and 4.2% with 2% to 5% of Americans experiencing BED in a 6-month period.[105] Although females are largely afflicted with eating disorders, it is estimated that 5% to 15% of people with anorexia or bulimia and 35% of those with BED are male.[105] Changes in the oral tissues are often one of the first signs of an eating disorder. Dental professionals should recognize the oral effects of eating disorders (Table 14–12 ■) and talk with the patient about these concerns.

Anorexia nervosa is typified by self-starvation and excessive weight loss. **Bulimia nervosa** usually consists of secretive cycles of binge eating extremely

■ **Table 14–11** Diet Suggestions to Reduce the Risk of Early Childhood Caries

- **Do not** allow babies to sleep with a bottle containing anything other than water.
- **Do not** allow infants to constantly drink from a sippy cup if it contains juice, milk, or a sweet beverage.
- **Do not** allow older children to use slowly dissolving hard candies, lollipops, or the like on a regular basis.
- **Do not** allow children to snack frequently throughout the day.
- **Do** clean an infant's teeth daily as soon as they erupt into the mouth.
- **Do** provide nutritious snacks like fruits and vegetables rather than sweets between meals.
- **Do** have regular meal and snack times, and minimize the number of between-meal snacks.
- **Do** give children sweets at dessert time when they can brush teeth immediately afterwards.

■ **Table 14–12** Signs and Symptoms of Eating Disorders

- Loss of tissue and erosive lesions on the lingual (**perimolysis**) and occulsal surfaces of teeth due to the effects of vomiting. These occur in 89% of people with bulimia nervosa. Erosion can occur as early as 6 months from the start of the condition.
- Changes in color, shape, and length of teeth. Teeth may become brittle and translucent.
- Palatal or pharyngeal trauma due to the use of blunt instruments to induce vomiting.
- Increased dentin hypersensitivity. In extreme cases the pulp may be exposed, leading to periapical infection or pulpal necrosis.
- Enlargement of the parotid salivary glands, dry mouth (xerostomia), and reddened, dry, cracked lips.
- Presence of dental caries.
- Unprovoked, spontaneous tooth pain.

Source: Hallett & O'Rourke, 2006.[102]

large quantities of food followed by purging through vomiting, laxative use, or overexercising. The average intake of food during a binge is 3,400 calories over an hour, with some individuals ingesting as much as 50,000 calories in 24 hours.[106] In contrast, **binge-eating disorder (BED)** involves periods of uncontrolled, continuous eating much like bulimia nervosa, but no purging is involved. Body weight may vary greatly in this group from normal to severely obese.[106]

All eating disorders require a multidisciplinary approach to care including physicians, psychiatrists, psychologists, nutritionists, and social workers. Initially,

patients often deny having an eating disorder. The dental professional's approach to the discussion must be empathetic and nonjudgmental to elicit the information necessary to lead into the discussion of eating disorders and their potential impact on oral and general health. Studies have demonstrated that dental practitioners are uncomfortable in discussing concerns and/or suspicions about eating disorders with patients. In response to this issue, the National Eating Disorders Association in cooperation with the Washington Dental Service Foundation developed a script for a suggested approach to this discussion (Table 14–13 ■).

■ **Table 14–13** Script for Discussing Eating Disorders with the Dental Patient

Introduce the issue . . .	• I am noticing (name the conditions) on your teeth, gums, tongue, throat, etc. • This is something I have seen in individuals who engage in (name the behavior: e.g. vomiting, consuming excessive soda, gastroesophageal reflux, etc.)
Ask for information . . .	• How do you think this condition might have occurred in your mouth?
Provide resources . . .	• Are you seeing a professional about these behaviors/condition(s)? • Because eating disorders impact your oral, mental, and physical health, it is very important to seek professional help from a counselor, medical doctor, nutritionist, support group, or some combination of these. For eating disorders information and treatment referrals, contact the National Eating Disorders Association at 800-931-2237 or visit www.NationalEatingDisorders.org.
Discuss next steps . . .	• While you are getting help for these behaviors and establishing healthier eating habits, I would like to suggest some options for improving your oral health (i.e., mouthguards, avoid brushing immediately after vomiting, the use of fluorides, etc.)

Source: Hallett & O'Rourke, 2006.[102]

The diagnosis of this disorder by the dental provider and the realization of the dental destruction caused by the disorder often convince patients to agree to treatment. The patient must be cautioned that, for dental rehabilitation to be successful, the underlying problem (the eating disorder and its causes) must be resolved.

Aging Issues

The aging patient is often faced with a variety of challenges that can undermine both oral health and nutritional status.[107] As a result, the elderly are considered particularly susceptible to malnutrition.[108] Compared with younger individuals, elders have a significantly decreased ability to respond to physiologic challenges. This impairment is particularly true of infectious disease because of the immunosenescence that occurs with aging. Sensory function decreases leading to impaired taste and smell, which can have an impact on the enjoyment of food and impact nutritional status.[109] Changes in the gastrointestinal system can affect the ability to digest, absorb, and use food properly. Functional problems, such as arthritis or vision difficulties, can affect the ability to prepare and eat food. Psychosocial problems such as loneliness, depression, lack of money, and poor access to food all can undermine good eating habits.

Problems in the oral cavity, such as xerostomia and loose teeth, have been considered major contributors to the poor eating habits of the elderly and may be a major contributor to malnutrition.[108,110,111] Several studies have shown that dentate status can affect eating ability and subsequent diet quality.[112–115] Individuals with one or two complete dentures had a 20% decline in diet quality compared with those with at least partial dentition in one or both arches.[116] Another study showed that, compared with those with 25 or more teeth, edentulous individuals consumed less fiber and carotene, fewer vegetables, but more cholesterol, saturated fat, and calories.[117] Dentures can affect taste and swallowing ability, especially if they are maxillary dentures. The denture covers those taste buds found on the upper palate. When the upper palate is covered, it becomes difficult to detect the location of food in the mouth. For this reason, dentures are considered to be the major cause of choking in adults.[118]

Xerostomia is common in the older population, in part because of xerostomic medications commonly taken. Xerostomia makes eating more difficult and increases the cariogenic potential of the diet.[119,120] It has also been associated with burning mouth syndrome and inadequate diet.[121]

Conversely, nutrition is an important factor in oral status.[122] In a sample population of 843 elderly people, there was a significant association between low levels of ascorbic acid and the prevalence of oral mucosal lesions.[123] Low calcium intake throughout life has been shown to contribute to osteoporosis. In turn, osteoporosis in alveolar bone is thought to be a contributing factor to the resorption of alveolar bone that ultimately results in tooth loss.[124] The alveolar process is composed primarily of trabecular bone, which is more labile to calcium imbalances than is cortical bone. Thus, the alveolar bone provides a potential labile source of calcium available to meet other tissue needs. Because the alveolar process is thought to undergo resorption before other bones, it is projected that changes detected in the alveolar process may eventually be used for early detection of osteoporosis.[125] Mandibular bone mass was correlated with total body calcium and bone mass of the radius and vertebrae in dentate and edentulous postmenopausal women with osteoporosis, with the highest correlation between total body and mandibular bone mass.[126] Thus, the mandible reflects the mineral status of the entire skeleton. Calcium intake in postmenopausal osteoporotic women was also correlated with mandibular density, supporting the hypothesis that low calcium intake may contribute to reduced bone density.[127,128] In a study of 329 healthy postmenopausal women, an inverse relationship was shown between bone mineral density and number of existing teeth, with those women who received dentures after the age of 40 having the lowest bone mineral density.[129]

Older patients should be carefully screened for nutritional risk factors, and should be educated about the importance of good nutrition to general and oral health.[130] If major nutritional problems are suspected, the patient should be referred to a nutritionist.[131,132] When new dentures are provided, patients should be counseled on how to adapt their usual diet to a softer consistency for the first few days after denture insertion. (Table 14–14 ■) provides dietary suggestions for older dental patients.

■ **Table 14–14**   Dietary Suggestions to Assist in Dental Concerns of Older People

Food Group	Difficulty Chewing or Swallowing	Impaired Taste or Appetite	Dry Mouth
Dairy products	Have cottage cheese, yogurt instead of hard cheeses.	Use flavored milk and yogurt. Add powdered milk to foods to increase protein and calorie intakes.	Add milk or yogurt to moisten dry foods.
Meats and proteins	Substitute fish, eggs, peanut butter, tofu for hard-to-chew meats. Cut into small pieces.	Chew thoroughly. Add herbs and spices instead of salt.	Add broths, gravies, and sauces.
Fruits and vegetables	Use cooked, canned fruits and vegetables. Cut into small pieces or puree foods.	Have ripe fruits and raw vegetables with skins.	Use soups and stews with high water content.
Grains	Avoid breads with hard crusts; use pasta, rice, cooked cereals.	Use whole grains such as rye and pumpernickel.	Moisten breads, cereals with milk or broths.
Other	Avoid seeds and nuts that tend to slip under dentures.	Wine before a meal may stimulate the appetite when used in moderation.	Use candy or gum with non-nutritive sweeteners instead of sucrose-containing products. Drink plenty of fluids.

Source: Hallett & O'Rourke, 2006.[103]

DENTAL AND NUTRITIONAL IMPLICATIONS OF COMMON CHRONIC CONDITIONS

Diabetes Mellitus

The dental patient with **poorly controlled diabetes** is at greater risk for developing oral infections and periodontal disease than the patient without diabetes.[133,134] The dentist and dental hygienist need to be aware of current approaches to diabetes management and should carefully monitor the patient's health status before initiating dental treatment.

The nutrition care plan generally requires that patients have meals and snacks of specific nutrient composition at regularly scheduled intervals, coordinated with medications, insulin or oral agents, and exercise. Dietary management has changed from the high-fat, low-carbohydrate diets of past decades to the more liberal use of complex carbohydrates and the reductions in fat recommended today.[135] A well-balanced diabetic diet should be low in cariogenicity, because the use of cariogenic fermentable carbohydrates should be infrequent. Frequent use of hard candies or other foods taken to counteract hypoglycemia are an indication that the diabetes is not well controlled. Patients with uncontrolled diabetes should be referred to their physician for further management. In the dental office, quickly assimilated carbohydrate sources, such as juices, cake frosting, soda, or glucose tablets, should be kept readily available in the event that a diabetic patient develops symptoms of hypoglycemia. (Table 14–15 ■) provides diet guidelines for the patient with diabetes mellitus.

Immunocompromising Conditions

Immunocompromised patients, such as those with cancer or AIDS, often have increased requirements for nutrients while having major physiologic and psychosocial

■ **Table 14–15** Diet Guidelines for the Patient with Diabetes Mellitus

- Have regular physician appointments to monitor health status and medications.
- See a registered dietitian for personalized diet guidance.
- Have regular meal and snack times. **Do not** skip meals, snacks, or medications.
- Have a balance of whole grains, proteins, fruits, vegetables, and dairy products in your meals and snacks.
- Have concentrated sweets (candy, cakes, cookies, etc.) only occasionally, because they contribute to rapid rises in blood sugar (consult a registered dietitian).
- Avoid the use of slowly dissolving hard candies, mints, breath mints and the like, because they can raise blood sugar and contribute to dental caries

impediments to eating. A recent cross-sectional study found that HIV-positive subjects had low ascorbate levels, suggesting that vitamin C requirements in those with HIV infection may be significantly higher than the RDA.[136]

Cancer often sets up a syndrome of weight loss and wasting in which both metabolism and nutrient losses increase. The cancer often causes severe anorexia, taste changes, and early satiety. The pain and discomfort of oral infections, such as the herpes simplex and oral candidiasis found in AIDS and chemotherapy patients, can also impair the desire and ability to eat.[137] Over half of all head and neck cancer patients are nutritionally compromised at initial diagnosis.[138] Radiation therapy increases eating difficulty by causing painful oral mucositis, dysphagia, and severe xerostomia.[139]

When providing dental treatment to patients suffering from cancer or AIDS, dental providers need to understand the nutrition principles underlying the care, so that dental services provided can be coordinated effectively with total care. The nutrition care plan initially focuses on providing high-caloric intake in frequent small meals. Liquid supplements may be used if optimal nutrition cannot be achieved via food alone. In more serious cases, patients may need enteral (tube) feedings or more advanced nutritional support. A high-calorie, high-protein diet will likely be high in sugars and total calories.[140] In these cases, the dental provider should not caution patients to reduce the frequency of eating, because this directive will contradict nutritional management goals. Rather, thorough cleaning after each eating event, and use of fluoride and xylitol-containing products should be stressed. This approach is standard protocol for immunocompromised patients as part of an aggressive preventive dental program.[141] Patients

with cancer should be cautioned, however, about the potential oral sequelae of an increased frequency of eating. Patients should also be cautioned to avoid the use of slowly dissolving hard candy, which is often used to mitigate the discomfort caused by the xerostomia. The most important monitoring tool for these patients is weight status. The patient should be queried at each visit about how their weight is being maintained. Involuntary weight loss of 10 pounds or more is a warning for the need for more-intensive care. (Table 14–16 ■) provides general diet guidelines for immunocompromised dental patients.

ORAL SURGERY AND INTERMAXILLARY FIXATION

The patient who has had oral surgery, whether therapeutic or as a result of trauma, needs special nutritional consideration.[142] An adequate diet before surgery is needed to support adequate postsurgical response. If food consumption will be impaired for a short period of time, the risk of nutritional deficiency is low. The risk of deficiency increases with length of eating impairment. The surgery itself can result in anorexia, inability to chew, and increased metabolic requirements.[143] After surgery, a patient may need a liquid diet for 1 or 2 days, but should progress as soon as possible to a soft diet of high nutritional quality until a normal diet can be resumed. In some cases, nutritionally complete liquid supplements may be appropriate and should be prescribed in consultation with the patient's dietitian and physician. Often patients prefer purees of normal foods over commercial liquid supplements.[144] Multivitamin and mineral supplements may be appropriate as well. Table 14–16 also provides examples of dietary suggestions for oral surgery patients.

■ **Table 14–16** General Diet Guidelines for Patients Needing Soft or Liquid Diet or Increased Calories

Food Group (Daily Amount)	Liquid Choices	Soft Choices	To Increase Calories
Dairy products and other calcium sources (at least 3 servings/day; a serving is 1 cup)	All forms of milk, milk shakes, instant breakfast drinks, soft custards, ice cream, yogurt, pudding	All forms of milk, milk shakes, instant breakfast drinks, soft custards, ice cream, yogurt, pudding Soft cheeses like cottage cheese	Double-strength milk mix: 1 cup nonfat dry milk powder and 1 quart whole milk Provides twice the protein, vitamins, and minerals, and 1.5 times the calories
Proteins (at least 5 ounces/day; one slice of meat is about 1 ounce; a usual serving of protein is 4–5 ounces)	Broth, strained cream soups, eggs in custard, strained or pureed meat or poultry in soups, plain yogurt, pudding	Eggs, cheese, milk and milk shakes, pea and bean soups, soups with tender meat, fish, poultry, chowders, tender meat in gravy	Hearty meat, fish, poultry, beans, tofu, peanut butter, stews, soups, chowders, meat, sauces, pot roasts Gravies and sauces added to most fish and poultry Eggs added to soups, sauces, and hot cereal
Fruits (at least 3 servings/day; a serving is 1/2 cup)	Fruit juices, nectars, ices, popsicles, applesauce, strained fruits	Fruit juices, ices, nectars, popsicles, applesauce, pureed or strained cooked fruits, canned fruits, fruit gelatins	Soft
Vegetables (at least 4 servings/day; a serving is 1/2 cup)	Vegetable juices, strained or pureed vegetables mixed with broth	Vegetable juices, strained or pureed vegetables mixed with broth Pureed, soft, canned, cooked vegetables	Soft, cooked vegetables, vegetable soups, stews, juices, sauces, and gravies Starchy vegetables such as potatoes, winter squash, creamed corn
Grains (at least 3 servings/day; a serving is one slice)	Soft bread with crusts removed softened in soup or milk; diluted cereals	Cooked cereals, soft breads, mashed potatoes, pasta, rice, crackers in soup	Creamy, hot cereals, noodles, pasta, bread Dry cereals added to soups and sauces Wheat germ added to cereals Breakfast drinks, custards, frappes, yogurt, etc. French toast, pancakes, bread pudding Avoid dry toast and hard crusty bread unless soaked in beverage or soup

SUMMARY

Nutritional status and dietary habits can affect and be affected by specific oral conditions. Comprehensive patient care requires that nutritional factors be considered in the etiology, progression, and sequelae of oral problems.[145,146]

Dental providers should routinely screen patients for nutritional issues, provide dentally oriented counseling, and refer patients to dietitians for further care. The nutritional implications in dental conditions are many and complex. No longer can dental professionals take the stance that nutrition is outside their scope of practice.

REFERENCES

1. Rugg-Gunn, A. J. (1993). Nutrition, dental development and dental hypoplasia. In *Nutrition and dental health.* New York: Oxford University Press, 15–35.
2. Alvarez, J. O. (1995). Nutrition, tooth development, and dental caries. *Am J Clin Nutr,* 61(Suppl):410S–16S.
3. Papas, A. S., Palmer, C. A., Rounds, M. C., Herman, J., McGandy, R. B., Hartz, S. C., Russell, R. M., DePaola, P. (1989). Longitudinal relationship between nutrition and oral health. *Ann NY Acad Sci,* 561:124–42.
4. U.S. Preventive Services Task Force. (1996). *Guide to clinical preventive services* (2nd ed.). Baltimore: Williams & Wilkins.
5. Food and Nutrition Board. (1989). *Recommended dietary allowances* (10th ed.). Washington, DC: National Academy Press.
6. Food and Nutrition Board. (2006). *Dietary reference intakes: The essential guide to nutrient requirements.* Washington, DC: National Institute of Medicine.
7. U.S. Department of Health and Human Services and U.S. Department of Agriculture. (2005). *Dietary guidelines for Americans, 2005* (6th ed.). Washington, DC: U.S. Government Printing Office.
8. American Dietetic Association. (1997). Weight management—position of ADA. *J Am Diet Assoc,* 97:71–74.
9. Meisler, J. G., & St. Jeor, S. (1996). Summary and recommendations from the American Health Foundation's Expert Panel on Healthy Weight. *Am J Clin Nutr,* 1996;63(Suppl 1): 474S–77S.
10. U.S. Department of Health and Human Services. (October 2000). *The practical guide: Identification, evaluation and treatment of overweight and obesity in adults* (NIH Publication No. 00-4084). Bethesda, MD: U.S. Department of Health and Human Services, National Institutes of Health, National Heart, Lung, and Blood Institute.
11. U.S. Department of Agriculture, Center for Nutrition Policy and Promotion. (2005). *MyPyramid* (Home & Garden. Bull. No. 252). Washington, DC: U.S. Government Printing Office.
12. Food and Drug Administration, Center for Food Safety and Applied Nutrition. (April 2005). Food labeling: Guidance for industry: A dietary supplement labeling guide. Retrieved 11/29/06 from http://www.cfsan.fda.gov/~dms/dslg-toc.html.
13. Food and Drug Administration, Center for Food Safety and Applied Nutrition. (December 22, 1999). Guidance for industry: Significant scientific agreement in the review of health claims for conventional foods and dietary supplements. Retrieved 11/30/06 from http://www.cfsan.fda.gov/~dms/ssaguide.html.
14. Den Besten, P. K. (1999). Mechanism and timing of fluoride effects on developing enamel. *J Public Health Dent,* 59(4):2226–30.
15. Seow, W. K., Young, W. G., Tsang, A. K., & Daley, T. (2005). A study of primary dental enamel from preterm and full-term children using light and scanning electron microscopy. *Pediatr Dent,* 27(5):37409.
16. Navia, J. M. (1970). Evaluation of nutritional and dietary factors that modify animal caries. *J Dent Res,* 49:1213–28.
17. Enwonwu, C. (1974). Role of biochemistry and nutrition in preventive dentistry. *J Am Soc Prev Dent,* 4:6–17.
18. DePaola, D. P., & Kuftinec, M. M. (1976). Nutrition in growth and development of oral tissues. *Dent Clin North Am,* 20:441–59.
19. Pindborg, J. J., Bhat, M., & Roed-Peterson, B. (1967). Oral changes in South India children with severe protein deficiency. *J Periodont,* 38:218–21.
20. Menaker, L., & Navia, J. M. (1974). Effect of undernutrition during the perinatal period on caries development in the rat; Changes in whole saliva volume and protein content. *J Dent Res,* 53:592–97.
21. Spanheimer, R., Zlatev, T., Umpierrez, G., & Digitolamo, R. (1991). Collagen production in fasted and food-restricted rats: Response to duration and severity of food deprivation. *J Nutr,* 121(4):518–24.
22. Alvarez, J. O., Caceda, J., Woolley, T. W., Carley, K. W., Baiocchi, N., Caravedo, L., & Navia, J. M. (1993). A longitudinal study of dental caries in the primary teeth of children who suffered from infant malnutrition. *J Dent Res,* 72(12):1573–76.
23. Alvarez, J. O., Eguren, J. C., Caceda, J., & Navia J. (1990). The effect of nutritional status on the age distribution of dental caries in the primary teeth. *J Dent Res,* 69:1564–66.
24. Johansson, I., Saellstrom, A. K., Rajan, B. P., & Parameswaran, A. (1992). Salivary flow and dental caries in Indian children suffering from chronic malnutrition. *Caries Res,* 26(1):38–43.

25. Alvarez, J. O., & Navia, J. M. (1989). Nutritional status, tooth eruption, and dental caries: A review. *Am J Clin Nutr,* 49:417–26.

26. Rami-Reddy, V., Vijayalakshmi, P. B., & Chndrassekhar-Reddy, B. K. (1986). Deciduous tooth emergence and physique of velama children of Southeastern Andrha Pradesh, India. *Acta de Odont Pediatr,* 7:1–5.

27. Delgado, H., Habicht, J. P., Yarbrough, C., Lechtig, A., Martonell, R., Malina, R. M., & Klein, R. E. (1975). Nutritional status and the timing of deciduous tooth eruption. *Am J Clin Nutr,* 38:216–24.

28. Alvarez, J. O., Lewis, C. A., Saman, C., Caceda, J., Montalvo, J., Figueroa, M. L., Izquierdo, J., Caravedo, L., & Navia, J. M. (1988). Chronic malnutrition, dental caries, and tooth exfoliation in Peruvian children aged 3–9 years. *Am J Clin Nutr,* 48:368–72.

29. Alvarez, J. O., Caceda, J., Woolley, T. W., Carley, K. W., Baiocchi, N., Caravedo, L., & Navia, J. M. A longitudinal study of dental caries in the primary teeth of children who suffered from infant malnutrition. *J Dent Res.* 1993 Dec; 72(12):1573–76.

30. Vogel, R. (1985). Oral fluids: Saliva and gingival fluid. In Pollack, R. L., & Kravitz, E., Eds. *Nutrition in oral health and disease.* Philadelphia: Lea & Febiger, 84–107.

31. Watson, R. R., & McMurray, D. M. (1979). Effects of malnutrition on secretory and cellular immunity. In Furia, T. E., Ed. *CRS—Critical reviews of food and nutrition.* Cleveland, OH: CRS Press.

32. Mandl, S., Schimmelpfennig, C., Edinger, M., Negrin, R. S., & Contag, C. H. (2002). Understanding immune cell trafficking patterns via in vivo bioluminescence imaging. *J Cell Biochem Suppl,* 39:239–48.

33. Aine, L., Backstron, M. C., Maki, R., Kuusela, A. L., Koivisto, A. M., Ikonen, R. S., & Maki, M. (2000). Enamel defects in primary and permanent teeth of children born prematurely. *J Oral Pathol Med,* 29(8):403–409.

34. Demarini, S. (2005). Calcium and phosphorus nutrition in preterm infants. *Acta Paediatr Suppl,* 94(449): 87–92.

35. Seow, W. K., Masel, J. P., Weir, C., & Tudehope, D. I. (1989). Mineral deficiency in the pathogenesis of enamel hypoplasia in prematurely born, very low birthweight children. *Pediatr Dent,* 11(4):297–302.

36. Sintes, J., & Miller, S. (1983). Influence of dietary iron on the dental caries experience and growth of rats fed an experimental diet. *Arch Latinoam Nutr,* 33:322–28.

37. Solomons, N. W. (1988). Zinc and copper. In Shills, M., & Young, V., Eds. *Modern nutrition in health and disease.* Philadelphia: Lea and Febiger, 238–50.

38. Pekarek, R., Sandstead, H., Jacob, R. (1976). Abnormal cellular immune responses during acquired zinc deficiency. *Am J Clin Nutr,* 29:745–49.

39. Frithiof, L., Lazavstedt, S., Eklund, G., Soderberg, U., Skarberg, K. O., Blomquist, J., Asman, B., & Eriksson, W. (1980). The relationship between bone loss and serum zinc levels. *Acta Med Scand,* 207:67–70.

40. Bendich, A., & Chandra, R. K. (1990). *Micronutrients and immune functions.* New York: New York Academy of Sciences.

41. DePaola, D., Faine, M., & Palmer, C. (1999). Nutrition in relation to dental medicine. In Shils, M., Olson, J, Shike, & M, Ross, A. C., Eds. *Modern nutrition in health and disease* (9th ed.). Philadelphia: Lea & Febiger.

42. deMenzes, A. C., Costa, I. M., & El-Guindy, M. M. (1984). Clinical manifestations of hypervitaminosis A in human gingiva: A case report. *J Periodontol,* 8:474–76.

43. Crandall, C. (2004). Vitamin A intake and osteoporosis: A clinical review. *J Womens Health.* 12(8):939–53.

44. Ostergaard, E., & Löe, H. (1975). The collagen content of skin and gingival tissues in ascorbic acid deficient monkeys. *J Period Res,* 10(2):103–14.

45. Nakamoto, T., McCroskey, M., & Mallek, H. M. (1984). The role of ascorbic acid deficiency in human gingivitis—a new hypothesis. *J Theor Biol,* 108(2):163–71.

46. Nishida, M., Grossi, S. G., Dunford, R. G., Ho, A. W., Trevisan, M., & Genco, R. J. (2000). Dietary vitamin C and the risk for periodontal disease. *J Periodontol,* 71(8):1215–23.

47. Staudte, H., Sigusch, B.W., & Glockmann, E. (2005). Grapefruit consumption improves vitamin C status in periodontitis patients. *Br Dent J,* 199(4):213–17.

48. Buzina, R. Aurer-Kozelj, J., Srdak-Jorgić, K., Bühler, E. & Gey, K. F. (1986). Increase of gingival hydroxyproline and proline by improvement of ascorbic acid status in man. *Int J Vitam Nutr Res,* 56(4): 367–72.

49. Wintergerst, E. S., Maggini, S., Hornig, D. H. (2006). Immune-enhancing role of vitamin C and zinc and effect on clinical conditions. *Ann Nutr Metab,* 50(2):85–94.

50. Charbeneau, T. D., & Hurt, W. C. (1983). Gingival findings in spontaneous scurvy. A case report. *J Periodontol,* 54(11):694–97.

51. DePaola, D., Faine, M., & Palmer, C. (1999). Nutrition in relation to dental medicine. In Shils, M., Olson, J., Shike, M., & Ross, A. C., Eds. *Modern nutrition in health and disease* (9th ed.). Philadelphia: Lea & Febiger.

52. Institute of Medicine. (1998). *Dietary reference intakes for thiamin, riboflavin, niacin, vitamin B_6, folate, vitamin B_{12}, pantothenic acid, biotin, and choline.* Washington, DC: National Academy Press.

53. Grobler, S. R., Senekal, P. J., & Laubscher, J. A. (1990). In vitro demineralization of enamel by orange juice, apple juice, Pepsi Cola and diet Pepsi Cola. *Clin Prev Dent,* 12:5–9.

54. Lussi, A., Jaeggi, T., & Zero, D. (2004). The role of diet in the aetiology of dental erosion. *Caries Res,* 38:34–44.

55. Milosevic, A., Kelly, M. J., & McLean, A. N. (1997). Sports supplement drinks and dental health in competitive swimmers and cyclists. *Br Dent J,* 182:303–308.

56. Dodds, M. W. J., Johnson, D. A., & Yeh, C. (2005). Health benefits of saliva: A review. *J Dent,* 33:223–33.

57. Parry, J., Shaw, L., Arnaud, M. J., & Smith, A. J. (2001). Investigation of mineral waters and soft drinks in relation to dental erosion. *J Oral Rehabil,* 28:766–72.

58. von Fraunhofer, J. A., & Rogers, M. M. (July–August 2004). Dissolution of dental enamel in soft drinks. *Gen Dent,* 52(4):308–12.

59. Navia, J. M. (1994). Carbohydrates and dental health. *Am J Clin Nutr,* 59(Suppl):719S–27S.

60. Winn, D. M., Brunelle, J. A., Brown, L. J., Selwitz, R. H., Kaste, L. M., Oldakowski, R. J., & Kingman, A. (1996). Coronal and root caries in the dentition of adults in the United States, 1988–1991. *J Dent Res,* 75(Spec Iss):642–51.

61. Kaste, L. M., Selwitz, R. J., Oldakowski, J. A., Brunelle, J. A., Winn, D. M., & Brown, L. J. (1996). Coronal caries in primary and permanent dentition of children and adolescents 1–17 years of age: United States, 1988–1991. *J Dent Res,* 75(Spec Iss):631–41.

62. Huumonen, S., Tjaderhane, L., & Larmas, M. (1997). Greater concentration of dietary sucrose decreases dentin formation and increases the area of dentinal caries in growing rats. *J Nutr,* 127(11):2226–30.

63. Tjaderhane, L., Hietala, E. L., & Larmas, M. (1994). Reduction in dentine apposition in rat molars by a high sucrose diet. *Arch Oral Biol,* 39(6):491–95.

64. Sreebny, L. M. (1982). Sugar availability, sugar consumption, and dental caries. *Comm Dent Oral Epidemiol,* 10:1–7.

65. Paes Leme, A. F., Koo, H., Bellato, C. M., Bedi, G., & Cury, J. A. (2006). The role of sucrose in cariogenic dental biofilm: New insight. *J Dent Res,* 85(10):878–87.

66. Rugg-Gunn, A. J., Hackett, A. F., Appleton, D. R., Jenkins, G. N., & Eastoe, J. E. (1984). Relationship between dietary habits and caries increments assessed over two years in 405 English adolescent school children. *Arch Oral Biol,* 29:983–92.

67. Burt, B. A., Eklund, S. A., Morgan, K. J., Larkin, F. E., Guire, K. E., Brown, L. O., & Weintraub, J. A. (1988). The effects of sugar intake and frequency of ingestion on dental caries increment in a three-year longitudinal study. *J Dent Res,* 67:1422–29.

68. LaChapelle, D., Couture, C., Brodeur, J. M., & Sevigny, J. (1990). The effects of nutritional quality and frequency of consumption of sugary foods on dental caries increment. *Can J Public Health,* 81:370–75.

69. Newbrun, E. (1992). Preventing dental caries: Current and prospective strategies. *J Am Dent Assoc,* 123: 19–24.

70. Scheinin, A., Mäkinen, K. K., & Ylitalo, K. (1976). Turku sugar studies vs. final report on the effect of sucrose, fructose, and xylitol diets on the caries incidence in man. *Acta Odontol Scand,* 34:179–216.

71. Tanzer, J. M. (1995). Xylitol chewing gum and dental caries. *Int Dent J,* 45:65–76.

72. Pollard, M. A., Imfeld, T., Higham, S. M., Agalamanyi, E. A., Corzon, M. E., Edgar, W. M., & Borgia, M. (1996). Acidogenic potential and total salivary carbohydrate content of expectorants following the consumption of some cereal-based foods and fruits. *Caries Res,* 30:132–37.

73. Kashket, S., Zhang, J., & Van Houte, J. (1996). Accumulation of fermentable sugars and metabolic acids in food particles that become entrapped on the dentition. *J Dent Res,* 75:1885–91.

74. König, K. G., & Schmid, P. (1968). An analysis of frequency-controlled feeding of small rodents and its use in dental caries experiments. *Arch Oral Biol,* 13:13–26.

75. Gustafson, B., Quensel, E., & Lanke, L. (1954). The Vipeholm dental caries study: The effect of different carbohydrate intake on caries activity in 436 individuals observed for five years. *Acta Odontol Scand,* 11:232–64.

76. Lingstrom, P., Birkhed, D., Ruben, J., & Arends, J. (1994). Effect of frequent consumption of starchy food items on enamel and dentin demineralization and on plaque pH in situ. *J Dent Res,* 73(3):652–60.

77. Mundorff-Shrestha, S. A., Featherstone, J. D. B., & Eisenberg, A. D. (1994). Cariogenic potential of foods, II. Relationship of food composition, plaque microbial counts, and salivary parameters to caries in the rat model. *Caries Res,* 28:106–15.

78. Rugg-Gunn, W., Edgar, M., & Jenkins, G. N. (1981). The effect of altering the position of a sugary food in a meal upon plaque pH in human subjects. *J Dent Res,* 60:867–72.

79. Edgar, W. M., & Bowen, W. H. (1982). Effects of different eating patterns on dental caries in the rat. *Caries Res,* 16:384–88.

80. Jensen, M. E., Harlander, S. K., & Schachtele, C. F. (1984). Evaluation of the acidogenic and antacid properties of cheeses by telemetric recording of dental plaque. In Hefferen, J. J., Koehler, H. M., & Osborn, J. C., Eds. *Food, nutrition and dental health* (Vol. V). Park Forest South, IL: Pathotox.

81. Nase, L., Hatakka, K., Savilahti, E., Saxelin, M., Ponka, A., Poussa, T., Korpela, R., & Meurman, J. H. (2001). Effect of long-term consumption of a probiotic bacterium, *Lactobacillus rhamnosus GG,* in milk on dental caries and caries risk in children. *Caries Res,* 35(6):412–420.

82. Ahola, A. J., Yli-Knuuttila, H., Suomalainen, T., Poussa, T., Ahlstrom, A., Meurman, J. H., & Korpela, R. (2002). Short term consumption of probiotic-containing cheese and its effect on dental caries risk factors. *Arch Oral Biol,* 47(11):799–804.

83. Bowen, W. H. (1994). Food components and caries. *Adv Dent Res,* 8:215–20.

84. Mundorff, S. A., Featherstone, J. D. B., & Bibby, B. G. (1990). Cariogenic potential of foods, I. Caries in the rat model. *Caries Res,* 24:344–55.

85. Jensen, M. E. (1985). Dental caries: A diet-related disease. *Curr Q,* 1:18–20.

86. Koulourides, T., & Chien, M. C. (1992). The ICT in situ experimental model in dental research. *J Dent Res,* 71:822–27.

87. DePaola, D. (1986). Executive summary: Scientific consensus conference on methods for assessment of the cariogenic potential of foods. *J Dent Res,* 65(Spec Iss):1540–43.

88. Curzon, M. E. J., & Pollard, M. A. (1996). Integration of methods for determining the acid/cariogenic potential of foods: A comparison of several different methods. *Caries Res,* 30:126–31.

89. Vogel, R., & Alvares, O. F. (1985). Nutrition and periodontal disease. In Pollack, R. L., & Kravitz, E., Eds. *Nutrition in oral health and disease.* Philadelphia: Lea & Febiger, 136–50.

90. Navia, J. M., & Menaker, L. (1976). Nutritional implications in wound healing. *Dent Clin North Am,* 20(3):549–67.

91. Alfano, M. C., Miller, S. A., & Drummond, J. F. (1975). Effect of ascorbic acid deficiency on the permeability and collagen biosynthesis of oral mucosal epithelium. *Ann NY Acad Sci,* 258:253–63.

92. Alfano, M. C., & Masi, C. W. (1978). Effect of acute folic acid deficiency on the oral mucosal permeability. *J Dent Res,* 57:312. Abstract 949.

93. Joseph, C. E., Ashrafi, S. H., Steinberg, A. D., & Waterhouse, J. P. (1982). Zinc deficiency changes in the permeability of rabbit periodontium to ^{14}C-phenytoin and ^{14}C-albumin. *J Periodont,* 53:251–56.

94. Alfano, M. C. (1976). Controversies, perspectives and clinical implications of nutrition in periodontal disease. *Dent Clin North Am,* 20:519–48.

95. Malleck, H. M. (1978). *An investigation of the role of ascorbic acid and iron in the etiology of gingivitis in humans.* (Doctoral Thesis). Cambridge, MA: Institute Archives, Massachusetts Institute of Technology.

96. Whitehead, N., Ryner, F., & Lindenbaum, J. (1973). Megaloblastic changes in the cervical epithelium. Association with oral contraceptive therapy and reversal with folic acid. *JAMA,* 226(12):1421–24.

97. Merchant, A. T., Pitiphat, W., Franz, M., & Joshipura, K. J. (2006). Whole grain and fiber intakes and periodontitis risk in men. *Am J Clin Nutr,* 83(6):1395–1400.

98. Beltran-Aguilar, E. D., Barker, L. K, Canto, B. A., Gooch, B. F., Griffin, S. O., Hyman, J., Jaramillo, F., Kingman, A., Nowjack-Raymer, R., Selwitz, R. H., & Wu, T. (2005). Surveillance for dental caries, dental sealants, tooth retention, edentulism, and enamel flourosis—United States, 1988–1994 and 1999–2002. *MMWR Morb Mortal Wkly Rep,* 54(03): 1–44.

99. Kelly, M., & Bruerd, B. (1987). The prevalence of baby bottle tooth decay among two Native American populations. *J Pub Health Dent,* 47:94–97.

100. Broderick, E., Mabry, J., Robertson, D., & Thompson, J. (1989). Baby bottle tooth decay in Native American children in Head Start Centers. *Pub Health Rep,* 104:50–54.

101. Kaste, L. M., & Gift, H. C. (1995). Inappropriate infant bottle feeding. *Arch Pediatr Adolesc Med,* 149:786–91.

102. Hallett, K. B., O'Rourke, P. K. (2006). Pattern and severity of early childhood caries. *Community Dent Oral Epidemiol,* 34(1):25–35.

103. O'Sullivan, D. M., & Tinanoff, N. (1993). Maxillary anterior caries associated with increased caries risk in other primary teeth. *J Dent Res,* 72:1577–80.

104. National Eating Disorders Association. (2002). Dental complications of eating disorders: Information for dental practitioners. Retrieved 11/26/06 from http://www.nationaleatingdisorders.org.

105. National Institute of Mental Health. (2001). *Eating disorders: Facts about eating disorders and the search for solutions* (NIH Publication No. 01-4901). Bethesda, MD: National Institutes of Health.

106. Zachariasen, R. D. (1995). Oral manifestations of bulimia nervosa. *Women Health,* 22(4):67–76.

107. Douglass, C. W., Jette, A. M., Fox, C. H., Tennstedt, S. L., Joshi, A., Feldman, H. A., McGuire, S. M., & McKinlay, J. B. (1993). Oral health status of the elderly in New England. *J Gerontology,* 48:M39–46.

108. Palmer, C. A. (1991). Nutrition and oral health of the elderly. In Papas, A., Niessen, L., & Chauncy, H. *Geriatric dentistry: Aging and oral health.* St. Louis: Mosby Year Book, 264–82.

109. Schiffman, S. S. (1991). Taste and smell losses with age. Contemporary Nutrition, General Mills Nutrition Department: 16:2:6–8.

110. Brodeur, J. M., Laurin, D., Vallee, R., & Lachapelle, D. (November 1993). Nutrient intake and gastrointestinal disorders related to masticatory performance in the edentulous elderly. *J Prosthet Dent,* 70(5):468–73.

111. Position of the American Dietetic Association: Oral health and nutrition (1966). *J Am Diet Assoc,* 96(2):184–89.

112. Slagter, A. P., Olthoff, L. W., Bosman, F., & Steen, W. H. (1992). Masticatory ability, denture quality, and oral conditions in edentulous subjects. *J Prosthet Dent,* 68(2):299–307.

113. Touger-Decker, R., Schaefer, M., Flinton, R., & Steinberg, L. (1996). Effect of tooth loss and dentures on diet habits. *J Prosthet Dent,* 75:831.

114. Sebring, N. G., Guckes, A. D., Li, S., & McCarthy, G. R. (1995). Nutritional adequacy of reported intake of edentulous subjects treated with new conventional or implant-supported mandibular dentures. *J Prosthet Dent,* 74:358–63.

115. Greksa, L. P., Parraga, I. M., & Clark, C. A. (1995). The dietary adequacy of edentulous older adults. *J Prosthet Dent,* 73:142–45.

116. Papas, A., Palmer, C., McGandy, R., Hartz, S. C., & Russell, R. M. (1987). Dietary and nutritional factors in relation to dental caries in elderly subjects. *Gerodontics,* 3:30–37.

117. Joshipura, K., Willett, W., & Douglass, C. (1996). The impact of edentulousness on food and nutrient intake. *J Am Dent Assoc,* 127:459–67.

118. Anderson, D. L. (1977). Death from improper mastication. *Int Dent J,* 27:349.

119. Dormenval, V., Budtz-Jorgensen, E., Mojon, P., Bruyere, A., & Rapin, C. H. (1995). Nutrition, general health status and oral health status in hospitalized elders. *Gerodontology,* 12(12):73–80.

120. Faine, M., Allender, D., Baab, D., Persson, R., & Lamont, R. J. (1992). Dietary and salivary factors associated with root caries. *Spec Care Dent,* 12(4):177–82.

121. Maresky, L. S., van der Bijl, P., & Gird, I., (March 1993). Burning mouth syndrome. Evaluation of multiple variables among 85 patients. *Oral Surg Oral Med Oral Pathol,* 75(3):303–307.

122. Mulligan, R. (1989). Oral health: Effect on nutrition and rehabilitation in older persons. *Top Geriatr Rehab,* 5:27–35.

123. Vaanen, M. K., Markkanen, H. A., Tuovinen, V. J., Kullaa, A. M., Karinpau, A. M., & Kumpusalo, E. A. (1993). Periodontal health related to plasma ascorbic acid. *Proc Finn Dent Soc,* 89(1–2):51–59.

124. Paganini-Hill, A. (1995). The benefits of estrogen replacement therapy on oral health. The Leisure World cohort. *Arch Intern Med,* 155(21):2325–29.

125. Whalen, J. P., & Krook, L. (1996). Periodontal disease as the early manifestation of osteoporosis. (Editorial). *Nutrition,* 12(1):53–54.

126. Kribbs, P. J., Chestnut, C. H., Ott, S., & Kilcoyne, R. F. (1990). Relationships between mandibular and skeletal bone in a population of normal women. *J Prosthet Dent,* 63(1):86–89.

127. Kribbs, P. J. (1990). Comparison of mandibular bone in normal and osteoporotic women. *J Prosthet Dent,* 63(2):218–22.

128. Houki, K., DiMuzio, M. T., & Fattore, L. (1994). Mandibular bone density and systemic osteoporosis in elderly edentulous women. *J Bone Miner Res,* 9 (Suppl):S211.

129. Krall, E. A., Dawson-Hughes, B., Papas, A., & Garcia, R. I. (1994). Tooth loss and skeletal bone density in healthy postmenopausal women. *Osteoporos Int,* 4:104–109.

130. American Academy of Family Physicians, American Dietetic Association and National Council on Aging. (1992). *Nutrition interventions manual for professionals caring for older Americans.* Washington, DC: Nutrition Screening Initiative.

131. Saunders, M. J. (1995). Incorporating the nutrition screening initiative into the dental practice. *Spec Care Dent,* 15(1):26–37.

132. Pla, G. W. (1994). Oral health and nutrition. *Prim Care Clin Off Pract,* 21(1):121–23.

133. Holdren, R. S., & Patton, L. L. (1993). Oral conditions associated with diabetes mellitus. *Diabetes Spectr,* 6(1):11–17.

134. Cleary, T. J., & Hutton, J. E. (1995). An assessment of the association between functional edentulism, obesity, and NIDDM. *Diabetes Care,* 18:1007–1009.

135. The DCCT Research Group. (1993). Nutrition interventions for intensive therapy in the diabetes control and complications trial. *J Am Diet Assoc,* 93:768–72.

136. Stephensen, C. B., Marquis, G. S., Jacob, R. A., Kruzich, L. A., Douglas, S. D., & Wilson, C. M. (2006). Vitamin C and E in adolescents and young adults in HIV infection. *Am J Clin Nutr,* 83(4):870–79.

137. Robertson, P. B., & Greenspan, J. S., Eds. (1988). *Perspectives on oral manifestations of AIDS: Diagnosis and management of HIV-associated infections.* Littleton, MA: PSG Publishing.

138. Bassett, M. R., & Dobie, R. A. (1983). Patterns of nutritional deficiency in head and neck cancer. *Otolaryngol Head Neck Surg,* 91:119–25.

139. Nikoskelainen, J. (1990). Oral infections related to radiation and immunosuppressive therapy. *J Clin Periodont,* 17(7):504–507.

140. Smith, T. J., Dwyer, J. T., & LaFrancesca, J. P. (1990). Nutrition and the cancer patient. In Osteen, R. T., Cady, B., & Rosenthal, P., Eds. *Cancer manual* (8th ed.). Boston: American Cancer Society, 485–97.

141. Dwyer, J. T., Efstathion, M. S., Palmer, C., & Papas, A. (1991). Nutritional support in treatment of oral carcinomas. *Nutr Rev,* 49:332–37.

142. Kendall, B. D., Fonseca, R. J., & Lee, M. (1982). Postoperative nutritional supplementation for the orthognathic surgery patient. *J Oral Maxillofac Surg,* 40:205–13.

143. Soliah, K. (1987). Clinical effects of jaw surgery and wiring on body composition: A case study. In *Dietetic currents* (Vol. 14). Columbus, OH: Ross Laboratories, 13–16.

144. Patten, J. A. (1995). Nutrition and wound healing. *Compend Continu Educ Dent,* 16(2):200–214.

145. Lokshin, M. F. (1994). Preventive oral health care: A review for family physicians. *Am Fam Physician,* 50(8):1677–84, 1687.

146. Karp, W. B. (1994). Nutrition update for the dental health professional. *J Calif Dent Assoc,* 22(8):26–29.

Chapter 15

Sugar and Other Sweeteners

Michelle L. Sensat

Jill L. Stoltenberg

OBJECTIVES

After studying this chapter, the student should be able to:

1. Define sugars, sweeteners, and sugar substitutes.
2. Identify the three sugars that are composed of glucose, fructose, or galactose.
3. Differentiate between cariogenic sugars and non-cariogenic sweeteners.
4. Describe the potential impact that excessive sugar intake has on dental and systemic health.
5. Explain the role of sugar in the caries process.
6. Suggest alternative sweetener options that are non-cariogenic on the basis of a working knowledge of comparative sweetness to sucrose.
7. Identify contraindications that may preclude someone from using a specific sugar substitute.
8. Describe the role of xylitol in the prevention of dental caries.
9. Explain how *Streptococcus mutans* bacteria initiate and propagate the caries process.
10. Describe preventive strategies to halt or decrease caries frequency in the high-risk or at-risk patient.

KEY TERMS

Sweeteners
Nutritive
Caloric sweeteners
Non-nutritive
Noncaloric sweeteners
Sugar substitutes
Monosaccharides
Disaccharides
Taste receptor cells
Taste buds
Saccharose
Common sugar
Saccharin
Cyclamate
Aspartame
Sucrose
Molasses
Fructose
Fruit sugar
High-fructose corn syrup
Hereditary fructose intolerance
Polyols
Sugar alcohols

INTRODUCTION

Sweeteners are sugars or substances added to foods and beverages that provide a pleasurable taste and, in some cases, added energy. Those that provide energy are termed "**nutritive**" or **caloric sweeteners** (i.e., sucrose, fructose, and sugar alcohols). Those that do not provide energy are called "**non-nutritive**" or **noncaloric sweeteners,** as well as "**sugar substitutes**" (i.e., acesulfame-K, aspartame, neotame, saccharin, and sucralose). (Table 15–1 ■) contains a list of nutritive sweeteners used in the food supply.

Sweetness is a stimulus that can be imparted by a wide variety of molecules. Sugars, amino acids, peptides, proteins, olefinic alcohols, nitroanilines, saccharin, chloroform, and many other organic compounds are capable of imparting a sweet taste.[1]

The term sugar, to most people, refers to the common crystalline, granular table sugar, or sucrose. However, sucrose is only one of many naturally occurring sugars found in the human diet. Chemically, sugars are a group of compounds composed of carbon (C), hydrogen (H), and oxygen (O) atoms, also known as carbohydrates.[2]

Naturally occurring sugars can be divided into two classifications of carbohydrates: simple sugars, or monosaccharides, and disaccharides. **Monosaccharides** contain 3 to 7 carbon atoms per monomer and include the following primary simple sugars in the human diet: glucose, fructose, and galactose. Mannose, another monosaccharide, also plays a minor role in the human diet.[2] (Figure 15–1 ■) shows examples of structural formulas for several naturally occurring sugars. These simple sugars are readily absorbed.[3] **Disaccharides** are two monosaccharides, or two monomers, that are joined together. Primary disaccharides in the human diet include sucrose (one glucose and one fructose), lactose (one galactose and one glucose), trehalose (two molecules of α-glucose, $1 \rightarrow 1$ linkage), and maltose (two molecules of α-glucose, $1 \rightarrow 4$ linkage).[2] (Figure 15–2 ■)

This chapter will discuss both nutritive and non-nutritive sweeteners, comparing contributions of each to commercial food products, their effects on the dental caries process, and their place in caries prevention.

TASTE PERCEPTION AND SENSATION

Total perception of food is complex. Multiple senses are at work: taste; olfaction (which includes smells, or aromas); touch, also called "mouth feel," from texture of food and fat content; and thermoreception and nociception, caused by strong spices and irritants.[4] There are generally four categories of primary stimuli with regard to taste: sweet, sour, salty, and bitter. One other primary taste, savory, also termed *umami,* is controversial.[4] Mixtures of these primary stimuli are found in complex foods.

■ **Table 15–1**   Nutritive Sweeteners in the Food Supply

Sweeteners (Other Names)*	Description
Monosaccharides	
Glucose/dextrose (dextrin, corn sugar)	Used in food processing and canned foods
Fructose (fruit sugar, levulose)	Produces laxative effect at intake of 20 grams or more
Disaccharides	
Sucrose (granulated, powdered, brown, turbinado [raw], invert sugar)	Sweetens and tenderizes baked goods
High-fructose corn syrup (HFCS)	Used in soft drinks
Corn syrup (corn sugar, corn syrup solids)	Used in candy, snack foods, ice cream, fruit drinks, nondairy creamers
Maltose (malt sugar or syrup)	Made from barley; used in malt flavored foods and alcoholic beverages
Molasses/sorghum/maple syrup	Used in breads and on pancakes, waffles
Honey (raw, comb, creamed)	Harvested from bees; not safe for infants
Lactose (milk sugar)	Used in whipped toppings and commercial baked goods

*All provide 4 kcal/g.

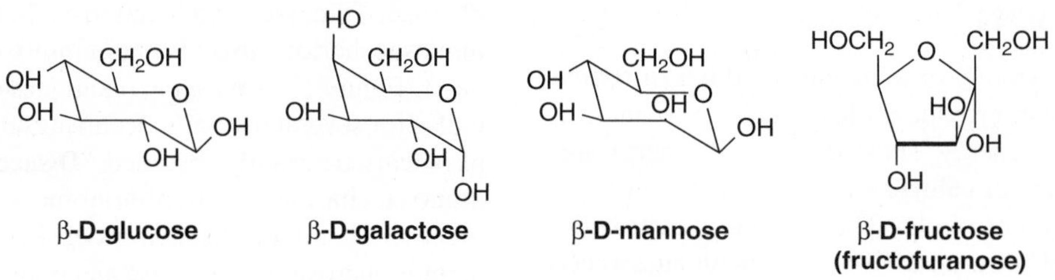

■ **FIGURE 15–1** Primary monosaccharides in foods.
(From Sigman-Grant, M., & Morita, J. (2003). *Am J Clin Nutr,* 78 (4 Suppl):817S.[1])

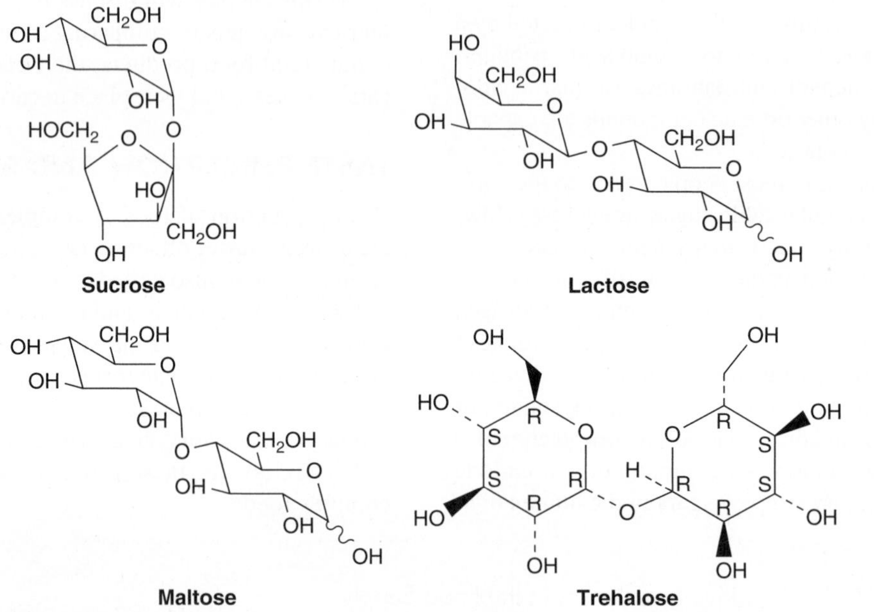

■ **FIGURE 15–2** Primary Disaccharides in Foods.
(From Sigman-Grant, M., & Morita, J. (2003). *Am J Clin Nutr,* 78 (4 Suppl):818S.[2])

The chemical detection of taste agents occurs in specialized epithelial cells called **taste receptor cells;** they are present in vertebrates as ovoid clusters or **taste buds.** Each taste bud contains 50 to 100 cells. These buds are found embedded within the non-sensory lingual epithelium, and are found within specialized connective tissues called papillae, including fungiform, foliate, and circumvallate papillae. Taste buds are also found in the palate, pharynx, and upper portion of the esophagus.[4]

Taste sensation is initiated by arrival of a stimulus at the taste buds. Recognition of the taste agent or agents occurs when receptor sites of the taste bud cells carry, by cranial nerves VII, IX, and X, messages to the brain that are then processed and recognized as either sweet, sour, salty, bitter, or some combination of these primary stimuli.[4]

HISTORY OF SWEETENERS

The first recorded sweetener was honey, used in the ancient cultures of Greece and China.[5] Honey later was replaced by **saccharose,** or **common sugar,** originally made from sugar cane. Early human cultures valued sweetness and considered it rare enough that they kept naturally available sweeteners from their regions for special religious or celebratory events. A large industry for sugar cane production in the Western Hemisphere was in place by the seventeenth century, and this industry supplied sweeteners to Europe. Napoleon's scientists developed sugar extraction from sugar beets when France was isolated from major shipping early in the nineteenth century.

During the World Wars, saccharose production largely came from sugar beets rather than sugar cane owing to ease of production. The search for other sweeteners led to new chemical developments. During World Wars I and II, **saccharin,** the first artificial sweetener, first manufactured in 1879 by Remsen and Fahlberg, became used widely because of its low production costs and the shortage of regular sugar.[5] As the economy recovered after the wars, sugar became more plentiful and affordable. Unfortunately, with the growing candy and fast food industry, obesity soon increased in Western societies. Since the 1950s, a push to use saccharin shifted from cost concerns to calorie reduction and weight control. Profitable market demand soon followed for reduced-calorie diet products, which contained reduced sugar or substitution of sugar with artificial sweeteners. Saccharin, however, was known not only for its sweetness, but its bitter aftertaste, so there was an interest to create new, better tasting reduced-calorie sweeteners.[5]

In the 1950s, a breakthrough was achieved with the development of **cyclamate.** It tasted better than saccharin and blended very well with it. Cyclamate, saccharin, and other additives were then mixed together and sold under the name Sweet'N Low, which became widely used in the United States. Cyclamate was used in tablet or liquid form as a tabletop sweetener and also as a sweetener in soft drinks.

The United States Food and Drug Administration (FDA), in 1970, banned cyclamate from all diet foods and fruits because of suspicion of induced cancer in laboratory animals.[6] In all other countries, however, it is still used today, particularly in combination with other sweeteners.

In 1981, **aspartame** was approved and marketed as NutraSweet. This allowed dairy products such as yogurt, to be sold as "diet" or "light," reduced-calorie foods for the first time.[7]

Saccharin, cyclamate, and aspartame were known as the "first-generation sweeteners." Second-generation sweeteners soon followed, including acesulfame-K, sucralose, alitame, and neotame, which differ widely in their key markets throughout the globe. (Table 15–2 ■) shows a list of current sweeteners and their key market areas.[7] These second-generation sweeteners, unfortunately, had limitations similar to those of the first-generation sweeteners. Their taste was often bitter, with a metallic aftertaste, and they provided an unrealistic mouth feel compared with regular sugar. Many synergic artificial sweeteners, that is, sweeteners that enhance each others' flavor, are now combined to improve the overall quality of sweetened products (i.e., a combination of acesulfame-K, aspartame, and others in soft drinks).[5]

Today, consumers' feelings are mixed concerning use of artificial sweeteners, largely because of earlier reports of cancer risks with these substances. In the 1980s, when many sweeteners were new to the market, there were several published reports of carcinogenic effects associated with use of artificial sweeteners. Their publication was unfortunate, because many of the

■ **Table 15–2**   Current Artificial Sweeteners and Their Key Market Areas

Sweetener	Key Market Areas
Acesulfame-K	North America, Europe, and Asia
Alitame	Oceania, South/Central America
Aspartame	North America, Europe, and Asia
Cyclamate	Europe and Asia
Neohesperidine DC	Europe and Japan
Neotame	United States
Saccharin	Asia, Europe, and United States
Stevioside	Asia
Sucralose	North America
Thaumatin	Europe and Asia

Source: Lindley, M. G. (1999). *World Rev Nutr Diet,* Basel, Karger, 85:45–51.[7]

reports lacked a sound scientific background or were poorly investigated.[5] Some scientific publications of that time also were not well researched and possessed erroneous statistical analyses of findings. In the last decade, the cancer and artificial sweetener link has not been discussed as frequently as in the early years, although some long-term studies with saccharin and cyclamate have been conducted and published.[5] There appears to be no resurgence in concern with regard to saccharin use, and popularity of new products has shifted demand to the newer, sweeter, and better tasting artificial sweeteners.

SUCROSE AND CONSTITUENTS

Sucrose is a nutritive sweetener and the most commonly used tabletop sweetener. It is a disaccharide (one glucose and one fructose) and provides 4 kilocalories/gram (kcal/g) (approximately 16 kcal per teaspoon) when consumed. Sucrose is manufactured from the processing of sugar cane or sugar beets, and through refinement, yellow-brown pigments are removed to produce the white crystalline form of common table sugar. **Molasses** is sucrose in its least refined state.[8] Sucrose, cane or beet sugar, is used in the following food items in descending order of frequency: bakery and cereal products; candy and other confectionary items; ice cream and dairy products; beverages; canned, bottled, and frozen foods; and other miscellaneous foods.[9]

A component of sucrose, **fructose,** is also often added to foods to synergize the sweetness potential of sucrose and some non-nutritive sweeteners.[10] As a monosaccharide, fructose provides 4 kcal/g when consumed. It makes up 50% of a sucrose molecule, the other 50% is glucose; is present in fruit, also known as **fruit sugar** or levulose; and is added to foods and beverages as **high-fructose corn syrup** (HFCS; 42%–55% fructose) or in a crystallized form.[8] Fructose has replaced sucrose in many foods and beverages because of its intense sweetness, reduced cost, and properties that enhance flavor, color, and product stability.[10] Corn syrups can be found in beverages, processed foods, cereal and baked goods, dairy products, and candy and other confectionary goods.[9]

Exact data on sugar consumption is hard to obtain because of limitations of data gathering. Two major surveys that are used to estimate a person's intake of food are the Continuing Survey of Food Intakes by Individuals and the National Health and Nutrition Examination Survey.[11] For the intake of sugars, the 24-hour dietary recall method is used most often. The major limitation with the data gathered is that these surveys rely on self-reported, retrospective, recall of dietary intake.[12] Furthermore, the data are cross-sectional and provide no information regarding previous or subsequent consumption beyond the days of the dietary intake recall, nor what an individual person might do if presented with alternative food choices.[2] Accuracy of self-reported food intake is also a problem.[13,14]

In an article published in 2003, the reported mean population intake of added sugars was approximately 80 grams, which equals a mean of 15.8% of total energy intake.[15,16] Average intake for children younger than 12 years was less than 19% of total energy, increased to approximately 20% of total energy for adolescents, and then decreased throughout adulthood.

Uses of Sucrose

Sucrose has, in addition to its sensory qualities, functional properties that make it desirable for use in the food industry. It is ideal in the following roles:

- *Sweetening agent:*   The character of the sweetness of a product can be varied according to the pH and temperature used to manufacture it, as well as by its interaction with other ingredients. Level of sweetness is important to the acceptance of certain foods.[17]
- *Flavor blender and modifier:*   In some foods, sucrose assists in blending flavors; in other foods, it reduces the acidic and/or sour taste (i.e., pickles).
- *Texture and bodying agent:*   Sucrose imparts a texture that is highly acceptable to consumers. It gives fullness and a distinctive mouth feel to foods and beverages.
- *Dispersing/lubricating agent:*   In dry packaged mixes, sucrose keeps other ingredients from packing too closely. This permits a better blending of the ingredients during food preparation.
- *Caramelization/color agent:*   Caramelization during cooking and baking produces a brown color, which provides a desirable, characteristic flavor and aroma to the food product.
- *Bulking agent:*   When sucrose is replaced by a noncaloric sweetener that may be hundreds of times sweeter, other ingredients must be added to replace the lost sucrose "bulk" to maintain the food's normal appearance and consistency.[18]

Evaluation of the Health Aspects of Sucrose

In the United States, sucrose (along with several other sweeteners) are considered generally recognized as safe (GRAS) ingredients, and other artificial sweeteners are categorized as food additives. These distinctions are defined by the 1958 Food Additives Amendment to the Federal Food, Drug, and Cosmetic Act.[8] The Food and Drug Administration must approve the safety of all food additives. The *Code of Federal Regulations* (21 CFR 171), revised in 2002, defines food additives and procedures necessary for evaluating the safety of these substances. When reviewing potential sweeteners as food additives, the FDA asks the following questions: (1) How is it made? (2) What are the properties of the sweetener in foods and beverages (i.e., product specifications)? (3) How much of the sweetener will be consumed, and will certain groups be particularly susceptible to the food additive? and (4) Is the sweetener safe and does it cause adverse effects to the individual or offspring, including cancer, or chronic toxicity?[8]

In recent years, intake of sugars was suggested to be associated with a variety of health issues, namely obesity, diabetes and glycemic response, hyperlipidemias, behavioral disorders, and dental caries.[8,19] After intense scrutiny, many supposed adverse health effects of sugars were found to lack a scientific foundation.[20] Sugars alone were not associated with obesity, hyperactivity in children, diabetes, and coronary heart disease.[21] A position statement by the American Dietetic Association clarifies this issue: "Consumers can safely enjoy a range of nutritive and nonnutritive sweeteners when consumed in a diet that is guided by current federal nutrition recommendations, such as the Dietary Guidelines for Americans and the Dietary References Intakes, as well as individual health goals."[8] Furthermore, the Institutes of Medicine suggest a maximum intake level of nutritive sweeteners to be less than 25% of total energy; otherwise dietary quality suffers.[8]

SUGARS AND DENTAL CARIES FORMATION

Substantial research implicates sugars (i.e., sucrose, glucose, fructose, maltose) and all fermentable carbohydrates as principal dietary substances that promote caries formation.[22-26] While the connection between sweet carbohydrates and dental decay has been observed for hundreds of years, two landmark animal studies and three human clinical studies have contributed to the understanding of the importance of sugar, along with bacterial biofilms, in the development of caries.

In 1955, the first animal study was conducted with laboratory rats in a gnotobiotic (germ-free) environment.[27] One group of rats was fed a cariogenic diet containing large amounts of sugar. The second group was fed the same diet; however, at the same time, specific microorganisms were introduced to the otherwise germ-free environment. Rats receiving the cariogenic diet alone did not develop caries; those with the cariogenic diet in the presence of bacteria did develop carious lesions (Table 15–3 ■). Observations at that time and since have clearly demonstrated that certain strains of microorganisms (i.e., *Streptococci mutans* and lactobacilli) are more caries-productive than others.

In another study using rats as subjects, the rats were fed a caries-producing diet by means of a stomach tube, with no food actually coming in contact with the teeth.[28] No caries resulted. When the same diet was fed orally and contacted the teeth, caries did occur. These two studies conclusively demonstrated that (1) bacteria are essential for caries development, regardless of diet, and (2) the action of sugar in the caries process is local, not systemic (Table 15–4 ■).

Several human studies have further clarified the animal studies. Two of the most often cited studies occurred at Hopewood House[29] in Australia and at Vipeholm in Sweden.[30]

■ Table 15–3   Dental Caries in Germ-Free Rats and Caries-Free Rats Inoculated with Known Bacterial Cells (Enterococci Predominating)

Group	Microbial State	No. of Rats	No. of Rats Developing Molar Caries
A	Germ free	9	0
B	Inoculated with enterococci plus others	13	13

Source: Copyright by the American Dental Association. Reprinted by permission. From Orland et al., (1955). *J Am Dent Assoc,* 50:259–272.[27]

■ **Table 15–4**   Caries in Rats Fed a Decay-Producing Diet via Normal and Stomach Tube Routes

Group	Methods of Feeding	No. of Rats	Avg. No. of Carious Molars	Avg. No. of Carious Lesions
A	Normal	13	5.0	6.7
B	Stomach tube	13	0	0

Source: Kite et al. American Society for Nutrition Sciences. (1950). *J Nutr,* 42:89–103.[28]

Hopewood House was an orphanage in Australia that housed up to 82 children. From its beginning, sugar and other refined carbohydrates were excluded from the children's diet. Carbohydrates were served in the form of whole meal bread, soybeans, wheat germ, oats, rice, potatoes, and some molasses. Dairy products, fruits, raw vegetables, and nuts were prominently featured in the typical menu. Dental surveys of these children from the ages of 5 to 11 years revealed a greatly reduced caries incidence compared with the state school population in that age group, even though the orphaned children's oral hygiene was poor, with about 75% suffering from gingivitis. When the children became old enough to earn wages in the outside economy, they deviated from the orphanage diet. A steep increase of decayed, missing, and filled teeth (DMFT) after the age of 11 years indicated that the teeth did not acquire any permanent resistance to caries (Figure 15–3 ■).

The Vipeholm study was conducted at a mental institution in the southern city of Vipeholm, Sweden. Adult patients on a nutritionally adequate diet were observed for several years and found to have a slow caries rate. The patients were then divided into different groups to compare the cariogenicity accompanying various changes in frequency and consistency of carbohydrate intake. Sucrose was included in the diet as toffee, chocolate, or caramel, in bread, or in liquid form. Caries increased significantly when foods containing sucrose were ingested between meals. In addition to the frequency of eating, the consistency of the sugar-containing food was very important. Sticky or adherent forms of food that maintained high sugar levels in the mouth for longer periods of time were much more cariogenic than forms that were rapidly cleared.

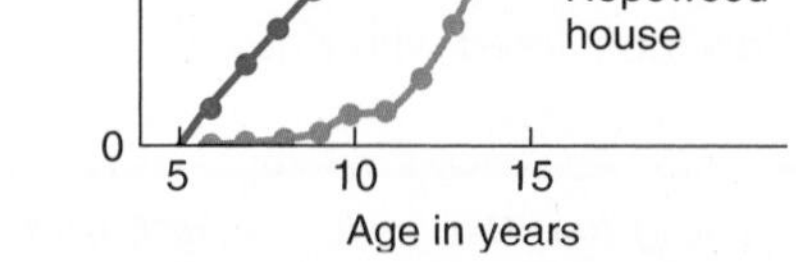

The Vipeholm study also demonstrated that it was possible to increase the average consumption of sugar from about 30 to 330 grams with little increase in caries, when the additional sugar was consumed at mealtime and in solution form.[30] Two important points about the design of the Vipeholm study are, excessive quantities and abnormal presentations of food were used, and, by today's standards, the study would not have received ethical clearance.

Additional evidence of sugar's link to dental caries comes from a genetic disease. Some people have a lowered caries incidence attributable to a condition known as **hereditary fructose intolerance** (HFI). After the intake of fructose, these persons experience nausea and vomiting, and sweat excessively; they may also develop malaise, tremor, coma, and convulsions. As a result, these individuals carefully avoid foods with fructose or sucrose that has fructose as one of the metabolic products. Those HFI individuals who have survived this disorder by successfully avoiding fructose or sucrose from any source are either caries-free or have very few caries.[31] The low prevalence of caries in HFI persons is an indication that starchy foods alone do not produce decay, whereas foods with sugar do produce decay.

What annual level of sugar consumption makes a diet highly cariogenic? A truly safe level has not been established, although animal and human studies that have

■ **FIGURE 15–3**   Plot of the mean number of decayed, missing, filled (DMF) teeth versus chronologic age in state schools in Australia and in Hopewood House.
(Reprinted by permission from Marthaler (1967). *Caries Res,* 1:21.)

examined the drop and recovery of plaque pH after consumption of specific foods has suggested an annual intake between 10 and 15 kg per person per year.[32]

Two similar epidemiologic studies of the caries prevalence in 12-year-olds and the per-capita sugar use have been done. The first, conducted in 47 countries, showed a statistically significant relationship between the availability of sugar and the number of DMFT.[33] When the daily per-capita supply of sugar was less than 50 grams, the DMFT index was less than 3.0 (Table 15–5 ■). More recently, a study in 90 countries showed a statistically significant relationship between the logarithm of DMFT and sugar consumption at a slope of 0.021 per kilogram per person per year.[34] It is interesting to note that this association disappeared when only the data from the 29 industrialized countries were analyzed. This finding indicates that factors other than sugar consumption (i.e., oral hygiene, professional care, fluoride use), should be considered when explaining variations in caries prevalence.

It is erroneous to think that oral hygiene and optimum fluoride exposure alone will protect teeth from deleterious dietary practices. It is also an oversimplification to believe that simply removing "sugar" from the diet is an adequate approach to preventing caries progression. The caries-promoting activity of carbohydrates and sweeteners vary according to frequency of intake as well as combined intake with other foods that may vary in protein or fat content.

Processed, high-starch snacks, whether gelatinized, baked, or fried, produce as much acid in dental plaque as sucrose alone, however at a slower rate.[35,36] Foods containing both cooked starch and sucrose have been shown to enhance caries potential.[37] Caries potential is enhanced because the starch brings the sucrose into closer contact with the tooth surface.[38] It is important to emphasize that added sugars can be part of a total diet when recommended intake guidelines are followed and when the sugars are eaten with meals, while avoiding food and beverage intake that contains sugars or starches between meals for caries prevention.[8,39]

The modern understanding of the dental caries process, called the chemoparasitic theory, was described by W. D. Miller in 1890.[40] Caries is caused by dissolution of teeth by acid produced during the metabolism of dietary carbohydrates by oral bacteria. The resultant lowered pH favors the growth of *S. mutans* and other acidogenic bacteria. The two primary bacteria involved in caries formation are *S. mutans* and lactobacilli.[41]

Plaque composition studies have established that persons who regularly consume dietary components with a high fermentable sugar content have increased proportions of *S. mutans* and lactobacilli in their dental plaque, tipping the delicate balance of the oral environment to a more acidic, demineralizing role.[42] Significant factors regulating homeostasis in the mouth include the integrity of the host defenses (i.e., salivary flow) and the composition of the diet.[43] Stimulation of salivary flow or suppression of sugar catabolism and acid production by the use of metabolic inhibitors and non-fermentable artificial sweeteners in snacks could assist in the maintenance of microbial homeostasis in plaque and thus a reduction in caries incidence.[42] For instance, use of fluorides, consumption of foods and beverages that contain non-fermentable sugar substitutes such as aspartame or polyols, stimulation of salivary flow after main meals by chewing sugar-free gum, and selection of a diet that favors remineralization (i.e., content high in calcium, phosphate, and protein) are all ways to prevent the lowered pH and breakdown of microbial homeostasis in dental plaque biofilms.[41,42]

■ **Table 15–5**   Sugar Supply and Caries Prevalence in 12-Year-Old Children of 47 Countries

DMFT Index	Sugar Supply (gram/person/day)		
	50	50–120	120
3.0	21 countries	9 countries	
3.0–5.0		9 countries	1 country
5.0		1 country	6 countries

DMFT, decayed, missing, filled teeth.
Source: Reprinted by permission from Sreebny, L. M. (1982). *Community Dent Oral Epidemiol,* 10:1–17.[33]

THE POLYOLS AS SWEETENERS

Several **polyols** are currently used as sugar substitutes owing to their sweet taste. They are not sugars; rather they are **sugar alcohols.** Each molecule resembles a sugar, with the exception that an alcohol grouping (-OH) is attached to each carbon atom of the polyol (Figure 15–4 ■). Polyols can have a chemical structure that is derived from monosaccharides (e.g., sorbitol, mannitol, xylitol, erythritol), disaccharides (e.g., isomalt, lactitol, maltitol), or polysaccharide-derived mixtures (e.g., maltitol syrup, hydrogenated starch hydrolysates [HSH])[8] (Table 15–6 ■). The sweetness of polyols varies considerably and only a few of them suffice as sugar substitutes.

Polyols have 40% of the caloric content of sucrose,[44] which is an advantage to those limiting caloric intake for weight control. Another advantage is that polyols have physical characteristics similar to sucrose, so their substitution in products does not alter the overall quality, size, and weight of the products to which they are added. However, one disadvantage to using polyols in baked goods is that browning (i.e., caramelization) does not occur.

Sorbitol

Sorbitol is a sugar alcohol (polyol) that occurs naturally in many fruits and berries. It is produced commercially from glucose and is on the GRAS list as a "bulk" sweetener for use in chewing gum, chocolates, jams and jellies, frozen confections, and other confectionaries.[8] It is only half as sweet as sucrose. Although considered noncariogenic, in solution it is slowly fermented by *S. mutans.*[45] In patients with reduced salivary gland

function, it has been shown to be cariogenic with prolonged use.[46] Sorbitol is not easily metabolized or absorbed from the gastrointestinal (GI) tract and may cause diarrhea if large quantities are ingested.[45]

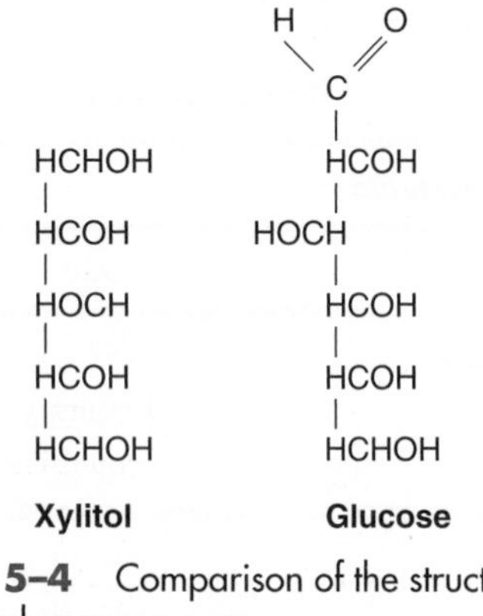

Mannitol

Mannitol is a naturally occurring polyol found in seaweed, but is also commercially obtained from the sugar mannose. Oral microorganisms metabolize this sweetener very slowly, so there is virtually no cariogenic activity with its use.[47] Mannitol is used as a dusting agent for chewing gum and as a bulking agent in powdered foods.[8]

Xylitol

Xylitol is the polyol that has received the greatest amount of attention by the dental profession for its anticaries benefits. Discovered in wood chips in 1890 and in wheat and oat straw in 1891, xylitol is produced commercially from birch trees and other hardwoods that contain xylan. Recently, in an effort to reduce production costs, biotechnology is being used to produce xylitol from corn cobs and from the waste of sugar cane or other fibers.[48–54]

Xylitol is used primarily in chewing gum, although it can also be found in mints, mouthrinses, and some dentifrices. Xylitol's sweetness approximates that of sucrose; however, it is about 10 times more costly to produce than sucrose.

Many studies have shown that xylitol creates a protective effect and reduces tooth decay in part by reducing levels of *S. mutans* found in plaque and saliva, and also by reducing the level of lactic acid produced by the bacteria.[45,49,55–59] In a double-blind cohort study in Belize, 1,277 schoolchildren were randomly assigned into nine treatment groups, consisting of four xylitol groups of differing doses, two xylitol–sorbitol groups of differing doses, two sucrose groups of differing doses, and one sorbitol group. When four blinded and calibrated dentist examiners carried out dental examinations at baseline, 16, 28, and 40 months, applying World Health Organization (WHO) criteria for caries detection, the most significant caries reduction was found in the group assigned to the highest xylitol concentration.[55] In a more recent study by Hildebrandt and colleagues, xylitol chewing gum was compared with a xylitol mouthrinse, and both were found to cause a similar reduction in oral *S. mutans* levels.[60]

Evidence is sufficient for clinicians to consider including xylitol-containing products for the prevention

■ **FIGURE 15–4** Comparison of the structural formula of a polyol and common sugar.

■ **Table 15–6**   Polyols and Novel Sugar Sweeteners

Type	kcal/g	Regulatory Status	Estimated Daily Intake (EDI) or Acceptable Daily Intake (ADI)	Description
Monosaccharide polyols or novel sugars				
Sorbitol	2.6	GRAS[a]–Label must warn about a laxative effect		50%–70% as sweet as sucrose; some individuals experience a laxative effect load of ≥50 g
Mannitol	1.6	Approved food additive; the label must warn about a laxative effect		50%–70% as sweet as sucrose; some individuals experience a laxative effect from a load of ≥20 g
Xylitol	2.4	Approved food additive for use in foods for special dietary uses		as sweet as sucrose; new forms have better free-flowing abilities
Erythritol	0.2	Independent GRAS determinations; no questions from FDA	EDI mean: 1 g/p/d; 90th percentile: 4 g/p/d	60%–80% as sweet as sucrose; also acts as a flavor enhancer, formulation aid, humectant, stabilizer, and thickener, sequestrant, and texturizer
D-Tagatose	1.5	Independent GRAS determinations; no questions from FDA	EDI mean: 7.5 g/p/d; 90th percentile: 15 g/p/d ADI 15 grams/60 kg adult/d	75%–92% as sweet as sucrose; sweetness synergizer; functions also as a texturizer, stabilizer, humectant, and formulation aid
Disaccharide polyols or novel sugars				
Isomalt	2	GRAS affirmation petition filed		45%–65% as sweet as sucrose; used as a bulking agent
Lactitol	2	GRAS affirmation petition filed		30%–40% as sweet as sucrose; used as a bulking agent
Maltitol	2.1	GRAS affirmation petition filed		90% as sweet as sucrose; used as a bulking agent
Trehalose	4	Independent GRAS determinations; no questions from FDA	EDI mean: 34 g/p/d; 90th percentile: 68 g/p/d	45% as sweet as sucrose; functions also as a texturizer, stabilizer, and humectant
Polysaccharide Polyols				
HSH[b]		GRAS affirmation petition filed		25%–50% as sweet as sucrose (depending on the monosaccharide composition)

[a]GRAS=Generally Recognized As Safe.
[b]Other names include hydrogenated starch hydrolysates and maltitol syrup (Adapted from *J Amer Diet Assoc* 2004:257.)[8]

of dental caries in high-risk populations (Figure 15–5 ■). However, sufficient dose and frequency of use must be followed to obtain the desired result, that is, a daily xylitol dose of 6 to 10 grams, 3 to 5 times per day, for a minimum contact time of 5 minutes. Xylitol's effectiveness

is greater at a higher frequency of consumption as well as a higher dose. The main side effect associated with consumption of polyols, including xylitol, is osmotic diarrhea, but only when consumed in very large quantities.[49] Nevertheless, those persons with preexisting

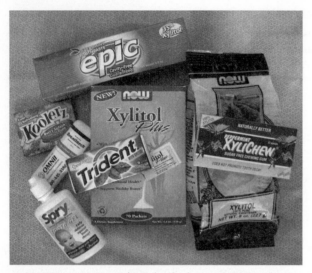

■ **FIGURE 15–5** Selected xylitol-containing products.

gastrointestinal disorders should consider this potential problem before starting a dosing regimen.

INTENSE SWEETENERS

With regard to primary preventive dental practices, non-cariogenic sweeteners and sugar substitutes used in foods, beverages, oral medications, mouthrinses, dentifrices, and candy are highly desirable for the prevention of dental caries and some adverse health effects. For these reasons, dental providers advocate their use.

Because of their intense sweetness compared with sucrose, these sweeteners are used in very small quantities and thus, in the long term, are more economical. The following section describes the most popular intense sweeteners currently used in the United States, ones currently being introduced into the market, and those used elsewhere in the world, but not yet approved for use in the United States (Table 15–7 ■).

■ **Table 15–7** Approved Non-nutritive Sweeteners

Type	*kcal/g*	*Regulatory Status*	*Other Names*	*Description*
Saccharin	0	Approved as sweetener for beverages and as a tabletop sweetener in foods with specific maximum amounts allowed	Sweet and Low, Sweet Twin, Sweet 'N Low Brown, Necta Sweet	200–700 times sweeter than sucrose; non-cariogenic and produces glycemic response; synergizes the sweetening power of nutritive and non-nutritive sweeteners; sweetening power is not reduced with heating
Aspartame	4[a]	Approved as a general-purpose sweetener	NutraSweet, Equal, Sugar Twin Sugar Twin (Blue box)	160–200 times sweeter than sucrose; non cariogenic and produces limited glycemic response
Acesulfame-K	0	Approved as a general-purpose sweetener	Sunett, Sweet & Safe, Sweet One	200 times sweeter than sucrose; noncariogenic and produces no glycemic response; synergizes the sweetening power of nutritive and non-nutritive sweeteners; sweetening power is not reduced with heating
Sucralose	0	Approved as a general-purpose sweetener	Splenda	600 times sweeter than sucrose; noncariogenic and produces no glycemic response; sweetening power is not reduced with heating
Neotame	0	Approved as a general-purpose sweetener	Not available at time of publication	8,000 times sweeter than sucrose; noncariogenic and produces no glycemic response; sweetening power is not reduced with heating

[a]This sweetener does provide energy; however, because of the intense sweetness, the amount of energy derived from it is negligible.
(From *J Amer Diet Assoc* 2004:258.)[8]

Saccharin

Saccharin is approximately 200 to 700 times sweeter than sucrose. It is non-nutritive and non-cariogenic. It is the oldest of the artificial sweeteners used in the United States and is marketed under the brand name of Sweet 'N Low. Each year, 8 million pounds of saccharin are used in food: 2 to 3 million pounds as tabletop sweetener, 1 to 2 million pounds in beverages, and 3 million pounds in personal care products. Despite a decline in usage since a peak in 1982, saccharin remains the largest volume, lowest cost intense sweetener used in the world today.[8,61]

Saccharin is approved for use as a food additive in foods and beverages, tabletop sugar substitutes, and gum. It can also be used in cosmetics and pharmaceuticals. Since 2001, products that contain saccharin no longer need to carry a warning about saccharin's association with cancer in laboratory animals. In 1977, the FDA proposed a ban on use of saccharin because it was reported to cause bladder cancer in laboratory rats. In 2000, the National Toxicology Program of the National Institutes of Health concluded that saccharin should be removed from the list of potential carcinogens, and in 2001 federal legislation allowed the warning label placed on products to be removed.[62] The FDA has approved saccharin in the following forms: ammonium saccharin, calcium saccharin, and sodium saccharin. In beverages, amounts cannot exceed 12 mg per fluid ounce, as a sugar substitute it cannot exceed the sweetening power of 1 teaspoon of sucrose (20 mg) for use in cooking or at the table, and in processed foods amounts cannot exceed 30 mg per serving.[8] The product label must list saccharin as an ingredient and state the amount contained per serving as indicated above.[63]

Aspartame

Aspartame, a dipeptide, is 160 to 220 times sweeter than sucrose. It is sold under the brand names Nutrasweet and Equal. Upon digestion, intestinal esterases hydrolyze aspartame to aspartic acid, methanol, and phenylalanine, which are components found naturally in fruits, vegetables, meats, and milk.[64] Metabolized aspartame provides 4 kcal/g, but because of its intense sweetness, only very small amounts are needed, so the amount of caloric intake is negligible.[8]

In 1981, the FDA approved aspartame as a sweetener in dry goods (i.e., tabletop sweetener, cold breakfast cereals, gelatins, and puddings) and in chewing gum.

In 1983, the approval was expanded to include carbonated beverages. In 1996, the FDA further approved aspartame as a "general purpose sweetener" for use in all foods and beverages. Over 100 nations have also approved aspartame for use as a sweetener.[8]

Aspartame is available in liquid, granular, encapsulated, and powder forms. Soft drinks account for over 70% of aspartame consumption, but it also is added to more than 6,000 foods, personal care products, and pharmaceuticals. The United States accounts for up to 75% of sales, leading the world in aspartame demand. One disadvantage of aspartame is that excessive heating causes decomposition and lessens aspartame's sweetening ability.[8] Another serious consideration is its ingestion by persons with phenylketonuria. Phenylketonuria is a homozygous recessive inborn error of metabolism in which individuals affected cannot metabolize phenylalanine. In persons with this rare condition, excessive intake of aspartame can cause higher plasma phenylalanine levels and many adverse effects.[65] The FDA requires that foods containing aspartame have the following label with prominent wording: "PHENYLKETONURICS: CONTAINS PHENYLALANINE."[66]

Acesulfame-K

Acesulfame-K (acesulfame potassium) is a non-nutritive sweetener approximately 200 times sweeter than sucrose.[8,45] It was approved by the FDA in 1988 for use in dry food products. In 1994, approval was expanded for use in yogurt, refrigerated desserts, syrups, and baked goods. Acesulfame-K is currently approved for use in foods, beverages, pharmaceuticals, and cosmetics in more than 30 countries.[45] Interestingly, 95% of the consumed sweetener is excreted unchanged in the urine, so consumption does not affect intake of potassium.[67] It can withstand high temperatures, making it ideal for cooking and baking, and is available in granular forms to blend with other nutritive and non-nutritive sweeteners.[8]

Sucralose

Sucralose, sold under the brand name Splenda, is a non-cariogenic and non-nutritive sweetener that is 600 times sweeter than sucrose. It is poorly absorbed (approximately 11% to 27%) and is largely excreted in the feces and urine unchanged. Sucralose was first approved in 1998 for use as a tabletop sweetener, and in a number of desserts, confections, and nonalcoholic beverages. In 1999, sucralose was approved as a general-purpose sweetener. In a review of more than 110 studies in humans and animals, this sweetener did not pose carcinogenic, reproductive, or neurologic risk to humans.[68]

Neotame

Neotame is a new product developed by the manufacturers of NutraSweet. It is very similar in structure to aspartame and has a highly intense sweetness with a clean taste. It is 7,000 to 13,000 times sweeter than sucrose and is heat stable for baking. It has been reported to be stable for use in carbonated soft drinks, powdered soft drinks, yellow cake, yogurt, and hot-packed still drinks.[69] Neotame was granted approval by the FDA in 2002 for use as a food additive and sweetening agent to enhance flavor in several food categories. It is not approved for use in meat and poultry.[8,70,71]

NON-NUTRITIVE SWEETENERS NOT APPROVED IN THE UNITED STATES

Alitame

Alitame is 2,000 times sweeter than sucrose, without the bitter or metallic taste of most high-intensity sweeteners.[72] Alitame is blended with other sweeteners to enhance the quality of sweetness. In 1986, a petition was submitted to the FDA for approval of alitame as a tabletop sweetener and for use in products including baked goods, beverages, and confections. As of January 2003, this petition was in the abeyance category, (i.e., deficiencies were found, a new petition must be submitted, and another review is necessary).[8] Currently, alitame is approved for use in foods and beverages in Australia, New Zealand, Mexico, People's Republic of China, and Columbia.[8]

Cyclamate

Cyclamate is more than 30 times sweeter than sucrose. It is currently in use by more than 50 countries worldwide; however, cyclamates were banned in 1969 by the FDA as a food ingredient when the saccharin/cyclamate mixture was shown to cause cancer in laboratory rats.[73] The concern was that it could be toxic in some individuals who metabolize cyclamate to cyclohexylamine.[74] In 1982, the Cancer Assessment Committee of the FDA determined that cyclamate was not carcinogenic. Although this conclusion was reaffirmed later in 1985 by

the National Academy of Sciences, the petition to reapprove cyclamate is still under review by the FDA.

Neohesperidine

Neohesperidine dihydrochalcone is 1,500 times sweeter than sucrose. It imparts a licorice flavor to foods and beverages, and can enhance the mouth feel of beverages. In the United States, it is GRAS as a flavor ingredient but not as a sweetener.[8]

Stevia (Steveoside)

Steveoside is derived from a shrub in South America and is 300 times sweeter than sucrose.[75] It provides an enhanced sweet taste but cannot be marketed or sold as a sweetener in the United States. The FDA has not been provided with enough evidence to safely say that it can be used as a food additive. Stevia can be sold as a "dietary supplement" in packets that resemble tabletop sweeteners. It should be emphasized that Stevia is not approved as a non-nutritive sweetener.[8,75]

Thaumatin

Thaumatin acts as a flavor enhancer and is a mixture of proteins which imparts an intensely sweet taste.[8] In the United States, thaumatin is GRAS as a flavor adjunct in a number of categories of foodstuffs.[8]

HEALTH CONSIDERATIONS

Obesity

Non-nutritive sweeteners have the potential to promote weight loss in those persons who are overweight and/or obese. Originally, the goal during development of the sweeteners was to provide a sweet taste to foods and beverages without providing energy (i.e., high caloric content) to persons wanting to control energy intakes.[8]

Diabetes and Glycemic Response

Sweeteners do not cause diabetes, but high intake of nutritive sweeteners in a susceptible individual should be avoided because it has been determined that high intake of fructose can lead to high blood lipid levels for persons with diabetes. A safer alternative is to use nonnutritive sweeteners whenever possible.[8]

Hyperlipidemias

Diets high in nutritive sweeteners have been shown to increase serum triacylglycerol and low-density lipoprotein cholesterol levels in short-term studies. Fructose has been found to be more hyperlipidemic than sucrose. For those controlling cholesterol levels, intake of this nutritive sweetener should be decreased whenever feasible.

Behavioral Disorders

Although once believed to be associated with excessive sugar consumption, hyperactivity is not the result of sugar intake in children.[8] It is important to note, too, that when the FDA approved use of non-nutritive sweeteners and accepted levels for consumption in children, no adverse effects were found if intake remained within the recommended guidelines.[8]

SUMMARY

A wide variety of chemicals can add to the sweetness of the human diet. Each sweetener has its benefits and its shortcomings. Nutritive sweeteners, which humans have used the longest, impart calories with their use, and they support dental decay with frequent oral contact. Nonetheless, sweetness will be highly sought and highly valued by humans. It is no wonder that the market demand for both nutritive and non-nutritive sweeteners is so high. Humans' affinity for sweet taste is established in utero and continues throughout one's lifetime. With the current push to prevent weight gain, dental caries, and control glycemic response in those who have diabetes, market demand will continue to drive the development of improved, sweeter, and more cost-effective non-nutritive alternatives to sucrose. Particularly with regard to xylitol as a phenomenon in the effort to prevent dental caries, consumers will see a push to develop more xylitol products for decay prevention as well as further efforts to cut costs associated with its manufacture.

ACKNOWLEDGMENT

The authors extend their gratitude to Robert J. Feigal, DDS, PhD, Professor, Division of Pediatric Dentistry, School of Dentistry, University of Minnesota, for his thoughtful review and helpful comments during the preparation of this chapter.

REFERENCES

1. Tamussi, P. (2006). The history of sweet taste: Not exactly a piece of cake. *J Mol Recognit,* 19:188–99.
2. Sigman-Grant, M., & Morita, J. (2003). Defining and interpreting intakes of sugars[1,2,3,4]. *Am J Clin Nutr,* 78 (4 Suppl):815S–26S.
3. Mc Murry, J. (1998). *Fundamentals of organic chemistry* (4th ed.). Pacific Grove, CA: Brooks/Cole Publishing Company.
4. American Society for Neurochemistry. (1999). Neural processing and behavior 48. Molecular biology of olfaction and taste (part seven). In Siegel, G. J., Albers, R. W., & Price, D. L., Eds. *Basic neurochemistry. Molecular, cellular and medical aspects* (6th ed.). Baltimore: Lippincott Williams & Wilkins, 1–7.
5. Bright, G. (1999). Low-calorie sweeteners—From molecules to mass markets. *World Rev Nutr Diet,* 85:3–9.
6. Cohen, S. M., Anderson, T. A., de Oliveira, L. M., & Arnold, L. L. (1998). Tumorigenicity of sodium ascorbate in male rats. *Cancer Res,* 58:2557–61.
7. Lindley, M. G. (1999). New developments in low-calorie sweeteners. *World Rev Nutr Diet,* 85:44–51.
8. American Dietetic Association. (2004). Position of the American Dietetic Association: Use of nutritive and non-nutritive sweeteners. *J Am Diet Assoc,* 104 (2):255–75.
9. U.S. Department of Agriculture. Economic Research Service. (2000). *Sugar and sweetener situation and outlook yearbook.* Beltsville, MD: U.S. Department of Agriculture.
10. Hanover, L., & White, J. (1993). Manufacturing, composition, and applications of fructose. *Am J Clin Nutr,* 5 (Suppl):724S–32S.
11. Briefel, R. (2001). Nutrition monitoring in the United States. In Bowman, B., & Russell, R. M., Eds. *Present knowledge in nutrition* (8th ed.). Washington, DC: ILSI Press, 617–35.
12. van Staveren, W., & Ocke, M. C. (2001). Estimation of dietary intake. In Bowman, B., & Russell, R. M, Eds. *Present knowledge in nutrition* (8th ed.). Washington, DC: ILSI Press, 605–16.
13. Macdiarmid, J., & Blundell, J. E. (1997). Dietary underreporting: What people say about recording their food intake. *Eur J Clin Nutr,* 51:199–200.
14. Hirvonen, T., Mannisto, S., Roos, E., & Pietinen, P. (1997). Increasing prevalence of underreporting does not necessarily distort dietary surveys. *Eur J Clin Nutr,* 51:297–301.
15. U.S. Department of Agriculture. Products from the CSFII/DHKS 1994–96, 1998, 2002. Retrieved December 23, 2006, from http://www.barc.usda.gov/bhnrc/foodsurvey/Products9496.html.

16. Murphy, S., & Johnson, R. K. (2003). The scientific basis of recent US guidance on sugars intake. *Am J Clin Nutr,* 78:827S–33S.

17. Schiffman, S. S., Sattely-Miller, E. A., Graham, B. G., Bennett, J. L., Booth, B. J., Desai, N., & Bishay, I. (2000, February). Effect of temperature, pH, and ions on sweet taste. *Physiol Behav,* 68 (4):469–481.

18. Davis, E. (1995). Functionality of sugars. Physicochemical interactions in foods. *Am J Clin Nutr,* 62 (Suppl):170S–77S.

19. Guthrie, J., & Morton, J. (2000). Food sources of added sweeteners in the diets of Americans. *J Am Diet Assoc,* 100:43–48, 51.

20. Schneeman, B. (1995). Summary of the proceedings of a workshop: Nutritional and health aspects of sugars. *Am J Clin Nutr,* 62 (Suppl):294S–96S.

21. Mardis, A. (2001). Current knowledge of the health effects of sugar intake. *Fam Econ Nutr Rev,* 13:87–91.

22. Rugg-Gunn, A. J. (1989). Diet and dental caries. In Murray, J. J., Ed. *The prevention of dental diseases* (2nd ed.). Oxford: Oxford University Press, 4–114.

23. Scheinin, A., & Makinen, K. K. (1975). Turku sugar studies I-XXI. *Acta Odontol Scand,* 33 (Suppl 70):1–349.

24. Koulourides, T., Bodden, R., Keller, S., Manson-Hing, L., Lastra, J., & Housch, T. (1976). Cariogenicity of nine sugars tested with an intraoral device in man. *Caries Res,* 10:427–41.

25. Kandelman, D. (1997). Sugar, alternative sweeteners and meal frequency in relation to caries prevention: New perspectives. *Br J Nutr,* 77 (Suppl 1):S121–28.

26. Sreebny, L. (1982). Sugar and human dental caries. *World Rev Nutr Diet,* 40:19–65.

27. Orland, F., Blayney, J., Harrison, R., Reyniers, J., Trexler, P., Ervin, R., Gordon, H., & Wagner, M. (1955). Experimental caries in germ-free rats inoculated with enterococci. *J Am Dent Assoc,* 50:259–72.

28. Kite, O., Shaw, J., & Sognnaes, R. (1950). The prevention of experimental tooth decay by tube-feeding. *J Nutr,* 42:89–103.

29. Marthaler, T. M. (1967). Epidemiological and clinical dental findings in relation to intake of carbohydrates. *Caries Res,* 1:222–38.

30. Gustafsson, B. E., Quensel, C. E., Lanke, L. S., Lundqvist, C., Grahnen, H., Bonow, B. E., & Krasse, B. (1954). The Vipeholm dental caries study. The effect of different levels of carbohydrate intake on caries activity in 436 individuals observed for five years. *Acta Odont Scand,* 11:232–264.

31. Newbrun, E., Hoover, C., Mattraux, G., & Graf, H. (1980). Comparison of dietary habits and dental health of subjects with hereditary fructose intolerance and control subjects. *J Am Dent Assoc,* 101:619–26.

32. Sheiham, A. (1991). Why free sugar consumption should be below 15 kg. per person per year in industrialized countries: The dental evidence. *Br Dent J,* 171:63–65.

33. Sreebny, L. M. (1982). Sugar availability, sugar consumption and dental caries. *Community Dent Oral Epidemiol,* 10:1–17.

34. Woodward, M., & Walker, A. R. P. (1994). Sugar consumption and dental caries: Evidence from 90 countries. *Br Dent J,* 176:297–302.

35. Grenby, T. H. (1991). Snack foods and dental caries. Investigations using laboratory animals. *Brit Dent J,* 171:353–61.

36. Mörmann, J. E., & Mühlemann, H. R. (1981). Oral starch degradation and its influence on acid production in human dental plaque. *Caries Res,* 15:166–75.

37. Mundorff, S. A., Featherstone, J. D. B., Bibby, B. G., Curzon, M. E. J., Eisenberg, A. D., & Espeland, M. A. (1990). Cariogenic potential of foods. 1. Caries in the rat model. *Caries Res,* 24:344–55.

38. Sgan-Cohen, H. D., Newbrun, E., Huber, R., Tenenbaum, G., & Sela, M. N. (1988). The effect of previous diet on plaque pH response to different foods. *J Dent Res,* 67:1434–37.

39. U.S. Department of Health and Human Services. (2000). *Nutrition and your health: Dietary guidelines for Americans* (5th ed.). (Home and Garden Bulletin No. 232). Washington, DC: U.S. Government Printing Office.

40. Miller, W. D. (1973). The microorganisms of the human mouth. In König, K. G., Ed. Basel, Switzerland: S. Karger.

41. Touger-Decker, R., & van Loveren, C. (2003). Sugar and dental caries. *Am J Clin Nutr,* 78 (Suppl):881S–92S.

42. Marsh, P. D. (2006). Dental plaque as a biofilm and a microbial community—Implications for health and disease. *BMC Oral Health,* 6 (Suppl 1):S14.

43. Marsh, P. D. (1989). Host defenses and microbial homeostasis: Role of microbial interactions. *J Dent Res,* 68:1567–75.

44. Lindley, M. G., Birch, G. G., & Khan, R. (1976). Sweetness of sucrose and xylitol. Structural considerations. *J Sci Food Agric,* 27:140–44.

45. Roberts, M. W., & Wright, J. T. (2002). Food sugar substitutes: A brief review for dental clinicians. *J Clin Pediatr Dent,* 27 (1):1–4.

46. Wennerhoim, K., Arends, J., Birkhed, D., Ruben, J., Emilson, C. G., & Dijkman A. G. (1994). Effect of xylitol and sorbitol in chewing-gums on mutans streptococci, plaque pH and mineral loss of enamel. *Caries Res,* 28:48–54.

47. Imfeld, T. (1993). Efficacy of sweetness and sugar substitutes in caries prevention. *Caries Res,* 27 (Suppl 1):50–55.

48. Bertrand, M. G. (1891). Rechercheszur quelques derives du xylose. *Bull Soc Chim Paris,* 5:554–57.

49. Ly, K. A., Milgrom, P., & Rothen, M. (2006). Xylitol, sweeteners, and dental caries. *Pediatr Dent,* 28:154–63.

50. Tada, K., Horiuchi, J., Kanno, T., & Kobayashi, M. (2004). Microbial xylitol production from corn cobs using *Candida magnoliae. J Biosci Bioeng,* 98:228–30.

51. Latif, F., & Rajoka, M. I. (2001). Production of ethanol and xylitol from corn cobs by yeasts. *Bioresour Technol,* 77:57–63.

52. Buhner, J., & Agblevor, F. A. (2004). Effect of detoxification of dilute-acid corn fiber hydrolysate on xylitol production. *Appl Biochem Biotechnol,* 119:13–30.

53. Dominguez, J. M., Gong, C. S, & Tsao, G. T. (1996). Pretreatment of sugar cane bagasse hemicellulose hydrolysate for xylitol production by yeast. *Appl Biochem Biotechnol,* 57–58:49–56.

54. Santos, J. C., Pinto, I. R., Carvalho, W., Mancilha, I. M., Felipe, M. G., & Silva, S. S. (2005). Sugarcane bagasse as raw material and immobilization support for xylitol production. *Appl Biochem Biotechnol,* 121–124:673–83.

55. Hayes, C. (2001). The effect of non-cariogenic sweeteners on the prevention of dental caries: A review of the evidence. *J Dent Educ,* 65 (10):1106–109.

56. Ashley, D., & Barbieri, S. (2005, December). The use of xylitol in caries prevention. *Access Mag,* 24–27.

57. Peldyak, J., & Mäkinen, K. K. (2002). Xylitol for caries prevention. *J Dent Hyg,* 76 (4):276–83.

58. Hansen, A. (2006, August). Xylitol: A dental phenomenon. *Access Mag,* 24–26.

59. Hildebrandt, G. H., & Sparks, B. S. (2000). Maintaining mutans streptococci suppression with xylitol chewing gum. *J Am Dent Assoc,* 131:909–16.

60. Hildebrandt, G. H., Lee, I., & Hodges, J. S. (2006, March). Reducing oral mutans streptococci levels with xylitol mouth rinse. *J Dent Res,* 85 (Spec Iss A). Abstract 1542.

61. Bizzari, S., Jackel, M., & Yoshida, Y. (1996). High intensity sweeteners. In *Chemical Economics Handbook.* SRI Consulting, Menlo Park, CA, United States.

62. Department of Health and Human Services: Public Health Service. National Toxicology Program. (2001, May 30). Announces the availability of the Report on Carcinogens, Ninth Edition. *Fed Reg* 66:29340-29342.

63. Food and Drug Administration. Food additives permitted in food or in contact with food on an interim basis pending additional study. 66(104). Saccharin, ammonium saccharin, calcium saccharin, and sodium saccharin. 21 CFR 180.37 (2002).

64. Ranney, R., Oppermann, J., Muldoon, E., & McMahon, F. (1976). Comparative metabolism of aspartame in experimental animals and humans. *J Toxicol Environ Health,* 2:441–51.

65. Wolf-Novak, L. C., Stegink, L. D., Brummel, M. C., Persoon, T. J., Filer, L. J., Jr., Bell, E. F., Ziegler, E. E., & Krause, W. L. (1990). Aspartame ingestion with and without carbohydrate in phenylketonuric and normal subjects. Effect on plasma concentrations of amino acids, glucose, and insulin. *Metabolism,* 39:391–96.

66. Food and Drug Administration. Food additives permitted for direct addition to food for human consumption: Aspartame. 21 CFR 172.804 (2002).

67. Walker, R. Acesulfame potassium: WHO food additives (Series 28). Retrieved December 6, 2007, from http://www.inchem.org/documents/jecfa/jecmono/v28je13.htm.

68. Food and Drug Administration. Food additives permitted for direct addition to food for human consumption: Sucralose. 21CFR 172.64 (1998).

69. Witt, J. (1999). Discovery and development of neotame. *World Rev Nutr Diet,* 85:52–57.

70. Garbow, J. R., Likos, J. J., & Schroeder, S. A. (2001). Structure, dynamics, and stability of β-cyclodextrin inclusion complexes of aspartame and neotame. *J Agric Food Chem,* 49:2053–60.

71. Neotame. (2002). Retrieved January 17, 2007, from http://www.neotame.com.

72. Auerbach, M., Locke, G., & Hendrick, M. (2001). Alitame. In Nabors, L., Ed. *Alternative sweeteners* (3rd ed.). New York: Marcel Dekker, 31–40.

73. Price, J., Biava, C., Oser, B., Vogin, E., Steinfeld, J., & Ley, H. (1967). Bladder tumors in rats fed cyclohexylamine or high doses of a mixture of cyclamate and saccharin. *Science,* 167:1131–32.

74. Kojima, S., & Ichibagase, H. (1966). Cyclohexylamine, a metabolite of sodium cyclamate. *Chem Pharm Bull,* 14:971.

75. Geuns, J. M. C. (2003). Phytochemistry: Stevioside. *Science Direct,* 64 (5):913–21.

Chapter 16

Professional Dental Hygiene Care

Kathleen O'Neill-Smith

Carolyn Horton Ray

OBJECTIVES

After studying this chapter, the student should be able to:

1. Describe the dental hygiene process of care.
2. Describe the integration of the dental hygiene process of care into the dental hygiene appointment.
3. Compare and contrast dental hygiene therapy for patients with and without attachment loss.
4. Describe the elements of the dental hygiene appointment.
5. Describe the use of the *CDT 2007–2008* in creating a dental hygiene care plan.

KEY TERMS

Comprehensive oral evaluation
Assessment
Periodic oral evaluation
Diagnosis
Planning phase
Implementation phase

INTRODUCTION

The American Dental Hygienists' Association (ADHA) recognizes that the dental hygiene process of care includes assessment, diagnosis, planning, implementation, and evaluation. The policy describes the dental hygiene process of care as:

- *Assessment:*   The systematic collection and analysis of data to identify client's (patient's) needs.
- *Diagnosis:*   The identification of client (patient) strengths and oral health problems that dental hygiene intervention can improve.
- *Planning:*   The establishment of realistic goals and the selection of dental hygiene interventions that can move the client (patient) closer to optimal health.
- *Implementation:*   The act of carrying out the dental hygiene care plan.
- *Evaluation:*   The measurement of the extent to which the client (patient) has achieved the goals as specified in the plan. Judgment to continue, discontinue, or modify the dental hygiene plan of care.[1]

The process of dental hygiene care for the patient requires the application of biologic and psychosocial concepts of health and human functioning. The dental hygiene appointment provides patient services that support total health through the promotion of optimal oral health. The American Dental Education Association (ADEA) Competencies for Entry into the Profession of Dental Hygiene describes the abilities expected of a dental hygienist entering the profession.[2]

The dental hygiene appointment may include assessments, diagnoses, preventive oral prophylaxis, therapeutic scaling and root planing, periodontal debridement, education and counseling, preventive and therapeutic modalities, and/or supportive care. Formulation of a dental hygiene diagnosis may be necessary to direct the dental hygiene treatment during the appointment and to deliver quality oral health care. Several steps must occur before a dental hygiene diagnosis can be determined.

ASSESSMENT

The appointment begins with a thorough assessment of the patient. The systematic collection and analysis of data are necessary to identify patient needs. In the dental hygiene process, *client* may refer to individuals, families, groups, or communities as defined in the ADHA Framework for Theory Development.[1]

In this chapter, the term *patient,* instead of *client,* will be used to address the specific one-on-one health provider interaction or relationship that occurs in the dental hygiene appointment.

Please note that the term *appointment* will be used to describe the integration of therapy used in the dental hygiene process of care. On the basis of the assessment, the dental hygienist can recognize deviation from health and intervene with appropriate therapy. The data collected during this process drive the treatment and care delivered to the patient. Assessment and analysis of risk factors provide information about a patient's periodontal disease susceptibility.[3–5] Recent evidence has identified certain risk factors that may make a patient more susceptible to periodontitis, and that may increase the extent and severity of the disease.[6]

The *CDT 2007–2008* is a manual published by the American Dental Association that provides a set of codes and accompanying definitions that reflect the commonly accepted dental procedures and can be used when billing dental insurance for procedures rendered. Although it is recognized that dental hygiene therapy is not driven by insurance codes, the dental provider must be aware of the utilization of the codes in treatment planning and implementation of therapy.

A **comprehensive oral evaluation** is always necessary to establish a baseline of medical and dental care. A comprehensive oral evaluation is a thorough assessment of the extraoral and intraoral hard and soft tissues, and may require interpretation of information acquired through additional diagnostic procedures. This **assessment** includes an evaluation for oral cancer, the patient's dental and medical history, and a general health assessment. "It includes the evaluation and recording of dental caries, missing or unerupted teeth, restorations, existing prostheses, occlusal relationships, periodontal conditions (including periodontal screening and/or charting), hard and soft tissue anomalies, etc." (D0150).[7]

If the patient is an established patient, then a **periodic oral evaluation** is performed. The purpose of an evaluation performed on a patient of record is to determine any changes in the patient's dental and medical health status since a previous comprehensive or periodic evaluation. This procedure includes an oral cancer evaluation and a periodontal screening and/or charting where indicated, and may require interpretation of information acquired through additional diagnostic procedures (D0120).[7]

Medical/Dental History

The concept that oral conditions can influence disease elsewhere in the body is not new; in fact, it can be dated back to the days of Hippocrates. Since the U.S. Surgeon General's report in 2001, awareness of the interaction between oral disease and systemic disease has increased.[8]

The mouth is no longer a separate entity from the body; what occurs in the mouth has disease implications for the entire body. Conditions such as cardiovascular disease, low-birth-weight infants and premature births, and respiratory tract infections have all been linked to periodontal disease.[9–13] Therefore, a thorough medical and family history must be taken and evaluated to identify predisposing conditions that may affect treatment, and patient management and outcomes. Such conditions include but are not limited to diabetes, hypertension, pregnancy, smoking, substance abuse, and medications, or other existing conditions that impact traditional dental therapy.[14] The dental provider must also thoroughly assess a patient's risk for certain oral diseases and conditions. There are a variety of health history forms available that include health conditions to be considered before oral health care treatment (Figure 16–1 ∎).

Vital Signs

During a dental hygiene appointment, the following vital signs need to be measured: blood pressure, pulse, and/or respiration (Table 16–1[15] ∎).

Respiration is the fundamental process of life in which oxygen is used to oxidize organic fuel molecules, providing a source of energy as well as carbon dioxide and water.[16] Measurement of the patient's respiration involves observation of the depth of breath, rhythm, quality, and any sounds associated with breathing. The following steps are performed to measure respiratory rate: (1) counting respirations immediately after counting the pulse; (2) maintaining the finger over the radial pulse; (3) counting respirations so that the patient is not aware, because the rate may be voluntarily altered; and (4) counting the number of times the chest rises in 1 clocked minute.[17] All findings are recorded in the patient's record.

Extraoral/Intraoral Examination

An examination is any investigation or inspection made for the purpose of diagnosis, which is usually qualified by the method used.[18] Extraoral examination should include direct observation and palpation of the head, neck, skin, face, and gait. Intraoral examination should include screening and evaluation of the oral mucosa, lips, floor of the mouth, tongue, salivary ducts, hard and soft palate, and oropharynx. The screening should also include detection of lesions and oral piercing.

Dental/Periodontal Examination

The dental examination will provide documentation of the exact location and condition of teeth, restorations, and dental caries.

The periodontal examination is the recognition of health, gingivitis, or periodontitis. This evaluation should include, but not be limited to, periodontal probing, presence of plaque biofilm and exudates, tooth mobility, and presence of clinical furcations.

∎ **Table 16–1**   AHA Blood Pressure Levels

The American Heart Association (AHA) recommended blood pressure levels are as follows:

Blood Pressure Category	Systolic		Diastolic
	(mm Hg)		(mm Hg)
Normal	Less than 120	and	less than 80
Prehypertension	120–139	or	80–89
High			
Stage 1	140–159	or	90–99
Stage 2	160 or higher	or	100 or higher

Source: Retrieved from http://www.americanheart.org. Reprinted by permission from www.americanheart.org. © 2008, American Heart Association, Inc.[15]

UNM Health History

Date_____

MEDICAL ALERT
_____

Name_____   _____   _____   _____
      Last   First   Initial   Soc. Sec. #   Home Phone   Business/Cell Phone

_____   _____   _____   _____   _____   _____
     Address   City   State   Zipcode   Occupation   Employer

Dr._____

_____   _____   _____   _____   _____   _____   _____
Birthdate   Sex   Height   Weight   Marital Status   Dentist's Name   Dentist's Phone

Dr._____

_____   _____   _____   _____
  Physician's Name   Phone #   Person to contact in case of emergency   Phone #

My last physical exam was on _____   Reason_____
                     Date

For the following questions check yes or no for the response that best applies. Your answers will be considered confidential. Please note that during your initial visit you will be asked some questions about your responses to this questionnaire and there may be additional questions concerning your health.

YES	NO	Patient Question	Provider's comments
		1. Are you in good health?	
		2. Are you now under the care of a physician?	
		3. Has there been any change in your general health within the past year?	
		4. Have you had any serious illness, operation, or been hospitalized in the past five years?	
		5. Have you had any problems with, or during, dental treatment?	
		6. Are you allergic, or had any reaction, to any medications, including local anesthetics?	
		7. Do you have any other allergies, such as metals, latex, food, pollen, etc.	
		Please check any of the following diseases or conditions you have experienced.	
		8. Damaged heart valves, artificial heart valves, shunts, heart murmur, or rheumatic fever	
		9. Cardiovascular disease such as heart trouble, heart attack, angina, high blood pressure, hardening of the arteries, stroke, etc.	
		10. Born with any heart problems	
		11. Sinus trouble, asthma, or hayfever	
		12. Fainting spells, seizures, epilepsy, or convulsions	
		13. Persistent diarrhea, weight loss, or vomiting	
		14. Diabetes	
		15. Hepatitis, yellow jaundice, cirrhosis, or liver disease	
		16. AIDS or HIV infection, Date of Diagnosis:_____ Current viral load count: _____ Current t-cell count or % _____	
		17. Thyroid problems (goiter)	
		18. Respiratory problems, emphysema, bronchitis, etc.	
		19. Arthritis or painful swollen joints	
		20. Stomach ulcer, hyperacidity, or other conditions	
		21 Kidney conditions or dialysis	
		22. Tuberculosis or positive TB skin test	
		23. Anemia or blood disorders	
		24. Gonorrhea, syphilis, herpes, or other similar diseases	
		25. Problems with mental health or nerves	

■ **FIGURE 16–1**   Sample health history form.

		26. Cancer	
		27. Prosthetic devices (joints, valves, hearing aid, implants) other than dentures	
		28. Use tobacco or snuff products	
		29. Diagnosed with alcoholism	
		30. Vision or hearing problems	
		31. Use recreational drugs	
		32. Pregnant or nursing a baby	
		33. Ever taken Redux or Ponimi "fen-phen"	
		Are you taking any medications, including any non-prescription medications or natural supplements? (birth control, calcium, ginseng, garlic, etc.)	

Medication Name:	Condition Used For	Dental Implications	Resource

I certify that I have read and understand the above questionnaire and that my medical condition may affect my dental health and treatment. I have answered the questions willingly, truthfully, and to the best of my ability.

_____   _____
Signature of Patient or Legal Guardian   Date

_____   _____
Signature of Student   Date

_____   _____
Signature of Dental Provider   Date

Vital Signs: Blood Pressure_____   Pulse_____   Respiration_____

■ **FIGURE 16–1**   (*Continued*)

Date:_____

Please describe any changes in your health since you last completed this form and any medication you are taking. Write NONE if there has been no change.

_____

_____

_____

_____

_____

Vital Signs: Blood Pressure_____ Pulse_____ Respiration_____

Patient or Parent/Guardian Signature:_____

Student Signature _____ Faculty/Dentist Signature:_____

Date:_____

Please describe any changes in your health since you last completed this form and any medication you are taking. Write NONE if there has been no change.

_____

_____

_____

_____

_____

Vital Signs: Blood Pressure_____ Pulse_____ Respiration_____

Patient or Parent/Guardian Signature:_____

Student Signature _____ Faculty/Dentist Signature:_____

Date:_____

Please describe any changes in your health since you last completed this form and any medication you are taking. Write NONE if there has been no change.

_____

_____

_____

_____

_____

Vital Signs: Blood Pressure_____ Pulse_____ Respiration_____

Patient or Parent/Guardian Signature:_____

Student Signature _____ Faculty/Dentist Signature:_____

Date:_____

Please describe any changes in your health since you last completed this form and any medication you are taking. Write NONE if there has been no change.

_____

_____

_____

_____

_____

Vital Signs: Blood Pressure_____ Pulse_____ Respiration_____

Patient or Parent/Guardian Signature:_____

Student Signature _____ Faculty/Dentist Signature:_____

■ **FIGURE 16–1**   (*Continued*)

(Reprinted by permission from University of New Mexico, Division of Dental Hygiene, Albuquerque, NM, 2008).

Self-Care Evaluation

Review of current self-care practices and evaluation of the patient's skill levels and knowledge of hygiene practices should be investigated and recorded in the patient record. The effectiveness of self-care should also be documented. Many dental indices are available for the dental hygienist to incorporate in the patient's disease control monitoring; they also aid in quantifying and evaluating disease and health.

Diagnostic Radiographs

Radiographs are used to confirm and diagnose the disease process. Radiographs should be of diagnostic quality and properly identified and dated. Information attained from the patient assessment is reviewed, and the findings are used in the dental hygiene diagnosis to establish realistic goals and treatment strategies.

DIAGNOSIS

A **diagnosis** is the determination of the nature of disease made from the study of the signs and symptoms.[19] Dental caries and periodontal disease are the two most common dental diagnoses.

Dental hygiene diagnoses were introduced in 1982 by S. Miller.[20] Miller suggested that the judgment and decision making done by dental hygienists involved the formulation of a dental hygiene diagnosis. The ADHA published *dhdx* in 2005. The position paper recognizes the necessity of the dental hygiene diagnosis for the development, implementation, and evaluation of the dental hygiene treatment plan. To provide comprehensive quality oral health care, dental hygienists must fulfill the professional obligation of formulating a dental hygiene diagnosis.[21,22]

The assessment phase of the dental hygiene process of care provides the dental hygienist with an abundant amount of information to analyze, synthesize, and interpret. Information attained from the patient assessment is used by the hygienist to derive a dental hygiene diagnosis. This term has a specificity that implies the treatment is limited to that which can be accomplished by qualified and licensed hygienists.

Historically, dental hygienists have documented findings of the assessment phase in the patient's records, along with the treatment therapy completed during the appointment. The dental hygiene diagnosis requires hygienists to take the process a step further by organizing

the documentation to include probable cause and potential resolution that can be achieved by their intervention (Figure 16–2 ■).

In collaboration with the dental hygiene diagnosis, dental diagnoses must be determined. When clinical attachment loss is noted on the comprehensive periodontal evaluation, radiographs should be used to confirm the degree of attachment loss. The extent and severity of gingival/periodontal disease can be determined with the criteria set forth by the American Academy of Periodontology (Table 16–2 ■)

Dental hygiene process of care.

Assessment Outcomes

Generalized bleeding on probing

50% plaque index

History of dental neglect

Localized 5- to 7-mm probing depths

30% attachment loss evident on x-rays

DHDX

Erythematous, enlarged marginal & papillary gingiva with BOP indicative of generalized, moderate gingivitis; localized areas of 5- to 7-mm attachment loss evident on radiographs, indicative of localized severe chronic periodontitis. Pt's hx would suggest inadequate plaque removal as 1° etiologic factor.

Possible DH Therapy

Periodontal debridement/periodontal scaling and root planing

Individualized oral hygiene instructions

Subgingival irrigation

Selective/coronal polishing

Appropriate periodontal maintenance appts.

DHDX, dental hygiene diagnosis; BOP, bleeding on probing; pt, patient; hx, history; 1°, first degree (primary); DH, dental hygiene; appts, appointments.

■ **FIGURE 16–2** Dental hygiene process of care. (Developed from the Commission on Dental Accreditation standards.)

■ **Table 16–2**   Classification of Periodontal Diseases and Conditions

I. Gingival Diseases
  A. Dental plaque-induced gingival diseases*
    1. Gingivitis associated with dental plaque only
       a. without other local contributing factors
       b. with local contributing factors (See VIII A)
    2. Gingival diseases modified by systemic factors
       a. associated with the endocrine system
          1) puberty-associated gingivitis
          2) menstrual cycle-associated gingivitis
          3) pregnancy-associated
             a) gingivitis
             b) pyogenic granuloma
          4) diabetes mellitus-associated gingivitis
       b. associated with blood dyscrasias
          1) leukemia-associated gingivitis
          2) other
    3. Gingival diseases modified by medications
       a. drug-influenced gingival diseases
          1) drug-influenced gingival enlargements
          2) drug-influenced gingivitis
             a) oral contraceptive-associated gingivitis
             b) other
    4. Gingival diseases modified by malnutrition
       a. ascorbic acid-deficiency gingivitis
       b. other
  B. Non-plaque-induced gingival lesions
    1. Gingival diseases of specific bacterial origin
       a. *Neisseria gonorrhea*-associated lesions
       b. *Treponema pallidum*-associated lesions
       c. streptococcal species-associated lesions
       d. other
    2. Gingival diseases of viral origin
       a. herpesvirus infections
          1) primary herpetic gingivostomatitis
          2) recurrent oral herpes
          3) varicella-zoster infections
       b. other
    3. Gingival diseases of fungal origin
       a. *Candida*-species infections
          1) generalized gingival candidosis
       b. linear gingival erythema
       c. histoplasmosis
       d. other
    4. Gingival lesions of genetic origin
       a. hereditary gingival fibromatosis
       b. other
    5. Gingival manifestations of systemic conditions
       a. mucocutaneous disorders
          1) lichen planus
          2) pemphigoid

          3) pemphigus vulgaris
          4) erythema multiforme
          5) lupus erythematosus
          6) drug-induced
          7) other
       b. allergic reactions
          1) dental restorative materials
             a) mercury
             b) nickel
             c) acrylic
             d) other
          2) reactions attributable to
             a) toothpastes/dentifrices
             b) mouthrinses/mouthwashes
             c) chewing gum additives
             d) foods and additives
          3) other
    6. Traumatic lesions (factitious, iatrogenic, accidental)
       a. chemical injury
       b. physical injury
       c. thermal injury
    7. Foreign body reactions
    8. Not otherwise specified (NOS)
II. Chronic Periodontitis†
  A. Localized
  B. Generalized
III. Aggressive Periodontitis†
  A. Localized
  B. Generalized
IV. Periodontitis as a Manifestation of Systemic Diseases
  A. Associated with hematological disorders
    1. Acquired neutropenia
    2. Leukemias
    3. Other
  B. Associated with genetic disorders
    1. Familial and cyclic neutropenia
    2. Down syndrome
    3. Leukocyte adhesion deficiency syndromes
    4. Papillon-Lefèvre syndrome
    5. Chediak-Higashi syndrome
    6. Histiocytosis syndromes
    7. Glycogen storage disease
    8. Infantile genetic agranulocytosis
    9. Cohen syndrome
    10. Ehlers-Danlos syndrome (Types IV and VIII)
    11. Hypophosphatasia
    12. Other
  C. Not otherwise specified (NOS)

(Continued)

■ **Table 16–2** *Continued*

V. Necrotizing Periodontal Diseases
    A. Necrotizing ulcerative gingivitis (NUG)
    B. Necrotizing ulcerative periodontitis (NUP)
VI. Abscesses of the Periodontium
    A. Gingival abscess
    B. Periodontal abscess
    C. Pericoronal abscess
VII. Periodontitis Associated With Endodontic Lesions
    A. Combined periodontic-endodontic lesions
VIII. Developmental or Acquired Deformities and
    Conditions
    A. Localized tooth-related factors that modify
        or predispose to plaque-induced gingival
        diseases/periodontitis
        1. Tooth anatomic factors
        2. Dental restorations/appliances
        3. Root fractures
        4. Cervical root resorption and cemental tears
    B. Mucogingival deformities and conditions around teeth
        1. Gingival/soft tissue recession
            a. facial or lingual surfaces

        b. interproximal (papillary)
        2. Lack of keratinized gingiva
        3. Decreased vestibular depth
        4. Aberrant frenum/muscle position
        5. Gingival excess
            a. pseudopocket
            b. inconsistent gingival marin
            c. excessive gingival display
            d. gingival enlargement (See I.A.3. and I.B.4.)
        6. Abnormal color
    C. Mucogingival deformities and conditions on
        edentulous ridges
        1. Vertical and/or horizontal ridge deficiency
        2. Lack of gingiva/keratinized tissue
        3. Gingival/soft tissue enlargement
        4. Aberrant frenum/muscle position
        5. Decreased vestibular depth
        6. Abnormal color
    D. Occlusal trauma
        1. Primary occlusal trauma
        2. Secondary occlusal trauma

*Can occur on a periodontium with no attachment loss or on a periodontium with attachment loss that is not progressing.
†Can be further classified on the basis of extent and severity. As a general guide, extent can be characterized as Localized = ≤ 30% of sites involved and Generalized = > 30% of sites involved. Severity can be characterized on the basis of the amount of clinical attachment loss (CAL) as follows: Slight = 1 or 2 mm CAL, Moderate = 3 or 4 mm CAL, and Severe = > 5 mm CAL.
Source: Armitage, G. C. (1999). Development of a Classification System for Periodontal Diseases and Conditions. *Annals of Periodontology,* 4:1–6.

A diagnosis and proposed treatment plan that is based on the results of the examination should be presented to the patient. Patients should be informed of the disease process, therapeutic alternatives, potential complications, the expected results, and their responsibilities in treatment. Consequences of no treatment should also be explained to the patient.[23]

PLANNING

During the **planning phase** of the dental hygiene process of care, dental hygiene therapy must be determined along with the establishment of realistic patient goals. The dental hygiene care plan serves as a component of the dental treatment plan (Figure 16–3 ■). It should be unique and customized on the basis of the findings of the assessment and diagnosis. The dental hygiene therapy, that is, self-care education, periodontal debridement, and so forth are all elements of the care plan.

The amount of time needed for the implementation of the therapy will guide the appointment planning.

Elements to be considered in planning appointment times are number of appointments needed, allocation of time for dental hygiene interventions, and the sequencing of appointments. Patient involvement is essential to ensure informed consent, and the setting of appropriate and realistic patient goals.

IMPLEMENTATION

The **implementation phase** of the dental hygiene process of care is when treatment begins. Implementation begins with preparing the operatory for the treatment, using proper infection control procedures, and selecting the materials, instruments, and equipment to be utilized. The treatment is then performed by providing oral prophylaxis, pain management, periodontal debridement, patient instruction, selective coronal polishing, and/or other procedures identified in the planning phase (Figure 16–4 ■).

Even though the recall/maintenance dental hygiene appointment is typically an "hour," the dental hygienist

**Dental hygiene care plan. (Developed from the Commission
on Dental Accreditation standards.)**

Assessment	Appt. 1	Appt. 2	Appt. 3	Appt. 4	Appt. 5	Appt. 6
Chief complaint						
Medical/dental history						
Vital signs						
Intra- and extraoral examination						
Dental charting						
Periodontal examination						
Plaque indices						
Gingival assessment						
Risk assessment						
Radiographs						
Planning						
DH diagnosis						
Informed consent						
Implementation						
Pain management						
Periodontal debridement/scaling						
Ultrasonic debridement						
Hand scaling						
Subgingival irrigation						
Application of chemotherapeutic agents						
Selective/coronal polishing						
Application of pit-and-fissure sealants						
Fluoride application						
Health education/preventive						
Counseling						
Brushing						
Interdental aids						

■ **FIGURE 16–3**   Dental hygiene care plan.
(Developed from the Commission on Dental Accreditation Standards.)

Nutritional counseling					
Infection control					
Desensitization					
Care of restorations					
Evaluation					
Reevaluation of oral/periodontal health					
Continuing care					
Recall					
Periodontal maintenance					
Referral(s)					

Note: DH, dental hygiene; appt., appointment.

■ **FIGURE 16–3** (*Continued*)

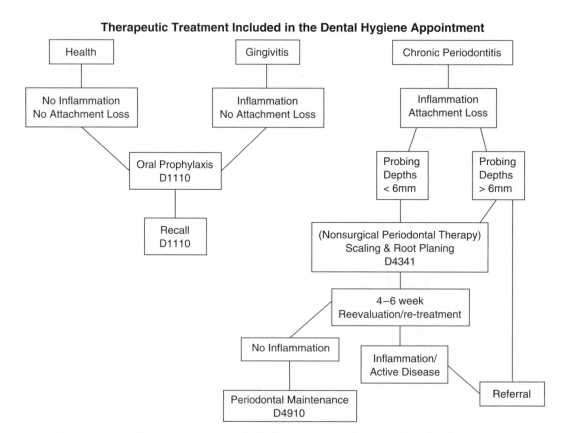

Therapeutic Treatment Included in the Dental Hygiene Appointment

■ **FIGURE 16–4** Therapeutic Treatment Included in the Dental Hygiene Appointment.

really has only about 50 minutes for the patient. The appointment can be divided into segments.[24]

- Assessment (15 minutes)
  - Patient history (update with blood pressure)
  - Clinical data collection (intra- and extraoral exam), periodontal and dental charting
  - Radiographs
- Diagnosis/planning/implementation (30 minutes)
  - Diagnosis
  - Treatment planning
    - Informed consent
  - Patient instruction
  - Instrumentation (use of hand and/or ultrasonic instruments for removal of bacteria)
  - Selective coronal polishing
  - Fluoride application
- Evaluation/reevaluation (5 minutes)
  - Re-treatment of localized active sites by instrumentation

- Application of chemotherapeutic agent as needed
- Dentist's examination if necessary
- Disinfection (10 minutes)
  - Break down of unit
  - Set up for next appointment
  - Re-schedule patient

(Table 16–3 ■) provides additional information about dental hygiene procedures and the process of diagnosis.

EVALUATION

Evaluation assesses the effectiveness and outcome of the completed treatment. The success of instrumentation is determined by evaluating the periodontal tissue after treatment and during the maintenance phase of therapy.[25] This evaluation will serve as the basis for determining whether the treatment was successful or if adjunct therapy is warranted.

■ **Table 16–3** Sample Treatment Options Based on Individual Dental Hygiene Diagnosis

Generalized Moderate Gingivitis (no attachment loss)

Procedures

Comprehensive oral examination (D0150)

FMR (D0210)

OHI (D1330)

Oral prophylaxis (D1110)

Selective polishing

Nutrition (D1310)

Smoking cessation (D1320)

Suitable maintenance interval

Generalized Slight Periodontitis (1- to 2-mm attachment loss)

Procedures (multiple appointments based on patient assessment and needs)

First appointment

Comprehensive oral health examination

FMR

OHI

Second appointment

Periodontal scale and root plane—4 quads (D4341)

Suitable periodontal maintenance appointment (D4910)

(Continued)

■ **Table 16–3** *Continued*

Generalized Moderate Periodontitis (3- to 4-mm attachment loss)

Procedures

First appointment

Comprehensive oral examination

FMR

OHI

Multiple appointments based on patient assessment and needs

Second appointment

Periodontal scale and root plane—2 quads (D4341)

Disease control/nutritional counseling (D1310)

Tobacco cessation (D1320)

Irrigation (D9630)

Suitable periodontal maintenance appointments (D4910)

Generalized Severe Periodontitis (5+-mm attachment loss)

Procedures

First appointment

Comprehensive oral examination

FMR

OHI

Multiple appointments based on patient assessment and needs

Second appointment

Periodontal scale and root plane (starting with worst quad)

Anesthesia

Disease control/nutritional counseling

Tobacco cessation

Irrigation (D9630)

Third appointment

Periodontal scale and root plane quad

Anesthesia

Disease control/nutritional counseling

Irrigation

Fourth appointment

Periodontal scale and root plane quad

Anesthesia

Tobacco cessation

Irrigation

Fifth appointment

Periodontal scale and root plane quad

Anesthesia

Disease control/nutritional counseling

■ **Table 16–3**   *Continued*

> Tobacco cessation
>
> Irrigation
>
> **Sixth appointment**
>
> Reevaluation
>
> Coronal polishing
>
> Localized chemotherapeutic agents (D4381)
>
> Desensitizing medicament (D9910)/(D9911)
>
> Referral for periodontal consult

FMR, focused medical review; OHI, oral hygiene instructions

SUMMARY

As an oral health educator, it is the responsibility of every dental provider to teach the patient that oral disease is a disease like any other and deserves treatment, and that interrelationships exist between the oral environment and every other system in the body. Having a chronic infection is a serious problem that should not be ignored. Although treating periodontal disease will not guarantee patients a lifetime of health, it is one step they can take toward a healthier life overall.[25]

Assessment, diagnosis, planning, implementation, and evaluation are the essential elements of the dental hygiene process of care. To meet each patient's distinct oral health care needs, the dental hygienist must formulate an individualized dental hygiene diagnosis and a comprehensive treatment plan. The dental hygiene process of care provides the criteria and mechanisms to establish such a plan.

ACKNOWLEDGMENTS

The authors express their sincere appreciation to Barbara Bennett and Becky Eden for their research guidance and time.

REFERENCES

1. American Dental Hygienists' Association. (1993). Policy 18–96, Glossary.
2. American Dental Hygienists' Association. (1993). Policy 16–93, Education.
3. Page, R., & Beck, J. (1997). Risk assessment for periodontal disease. *Int Dent J*, 47:61.
4. Genco, R. J. (1999). Overview of risk factors for periodontal disease and implications for diabetes and cardiovascular diseases. *Compendium*, 19 (Suppl):40.
5. Genco, R. J. (1996). Current view of risk factors for periodontal diseases. *J Periodontol*, 7:1041.
6. Newman, M. G., Korman, K. S., & Holtzman, S. (1994). Association of clinical risk factors with treatment outcomes. *J Periodontol*, 65:489–97.
7. American Dental Association. (2007). *CDT current dental terminology 2007–2008.* Chicago: American Dental Association Health Foundation.
8. U.S. Department of Health and Human Services, Centers for Disease Control and Prevention. (2001). *Healthy people 2000—Final review.* Retrieved 3/07 from http://www.cdc.gov/nchs/data/hp2000/hp2k01.pdf.
9. Herzberg, M. C., & Meyer, M. W. (1996). Effects of oral flora on platelets: Possible consequences in cardiovascular disease. *J Periodontol*, 67 (10):1138–42.
10. Loesche, W. J. (1994). Periodontal disease as a risk factor for heart disease. *Compend Contin Edu Dent*, XV (8):976–91.
11. Loesche, W. J., Schork, A., Terpenning, M. S, Chen, Yin-Miar, Dominguez, B. L., Grossman, N. (1998). Relationship between dental disease and coronary heart disease in elderly U.S. veterans. *J Am Dent Assoc 1998*, 129:301–11.
12. Slavkin, H. C. (1997). First encounters: Transmission of infectious oral disease from mother to child. *J Am Dent Assoc*, 128:773–78.
13. Gurenlian, J. R. (2006). Inflammation: The relationship between oral health and systemic disease. Retrieved 3/07 from http://www.adha.org/ce_courses/course13/index.html. (Course 13-Special supplement to Access, April, 2006).

14. American Academy of Periodontics. (2001). Treatment of plaque-induced gingivitis, chronic periodontitis, and other clinical conditions. (Position Paper). *J Periodontol,* 72:1790–800.

15. American Heart Association. (2007). What is high blood pressure? Retrieved 3/07 from http://www.americanheart .org/presenter.jhtml?identifier=2112.

16. Medical Economics. (1995). *PDR Medical Dictionary* (1st ed.). Montvale, NJ: Medical Economics, 1532.

17. Wilkins, E. M. (1999). *Clinical practice of dental hygiene* (8th ed.). Philadelphia: Lippincott Williams & Wilkins, 111.

18. Medical Economics. (1995). *PDR Medical Dictionary* (1st ed.). Montvale, NJ: Medical Economics, 607.

19. Medical Economics. (1995). *PDR Medical Dictionary* (1st ed.). Montvale, NJ: Medical Economics, 474.

20. Miller, S. (1982, July/August). Dental hygiene diagnoses. *RDH,* 46.

21. American Dental Hygienists' Association. (2005, June). Dental hygiene diagnosis: dhdx. (Position Paper). Chicago: American Dental Hygienists' Association.

22. Wilkins, E. M. (1999). *Clinical practice of the dental hygienist* (8th ed.). Philadelphia: Lippincott Williams & Wilkins, 32.

23. American Academy of Periodontology. (1999). International workshop for a classification of periodontal diseases and conditions. *Ann Periodontol,* 4 (1):1.

24. Wolfe, H. F., & Hassell, T. M. (2006). *Color atlas of dental hygiene periodontology.* New York and Stuttgart: Thieme Medical Publishers.

25. Scientific America. (2006). Interview with Majorie K. Jeffcoat. *Oral and whole body health.* Scientific America, Inc. New York, NY, 23.

Chapter 17

Health Education and Promotion Theories

Mary Catherine Hollister

OBJECTIVES

After studying this chapter, the student should be able to:

1. Define patient autonomy.
2. Explain the elements of the major health education theories.
3. Apply appropriate health education models to cases.
4. Identify principles of adult learning.
5. Use motivational interviewing techniques to devise a patient education strategy.

KEY TERMS

Health education
Patient education
Patient autonomy
Health belief model
Transtheoretical model and stages of change
Precontemplation stage
Contemplation stage
Preparation
Action stage
Maintenance stage
Termination stage
Consciousness raising
Vicarious learning
Self-efficacy
Self-evaluation
Environmental evaluation
Counter-conditioning
Contingency management
Precontemplator
Termination
Theory of reasoned action
Behavioral beliefs
Normative beliefs

(continued)

KEY TERMS (CONTINUED)
Social learning theory
Social cognitive theory
Self-efficacy
Locus of control
Internal LOC
External LOC

Multidimensional locus of control
Salutogenesis
Salutogenesis model
Stressor
Generalized resistance resources
Sense of coherence
Motivational interviewing

INTRODUCTION

In American society today, health information abounds. Anyone with exposure to media has heard about the dangers of smoking, methods to control weight, and the bad effects of high cholesterol levels; the individual also knows that every healthy diet should contain whole grains and lots of fruits and vegetables. If information alone changed health behaviors, our society would be full of fit, non-smoking individuals with normal blood pressure and cholesterol levels.

Because the most common oral diseases, dental caries and periodontal diseases, are preventable, an informed, motivated patient, practicing basic preventive techniques is likely to have good oral health for life. Other risk factors such as medical condition, history of disease, access to dental care, and other factors will contribute to disease, but lifestyle choices such as tobacco use, dietary choices, and oral hygiene practices play a significant role in oral health. Unlike family history, use of medications, and other factors that may affect oral health, lifestyle choices are under the patient's control. Therefore, it is the dental professional's responsibility to assist the patient in adopting healthy lifestyle choices that will promote good oral health. The most common method of assisting a patient with lifestyle choices is through health education.

Health education, also called **patient education,** too often consists of information only. The dental professional provides the patient information orally and in writing, through pamphlets, Web sites, or other printed materials. The dental professional then considers the "job done." The obligation of patient education has been fulfilled. It is the patient's responsibility to take that information and change behaviors. This approach may be effective with a very small number of patients, but most patients nod and smile and go back to business as usual. Patients do indeed need accurate information to make a behavior change, but information alone is usually not sufficient to bring about a behavior change.[1]

HISTORY OF HEALTH EDUCATION

Early health education often took a paternalistic approach. Providers focused on a prescribed regimen and dictated behaviors to patients. The provider was considered the expert who imparted knowledge to the patients. Patients were expected to absorb that knowledge and change behaviors accordingly. Those patients who did not follow provider recommendations were often considered non-compliant and were subject to more "expert-to-patient" education.[1] Over the years, the understanding of patient education has changed. Current health education theories recognize the importance of patient autonomy. **Patient autonomy** has been defined as the capability and right of patients to control the course of their own medical treatment and participate in the treatment decision-making process.[2] Patient autonomy is of prime consideration in giving informed consent for clinical procedures. But, in addition to consent for clinical procedures, the provider must involve the patient in the entire decision-making process. This means recognizing patient autonomy in providing patient education.

In recognizing patient autonomy, the provider allows the patient to decide the most relevant health issues to be addressed and encourages the patient to take an active part in both health behaviors and health management.[1,3] Enlisting the patient as an active participant, allowing the patient to have autonomy in deciding the best course of action to take, and helping the patient achieve those goals have proven to be much more successful in bringing about healthy lifestyle choices than the previous method of "expert-to-patient" information exchange.[1,3]

It may seem obvious that all patients want good oral health, so decisions about healthy practices and treatments will be similar in most patients. Upon closer examination, this may not be as black and white as it seems. Consider two patients with slightly yellow anterior teeth and one carious lesion on an upper first molar requiring a two-surface restoration. The first patient is a sales representative who is very concerned about the appearance of his smile. Therefore, less-esthetic amalgam posterior restorations and anterior veneers may be his treatment of choice. The second patient is very environmentally conscious and is unwilling to accept mercury-containing amalgam restorations. She may accept less-esthetic anterior teeth and request no treatment for the anterior teeth and a resin posterior restoration.

The theories below differ in approach and basic philosophies, but all theories currently being embraced in health education recognize the importance of patient autonomy and self-determination. It is important to note that each of the theories discussed have strengths and weaknesses. Each may be appropriate in certain situations; no single theory will be useful in every circumstance.

HEALTH BELIEF MODEL

First proposed in the 1950s by Hockbaum and adopted in the 1970s by the U.S. Public Health Service, the **Health Belief Model** (HBM) was one of the first attempts to view health in a social context (Figure 17–1 ■). The theory was a milestone in health education, because it placed a high value on the attitudes of the learner and recognized the importance of the learner's readiness to enact meaningful behavior change.

The underlying principle of the HBM implies that individuals with better information make better health decisions. Hochbaum eloquently stated that "you will find it worthwhile to keep an open mind. If you are prepared to accept new concepts, you will understand yourself much better; with a better understanding of how and why you make your choices, you will be much better able to make them intelligently, independently, and maturely."[4]

The HBM is a staged theory, with each step in the decision process dependent on the previous decision or belief. Briefly, individuals must first believe they are susceptible to a condition; second, they must believe the condition is serious; third, they must believe there is a successful intervention for the condition; and last, they must overcome all barriers to using the intervention. Each step is contingent on the previous belief.

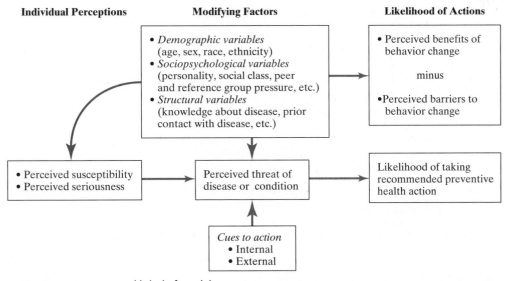

■ FIGURE 17–1 Health belief model.
(From Nathe, C. (2005). *Dental public health* (2nd ed.). Upper Saddle River, NJ: Prentice Hall.)

Oral Health Applications

Studies have shown good correlation between current actions and beliefs and correlating stages in the model. Cross sectional research has found reliable correlations between oral hygiene behaviors and appropriate HBM stages.[5,6] However research has not supported the HBM as a model that will produce predictable changes.[7–8,9] One possible explanation for the apparent contradiction is that, in cross-sectional studies, behavior is measured *after* the change has occurred. After a change occurs, individuals are likely to report that, as their beliefs changed, so did behaviors. However, changing beliefs, just like increased information, may not be sufficient for behavior change. That may explain why research has not confirmed the predictive value of the HBM.

The strength of the HBM is that it acknowledges the patient's values and attitudes toward health behaviors. Limitations are that increased information and changing beliefs may not be sufficient to cause behavior change, and that behavior changes rarely follow a logical, stepwise progression.[3]

TRANSTHEORETICAL MODEL AND STAGES OF CHANGE

The **transtheoretical model and stages of change** developed by Prochaska, Norcross, and DiClemente is based on an individual's readiness to adopt a new health behavior (Figure 17–2 ■). Like HBM, stages of change represent distinct beliefs and levels of readiness, but unlike HBM, stages of change include methods for assessing stages and helping patients progress through those stages. The transtheoretical theory states that, as individuals move through a series of readiness stages, each stage is characterized by certain behaviors and attitudes. Assessing an individual's stage allows health care workers and educators to tailor the intervention appropriate to the person's stage of readiness.[10] Key to applying the theory in a health education setting is accurate identification of an individual's stage of readiness to learn and to make behavior changes. Individuals may skip over stages or lapse to previous stages, but an awareness of the patient's current stage of readiness allows the counselor to provide appropriate assistance in moving toward healthier lifestyle choices.

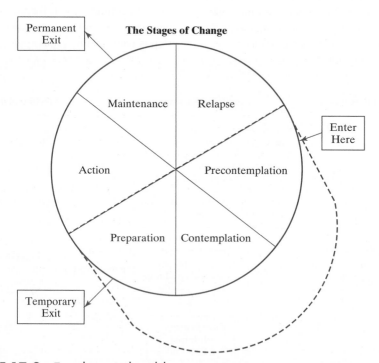

■ **FIGURE 17–2** Transtheoretical model.

The six stages of change are precontemplation, contemplation, preparation, action, maintenance, and termination. In the **precontemplation stage,** an individual has little or no interest and no intention of changing a behavior. In the **contemplation stage,** the individual is considering making a change within the next 6 months. The individual will examine the pros and cons of making a change, carefully weighing the benefits of changing versus the costs of changing. In the next stage, **preparation,** the individual is ready to make the change and actively makes plans to enact the change. In the **action stage,** the change has been adopted, and in the **maintenance stage,** the change has been continuous for at least 6 months. The **termination stage,** often not attained, represents a stage in which the change is permanent, to the extent that it is as if the previous behavior never existed. Those in true termination are unlikely to return to the previous behavior.[10,11]

Individuals move through the stages using a process of decisional balance. They may weigh the benefits and costs, or pros and cons, of the change. Benefits may include health, emotional, or social gains. Costs may be represented by obstacles such as social pressures, addiction that creates a physical dependence on the habit, or merely a desire to continue the behavior. As the scale tips more toward the benefit end of change, the individual may move to the next step. Self-efficacy (explained more fully in the social cognitive theory section below) develops as individuals begin to believe a change in behavior is likely to affect an outcome. Because the individuals believe that a change is possible, that they have the ability to enact the change, and that their actions will affect health outcomes, a move to a more advanced stage is likely.[10,11]

The strength of the theory is that it allows the provider or counselor to provide the precise intervention for which the participant is ready. At each stage the goal of the counselor is to assist the learner to identify benefits in the behavior change and overcome obstacles that would prevent the change. In this way, the counselor helps tip the decisional balance in favor of the change. The counselor does not dictate behavior change, rather the counselor and the learner identify relevant, immediate areas of concern, negotiate goals, and agree on short-term behaviors.[10,11]

Health care providers can help learners move through the stages using multiple mechanisms. Consciousness raising, vicarious learning, self-efficacy, self-evaluation, and environmental evaluation are useful in the precontemplation, contemplation, or preparation stage. **Consciousness raising** can alert the individual to a severe health problem and possible outcomes. Media campaigns, television programs, or celebrity illnesses may have a great impact on the public's consciousness of a disease or condition, and may affect the willingness to advance to a higher stage of readiness.[11] **Vicarious learning** occurs when individuals observe poor outcomes in others, thereby learning without actually experiencing that poor outcome. **Self-efficacy** is gained as the learner gains confidence that personal actions have an affect on outcomes. **Self-evaluation** and **environmental evaluation** assess personal habits and social environments that might affect a personal habit. Each of these strategies promotes autonomy in the learner and promotes a partnership between the counselor and the learner in health behavior modification.[11]

In the action and maintenance stages, strategies such as counter-conditioning and contingency management may be useful. By substitution of one habit for another, **counter-conditioning** may empower an individual to develop a healthy alternative for an unhealthy habit. **Contingency management** such as preplanning strategies for managing high-stress circumstances and rewarding positive changes may be most useful for helping individuals who have reached these higher stages. Those in the termination stage may provide assistance or counseling to those trying to change the behavior.[11]

Oral Health Application

Research has recorded the validity of stages of change and decisional balance in oral care behaviors. More research is needed to test the accuracy of the model in predicting altered behaviors for oral health care.[12] Currently, tobacco cessation is the most frequently used application of stages of change with regard to oral health, and has been verified through longitudinal research.[13,14] When used in tobacco counseling, the clinician must first establish the patient's readiness to change stage. A person who has no intention of stopping tobacco use would be a **precontemplator.** For this patient a brief session of counseling, offering information on the health consequences of using tobacco, and offering support at a future date, should the patient decide to quit, would be appropriate. A person in this stage may not be willing to set a quit date or develop quitting strategies. A patient in the contemplation stage would be considering quitting and may be willing to set a quit date. Offering support through counseling, information, quit aides, or identifying quitting resources such as classes or support groups would be appropriate for someone at this stage. This patient is moving toward making a change, so frequent encouragement and information about the benefits of the change may help tip the decisional balance in favor of proceeding to the next stage.

The patient in the preparation stage is ready to make the change. This person may enroll in a cessation class or purchase nicotine gum or patches. This patient should be willing to set a quit date and develop contingency plans to overcome cravings or trigger behaviors. Assistance for this patient may be writing the quit date in the chart, identifying plans for replenishing gum or patches, helping develop plans to overcome stressful situations that may trigger the desire for tobacco, and offering verbal encouragement.

A person in the action stage may be enrolled in a cessation class, be using a pharmaceutical resource, and would have stopped using tobacco products for 1 to 2 months. For this patient, frequent contacts to encourage continued abstinence, providing additional quit aides, completing a dental examination and prophylaxis, or other measures to support the current change is the most beneficial. Patients in maintenance who have continued the behavior change for more than 6 months may be willing to help others overcome tobacco addiction through peer counseling. This would also be appropriate for individuals in **termination,** although many tobacco users never reach this stage.

Prochaska, Redding, and Evers,[13] primary proponents of stages of change, tested a staged intervention against a standard self-help cessation program, by following participants for 18 months. Results were similar at 12 months. At 18 months the staged group moved ahead. Behaviors and attitudes about smoking and readiness often match the appropriate stage in cross-sectional studies. A program evaluation at a clinic for the medically underserved questioned smokers to assess their stage of change. Smokers who planned to quit within 6 months scored higher on statements consistent with quitting than did smokers who were not planning to quit. Decisional balance scores of those planning to quit indicated more concerns over negative consequences of smoking.[14,15]

The effectiveness of health behavior changes that are based on this theory as the sole basis of interventions has been mixed. Longitudinal analysis of smoking cessation programs found similar results in programs based on stages of change and other cessation strategies.[15,16] A systematic review of clinical trials based on stages of change interventions found the approach ineffective in school-aged children.[17] Cross-sectional and prospective analysis of a workplace smoking cessation program showed similar results. Behaviors and attitudes significantly correlated with the appropriate stage of change. However, the theory failed to predict progression through the stages at the 1- and 2-year follow-up.[18] These mixed results demonstrate that no single theory can be used in all situations. Each theory has relative merits in different situations. The challenge is to apply the appropriate theory in appropriate situations.

Stages of change is an important theory, because it encourages the learner to consider pros and cons of making a change, and it encourages counselors to meet individuals at their particular state of readiness. Identification of the appropriate readiness to learn a stage forms the foundation of motivational interviewing, which is discussed in the following chapter on tobacco cessation.

THEORY OF REASONED ACTION

Theory of reasoned action stresses the importance of attitudes and intentions to change a behavior (Figure 17–3 ■). According to this theory, the most important determinant of behavior is intention. Very few actions that produce

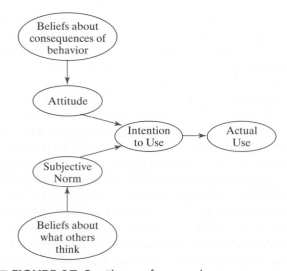

■ **FIGURE 17–3**   Theory of reasoned action.

a healthy outcome happen without ample knowledge and full intention to practice the healthy behavior. Two cognitive processes are at work to develop healthy behaviors: (1) belief about what significant others think is important, and (2) personal motivation to comply with those significant people. Other external variables that will influence attitudes and, thus, behaviors are internally processed within the context of significance.[19]

According to this theory, people make rational decisions based on knowledge, values, and attitudes. Therefore, a person's *intent* to perform a certain action is the most immediate and relevant predictor of carrying out that action. There are two kinds of beliefs that shape intentions: behavioral beliefs and normative beliefs.[20]

Behavioral beliefs are those attitudes held by the individual alone. A person forms attitudes based on relative risks, benefits, and possible outcomes. Therefore, personal knowledge and perception of importance to personal health influence behavioral beliefs. **Normative beliefs** are those held by other people who influence the individual. If a certain behavior is expected or is the social norm, or is expected by someone of importance to the individual, those expectations will have a bearing on an individual's intentions and, therefore, behavior.[20] Social norms may be formed in families, local communities, or larger societal communities. Celebrities' actions or experiences may influence social norms and, thus, health behaviors. When President Ronald Reagan was diagnosed with colon cancer, there was a sharp increase in tests for that disease. However, the effect was not sustained, and testing returned to previous levels within 6 months after the media attention dropped.

If the dental professional takes time to determine the social norms of a particular patient, the provider can use positive societal norms to assist a patient in adopting those positive behaviors as seen in the following example.

A 21-year-old woman who is 6 months pregnant with her first child presents for routine dental care. She has little knowledge of oral care for infants. She has a friend who gave her child a nighttime bottle with no ill effects, so she plans to do the same. However, she saw a television show on early infancy and learned the mother's oral status, as well as nighttime bottle-feeding, could cause severe tooth decay. She wants her baby to have a beautiful smile, and wants her friends and family to think she is a good mother.

This woman's desire to be a good mother and please her friends and family are powerful motivators to learn how to care for her child. The television show on baby care may set social norms for her to follow. Knowing that she values her family and friends' opinions, the dental provider may ask about other oral health practices among her family members or friends. If she describes a person who followed healthy practices, the provider may suggest she consult that person for advice. Because she has indicated that she gathers health information from television, the provider may also suggest other reputable media sources of information and advice.

A limitation of this theory is the reliance on intentions, which may not accurately predict actual behavior change. Intentions will only predict behavior if they are stable and consistent. When faced with an unexpected obstacle, individuals may change their intentions and therefore not carry out the intended behavior. Another limitation of this theory is that intentions must be matched very closely to the behavior to have predictive power.[20]

Social norms and community expectations are powerful predictors of individual behavior, according to this theory. Used in a community intervention, the theory may be better able to predict the behavior of the collective community, than of the individual. Social norms do not change as readily as individual choices. Therefore, social norms are more stable and provide strong normative beliefs to those in a close community.[20]

This theory helps explain an individual's perceptions of normal and expected behavior. The theory seems to be most successful in predicting behaviors that are completely within the individual's control and in which intentions remain stable, such as daily oral hygiene practices. Extraneous factors outside of the individual's control, such as fatigue or change of environment, may quickly change intentions and therefore change behavior and outcome.

Oral Health Applications

The theory of reasoned action has proven to be effective in influencing oral hygiene in young adults. The social expectations of the group had a strong influence on oral hygiene behavior.[20] Applying this concept to patient education, a teenager may consistently practice oral hygiene at home, but a change in environment such as moving to student housing at college may change intentions and behavior. Changes in the social norms or expectations of peers, change in routine, or fatigue associated with student life might affect oral hygiene routines.[21]

Community or cultural expectations may play a large role in affecting oral health behaviors. In communities where large numbers of children have early childhood caries, seeing children with crowned anterior teeth, extracted anterior teeth, or active decay may be regarded as a normal part of childhood. Changing the populations' expectations of acceptable oral health may make a noticeable impact on oral health and dietary behaviors.

If severe caries (Figure 17–4 ■) are accepted as a normal part of childhood, caregivers may not attribute personal actions to oral diseases. The counselor must assess the patient's/caregiver's dental knowledge and values to devise an effective health education plan. This approach could be applied to a local Head Start daily toothbrushing program. This program is mandated by the Head Start performance standards, and will be a consistent resource for Head Start students and parents. Dental professionals involved in these programs may apply the theory of reasoned action to encourage daily brushing, thereby creating a behavioral norm for the family. Social norms of daily brushing and use of fluoridated toothpaste that become firmly established within a family can have lasting effects, long after the children leave the Head Start program.

SOCIAL LEARNING THEORY

Social learning theory (SLT) states individuals do not learn or change behavior in a linear fashion. Rather changes take place bidirectionally; environment, information, and behavior all affect one another (Figure 17–5 ■).

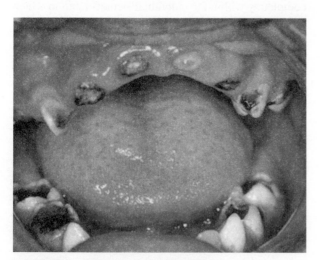

■ FIGURE 17–4 Early childhood caries.
(Courtesy of Dr. Lezley McIlveen, Department of Dentistry, Children's National Medical Center, Washington, DC.)

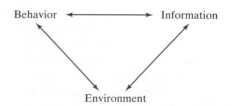

■ FIGURE 17–5 Social learning theory.

As an individual learns more, behaviors and environment may change, causing more knowledge to be gained, which in turn, reinforces behavior and healthy environments. This reciprocal determinism is key to understanding the theory. Behaviors do not move along a predictable continuum. Each element reinforces another as behavior is learned, practiced, reinforced in certain environments, and refined.[21]

Social learning theory was a product of behavioralists such as B. F. Skinner and others who believed behavior was a direct result of conditioning.[22] Psychologist Albert Bandura agreed with the basic tenets of the theory, but placed a focus on personal agency and actions, rather than pure conditioning. To refocus the theory away from a pure behavioralist view, Bandura renamed the theory **social cognitive theory** (SCT).[23] Self efficacy, the main construct of the SCT, is the belief that one's personal actions will have an impact on outcome. Individuals with high **self-efficacy,** practice forethought and planning, develop contingency plans, and put effort into overcoming obstacles. Self-efficacy is gained as information, behavior, and environment interact in a reciprocal manner. Lapses are a part of the learning process as the individual uses personal choices to develop behaviors consistent with individual choice and lifestyle.[24,25]

Self-efficacy is gained through several mechanisms. Enactive attainment, or experiencing success, is the most powerful method. As an individual gains new knowledge and puts that knowledge to use, the individual can personally experience the outcome resulting from the actions. Vicarious learning is another method. Individuals do not have to experience the effects of poor health choices if they can learn from others' experiences. The third method of gaining self-efficacy is through verbal persuasion. Affective states such as pain or fatigue will deter self-efficacy.

Enactive attainment, or performance accomplishment, allows the learner to experience the results of actions.

Providers may assist this experience by encouraging the learner to model behaviors (participant modeling) or suggesting a trial period. Learners may not only experience a successful outcome, they may also develop coping skills for stressful situations, or times when the desired behavior is difficult to continue. During a trial period the learner may also develop unique methods of implementing suggested behaviors.[26]

Vicarious learning through modeled behavior allows the patient to develop expectations based on others' experiences. It also allows patients to learn of poor outcomes without actually experiencing them. A patient who has lost a tooth due to severe caries may be motivated to change behaviors to prevent losing more teeth. A patient who has not actually experienced tooth loss may adopt healthy practices to prevent tooth loss by hearing of someone else's behaviors and resulting outcome.[27]

Modeled behavior is not as powerful at changing behavior as personal experience, so repeated encounters with the patient to encourage changes may be needed. Successes gained through repeated efforts by the model may be more influential than behaviors changed with ease. This concerted effort demonstrates the possibility of overcoming obstacles through planning and forethought, even in stressful situations. Modeling may be more successful if the model has similar characteristics to the patient, thus increasing the relevance of the model to the patient.[27]

Verbal persuasion will be a necessary follow-up for those attempting to sustain a changed behavior. Persuasion will include assisting the patient to develop goals, determine expectations of outcomes, and formulate strategies for coping with challenging situations. Simply telling a patient what to expect is much less powerful than actual experience or personal testimonies. But verbal persuasion is an important component for tailoring a program to a particular patient and encouraging successful changes.[27]

One example is seen in the following situation. A 42-year-old male presents with severe generalized gingivitis and isolated 4-mm pockets. The patient has a family history of type 2 diabetes and hypertension, although the patient has neither condition. Upon questioning, the provider learns that the patient's father experienced loose teeth, resulting in full dentures at an early age. The patient wants to keep his teeth.

The dental provider can use vicarious learning to explain to the patient how periodontal disease may have been the reason for his father's tooth loss. The provider can teach proper oral hygiene techniques to control gingivitis and schedule subsequent appointments to treat the early periodontitis. At a subsequent appointment, the patient has experienced improved gingival health because of his oral hygiene efforts. Verbal persuasion will attribute the improved oral status to the patient's practices. Thus the provider has allowed the patient to experience success through his own efforts (enactive attainment), allowed him to learn of poor outcomes through his father's experience (vicarious learning), and pointed out that the results are a direct result of his efforts (verbal persuasion).

Health behaviors will change as individuals gain knowledge, practice new skills, and experience changing environments. For example, a person may learn about nutrition from a medical provider or dietitian. The individual may then try out a new recipe or food. The individual may also attend a nutrition class, which in turn provides exposure to others who will share knowledge and experiences. Altered behaviors may produce desired results of overall well-being or weight loss. Frequent contacts with the dietitian or attending nutrition classes provides opportunities for verbal persuasion to continue encouragement of new behaviors. Personal testimonies provide vicarious learning for class members. A continuous process of knowledge, experiences, and environment slowly changes the individual's understanding and behaviors. This process can be very slow, requiring frequent reinforcement of positive changes. Over time self-efficacy is gained as the individual finds that changed behaviors can produce desired results.

Self-efficacy has been an accurate predictor of oral health in both cross-sectional and longitudinal studies.[28–30] It has been shown to be a significant predictor of behavior in conditions such as diabetes management and oral health.[28,29] Qualitative analysis of dental attitudes indicated that cognitive experiences, supportive and emotional dimensions, as well as childhood experiences influence dental attitudes and behaviors.[27] Dental self-efficacy was found to be a determinant in oral health and oral hygiene among diabetes patients and for general oral health in elderly patients.[28,29] Self-efficacy has been shown to be consistent with improvements in oral hygiene over time, but the benefit may be short term only. Periodontal patients showed improvements in oral hygiene and dental self-efficacy 6 months after the initial intervention, but differences were lost over time.[28] Researchers have proposed that self-efficacy may be a useful part of a multidimensional model to predict Early Childhood Caries (ECC).[30]

A limitation of self-efficacy is that it tends to be domain-specific, and similar domains may influence one another. For example, as a person gains knowledge about plaque control, self-efficacy may increase in the areas of personal hygiene in general. However, that self-efficacy may not extend to other health domains. An individual can have high expectations that oral health is attainable through personal oral hygiene, but low expectations in other health areas.[28] Therefore, a patient may be confident in his or her ability to practice daily oral hygiene but has little confidence in having regular dental professional care. Such a patient may brush and floss daily but seek only emergency dental care.

LOCUS OF CONTROL

Like social cognitive theory, locus of control (LOC) is an extension of SLT. As in SLT, environment, knowledge, and behavior interact to affect lifestyle choices. Developed by Wallston, Wallston, and Kaplan in the mid-1970s, **locus of control** deals with perception of personal control over those elements and pertinent health issues. **Internal LOC** occurs when individuals think their personal actions determine health status. **External LOC** means individuals perceive others in control of health decisions and health status. External sources may be fate, chance, luck, God, or powerful others.[31] Unlike self-efficacy, which is domain-specific, LOC tends to be more global. As such, a person with internal LOC would perceive control over health status regardless of the health condition, and an individual with external LOC would consider outside forces as influential in any health issue.

The theory has been refined since its introduction. As originally presented and in much subsequent research, LOC has been considered a global orientation to health behavior. Scales to measure LOC were designed to be mid-level in specificity so they could be used to predict behaviors or outcomes for any condition. Validation of the theory, however, has found this approach to be problematic, because healthy people respond differently to the questions on the scales than do chronically ill individuals.[32] Several researchers have used the basic scales, but they found the scales needed to be modified to measure specific diseases or conditions such as diabetes,[32] headaches,[33] and adolescent depression.[34] This was successful within the context used in individual studies. However, because each study adapted the scales differently, little comparison between studies was possible. Development of the **multidimensional locus of control**

scale helped address this issue and makes the scale appropriate for specific conditions.[32]

Oral Health Applications

Locus of control has been found to be predictive for children's dental health. Researchers found that children of mothers who had more external LOC were at higher risk for developing dental caries.[35] In contrast, other research has found little association between mothers' LOC, children's health status, and use of preventive health services.[36] This theory continues to be refined for use in various populations and conditions.

SENSE OF COHERENCE

Antonovsky took a very different tact in health promotion and disease prevention. Antonovsky's central premise is that it is more useful to study health than to study disease. He referred to this method of study as "salutogenesis," the beginnings of health. **Salutogenesis** defines health in terms of a continuum of ease to disease and the conditions surrounding the individual which provide coping resources. Antonovsky's objection to the study of pathogenesis is that it tends to dichotomize people into either a "healthy" or "ill" state. He contends there is a continuum of "ease" or perfect health with no limitations to "dis-ease" or severe disease or disability resulting in severe limitations of daily life. Most individuals exist somewhere in between these two extremes.[37]

The **salutogenesis model** closely examines the role of stressors and tension as contributing factors for health and disease. A **stressor** is defined as a source of disturbance that upsets a sense of equilibrium. This disturbance may come from external or internal sources such as illness, hereditary factors, job stress, or lack of personal control. Many sources of stimuli are handled routinely as an individual and are not stressors. Stressors produce tension, and it is the perception of stress and the tension response that has an affect on an individual.[38]

To deal with and possibly to use stressors to enhance the life experience, people build a network of **generalized resistance resources** (GRRs). A GRR is more than a specific coping skill for a particular event. Rather, GRRs include all available resources at an individual level, a community, and a cosmic level that enable people to manage daily stressors as well as cataclysmic events. A network of GRRs may contain a person's heredity, education, knowledge, finances, physical resources, values, attitudes, or faith.

Generalized resistance resources can help an individual avoid stressors, as in practicing good health habits, or avoiding dangerous situations. They may also enable a person to effectively manage a stressor and avoid psychologic, emotional, or physical impairment. An examination of the list of GRRs shows that they encompass a broad range of elements. Included are biologic elements such as the immune system, cognitive elements such as knowledge, material resources such as personal income or medical insurance, social factors such as support and social norms, and macro-social support such as a belief in divine purpose.[38]

A GRR has an element of farsightedness. This quality allows an individual to envision coping strategies and anticipate the response of the environment. The coping strategy is not the actual behavior but the planned behavior. This strategy may give an individual a measure of personal control, but the actual response or behavior may be limited by circumstances such as physical ability or material resources.[38]

Sense of coherence (SOC) is the main construct of salutogenesis, and is central to a salutogenic orientation to health and disease. **Sense of coherence** is a method of seeing the world and one's place in it. It is cognitive, perceptual, and social. Individuals who have a strong network of GRRs will develop an overall SOC that is global in perspective, that is, SOC can be used in any situation to deal with a number of various stressors. Individuals with an SOC find problems manageable, comprehensible, and meaningful. Stressors are manageable if the individual has sufficient resources to handle the situation and the means to use those resources. Stressors are comprehensible if they are predictable or make sense, and meaningful if the individual is willing to expend time and energy to deal with those stressors.[38]

Oral Health Applications

Researchers have found that a mother's SOC significantly associated with several oral health indicators in adolescents.[38] Strong maternal SOC was associated with gingival health, overall number of caries, number of anterior caries, and professional dental visits. No longitudinal studies have been conducted to measure the long-term impact of SOC on oral health. From a pathogenic perspective, a clinician will diagnose a condition and work to cure it. From a salutogenic perspective, a clinician can work with a patient on goal-oriented behavior that will strengthen the SOC, thereby moving the patient

toward the "ease" end of the ease/dis-ease continuum. Sense of coherence will move a person toward consistency and stability.[38] The following case is a perfect example.

A 35-year-old female patient presents with multiple carious lesions. She says her family has "soft teeth," so she thinks her decay rate is completely out of her control. She also has difficulty controlling her weight and attributes her body size to her family history. Upon questioning, the dental provider discovers the patient has very good oral hygiene skills, but she lacks knowledge about nutrition related to oral health. She has been trying to lose weight and has been slowly sipping on a sugar-sweetened soft drink throughout the day.

The dental provider can increase the patient's SOC by identifying resources available to her for improved health. The patient has information available through the dental office, Internet, and printed resources. She has dental insurance, so she is able to receive all her restorations and regular preventive visits thereafter. She has established a trusting relationship with the dental provider, so she is willing to accept advice. By identifying resources, the provider has helped make oral health manageable. When the patient understands that decay is the result of personal behavior, the oral health becomes comprehensible. Through conversations with the patient, the provider has learned that oral health is very important to the patient, but she felt that tooth loss was inevitable. She now believes that she can save her teeth; therefore, she now feels her oral health is meaningful, and is willing to expend time and effort needed to ensure good oral health.

Each theory has its strengths and limitations (Table 17–1 ■). No single theory will apply to all situations. Often combining pertinent elements of several theories will produce the best results. Researchers have suggested that multidimensional models may prove to be the most effective, particularly for conditions with multiple risk factors such as early childhood caries.[39]

Before deciding on a course of behavior modification for an individual, the dental professional must consider the patient's values and beliefs, readiness to change, perception of control, perception of the effectiveness of personal actions, behavioral and social norms, as well as available resources. If the dental professional is considering proposing a change of policy for a community, school, or other group of people, the primary considerations may be social norms, community resources, and level of knowledge.

■ **Table 17-1** Summary of Health Behavior Models

Theory	*Major Elements*
Health Belief Model	1. Perceived susceptibility 2. Perceived seriousness 3. Perceived effectiveness of the intervention 4. Perceived ability to overcome obstacles
Transtheoretical stages of change	Behavior changes move through a predictable set of stages including: 1. Pre-contemplation 2. Contemplation 3. Preparation 4. Action 5. Maintenance 6. Termination
Theory of reasoned action	1. People make rational decisions based on knowledge, values, and attitudes. 2. Intentions and behavior changes are affected by behavioral beliefs and normative beliefs.
Social learning theory (SLT)	Change is effected through knowledge, environment, and behavior.
Social cognitive theory (SCT) (Self-efficacy)	1. Extension of SLT places an emphasis on personal actions. 2. Self-efficacy is the belief that personal actions will affect outcomes. 3. Self-efficacy is gained through enactive attainment, vicarious learning, and verbal persuasion. 4. As self-efficacy increases, individuals plan for contingencies, and persevere through difficulties.
Locus of control (LOC)	1. Extension of SLT places an emphasis on perception of personal control. 2. Internal LOC: Personal actions determine health status. 3. External LOC: Others strongly influence health status.
Sense of coherence (SOC)	1. Health lies on a continuum of ease to dis-ease. 2. Stressors move an individual to the dis-ease end of the continuum. 3. Individuals develop a network of general resistance resources that reduce stressors. 4. Individuals with high SOC find stressors manageable (they have the resources to cope), comprehensible (stressors make sense), and meaningful (willing to spend resources to deal with the stressor).

IMPLEMENTING HEALTH EDUCATION MODELS

Once the dental professional has mastered the concepts of health education theories, the challenge is to effectively implement those theories for various target audiences. Implementation will be very different for children, teens, adults, communities, or other groups. The setting of the intervention may also affect the implementation scheme. For example, different strategies may be needed in changing behaviors of independently living seniors, as opposed to seniors with similar abilities who reside in an assisted-living facility or a nursing home. The following section addresses implementation of learning theories for various target audiences.

ADULT HEALTH EDUCATION

Adults have unique learning needs influenced by a wealth of experience and established practices that work. The goals of this section are to introduce some concepts about adult learning and to give some suggestions for using the previously discussed health education models for adult patient education.

Adults come to health providers with well-established habits and preexisting knowledge. Adults have achieved a concept of self-direction gained by knowledge and experience accumulated throughout their lives from various sources. As such, adults must be considered autonomous and self-directed. In a situation in which a self-directing adult is not perceived as autonomous, tension and resentment may develop and education may not be effective.[40]

Adults have been taught in school, had education from health care providers, and have practiced health behaviors. Their current practices are a result of incorporating knowledge into practices that work for them. Adults will seldom change a behavior just from gaining new knowledge. When participating in an educational activity, adults know what goals they want to achieve. Therefore, information should be presented in a results-oriented manner so that adults will have a valid reason to change behaviors. Even with expanded knowledge, adults will need some help putting new knowledge into practice.[41]

A key point of adult learning is *relevance.* This concept means adults must understand why new information or a changed behavior is needed before true learning will take place. Self-directing adults must be considered partners in learning; successful counselors will consider the adult's values, preferences, and biases of previous knowledge and experience. Adults must be ready to learn and may only learn those things that they perceive to be a benefit to daily life. The second key point is, information must be practical, which means the information presented meets the patient's readiness to learn and can be put to immediate use.[41]

Putting these concepts to work in a health education situation, the provider must, through talking with and observing the patient, determine the patient's interests, attitudes, and current knowledge. The provider must also assess what the patient is ready to learn and what information can be put to immediate use. Determining appropriate topics of education at any point in time may be tricky, because the counselor must first determine what those topics are. The counselor will have to interview the patient to determine current level of knowledge, interests, and needs. The counselor must also refrain from giving the patient *everything*! If information is relevant and practical, it is more likely that the patient will try out the knowledge, observe success, and gain self-efficacy. Using these techniques empowers the patient, honors the patient's autonomy, and allows the patient to gain self-efficacy. An example could be that a patient presents for emergency dental care for relief of pain. The dental provider provides the emergency treatment, proceeds to counsel the patient on additional oral health needs, and recommends a comprehensive dental examination. The provider may make the counseling relevant by linking oral health to other concerns of the patient such as possible diabetes or cardiovascular complications.

The provider ensures the counseling is practical information by ensuring the patient has the means necessary to use the information immediately. Questions regarding insurance status, previous use of the dental health care system, and previous dental health experiences may allow the provider to help the patient act immediately on the recommendation.

A patient with more self-efficacy is more likely to continue learned behaviors or complete complex treatment plans.[28,29]

How could adult education techniques be used in oral health? Patients are empowered to be partners in care. To accomplish this, providers must concentrate on individual assessments of knowledge and interest. Discussing past dental experiences, oral health expectations, and previous successes can help the patient and provider identify treatment goals. This process will not be the same for every patient! Understanding that all education for adults must meet their immediate needs (relevance) and be put to immediate use (practical) will encourage patients to be an active participant in their health care.

Providers may be reluctant to allow patients to dictate treatment planning. Patients may not understand the need for certain treatments or sequences of planned procedures. Goals must be negotiated between the provider and the patient. Patient education may be more successful if the following principles of adult education are used: need to know, patient as decision maker, acknowledgment of previous experiences, meeting patients at their level of readiness to learn, and providing relevant and practical information. This approach allows providers and patients to work together in achieving healthy choices for better oral health.

One example could be a patient with type 2 diabetes who presents with a draining abscess, but the tooth is not causing any pain. Because of the lack of pain or interference with daily activities, the patient does not want to have the tooth treated. The provider may make education *relevant* by advising the patient on the impact of chronic infection on blood sugar. The provider may make the education practical by addressing other issues of concern to the patient such as anxiety, cost of treatment, or other perceived barriers to care. The patient then becomes a full partner in setting treatment goals. The patient can make fully informed decisions and is more likely to follow comprehensive treatment.

MOTIVATING PATIENTS

Learning is a dynamic process that involves motivation to learn, retention of knowledge, reinforcement of knowledge, and transference. All learners must have a motivation to accept new information or skills. Once the learner has a degree of incentive to learn or change behavior, the information or skills must be presented in a manner that will allow the learner to retain the knowledge and reinforce skills. Positive reinforcement occurs with a positive outcome and may lead to increased self-efficacy. Negative reinforcement occurs with a bad outcome and may come from the instructor or from natural results of behavior. For example, a dental provider may instruct a patient to floss daily. If the patient does not adopt that behavior, and the gum tissue continues to bleed, that is a negative consequence of the patient's behavior. It is then the provider's responsibility to persuade the patient

to continue daily flossing so that positive results can be achieved.[41]

Transference occurs when new knowledge or skills are applied to a different setting. Transference may be evident if a young mother learns about brushing and flossing, and then teaches her children similar practices.

As in presenting education to adults, motivating the adult learner requires certain considerations. Six sources of adult motivation are as follows:

- *Social relationships:* Changing behavior to meet people or improve social activities.
- *External expectations:* Desire to please someone in authority.
- *Social welfare:* Desire to improve society.
- *Personal advancement:* Improvement on the job or achievement of a personal goal.
- *Escape stimulation:* Avoidance of boredom.
- *Cognitive interest:* Learning for the sake of learning.

Adults also have many barriers to learning. These barriers may include lack of time, interest, money, confidence, or failure to see the need to change. The challenge of the health educator is to minimize barriers and increase the reason for learning. A specific method of achieving this goal is through the use of motivational interviewing.

MOTIVATIONAL INTERVIEWING

As discussed in the previous section, learners and providers must be partners. This is a departure from the counseling style of provider as expert and patient as novice. The patient is the expert on identifying needs and concerns, and their state of readiness to learn and change behaviors. The provider is an expert on the health condition and effective interventions. The provider must meet the patient at an appropriate level to assist behavior changes. A technique known as **motivational interviewing** (MI) has successfully used the principles of adult education, readiness to learn, and self-efficacy to empower patients to adopt healthy lifestyle changes.[42] Motivational interviewing focuses on patients' readiness to learn and change, and helps engage patients to motivate them to progress along the stages of change model.

Motivational interviewing is defined as patient-centered counseling that helps the patient resolve conflicts and ambivalence. Behavior changes are encouraged by encouraging patients to set personal goals as negotiated with the health care provider.[43] To effectively use MI, the provider needs to understand the spirit of MI. Techniques, length of interviews, and number of encounters may vary, but the essence of MI is described in the key points outlined below:

1. Motivation to change is initiated by the patient, not the provider.
2. It is the patient's responsibility to determine conflict or ambivalence between different courses of action.
3. Direct persuasion is not effective in changing behavior.
4. Counseling style is quiet and encourages patient participation.
5. Counselor must assist patient to examine conflict or ambivalence.
6. Readiness to change is not stagnant or an innate trait, but constantly fluctuates.
7. The counseling relationship is a partnership.[42]

Through interviews and observations, the learner and counselor work together to decide topics of immediate concern. The counselor must avoid the temptation to overload the patient with information. The patient will have more than one encounter with medical professionals. These multiple encounters offer the opportunity to expand education and improve health behaviors.

How do you determine the patient's current needs? Questions to the patient can reveal much about the patient's current level of knowledge and interest. Some possible questions to pose regarding dental needs and oral hygiene practices include the following:

- What concerns do you have about your mouth?
- Tell me about your past experiences with dental treatment.
- What methods have you used in the past to clean between your teeth?
- What do you know about how to prevent gum (periodontal) disease?

Frequently, individuals with severe dental disease will report no dental problems. If a brief look in the patient's mouth reveals obvious dental disease and the patient reports no problems, the counselor should stop after the first two questions and focus on the need for good oral health, possibly touching on the association between chronic oral infections and diabetes mellitus or cardiovascular complications. That would be an example of giving only relevant information. For a better understanding of MI, it may be useful to recognize characteristics of counseling that are *not* MI. Motivational interviewing has not taken place if the counselor:

1. Argues that the patient has a problem in need of change.
2. Offers direct advice without determining the patient's interest in change.
3. Adopts a superior attitude to the patient.
4. Does most of the talking.
5. Labels the patient.
6. Uses coercion.[43]

ORAL HEALTH APPLICATION

The benefits of MI were demonstrated in a group of mothers of young children at high risk for developing caries. Traditional health education was compared with MI techniques in changing oral health behaviors. Mothers in a control group received written information and viewed a videotape. Mothers in the experimental group received one session of MI and six follow-up calls within the first year. There were no clinical interventions for either group in the first year. After 2 years, the children in the experimental group had significantly fewer new caries than children in the control group. The researcher concluded that the MI techniques had a protective effect for early childhood caries.[42]

SUMMARY

Health education is complex and challenging. Providers must assess the learner's knowledge, interest, and values, must then identify the appropriate learning approach, and then design a personal oral health plan for the patient. This may seem overwhelming and not realistic within the available patient treatment time. However, after the provider has become comfortable with the various learning theories, determining patient needs and designing patient education becomes a natural part of the oral health appointment.

REFERENCES

1. Radely, A. (1994). *Making sense of illness: The social psychology of health and disease.* London; Sage Publications.
2. Ascension Health. (2006). Healthcare ethics. Autonomy. Retrieved November 3, 2006, from http://www.ascensionhealth.org/ethics/public/isssues/autonomy.asp.
3. Susser, M. (1987). *Epidemiology, health and society.* New York: Oxford University Press.
4. Hochbaum, G. (1970). *Health behavior.* Belmont, CA: Wadsworth Publishing, 70.
5. Pine, C.M., McGoldrick, P.M., Burnside, G., Curnow, N.M., Chesters, R. K., Nicholson, J., Huntington, E. (2000). An intervention programme to establish regular toothbrushing: Understanding parents' beliefs and motivating children. *Int Dent J,* Suppl:312–23.
6. Nakazono, T. T., Davidson, P. L., & Anderson, P. M. (1997). Oral health beliefs in diverse populations. *Adv Dent Res,* 11:235–44.
7. McCall, K. D., Glasgow, R. E., & Gustafson, C. (1985). Predicting levels of dental behaviors. *J Am Dent Assoc,* 111:601–605.
8. Weisenburg, N., Kegeles, S. S., & Lund, A. K. (1980). Children's health beliefs and acceptance of dental preventive activity. *J Health Soc Behav* 21(1):59–74.
9. Groner, J. A., Ahijevych, K., Grossman, L. K., Rich, L. N. (2000). The impact of a brief intervention on maternal smoking behavior. *Pediatrics,* 105:267–71.
10. Prochaska, J. O., Norcross, J. C., & DiClemente, C. C. (1994). *Changing for good.* New York: Avon Books.
11. Prochaska, J. O., Redding, C. A., & Evers, K. E. (1997). *Health behavior and education.* San Francisco; Jossey-Bass.
12. Bertrand, J. T., & Anhang, R. (2006). The effectiveness of mass media in changing HIV/AIDS-related behaviour among young people in developing countries. *World Health Organ Tech Rep Ser,* 938:205–41.
13. Tillis, T. S., Stoch, D. J., Cross-Poline, G. N., Annan, S. D., Astroth, D. B., & Wolfe, P. (2003). The transtheoretical model applied to an oral self-care behavior change: development and testing of instruments for stages of change and decisional balance. *J Dent Hyg,* 77:16–25.
14. Gil, K. M., Schrop, S. L., Kline, S. C., Kimble, E. A., McCord, G., McCormick, K. F., & Gilchrist, V. (2002). Stages of change analysis of smokers attending clinics for the medically underserved. *J Fam Pract,* 51:1081.
15. Lawrence, T., Aveyard, P., Evans, O., & Cheng, K. K. (2003). A cluster randomised controlled trial of smoking cessation in pregnant women comparing interventions based on the transtheoretical (stages of change) model to standard care. *Tob Control,* 12:168–77.
16. Carlson, L. E., Taezner, P., Koopmans, J., & Casebeer, A. (2003). Predictive value of aspects of the Transtheoretical Model on smoking cessation in a community-based, large-group cognitive behavioral program. *Addic Behav,* 28:725–40.
17. Aveyard, P., Cheng, K. K., Almond, J., Sherratt, E., Lancashire, R., Lawrence, T., Griffin, C., & Evans, O. (1993). Cluster randomised controlled trial of expert system based on the transtheoretical ("stages of change") model for smoking prevention and cessation in schools. *British Med J,* 319:948–53.
18. Herzog, T. A., Abrams, D. B., Emmons, K. M., Linnan, L. A., & Schadel, W. G. (1999). Do processes of change predict smoking stage movements: A prospective analysis of the transtheoretical model. *Health Psychol,* 18:369–75.
19. Ajzen, I., & Fishbein, M. (1980). *Understanding attitudes and predicting social behavior.* Englewood Cliffs, NJ: Prentice Hall.
20. Tedesco, L. A., Keffer, M. A., Davis, E. L., & Christersson, L. A. (1992). Effect of a social cognitive intervention on oral health status, behavior reports, and cognitions. *J Periodontol,* 63:567–75.
21. Hollander, E. P., & Hunt, R. G., Eds. (1976). *Current perspectives in social psychology* (4th ed.). London: University Press.
22. Collier, G., Minton, H. L., & Reynolds, G., Eds. (1991). *Currents of thought in American social psychology.* New York: Oxford Press.
23. Bandura, A. (1986). *Social foundation of thought and action: A social cognitive theory.* Englewood Cliffs, NJ: Prentice Hall.
24. Bandura, A. (2001). Social cognitive theory: An agentic perspective. *Annu Rev Psychol,* 52:1–26.
25. Bandura, A. (1997). *Self efficacy: The exercise of control.* New York: Freeman.
26. Bandura, A. (1977). Self-efficacy: Toward a unifying theory of behavioral change. *Psycholog Rev,* 84:191–215.
27. Syrjala, A. M., Knuuttila, M. L., & Syrjala, L. K. (2001). Self efficacy perceptions in oral health behavior. *Acta Odontol Scan,* 59:1–6.
28. Syrjala, A. M., Kneckt, M. C., & Knuuttila, M. L. (1999). Dental self-efficacy as a determinant to oral health behaviour, oral hygiene and HbA1c level among diabetic patients. *J Clin Periodontol,* 26:616–21.
29. Kiyak, H. A. (1996). Measuring psychosocial variables that predict older persons' oral health behaviour. *Gerodontology* 13:69–75.
30. Litt, M. D., Reisine, S., & Tinanoff, N. (1995). Multidimensional causal model of dental caries development in low-income preschool children. *Pub Health Rep,* 11: 607–17.
31. Wallston, K. A., Stein, M. A., & Smith, C. A. (1994). Form C of the MCHL scales: A condition specific measurement of locus of control. *J Pers Assess,* 63:534–53.
32. Ferraro, L. A., Price, J. H., Desmond, S. M., & Roberts, S. M. (1987). Development of a diabetes locus of control scale. *Psychol Rep,* 61:763–70.

33. Vandecreek, L., & Odonnell, F. (1992). Psychometric characteristics of the headache-specific locus of control scale. *Headache,* 32:239–41.

34. Whitman, L., Desmond, S. M., & Price, J. H. (1987). Development of a depression locus of control scale. *Psychol Rep,* 60:583–89.

35. Reisine, S., & Litt, M. (1993). Social and psychological theories and their use for dental practice. *Int Dent J,* 43 (3 Suppl 1):279–87.

36. Amen, M. M., & Clark, V. J. P. (2001). The influence of mothers' health beliefs on the use of child health care services and mothers' perception of child health status. *Issues Compr Pediatr Nurs,* 24:153–63.

37. Antonovsky, A. (1979). Health stress and coping. San Francisco: Jossey-Bass.

38. Freire, M. C., Hardy, R., & Sheiham, A. (2002). Mothers' sense of coherence and their adolescent children's oral health status and behaviours. *Community Dent Health,* 19:24–31.

39. Atherton, J. S. (2005). Knowles' andragogy: An angle on adult learning. Retrieved October 9, 2006, from http://www.learningandteaching.info/learning/knowlesa .htm.

40. Leib, S. (1991). Principles of adult learning. Retrieved November 27, 2006, from http://honolulu.hawaii.edu/ intranet/committees/FacDevCom/guidebk/teachtip/ adults-2.htm.

41. Weinstein, P., Harrison, R., & Benton, T. (2006). Motivating mothers to prevent caries: Confirming the beneficial effect of counseling. *J Am Dent Assoc,* 137:789–93.

42. Rollnick, S., & Miller, W. Motivational interviewing: What is it? Retrieved November 27, 2006, from http://www.motivationalinterview.org/clinical/whatismi .html.

Chapter 18

Tobacco Cessation

Joan M. Davis

OBJECTIVES

After studying this chapter, the student should be able to:

1. Describe population characteristics of tobacco users in the United States and the resultant morbidity and mortality.
2. Describe the oral diseases and lesions related to the use of tobacco, both smoked and smokeless.
3. Describe the different types of tobacco and their uses, emphasizing the harmful toxins, carcinogens, and nicotine levels in both smoked and smokeless tobacco.
4. Describe the process of nicotine addiction as a chemical dependence, as well as the behavioral and social aspects of the addiction process.
5. Identify the specific FDA-approved pharmacotherapies available for tobacco cessation, including nicotine-replacement therapy and oral medication, emphasizing the appropriate assessment of the dependence level to nicotine and the most beneficial use of available medications.
6. Identify the various components of an effective tobacco-cessation intervention using the Public Health Service Guideline, stages of change model, and motivation for behavior change.
7. Describe the specific components of a tobacco-cessation intervention in the dental office setting, emphasizing the specific roles of the dental team for a comprehensive program.
8. Identify the elements of successful tobacco-prevention strategies in the office and community settings.

KEY TERMS

Second-hand smoke
Smoked
Smokeless (spit) tobacco
Dose response
Main-stream smoke
Side-stream smoke
Bidis
Kreteks
Clove cigarettes
Water pipes
Moist snuff
Packets
Chew tobacco
Reverse-smoking
Substance dependence
Nicotine withdrawal
Fagerstrom test for nicotine dependence

INTRODUCTION

Dental providers have a unique opportunity to see basically healthy individuals, often throughout their entire lives. This regular, long-term contact provides the clinician with the opportunity to identify tobacco use, and provide appropriate tobacco intervention based on both clinical findings and a supportive, patient-centered relationship. For those patients who have not initiated tobacco use or quit using tobacco, the clinician has the opportunity to encourage a tobacco-free life.

TOBACCO USE: MORBIDITY, MORTALITY, AND U.S. POPULATION TRENDS

Tobacco use continues to be the primary cause of preventable death and disease in the United States, with approximately 438,000 premature deaths attributed to smoking annually.[1] Of these estimated premature deaths, 39.8% were attributed to cancer, 34.7% to cardiovascular disease, and 25.5% to respiratory disease. Lung cancer, chronic obstructive pulmonary disease (COPD), and ischemic heart disease are the top three causes of death due to smoking.[1] The 2004 Surgeon General's general report provided definitive evidence that smoking was a causative factor for numerous diseases in addition to lung cancer (Table 18–1 ■), including but not limited to the following cancers: laryngeal, oral, pharynx, esophageal, pancreatic, bladder and kidney, cervical, endometrial, stomach, and acute leukemia.[2] In the Surgeon General's *Report on the Health Consequences of Smoking,* Department of Health and Human Services Secretary Thompson states that smoking remains the leading preventable cause of death in this country. It continues to cost our society too many lives, too many dollars, and too many tears.

Fortunately, tobacco use in the United States has fallen from 42% of adult smokers 18 years and older (51.9% males, 33.9 % females) in 1965 to 20.9% of adult smokers (23.9% males, 18% females) in 2005; in addition, 2.3% reported using smokeless tobacco in 2005, a 49% decline.[3] It is estimated that the decline in smoking over the past 50 years has resulted in the reduction of approximately 40% of deaths due to lung cancer in males.[4] A breakdown of characteristics of the estimated 45.1 million people 18 years or older who report smoking every day can be found in (Table 18–2 ■). Unfortunately, the decline in adult smoking has leveled off over the past 2 years, and may indicate that the *Healthy People 2010* objectives to reduce adult smoking levels to 12.0% and smokeless levels to 0.4%[5] may not be realized. More public health efforts are needed to prevent initiation of tobacco use; a need also exists for expanded cessation and policy measures focused on the populations with the highest percentage of smoking, those with a general education diploma at 43.2%, those below the poverty level at 29.9%, and American Indian/Alaska Indian native populations.[3,6]

Initiation of tobacco use continues to occur primarily before the age of 18 years, with 54.3% of students in grades nine through twelve reporting having tried cigarette smoking sometime in their lives.[7] Although youth rarely encounter the known chronic health effects as a result of smoking, this risk behavior may lead to the establishment of a life-long use of tobacco, leading to a much higher risk of developing smoking-related diseases.

■ **Table 18–1** The Health Consequences of Smoking from the 2004 Surgeon General's Report[2]

Disease and Adverse Health Effects

Cancer: Laryngeal, Oral, Pharynx, Esophageal, Pancreatic, Bladder and Kidney, Cervical, Endometrial, Stomach, and Acute leukemia

Cardiovascular Diseases: Abdominal aortic aneurysm, Atherosclerosis, Cerebrovascular disease, Coronary heart disease

Respiratory Diseases: Chronic obstructive pulmonary disease, Pneumonia, Respiratory effects in utero (reduced lung function) and in children and adolescents, Poor asthma control

Reproductive Effects: Fetal death and stillbirths, Reduced fertility in women, Low birth weight, Preterm delivery, Abruptio placentae

Other Effects: Increased risk for cataracts, Diminished health, Hip fractures, Low bone density, Peptic-ulcer disease

■ **Table 18–2** Characteristics of Adults Over 18 Years Who Are Current Smokers in 2005 from the National Health Interview Survey, United States, 2005[3]

Characteristics	
Race/Ethnicity	
White	21.9%
Black	21.5%
Hispanic	16.2%
American Indian/ Alaskan Native	32.0%
Asian	13.2%
Education	
0–12 yrs (no diploma)	25.5%
9–11 yrs	32.6%
GED diploma	43.2%
High school grad.	24.6%
Assoc. degree	20.9%
Some college	22.5%
Undergrad degree	10.7%
Graduate degree	7.1%
Age	
18–24	24.4%
25–44	24.1%
45–64	21.9%
> 65	8.6%
Poverty Status	
At or above	20.6%
Below	29.9%
Total	20.9% (45.1 million)

In the Youth Risk Behavior Surveillance 2005 survey, 23% of high school students reported current cigarette use (22.9% male, 23.0% female), and 8% reported using smokeless (13.6% males, 2.2% females) in the past 30 days.[7,8] As with the tobacco-use trend reported in adult data, reported youth tobacco use has also declined, but is unlikely to reach the *Healthy People 2010* goal of less than 16%.[5] A disturbing recent trend of tobacco initiation and use has been observed in 18- to 25-year-olds and college students, with 32.9% reporting that they are currently engaged in cigarette smoking.[9] This recent trend may reflect the restriction on advertising or selling tobacco products to minors and the tobacco industry's shift in advertising to college students.

The harm of tobacco smoke is not limited to those who are actually lighting up and smoking. **Second-hand smoke** is responsible for premature death and disease for non-smokers who are exposed to it. It is estimated that 22 million children and 30% of indoor workers are exposed to the hundreds of toxins found in second-hand smoke, which causes an increased risk of acute respiratory infection, ear infections, and more severe asthma in children, as well as coronary heart disease and lung cancer in non-smoking adults exposed to second-hand smoke.[10] Indoor air laws are designed to protect the health and welfare of both workers and patrons, not to limit the rights of others. Smoke-free initiatives are evidence-based health and safety initiatives and need to be supported.

TOBACCO-RELATED ORAL DISEASES AND LESIONS

The Directors for the National Cancer Institute and the National Institute for Dental Research emphasized that helping patients to stop using tobacco may be the single most important service dental professionals can provide for their patients' health. The physical consequences of using **smoked** and/or **smokeless (spit) tobacco** on the oral cavity are numerous and potentially life-threatening (Table 18–3 ■). Although the oral effects of smoked and smokeless tobacco are sometimes presented together; the actual tissue changes, damage, or disease caused by each type of tobacco are often unique to the specific form of tobacco used. All forms of tobacco contain the addictive drug nicotine, as well as cancer-causing nitrosamines; however, when tobacco is burned, an additional 4,000+ chemicals are generated and inhaled with each puff, causing a greater level of harm. The vast majority of reported health consequences of tobacco use are referring to smoked, not smokeless, tobacco.[2] For example, tobacco that is smoked has been clearly shown to be a causative factor in the development of periodontitis,[12] whereas smokeless tobacco has not. It is important to remember, though, that there is no safe or harmless tobacco product. All forms of tobacco are harmful and can lead to chemical dependence; therefore, one form should not be substituted for another.

Oral Cancer/Precancerous Lesions

In 2006, 30,990 new cases of oral (tongue, mouth, pharynx, other oral cavity) and pharyngeal cancers, with approximately 7,430 deaths due to oral cancer, were

■ **Table 18–3** Oral Lesions and Conditions Related to Tobacco Use

Oral cancer (smoked & smokeless)
Leukoplakia (smoked)
      Homogeneous leukoplakia
      Nonhomogeneous leukoplakia (precancer):
            Verrucous leukoplakia
            Nodular leukoplakia
            Erythroleukoplakia
Other tobacco-induced oral mucosal conditions
      Snuff dipper's lesions (smokeless only)
      Smoker's palate (nicotine stomatitis) (smoked only)
      Smoker's melanosis
Tobacco-associated effects on the teeth and supporting tissues
      Tooth loss (premature mortality)
      Staining
      Abrasion
      Periodontal diseases:
            Periodontitis (smoked)
            Focal recession (smokeless)
            Necrotizing ulcerative gingivitis (smoked)
Other tobacco-associated oral conditions
      Gingival bleeding
      Calculus
      Halitosis/Malodor
      Leukoedema
      Chronic hyperplastic candidiasis (candidal leukoplakia)
      Median rhomboid glossitis
      Hairy tongue
Possible association with tobacco
      Oral clefts
      Dental caries
      Lichen planus
      Salivary changes
      Taste and smell

Adapted from *Tobacco Effects in the Mouth*, NIH pub. No. 96-3330. June 1996.

estimated to occur in the United States.[13] Fortunately, the rate of deaths from oral and pharyngeal cancer has steadily declined over the past 20 years,[14] possibly because of the concurrent overall decrease of smoking from 42% in 1964 to 20.9% in 2005.[3] The primary risk factors for the development of oral cancer for both young and older adults is cigarette smoking and excessive use of alcohol,[15–18] accounting for more than 75% of oral cancers.[15] Rodriguez reviewed various risk factors in 137 cases of oral cancer in patients below the age of 46, and found that smoking accounted for 77% of all reported oral and pharyngeal cancers, alcohol consumption for 52%, and the combined effect of heavy smoking and drinking for 83% of the cancers in the study.[19] Smokers are more likely to develop leukoplakia than nonsmokers.[20] There also exists a clear dose response; the more a person smokes or uses any type of tobacco product, the more likely a form of leukoplakia will develop. Fortunately, most leukoplakias, which are premalignant lesions, will resolve if smoking is discontinued.[2,20]

Smokeless tobacco poses an oral cancer risk because of the presence of tobacco-specific nitrosamines found in all tobacco products and is able to cause smokeless tobacco-specific leukoplakia called Snuff Dipper's Pouch.[11,21] Although early research reported smokeless tobacco greatly increased the risk of oral cancer with long-term use,[22] later research has introduced the idea that smokeless tobacco poses a lower risk than smoked tobacco.[23,24] The level of risk from using smokeless tobacco depends a great deal on how much is used and how long it is used, and on the specific type of smokeless tobacco, which contains a range of nitrosamines depending on the product.[23] As stated before, there is no safe form of tobacco, and it should never be suggested that someone replace one form of tobacco with another as a harm-reduction strategy: Tobacco kills. Dental health care providers are ethically bound to screen for oral cancer on every adult patient on a regular basis, and to provide appropriate tobacco interventions to help all tobacco-using patients to quit, no matter what form they use.[25]

Periodontal Diseases

The majority of adults in the United States suffer from some level of mild-to-moderate periodontitis with 5% to 20% suffering from severe periodontitis.[26,27] Of those adults with periodontitis, it is estimated that 42% (6.4 million) of the cases can be attributed to cigarette smoking and 11% (1.7 million) to smokers who had already quit but show past damage. For those periodontal patients who continue to smoke, it is estimated that 75% of their periodontitis is attributed to smoked tobacco.[28] Even when gender, age, and plaque index was controlled for, smoking remained the primary contributing factor for the presence of established periodontal disease.[29] As with the risk of oral cancer, the level of periodontal destruction is exposure-dependent. The number of cigarettes plus the number of years smoked, known as **dose response,** often will be an indicator for the level of periodontal destruction.[29,30] In addition, smokers have greater probing depths, gingival recession, loss of attachment, and bone loss than nonsmokers.[29–33] Cigarette smoking is a potential contributing factor in necrotizing ulcerative gingivitis,[34] possibly doubles the risk of root canal therapy,[35] and may increase healing complications after placement of endosseous dental implants.[36,37]

The exact mechanism of tobacco smoke and the impact on periodontal health are not known, but research is pointing to the chemicals in tobacco smoke altering the host immune response (Table 18–4 ■).[38–46] A strong host response is essential for the body to fight the bacterial assault and prevent or fight the breakdown of the immune response, resulting in gingivitis and progression to periodontitis. Smoking alters the body's ability to mount a host response at both the local and systemic levels by

■ **Table 18–4** *Potential* Negative Impact on Periodontal Tissues from Smoked Tobacco[39–47]

- Change in vasculature—reducing immune response
- Suppression of hemorrhagic responsiveness (bleeding)
- Reduction of oxygen in the periodontal pocket—affecting composition of subgingival flora
- Interference with cytokine production—inhibiting the immune response
- Increase in protelytic enzymes—leading to periodontal destruction
- Compromised PDL attachment to root surface—poor healing following periodontal therapy
- Decrease in lymphocyte production

changes in vasculature;[38] these changes manifest as reduced bleeding upon probing, potentially causing misinterpretation of periodontal health;[39] reduction of oxygen in the periodontal pocket, which may alter subgingival flora;[40] interference with production of cytokines, thus inhibiting the systemic immune response;[41] an increase in proteolytic enzymes, resulting in periodontal destruction;[42–44] compromised periodontal ligament attachment to the root surface after root planning;[45] and a decrease in lymphocyte production.[46] Patients who smoke not only are more likely to present with moderate or advanced periodontitis but will often respond poorly to non-surgical periodontal therapy[47] and periodontal re-care therapy[48] compared with non-smokers or smokers who have quit. Fortunately, many of the soft-tissue changes associated with smoking, such as an increase of blood flow and gingival crevicular fluid, return to the status of a non-smoker over time.[49] Bone loss, on the other hand, remains as a historical marker of past tobacco use. Patients should be asked not only if they currently use tobacco but if they have ever used it, so as to better understand the current level of periodontitis and to provide relapse-prevention information. The research is clear: Cigarette smoking is a major risk factor for periodontitis and is considered to have a strong causal association to the development of this chronic disease.[12,28–46]

Smokeless Tobacco and Periodontal Disease

The use of smokeless tobacco directly affects the oral tissue where the snuff or chew tobacco directly touches the mouth. The consequences of the gingival and mucosal tissue being covered with tobacco, which releases nicotine, cancer-causing nitrosamines, and a high level of sweetening agents, results in a significantly greater amount of recession and attachment loss, possibly due to chemical injury rather than bacterial assault. It is believed that there exists no clear demonstrated association between use of smokeless tobacco and generalized severe periodontitis.[50–52] However, in a recent study, Fisher

reviewed population-based records of 12,932 adults in the National Health and Nutrition Examination Survey III study and found that the smokeless-tobacco users were twice as likely as non-tobacco users to have evidence of severe active periodontal disease, controlling for smokers.[53] More research is needed to examine the relationship between smokeless tobacco and generalized periodontal disease to further clarify this point. The American Academy of Periodontology strongly recommends inclusion of tobacco cessation in periodontal therapy.[54]

TOBACCO TYPES, TOXINS, AND CARCINOGENS

Understanding the cause of the numerous systemic and oral consequences of tobacco use requires the ability to identify the types of tobacco on the market, how they are used, and what toxic components each contain. Although all forms of tobacco are harmful, the tobacco type, amount used, and duration of use can have a great impact on the risk for disease.[2]

The most common form of tobacco use in the United States is cigarette smoking at 20.9%, with cigar smoking next at 2.3%,[3] and pipe smoking at 1.4%.[55] Smoked tobacco inhaled by the consumer (**main-stream smoke**) contains an estimated more than 3,800 compounds and more than 60 carcinogens, including tobacco-specific nitrosamines (Table 18–5 ■),[56–58] whereas **side-stream smoke** (also known as involuntary exposure to tobacco smoke, environmental tobacco smoke, or second-hand smoke) has most of the same toxins (ammonia, nitrogen oxides, and chemical carcinogens). However, that exposure may be up to 100 times higher than main-stream smoke.[59] Second-hand smoke not only poses significant health risks[10] but may also result in an increase in periodontitis.[60] The chemically complex mixture of toxins, carcinogens, and inert substances is a result of the combination of the tobacco leaf, pesticides used to grow the plant, the curing or fermenting process, additives, and the burning process. Even with the introduction of low-tar, filtered cigarettes in the late 1950s, smoking-related

■ **Table 18–5**   A Sampling of the Carcinogens/Toxins Found in Tobacco Smoke[58–60]

Nitrogen, oxygen, carbon dioxide, carbon monoxide, water, argon, hydrogen, ammonia, nitrogen oxides, hydrogen cyanide, hydrogen sulfide, methane, isoprene, butadiene, acetylene, benzene, toluene, styrene, formic acid, acetic acid, propionic acid, methyl formate, formaldehyde, acetaldehyde, acrolein, acetone, methanol, furan, pyridine, picolines, 3-vinylpyridine, nicotine, anatabine, naphthalene, tobacco specific N-nitrosamines . . .

morbidity and mortality did not decrease as a result.[2,61] Although filtered cigarettes deliver lower tar and nicotine, as measured by a "smoking machine," smokers compensate for the lower nicotine dose by inhaling more deeply, covering filter vents, and smoking more.[61]

Newer trends in smoked-tobacco use among high school students include the use of bidis (pronounced "bee-dees") at 2.6%, kreteks (pronounced "cree-teks") at 2.3%,[62] water pipes, and flavored cigarettes. **Bidis** are small, hand-rolled cigarettes imported from India or Southeast Asia. This hand-rolled "poor man's cigarette" is made from flakes and dust of dark tobacco leaves with vanilla, licorice, strawberry, cinnamon, or mango flavoring added to give a sweet taste and mask the strong tobacco smoke. These flavored, unfiltered cigarettes are attractive to youth, because they are relatively inexpensive compared with cigarettes. Bidis are sold in tattoo parlors, on the Internet, and at other venues that may not enforce regulations such as those adhered to by more traditional tobacco retail locations.

Kreteks, or **clove cigarettes,** are imported from Indonesia and contain a mixture of tobacco, cloves, and other additives. Although little research has been conducted on the physical effects of clove cigarettes, people who smoke them have been found to inhale deeper and therefore are provided with basically the same level of nicotine as that from regular cigarettes. Both bidis and kreteks deliver more nicotine, carbon monoxide, and tar than standard cigarettes,[63,64] and pose possible health risks. **Water pipes** (hookahs, narghile, shisha, or arghile), originating in Africa and Asia, are becoming popular among college students and others in the United States.[65] The water pipe contains a bowl in which fermented tobacco and flavorings are burned with the use of charcoal. The hookah smoke bubbles through water and is then breathed in via tubes, often by multiple users. Although users feel that the water "filters" out the toxins, hookah smoke has been shown to contain many of the same toxins found in cigarette smoke.[66] Unfortunately, youth and young adults are trying alternative tobacco and herbal products, believing that they are not as harmful as regular cigarettes (Figure 18–1 ■). When these products are formally tested, they often yield higher amounts of tobacco toxins. Therefore, the provider must ask youth and young adults if they are using any tobacco products rather than just asking "Do you smoke?" to better assess their use and become familiar with how tobacco is used in the community.

The use of smokeless tobacco has continued to decline in the United States among individuals 18 years old and over at 2.3% (men at 4.5% and women 0.2%),[3] but its use remains high (at 8%) in those under the age of 18 years.[7] In recent years, however, the tobacco industry has marketed the use of spit tobacco for smokers who are not allowed to smoke and may choose another type of tobacco use. As with smoked tobacco, smokeless comes in many and varied forms (Figure 18–2 ■). All smokeless tobacco contains tobacco-specific cancer-causing nitrosamines[67–69] and nicotine, which are "free" or available for absorption by the body in the presence of base chemicals (sodium carbonate and ammonium carbonate), added by the tobacco companies. The higher the pH, the greater is the available nicotine and therefore the greater potential effect on the brain (approximately one can of snuff equals four packs of cigarettes). Introductory spit products, such as Bandits (US Tobacco Co.) have a lower pH and more flavoring than Copenhagen (US Tobacco Co.) or Kodiak (Genuine Tobacco Co.), thus allowing youth or novices to experiment on flavored, low-nicotine products to adjust to using them before graduating to more potent and addictive products.[70,71] The two main forms of smokeless tobacco used in this country are snuff and chewing tobacco.

Snuff is finely ground tobacco sold in three forms: moist (fine or long cut), packets or sachets, and dry. **Moist snuff** comes in round flat tins; the user takes a pinch between two fingers and places the "dip" somewhere in the vestibule area in the buccal mucosal fold. Saliva then bathes the dip, forming tobacco juice, which is swallowed or spit, hence, the term "spit tobacco." Snuff is also sold in **packets** designed to contain the loose, fine-cut moist snuff to make it more acceptable to users who may be just trying it out or do not want to be seen using loose tobacco.

Chew tobacco comes in loose leaves, in a twist of tobacco leaves, or in a block of tobacco from which the user cuts off a chunk or "plug" of tobacco. Contrary to the name, chew tobacco is not chewed but rather placed in the oral cavity, usually in the vestibule area, to allow the nicotine to diffuse through the buccal mucosa. Chew tobacco contains between 30% to 40% fermentable carbohydrates compared with 2% in snuff.[72] This high level of sugar, repeatedly placed in one location in the mouth, has been shown to lead to 4 times more root caries being reported in tobacco chewers than in snuff users or smokers.[73] In addition to the presence of nitrosamines, chew tobacco contains *Bacillus* species, which produce organic

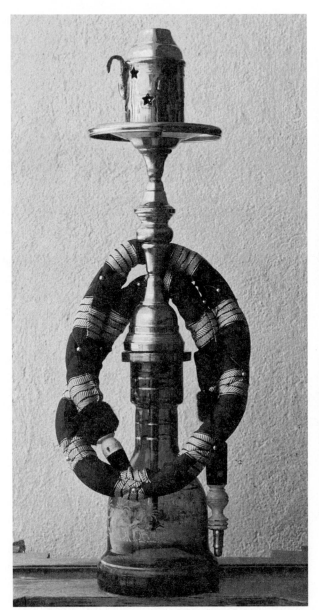

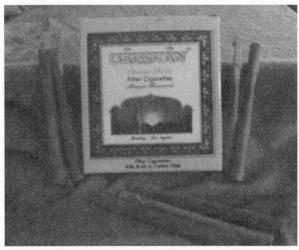

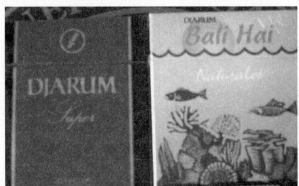

■ **FIGURE 18–1**   Alternate forms of tobacco: (A) Hookah; (B) Bidi (beedies or beadies); (C) Kreteks.
(A, Arthur Pawlowski © Dorling Kindersley)

toxins and may lead to the development of localized tissue damage in chewers.[74] And finally, cigars, chew, and snuff tobacco products have been shown to contain abrasive particles (silicone dioxide or silica), possibly leading to dental attrition.[75]

A culturally aware approach is an important aspect with all patient care, but especially when providing

tobacco-cessation interventions for patients from other cultures. Tobacco is commonly used all over the world in pastes and powders, as desserts, in toothpaste, in small packets (Swedish snuff, "snus"), and mixed with slaked lime, spices, ash, and/or fungus, which can be smoked, smoked on the burning end (**reverse-smoking**), sucked on, chewed, or wiped on the teeth and gingiva. It is not

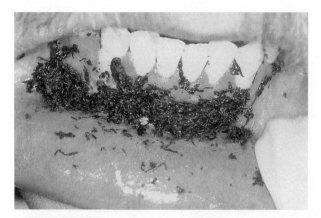

■ **FIGURE 18–2**   Snuff.

unusual for women to be regular users of these products; they may freely give tobacco to their children to use.[76] One of the more common alternative tobacco practices found in the United States is chewing betel-quid and areca-nut chewing. With this Indian import, an areca-nut paste is mixed with slack lime and tobacco and then wrapped in a betel leaf called a betel-quid (numerous other names and ingredients are used in other parts of Southeast Asia). Alone, the use of areca-nut products poses a high risk of developing oral cancer. When combined with tobacco (known as "Gutka"), the risks of leukoplakia, oral submucous fibrosis, oral cancer, and abnormal reproductive health outcomes are increased.[77,78] Clearly, an open-ended inquiry, such as "Tell me about your tobacco use," will best determine how to customize a tobacco intervention. In addition, all tobacco-related health effects identified in the oral examination should be incorporated into the cessation message, thus making the quit message personally meaningful.

NICOTINE USE: A BIOCHEMICAL DEPENDENCE

The use of tobacco is a complex, multifactorial human behavior that encompasses biochemical, behavioral, and social components.[79] With a single puff of smoked tobacco or plug of smokeless tobacco, nicotine enters the bloodstream through the lungs or oral mucosa and travels throughout the body. When this powerful psychoactive drug (subjectively affecting mood and feelings) binds to the nicotinic acetylcholine receptors in the brain, autonomic ganglia, and the neuromuscular junction, a cascade of biochemicals are released including acetylcholine, dopamine, serotonin, norepinephrine, β endorphin,

glutamate, pituitary hormones, and vasopressin.[80,81] This nicotine-initiated biochemical release results in numerous body systems being affected including (1) cardiovascular system, increasing heart rate and blood pressure and vasoconstriction in extremities; (2) respiratory system; (3) skeletal motor, causing feelings of relaxation; and (4) gastrointestinal system, through stimulation of the afferent chemical receptors and the autonomic nervous system.[80,81] The steady infusion of nicotine and sodium found in smokeless tobacco has been linked to the possible acceleration of coronary disease and vascular disease.[82] In addition, nicotine suppresses the appetite and increases body metabolism, often leading to an artificially lower weight for tobacco users. Once tobacco use is discontinued, an average of 5 to 10 pounds is gained, thus returning the individual to a non-nicotine or normal weight.[83]

The extent to which nicotine affects the central nervous system is determined by what method and how much tobacco is used. Inhaled tobacco smoke quickly moves from the lungs to the brain in approximately 7 seconds. The 1 to 2 mg of bioavailable nicotine remains in the system for 20 to 30 minutes and then rapidly drops off, cueing the user to replenish the nicotine with another cigarette. This peak-and-valley pattern explains the need for smokers to use tobacco every 1 to 2 hours depending on their level of dependence. Smokeless tobacco slowly diffuses through the mucous membrane and clears the system slowly, giving a more stable infusion of nicotine.[80] Because of the slow diffusion, smokeless tobacco users may smoke when they first wake to rapidly replenish the drug and then use smokeless tobacco to maintain a constant dosing of the drug.

The release of dopamine causes a sense of well-being, relaxation, and stress reduction, whereas release of norepinephrine (adrenaline) causes a sense of heightened alertness. These effects reward and reinforce the continued use of the tobacco, leading to nicotine dependence. For the first-time user, this powerful drug can cause dizziness, nausea, vomiting, and headache (toxicity). However, with repetition and increase in the amount used (dosing), these negative effects disappear, and a tolerance or desensitization of the neuroreceptors develops, requiring an increased and steady use of nicotine to obtain the desired effect.[80] In addition, with the continued use and increased dose of nicotine, the brain adapts to this chemical assault by significantly increasing (upregulating) the number of nicotinic neuroreceptors by 50% within a few weeks.[84,85] Unfortunately, the creation of additional receptors and desensitization of existing nicotinic receptors, combined with the memory of positive reinforcement from endorphin release, produces a powerful craving, a strong drive to use the substance, and avoidance of withdrawal if not given the needed dose of nicotine. The cravings and avoidance of withdrawal drive a user to sustain or increase the amount and/or frequency of tobacco use, thus establishing chemical and behavioral dependence, even when presented with compelling health consequenses.[86,87]

Now considered a chronic, relapsing, progressive disease, a formal diagnosis of **substance dependence** is made if a user meets three of the six major criteria (Table 18–6 ■) in the Diagnostic Criteria from *Diagnostic Statistical Manual of Mental Disorders, Fourth Edition.*[88] Habitual self-administration, the development of tolerance, compulsive drug-taking behavior, and withdrawal are central components for the diagnosing of substance dependence disorders for alcohol, cocaine, heroin, and nicotine. **Nicotine withdrawal** symptoms include depressed mood, insomnia, irritability, anxiety, difficulty concentrating, restlessness, decreased heart rate, and an increase in appetite.[88]

Not all tobacco users become dependent and may smoke or chew at will or in very small amounts, or only on weekends: social smokers or "chippers" (one to five cigarettes a day.) Breslau reported approximately 50% of daily smokers, who had smoked for a month or more, meet the criteria for nicotine dependence.[89] Although a patient may use limited amounts or is not currently dependent, even a small amount of tobacco exposes the individual to carcinogens, toxins, and nicotine; therefore, the user should be encouraged to quit.[90]

Current research points to a genetic basis for tobacco-use behavior and the likelihood of relapse once tobacco use is discontinued. This genetic disposition may explain why some people can quit seemingly at will and why others cannot seem to quit no matter how hard they try. Knowing if a patient is genetically predisposed to nicotine use may aid in developing appropriate behavioral and pharmacotherapy interventions for dependent patients who find it difficult to quit.[91,92]

TOBACCO USE: A BEHAVIORAL AND SOCIAL ADDICTION

Equally important to the chemical dependence of nicotine is the repetitive, habitual actions connected with each puff or dip, and the reinforcing experience of relaxation and sense of well-being. Each cigarette is a drug-delivery system containing approximately 1 to 2 mg of bioavailable nicotine, with inhalation through the lungs being a very effective mechanism to deliver this drug to the brain.[80] Tobacco companies enhanced this deadly delivery system by adding ammonia to cigarettes in the 1970s to raise the pH and increase the available nicotine, creating a better "hit" and subsequent positive reinforcement.[93] With approximately ten puffs taken per cigarette, a one-pack-per-day smoker will repeat the administration of nicotine 200 times each day to maintain relatively stable levels of the drug to satisfy cravings or avoid withdrawal symptoms.[94] The repetitions are often connected to specific activities performed each day, such as getting out of bed, having a cup of coffee, driving, spending time with friends or in a favorite activity, and after eating—resulting in cigarettes being habitually connected to every aspect of life's activities. The ritual of handling, placing, and using the tobacco is often reported to be as pleasurable as the effects of the nicotine, and should be

■ **Table 18–6**   Nicotine Dependence as a Mental Disorder*

1. Tolerance
2. Withdrawal
   A. daily use for at least several weeks
   B. depressed mood, insomnia, anxiety, irritability, restlessness, difficulty concentrating, restlessness, decreased heart rate, increase in appetite, weight gain
3. Repeated unsuccessful quit attempts
4. Reduced social activities or interactions due to tobacco use
5. Continued use despite knowledge of adverse effects
6. Using more tobacco than intended

Three or more of the following criteria must be met in order to establish dependence.
Adapted from the *Diagnostic and Statistical Manual of Mental Disorders,* 4th edition, Text Revisions. (Copyright 2000). American Psychiatric Association (DSM-IV-TR).[94]

considered when developing a cessation plan. Helping patients overcome this multifactorial addiction by necessity involves behavioral and pharmacologic assistance.

Pharmacotherapy for Treatment of Nicotine Dependence

The U.S. Public Health Service's (PHS) clinical practice guideline *Treating Tobacco Use and Dependence* (2000) established the importance of treating nicotine addiction as a disease, and recommended the use of appropriate cessation medications and behavioral interventions based on the patient's level of dependence and need. This resource provides an in-depth discussion and reference material on cessation medications, and can be found at http://www.ncbi.nlm.nih.gov/books/bv.fcgi?rid=hstat2 .chapter.7644.

Dental and medical professionals can have a significant impact on tobacco quit rates and should be actively involved in helping patients quit. Smokers trying to quit on their own succeed approximately 3% to 5% of the time.[95] The PHS guideline reports that a brief cessation intervention by a health care provider combined with appropriate medication may increase the success of maintaining abstinence to 30%.[79] With approximately 70% of the estimated 45 million smokers in the United States indicating that they would like to quit[3,94] and at least 50% of those smokers visiting their dentist's office each year, the potential impact dental clinicians could have on tobacco-related oral and general health is immense.[96]

The discussion and recommendation of appropriate pharmacotherapies to help manage withdrawal symptoms for those who are nicotine-dependent is an important aspect of a cessation intervention. Tobacco cessation medications are safe and effective, and have been shown to double the chances of a successful quit attempt.[70,79,97–99] Although the various cessation medications are effective, they may not be equally helpful to all users.[82] For example, women may not respond as well to nicotine-replacement therapy as men.[100] And for the most part, although pharmacotherapy can assist in quit attempts, medications alone have not been shown to sustain initial cessation rates at the 6-month interval.[101,102] As a multifactorial chronic relapsing disease, the combination of both behavioral and pharmacologic assistance is required to increase the chances of long-term success.[79]

First-Line Medications

The U.S. Federal Drug Administration (FDA) has approved several medications for over-the-counter (OTC) or prescription use in the treatment of nicotine dependence. First-line medications are approved for tobacco cessation (Table 18–7 ■). Second-line medications are used for tobacco cessation but are not FDA-approved for that use (i.e., off-label use).

Nicotine replacement therapies (NRT) are medications that provide nicotine in various forms intended to lessen or relieve withdrawal symptoms, but they have not been shown to relieve cravings. Although it seems counter-intuitive to treat nicotine addiction with nicotine, the administration of "pure" nicotine removes the exposure to tobacco's nitrosamines and toxins while behavioral changes are being made during the quit process. When used properly, NRT can provide approximately 30% to 80% of the nicotine normally obtained from tobacco, giving the user control over the amount of nicotine needed for cessation.[80,82,103,104] The patient must

■ **Table 18–7** Prescription and Over-the-Counter Tobacco-Cessation Medications*

Type	Form	Common Brand Name(s)	Availability
Nicotine Replacement Therapy	Gum	Nicorette®	Over-the-counter (OTC)
	Patch	Nicoderm®, Habitrol®, Prostep®, Nicotrol®	OTC and prescription
	Inhaler	Nicotrol®	Prescription
	Nasal Spray	Nicotrol®	Prescription
	Lozenge	Commit®**	OTC
Bupropion SR	Pill	Zyban®, Wellbutrin®	Prescription
Varenicline	Pill	Chantix®**	Prescription

*Approved by the Food and Drug Administration (FDA) and addressed in the 2000 PHS Guidelines.
**Received FDA approval on October 31, 2002, therefore not addressed in the 2000 PHS Guidelines.
Accessed 12/28/06 www.cdc.gov/tobacco/educational_materials/cessation

be advised to follow the label directions carefully, because (1) an excess of nicotine-replacement may cause toxicity and (2) too little nicotine will provide insufficient amounts available to ease withdrawal symptoms.[104] In either case, improper use of the medication is common and often leads to a return to tobacco use, called a relapse. This "failure" may give the tobacco user a sense that the pharmacotherapy did not work, leaving them reluctant to try again.

Pregnant and lactating women should be encouraged to quit tobacco without using cessation medications. However, when the benefits to the mother and child exceed the risks of cessation medications, a medical consult should be obtained for optimal care.[79]

Forms of NRT

OTC Nicotine Gum (Nicotine Polacrilex; 2 mg or 4 mg)   Nicotine gum was the first NRT approved for tobacco cessation by the FDA in the 1980s and has been shown to double the odds of a successful cessation attempt.[105] Unfortunately, this product is chewed like regular gum by many users, leading to nicotine toxicity (stomach ache, nausea) and is often discontinued. The patient should be instructed to (1) chew the gum a few times until a peppery/mint flavor is tasted; (2) place the gum in the vestibule area until the peppery taste is gone; (3) repeat this cycle for approximately 20 to 30 minutes, and (4) not use more than 20 pieces of 4-mg gum or 30 pieces of 2-mg gum. The level of nicotine peaks in the blood stream in about 20 to 30 minutes. Patients should be advised to avoid coffee, juices, and soft drinks 15 minutes before and while they use the gum, because a low, or acidic, pH will interfere with the nicotine absorption through the mucous membrane. Patients with temporomandibular joint problems or dentures have reported difficulties chewing the gum and may benefit from using the nicotine lozenge.

OTC Nicotine Lozenge (Nicotine Polacrilex with Aspartame; 2 mg or 4 mg)   The nicotine lozenge (Commit®), much like the gum, is an effective nicotine-replacement delivery system for tobacco users with low or high nicotine dependence.[106] The lozenge delivery system is easy to use (no chewing/parking) and delivers the complete dose of nicotine. As with nicotine gum, acidic beverages may interfere with the absorption of nicotine. Patients should be advised to avoid food, juice, coffee, or soft drinks 15 minutes before or during the use of the lozenge.

Sublingual lozenges are nicotine-containing tablets placed under the tongue; they are available in other countries, but are not yet available in the United States.

OTC Nicotine Transdermal Patch (7 mg, 14 mg, and 21 mg, or 15 mg)   The nicotine transdermal patch (Nicoderm CQ®, Nicotrol®) has been shown to be a safe and effective form of NRT, which works by diffusing a steady dose of nicotine through the skin.[107] The nicotine level peaks in about 4 to 8 hours and is maintained for 15 to 24 hours. Patients may experience mild skin irritation, but this side effect often will resolve in a few days, or the patch may be moved to different locations. Insomnia has been reported with the transdermal patch and may indicate that the dose should be lowered.

Prescription Nicotine Inhaler   The nicotine inhaler consists of a small cartridge that attaches to a cigar-like mouthpiece; it has been shown to be safe and effective in helping tobacco users quit.[79] The nicotine is not actually inhaled, but is "puffed" into the mouth where the medication is held, and then diffused through the oral mucosa. This system mimics the behavior of smoking and may meet the emotional need of a smoker to place something in the mouth. Mouth and throat irritation, coughing, and rhinitis are common but temporary side effects of this NRT.

Prescription Nicotine Nasal Spray   Nicotine nasal spray is administered directly into the nasal cavity, delivering a rapid dose of nicotine, which may benefit highly addicted users. The nasal spray has been reported to cause local irritations and congestion in about 94% of the users. Because of the more immediate dose of nicotine, this form of NRT poses a risk of addiction developing in about 15% to 20% of patients using the nicotine nasal spray.[79]

Proper Dosing of Nicotine Replacement

The proper amount and type of NRT to recommend to a patient is highly dependent on several factors, including (1) type of tobacco used, (2) amount of tobacco used, (3) level of nicotine dependence, (4) former experience with cessation medications, (5) medical contraindications, and (6) patient preference. Because each cigarette provides the user with 1 to 2 mg of available nicotine, then a reasonable amount or dose to recommend may be 1 mg of NRT to one cigarette smoked or one plug of smokeless used, which is basically the recommendation for use on NRT package instructions. As with all medications, the dosing should be adjusted for individual differences and needs. For example, if an individual smokes five cigarettes a day, using a 21-mg patch could easily cause nicotine toxicity. If a person smokes two packs a day, then a 7-mg patch would not be an adequate replacement. A smokeless-tobacco user may benefit from using the gum or lozenge to place in the mouth instead of a plug. A smoker may prefer the nicotine inhaler to give him the feel of something in his hands and mouth, and a chipper may prefer a 2-mg lozenge to use as needed. NRT offers the option of using them on a fixed schedule or as-needed.

A combination of NRTs may be a beneficial option by providing an ad libitum delivery of nicotine. For example, a nasal spray, gum, lozenge, or inhaler may be used with the patch, which delivers a slower, steady amount of nicotine, or with oral medications (bupropion and varenicline). This combination of medications allows for individualizing medications according to the patient's needs and preferences, which may yield higher quit rates.[97,98,108] The amount and form of NRT should be carefully considered and reduced at the first sign of toxicity.

Another important factor in determining the level and type of NRT is the degree of nicotine dependence. The **Fagerstrom Test for Nicotine Dependence** (FTND) consists of six basic questions on smoking behavior and has been widely used to assess the level of dependence.[109] The Heaviness of Smoking Index is a shorter, two-question survey that was adapted from the FTND and yields a quick indication of the level dependence:[110]

1. How soon after you wake up do you smoke your first cigarette?
   a. Within 5 minutes?
   b. 6–30 minutes?
   c. After 60 minutes?

2. How many cigarettes per day do you smoke?
   a. 10 or less
   b. 11–20
   c. 21–30
   d. 31 or more

If the person smokes within 30 minutes or less after waking and/or smokes 21 or more cigarettes per day, he is considered highly dependent. Because smokeless tobacco is used differently than smoked tobacco, the FTND was adapted for smokeless-tobacco use.[111] Like the FTND, the Fagerstrom Test for Nicotine Dependence—Smokeless Tobacco reports that the primary indicator of the level of dependence is related to how soon the smokeless tobacco is used when the user wakes

and if the tobacco juice is swallowed. Knowing the level of tobacco dependence will assist the clinician and patient in developing a cessation plan that includes appropriate behavioral responses and levels of medications necessary to address anticipated cravings and withdrawal symptoms.

Non-NRT Cessation Medications

Prescription bupropion SR (Zyban®), also marketed as an antidepressant (Wellbutrin®), was approved for smoking cessation by the FDA in 1997; it has been shown to be safe and approximately doubles cessation rates.[79,98,112] Although the exact mechanism is unknown, bupropion is believed to act on the neuroreceptors to mimic the effects of nicotine on dopamine and norepinephrine production, and to lessen withdrawal symptoms as well as delay weight gain.[112,113] This non-nicotine medication is taken in pill form and should be started 1 to 2 weeks before the quit date. Bupropion SR should not be prescribed for patients with a history of alcoholism, eating disorders, or seizure disorders, or for those using monoamine oxidative inhibitors.[79]

Prescription varenicline (Chantix®) was approved in 2006 by the FDA for smoking cessation and was designed specifically as a cessation medication. This unique cessation aid, taken in pill form, is designed to relieve both cravings and withdrawal symptoms. Varenicline is a partial agonist that binds to nicotinic acetylcholine receptors, thus blocking nicotine's stimulation of the release of dopamine and the subsequent rewarding effect sought by tobacco users. Initial research has shown this new medication to be relatively safe, non-addictive, and more effective than a placebo[114] or bupropion.[115] Varenicline helps with cessation attempts and holds great promise for those who have had difficulty in quitting by aiding in long-term abstinence (maintenance) with continued use.[116] (A cautionary note: some patients may experience depressive or suicidal thoughts while using varenicline. This potentially hazardous side-effect is currently under review by the FDA.)

Second-Line Therapies

Prescription clonidine, nortriptyline, and rimonabant have been used for nicotine-dependence treatment but are not approved by the FDA for smoking cessation. The PHS guideline does not recommend the use of second-line medications for use in normal clinical cessation therapy.

ALTERNATIVE CESSATION METHODS

Acupuncture, herbal remedies, hypnosis, auriculotherapy, and numerous other tobacco-cessation methods, although popular, are not evidence-based. Until these methods have independent supporting research to back their claims, they should not be formally recommended as cessation methods.[79] However, these methods may increase a user's belief that they can succeed (self-efficacy) and ultimately may help that individual.

COMPONENTS OF AN EFFECTIVE TOBACCO-CESSATION INTERVENTION

Dental health care providers assess risk through health histories, radiographs, and clinical evaluations, thereby developing treatment plans and providing oral health interventions as a regular and normal part of the oral care appointment. The inclusion of tobacco assessment and cessation is not only appropriate but an ethical obligation on the part of every clinician. With tobacco use being the primary cause of oral cancer and periodontitis, not to mention the number one cause of preventable death and disease in this country, every effort must be made to make tobacco cessation a normal part of dental care and a component of public health outreach.

Substantial evidence shows that even a brief tobacco-cessation intervention (TCI) provided by a health care provider can be effective in helping a patient successfully quit.[117] The more time oral professionals spend providing a TCI, the greater the benefit to the patients will be, resulting in an increase in successful quit rates.[79] Unfortunately, oral professionals continue to report barriers to offering tobacco interventions such as lack of time, training, and reimbursement, and they continue to offer limited TCIs.[118–120] Conversely, patients view tobacco interventions as a part of overall health care and expressed satisfaction when TCIs were provided.[121,122]

It is important to approach any behavioral change with sensitivity, and to adapt the message and evidence of tobacco-related oral disease to the patient (Table 18–8 ■). The concept of active listening, adapting the needed behavioral change to the person, and then helping the patient adopt the change is at the core of what is called motivational interviewing.

The PHS Guidelines' 5 A's

The gold standard for tobacco interventions worldwide is the PHS guideline *Treating Tobacco Use and Dependence.* The centerpiece of this seminal (original) document is the use of the 5 A's (ask, advise, assess, assist, arrange) and the 5 R's (relevance, risks, rewards, roadblocks, repetition). In recent thought, a more behavioral approach may be useful by placing "assess" before "advise" to understand the personal issues surrounding tobacco use before informing the patient that he needs to quit. Therefore this discussion will place assess before advise.

Ask

Asking if a patient uses tobacco is the first step in establishing oral health risks when interviewing a patient during an initial appointment or subsequent appointments. Establishing tobacco use can be done with questioning or by adding tobacco-use questions on the health history (Table 18–9 ■). A verbal follow-up and clarification can "assess" the behavioral and emotional issues associated with the tobacco use.

Assess

Taking into account the behavioral factors, emotional factors, level of addiction, past quit attempts, and current sense of willingness and ability to quit are all important

■ **Table 18–8**   The Primary Components of Motivational Interviewing

- Give clear advice
- Help remove perceived barriers
- Provide realistic choices
- Decrease the desirability of the poor choice/habit
- Practice empathy with the patient
- Provide positive feedback
- Clarify goals stated by the patient
- Actively help the patient succeed

Motivational Interviewing: Preparing People to Change Addictive Behavior by Miller and Rollnick, Guilford Press, 1991.

■ **Table 18-9**   Example of a Health History of Tobacco Use Assessment

ARE YOU USING?

1. YES or NO

    a. Any tobacco product: cigarettes (# per day_____) / cigar / snuff / pipe / bidi

    b. If YES, how long have you been using tobacco products? _____ years.

    c. How soon do you use tobacco when you wake up in the morning?
        Within: __ 5 min __10 min __20 min __ 30 min +

    d. Are you interested in reducing or quitting tobacco use? YES NO

    e. Would you like help in reducing/quitting: ____ now ____ this month ____ later
        ____ not interested right now

    f. If you have tried to quit, what have you tried or used? _____
        (This should give a fairly good idea of the patient's current *stage*.)

in providing a TCI. The use of the stages-of-change model can aid in assessing readiness to quit, thus guiding the clinician in what and how much to share with the tobacco user.

The Stage-of-Change Model in TCI   A possible TCI based on the stages of change involves the following five concepts:

- *Pre-contemplation:* Not willing to quit or even think about it.
- The TCI measures are as follows:
  - Provide a pamphlet and let the patient know you are there to help when the patient is ready to quit.
  - Use motivational intervention, that is, the PHS 5 R's.
  - Relate any evidence of tobacco-related disease during patient care to a quit message.
  - Note intervention in patient chart (intervention takes about 1 to 2 minutes).
- *Contemplation:* Willing to quit in the next 6 months, may be stuck in this stage for years, may have several previous failed quit attempts.
- The TCI measures are as follows:
  - Give pamphlet, briefly review pharmacotherapy option, provide information about state/federal quitlines (1-800-QUIT-NOW or www.smokefree .gov).
  - Offer future assistance when patient is ready.
  - Relate any evidence of tobacco-related disease during patient care.
  - Note intervention and stage in chart (takes about 1 to 2 minutes).
- *Preparation:* Willing to quit within the next month, ready to set a quit date.
- The TCI measures are as follows:

- Provide emotional support, and affirm benefits of not using tobacco stated by patient.
- Explore different options to aid the patient to quit.
- Explain pharmaceutical options; determine best fit.
- Refer patient to a tobacco quitline/online support.
- Provide printed resource materials (cessation workbook).
- Encourage development of a support system (family, friends).
- Help to set a quit date and note date in patient chart for future follow-up.
- Allow the patient to select the quit plan—write it out, copy the plan, and place it in the chart (takes approximately 20 minutes).
- *Action:* Has recently quit within the past 6 months.
- The TCI measures are as follows:
  - Provide emotional support, affirm benefits of not using tobacco stated by patient.
  - Review pharmaceuticals, if any, being used; support proper use.
  - Refer patient to a tobacco quitline/online support if patient has not accessed these resources.
  - Encourage use of the support system (family, friends).
  - Note quit date and patient's progress in chart.
  - Provide words of encouragement to continue (takes approximately 2 to 3 minutes).
- *Maintenance:* Has abstained for at least 6 months (relapse prevention).
- The TCI measures are as follows:
  - Provide verbal support; point out any positive oral-health effects.
  - Help patient develop strategies to prevent relapse (takes approximately 1 minute).

Advise

All tobacco users should be encouraged to quit—how the statement is posed can either create resistance or an opportunity for change. One approach may be an open-ended question such as "Today is a great day to quit. How do you feel about that?" as opposed to "You need to quit smoking." One approach opens the door for discussion; the other encourages a defensive response. Clearly, with a TCI, the stages model, 5 A's, and 5 R's blend together depending on the response of the patient. Knowing all aspects of an intervention provides the clinician with the understanding and tools to provide an appropriate service without alienating the tobacco user.

Assist

This concept has been covered under the action stage. Briefly, assist should include pharmacotherapy discussion, recommendation of over-the-counter nicotine replacement therapies, or writing of a prescription, referral to the phone quitline or online resources, preparation of a personalized quit plan, and provision of resource materials and self-help pamphlets.

Arrange

This concept involves the clinician "arranging" or providing follow-up on a TCI for a person who is ready to quit and has set a quit date. A simple follow-up letter, post card, or call has been shown to boost the success of a quit attempt.[79]

PHS's 5 R's

The 5 R's are used at the pre-contemplation or contemplation stage with the patient who is not ready to quit but has entered into some level of discussion. The use of motivational interviewing techniques can help avoid making the patient defensive when talking about the benefits of quitting. Offering unwanted information should be avoided, thus laying a basis of future discussions at recare appointments. The motivational messages of the 5 R's are as follows:

- *Relevance:*   Tailor specific health information (periodontal disease, stain, leukoplakia) to the patient's health status.
- *Risks:*   Explore if the patient knows and understands the health risks associated with tobacco use.
- *Rewards:*   Have the patient identify the benefits of quitting: improved health, better-tasting food,

saving money, fresher breath, and better-smelling clothing and hair.
- *Roadblocks:*   Have the patient identify possible barriers to quitting: withdrawal symptoms, fear of failure, depression, weight gain, lack of support, loss of friends.
- *Repetition:*   Use the 5 R's and motivational interviewing techniques each time a tobacco user receives dental treatment—keep the intervention short and focused. Actively listen to the patient; reflect his feelings, frustrations, and goals back to him. Allow the patient to choose a realistic quit plan that will work for him. Avoid "educating" the patient. Stress benefits of quitting.

An effective approach may be to say "Mrs. Jones, we have found evidence of moderate-to-severe periodontitis in your mouth, which may be a cause of your malodor. Periodontitis is a bacterial infection that your body has been unable to fight, most likely because of the toxins and carbon monoxide found in your tobacco smoke. Without a strong immune system, the ongoing bacterial infection will put you at an increased risk for losing your teeth—even with regular cleanings and good home care." The patient will need time to consider this information. Motivation to change often comes from very personal reasons and may not be related to the fear of cancer or lung disease. Effective TCI are a learned and practiced skill that must consider numerous issues, not to mention the time and office support needed to accomplish this essential service.

LEVELS OF A TCI

Over the last 20 years, numerous strategies have been presented to aid clinicians in consistently and effectively providing TCI. The PHS guideline suggests using a brief (a few minutes) or an intensive (20+ minutes) intervention, reporting that with all levels of intervention the success of a cessation attempt increases with more time spent.[79] The dental setting possibly offers clinicians more flexibility to offer varying levels of intervention.

Brief Intervention (1+ minute)

The American Dental Hygienists' Association has promoted the Smoking-Cessation Initiative by using the Ask, Advise, Refer System to encourage each patient who receives a tobacco intervention. The clinician is directed to ask about tobacco use, advise the patient to quit, and then give resource information, emphasizing the use of the state or federal quitline (1-800-QUIT-NOW or www.smokefree.gov). The advantage to this system is that it provides a clear plan of action for use in a limited period of time. An adaptation to this model may be asking and quickly assessing the patient's stage via the health history, then advising them to quit, and offering help when they are ready to quit. Quitline information and an informational pamphlet could then be placed in a bag with the toothbrush and paste. This is an effective TCI strategy, if the patient is not interested in setting a quit date and leaves open potential for continued discussion at future re-care appointments.

Moderate Intervention (5 to 10 minutes)

A moderate intervention may be necessary for those individuals who have thought about previous conversations with the clinician, want more information on medications and resources, want more detail on how tobacco is affecting them, and are interested in moving forward towards a future quit attempt. Cessation is a process, as is helping a patient quit. If trust and a sense of support are cultivated, the clinician will have numerous opportunities to offer the information and support that the patient is ready to hear. This process may cover several years before the patient is ready to set a quit date. Success is a successful quit, but success also encompasses the process of moving the patient towards that goal. Dental hygienists are well placed to spend the extra time needed during a re-care appointment while still staying on time.

Intensive Intervention (20+ minutes)

For those individuals who are ready to quit, need help creating a quit plan, or are highly addicted and have tried everything and failed, an intensive intervention may be indicated. The more time the provider spends with the patient, the more successful the quit attempt will be.[79] The intensive intervention should focus on past quit attempts, assessment of the patient's belief in being able to succeed, medications, barriers, establishing a support system, and a patient-developed quit plan. Few clinicians are able to create 20 minutes in an already tight schedule. Options to assist the patient may be to run over into the next appointment or to schedule another appointment for that specific purpose, even though dental insurance at this time does not cover that service. Another option is to refer the patient to a tobacco-counseling program or support group. There are several institutions now offering tobacco-dependence specialist certification. Dental health professionals may pursue this specialty to better serve the community and the patients in their practices.

ESTABLISHING A TCI PROGRAM

The dental office is composed of numerous individuals in different roles, with all members working together as a team to provide quality patient care. This principle is especially true for the integration of tobacco-cessation interventions.[123]

A successful TCI program consists of several basic components that need to be put in place: (1) acquiring information on local cessation resources from the local health department or hospital, and obtaining tobacco quitline numbers and no- or low-cost cessation pamphlets; (2) obtaining tobacco-cessation training/orientation for the office staff; (3) establishing a clear working relationship with the dentist concerning the level of TCI to be offered and how to recommend medications and determine the level of follow-up; and (4) maintaining and evaluating the effectiveness of the TCI program by reviewing patient's and staff's verbal reaction.

Step One

The collection of tobacco-cessation resources and services is very important when offering cessation interventions. The *ADA Guide to Dental Therapeutics*[124] and the PHS guideline *Treating Tobacco Use and Dependence*[79] are two important resources available to guide dental clinicians when recommending and/or prescribing pharmacotherapies.

Excellent sources for low- or no-cost tobacco-cessation materials include the local health department, the American Cancer Association, and the American Lung Association. The Centers for Disease Control and Prevention (CDC) also offers extensive educational and patient-cessation pamphlets, videos, and posters, which can be ordered at http://www.cdc.gov/tobacco.

Another important cessation resource is the tobacco quitline, which has been proven to be effective in helping tobacco users quit[125,126] and can be a time-saving tool for a busy office. Most state quitlines offer both reactive (the tobacco user calls the quitline) and proactive (the clinician faxes, with signed permission, a request for the quitline to call the tobacco user).

For example, (1) the hygienist provides a TCI; (2) the patient agrees to be contacted by the nicotine-dependence specialist from the state's quitline, and signs the form requesting the service and giving permission for the dental office to fax in the request; (3) the receptionist faxes the request; and (4) the patient is called several times by a trained specialist over the next several weeks. This service greatly enhances and expands the TCI provided by the dental staff.

In preparation for offering a TCI, the existing health history should be evaluated and revised to collect data on tobacco use, level of dependence, and readiness to quit. This review will save the clinician a substantial amount of time and greatly aid with assessment. Another component of a new service is the insurance code for reimbursement. Although there is an ADA code for tobacco cessation (D1320 – cdt/4, 2002), insurance does not cover cessation services at this time.

Step Two

As with anything new, starting or enhancing a TCI program must include the support and buy-in from all dental team members. Unfortunately, many providers still feel as though they lack the training or experience to provide cessation services. Dental team members are able to increase their sense of self-efficacy and clinical ability through the many excellent continuing education courses, in-services, journal articles, and self-instruction materials.[127–132]

Step Three

The scope of the office TCI protocol should be established before patients are offered cessation services. Patients are not served well if the dental hygienist provides an effective TCI during the re-care appointment, resulting in the patient being interested in quitting using bupropion, but the attending dentist discusses only the needed restorations, feeling uncomfortable prescribing an antidepressant (bupropion SR) for cessation. The roles and scope of services need to be established for each dental team member according to the following sample distribution of responsibilities:

- *Dentist:*   Diagnose, conduct TCI, and prescribe medications.
- *Dental hygienist:*   Perform comprehensive oral assessment, diagnose (depending on state statute),

conduct TCI, make referral, recommend OTC medications, make chart notations, and follow-up at re-care appointments.
- *Dental assistant:*   Provide resource materials and make chart notation of TCI.
- *Receptionist:*   Send referral/fax request to quitline, make formal follow-up, and schedule time for TCI.

As with any services, the TCI program should be evaluated for staff and patient acceptance as well as effectiveness. Staff meetings and patient comments as well as self-reports of quit attempts and successful quits can all aid in evaluation. This evaluation could be done informally or during staff meetings.

TOBACCO-PREVENTION STRATEGIES—IN-OFFICE AND COMMUNITY

Ideally, the most effective way to avoid tobacco-related disease and death is by preventing the use of tobacco in the first place. In the dental office/clinic, several positive steps can be taken to send a tobacco-free message such as, providing only magazines that do not contain tobacco advertising; posting a sign that invites patients to ask about smoking-cessation assistance; providing informational material on the benefits of quitting and quitlines in the waiting room; and asking youth (10 years and older) if they have tried any tobacco products, followed by support for their decision to not use them. All of these actions send a message that the dental staff is concerned about tobacco use and that help is available.

On a community, state, and federal level, dental professionals have many opportunities to become proactive in efforts to prevent tobacco use, as well as to eliminate public exposure to second-hand smoke. In the 2000 report of the Surgeon General, *Reducing Tobacco Use,*[70] the CDC identified four primary strategies that have been proven to reduce youth tobacco initiation and discontinuance of tobacco products.

1. Provide effective educational tobacco-prevention strategies for youth. School educational programs should emphasize refusal and decision-making strategies. Public health messages should include hard-hitting counter-advertising venues such as those found in the *TRUTH* campaign at http://www.thetruth.com.

2. Provide tobacco-cessation assistance adapted to the needs of youth.

3. Enact regulatory and policy measures restricting youth access to tobacco products and eliminate smoking in public spaces. These measures counter the generally held assumption that "smoking is OK because it is legal and everybody is doing it."

4. Raise taxes on tobacco products. This action restricts access by youth because of the high cost.

According to the Surgeon General's report, effective tobacco-prevention programs take a comprehensive approach, including those that contain policy, regulatory, educational, and cessation components. Clearly, this scope of action requires collaboration among many private, governmental, public health, and business entities. The CDC offers extensive resources including fact sheets, educational DVDs, posters, printed material, research articles, and links to organizations actively involved in tobacco prevention at http://www.cdc.gov/tobacco. Dental professionals are strategically positioned to provide not only one-on-one cessation interventions, but they can provide valuable professional input on a political and organizational level to work toward a tobacco-free society.

SUMMARY

Every dental patient who uses tobacco is at an increased risk for general and oral diseases including cardiovascular disease, oral cancer, and periodontitis. The complex behavioral and physiologic components of addiction make the process of assisting a tobacco user difficult but necessary. Understanding that tobacco interventions may need to be provided over an extended period of time with periods of relapse and remission should help the dental provider be emotionally prepared to avoid feelings of failure, if the patient refuses cessation information or relapses back to tobacco use. A successful quit rests with the patient, not with the clinician.

Fortunately, tobacco-cessation interventions by dental clinicians can and do make a difference. The combination of behavioral, pharmacotherapy, and follow-up has been shown to increase the tobacco user's ability to successfully quit from 3% to 5% on their own to 30% or more with clinician assistance. Dental health care professionals have the knowledge, opportunity, and ethical responsibility to offer an appropriate, patient-centered tobacco-cessation intervention as normal patient care.

REFERENCES

1. Centers for Disease Control and Prevention. (2005). Annual smoking-attributable mortality, years of potential life lost, and economic costs—United States: 1997–2001. *MMWR Morb Mortal Wkly Rep,* 54:626–28.

2. U.S. Department of Health and Human Services. (2004). *The health consequences of smoking—A report of the Surgeon General.* Rockville, MD: Public Health Service, Centers for Disease Control, Center for Health Promotion and Education, Office on Smoking and Health.

3. Centers for Disease Control and Prevention. (2006). Tobacco use among adults—United States, 2005. *MMWR Morb Mortal Wkly Rep,* 55:1145–48.

4. Thun, M. J., & Jemal, A. (2006). How much of the decrease in cancer death rates in the United States is attributable to reductions in tobacco smoking? *Tob Control,* 15:345–47.

5. U.S. Department of Health and Human Services. (2000). *Healthy People 2010.* Washington, DC: U.S. Government Printing Office. Retrieved 11/9/06, from http://www.healthypeople.gov/.

6. National Center for Health Statistics (2005). *Health, United States, 2005 with chartbook on trends in the health of Americans.* Hyattsville, MD: National Center for Health Statistics.

7. Centers for Disease Control and Prevention. (2006, June). Youth risk behavior surveillance—United States, 2005. *MMWR Morb Mortal Wkly Rep,* 55 (No. SS-5):1–108.

8. Centers for Disease Control and Prevention. (2006). Cigarette use among high school students—United States, 1991–2005. *MMWR Morb Mortal Wkly Rep,* 55:724–26.

9. Rigotti, N. A., Lee, J. E., & Weshler, H. (2000). U.S. college students' use of tobacco products. *JAMA,* 284:699–705.

10. U.S. Department of Health and Human Services. (2006). *The health consequences of involuntary exposure to tobacco smoke—A report of the Surgeon General.* Atlanta, GA: U.S. Department of Health and Human Services, Centers for Disease Control.

11. Mecklenburg, R. E., Greenspan, D., Kleinman, D. V., Manley, M. W., Niessen, L. C., Robertson, P. B., & Winn, D. E. (1996). *Tobacco effects in the mouth* (NIH Publication No. 96-3330). Bethesda, MD: U.S. Department of Health and Human Services, Public Health Service, National Institutes of Health.

12. Gelskey, S. C. (1999). Cigarette smoking and periodontitis: Methodology to assess the strength of evidence in support of a causal association. *Community Dent Oral Epidemiol,* 27(1):16–24.

13. American Cancer Society. (2006*). Cancer facts and figures 2006.* Atlanta, GA: American Cancer Society.

14. National Cancer Institute. (2006). *5-Year rate changes—Mortality United States, 1999–2003 all ages, both sexes,*

all races (incl. Hispanics). Bethesda, MD: U.S. Department of Health and Human Services, National Institutes of Health, National Cancer Institute. Retrieved 11/6/06, from http://statecancerprofiles.cancer.gov.

15. Blott, W. J., Mclaughlin, J. K., Winn, D. M., Austin, D. F., Greenberg, R. S., Preston-Martin, S., Berstein, L., Schoenberg, J. B., Stemhagen, A., & Fraumeni, J. R., Jr. (1988). Smoking and drinking in relation to oral and pharyngeal cancer. *Cancer Res,* 48:3282–87.

16. Danaei, G., Vander Hoorn, S., Lopez, A. D., Murray, C. J., & Ezzati, M. (2005). Causes of cancer in the world: Comparative risk assessment on nine behavioural and environmental risk factors. *Lancet,* 366:1784–93.

17. La Vecchia, C., Tavani, A., Franceshi, S., Levi, F., Corrao, G., & Negri, E. (1997). Epidemiology and prevention of oral cancer. *Oral Oncol,* 33:302–12.

18. Llewellyn, C. D., Linklater, K., Bell, J., Johnson, N. W., & Warnakulasuriya, K. A. (2002). Squamous-cell carcinoma of the oral cavity in patients aged 45 years and under: A descriptive analysis of 116 cases diagnosed in the South East of England from 1990–1997. *Oral Oncol,* 39:106–14.

19. Rodriguez, T., Altieri, A., Chatenoud, L., Gallus, S., Bosetti, C., Negri, E., Franceschi, S., Levi, F., Talamini, R., & La Vecchia, C. (2004). Risk factors for oral and pharyngeal cancer in young adults. *Oral Oncol,* 40:207–13.

20. Banoczy, J., Ginter, Z., & Dombi, C. (2001). Tobacco use and oral leukoplakia. *J Dent Educ,* 65(4):322–27.

21. Silverman, S., Gorsky, M., & Lozada, F. (1984). Oral leukoplakia and malignant transformation. *Cancer,* 53:563–68.

22. Department of Health and Human Services. (1986). *The health consequences of using smokeless tobacco* (NIH Publication No. 86-2874). Bethesda, MD: Department of Health and Human Services.

23. Bates, C., Fagerstrom, K., Jarvis, M., Kinze, M., McNeil, A., & Ramstrom, L. (2003). European Union policy on smokeless tobacco: A statement in favor of evidence-based regulation for public health. *Tob Control,* 12:360–67.

24. Accortt, N., Waterbor, J. W., Beall, C., & Howard, G. (2005). *Cancer Causes Control,* 16:1107–15.

25. Silverman, S. (2001). Demographics and occurrence of oral and pharyngeal cancers. *J Am Dent Assoc,* 132:7S–11S.

26. Burt, B. (2005). Epidemiology of periodontal diseases—Position paper. *J Periodontol,* 76:1406–19.

27. Borrell, L. N., Burt, B. A., & Taylor, G. W. (2005). Prevalence and trends in periodontitis in the USA: From the NHANES III to the NHANES, 1988–2000. *J Dent Res,* 84:924.

28. Tomar, S., & Asma, S. (2000). Smoking-attributable periodontitis in the United States: Findings from NHANES III. *J Periodontol,* 71:743–51.

29. Calsina, G., Ramon, J. M., & Echeverria, J. J. (2002). Effects of smoking on periodontal tissues. *J Clin Periodontol,* 29:771–76.

30. Bergstrom, J. (2003). Tobacco smoking and risk for periodontal disease. *J Clin Periodontol,* 30:107–13.

31. Jansson, L., & Lavstedt, S. (2002). Influence of smoking on marginal bone loss and tooth loss—A prospective study over 20 years. *J Clin Periodontol,* 29:750–56.

32. Bergstrom, J. (2003). Influence of tobacco smoking on periodontal bone height—Long-term observations and hypothesis. *J Clin Periodontol,* 31:260.

33. Krall, E. A., Garvey, A. J., & Carcia, R. I. (1999). Alveolar bone loss and tooth loss in male cigar and pipe smokers. *J Am Dent Assoc,* 130:57–64.

34. Kowolik, M. J., & Nisbet, T. (1983). Smoking and acute ulcerative gingivitis. *Br Dent J,* 154:241–42.

35. Krall, E. A., Abreau Sosa, C., Garcia, C., Nunn, M. E., Caplan, D. J., & Garcia, R. I. (2006). Cigarette smoking increases the risk of root canal treatment. *J Dent Res,* 85:313–37.

36. Schwartz-Arad, D., Samet, N., Samet, N., & Mamlider, A. (2002). Smoking and complications of endosseous dental implants. *J Periodontol,* 73:153–57.

37. Nociti, F. H., Neto, J. B. C., Carvalho, M. D., Sallum, E. A., & Sallum, A. W. (2002). Intermittent cigarette smoke inhalation may affect bone volume around titanium implants in rats. *J Periodontol,* 73:982–87.

38. Kinane, D. E., & Chestnutt, I. G. (2000). Smoking and periodontal disease. *Crit Rev Oral Biol Med,* 11(3):356–65.

39. Bergstrom, J., & Bostrom, L. (2001). Tobacco smoking and periodontal hemorrhagic responsiveness. *J Clin Periodontol,* 30:107–13.

40. Hanioka, T., Tanaka, M., Takaya, K., Matsumori, Y., & Shizukuishi, S. (2000). Pocket oxygen tension in smokers and non-smokers with periodontal disease. *J Periodontol,* 71:550–54.

41. Ryder, M. I., Saghizadeh, M., Ding, Y., Nguyen, N., & Soskoline, A. (2002). Effects of tobacco smoke on the secretion of interleukin-1β, tumor necrosis factor-α, and transforming growth factor β from peripheral blood mononuclear cells. *Oral Microbiol Immunol,* 17:331–36.

42. Giannopoulou, C., Cappuyns, I., & Mombelli, A. (2003). Effect of smoking on gingival crevicular fluid cytokine profile during experimental gingivitis. *J Clin Periodontol,* 30:996–1002.

43. Kamma, J. J., Giannopoulou, C., Vasdekis, V. G. S., & Mombelli, A. (2004). Cytokine profile in gingival crevicular fluid of aggressive periodontitis: Influence of smoking and stress. *J Clin Periodontol,* 31:894–902.

44. Mantyla, P., Stenman, M., Kinane, D., Salo, T., Suomalainen, K., Tikanoja, S., & Sorsa, T. (2006). Monitoring periodontal disease status in smokers and nonsmokers using a gingival crevicular fluid matrix metalloproteinase-8-specific chair-side test. *J Periodont Res,* 41:503–12.

45. Gamal, A. Y., & Bayomy, M. M. (2002). Effect of cigarette smoking on human PDL fibroblasts attachment to

periodontally involved root surfaces in vitro. *J Clin Periodontol,* 29:763–70.

46. Johnson, G. K., & Hill, M. (2004). Cigarette smoking and the periodontal patient. *J Periodontol,* 75:196–209.

47. Labriola, A., & Needleman, I. (2005). Systematic review of the effect of smoking on nonsurgical periodontal therapy. *Periodontology 2000,* 37:124–37.

48. Meinberg, T. A., Canarsky-Handley, A. M., McClenahan, A. K., Poulsen, D. D., Marx, D. B., & Reinhardt, R. A. (2001). Outcomes associated with supportive periodontal therapy in smokers and non-smokers. *J Dent Hygiene,* 75:15–19.

49. Morozumi, T., Kubota, T., Sato, T., Okuda, K., & Yoshie, H. (2004). Smoking cessation increases gingival blood flow and gingival crevicular fluid. *J Clin Periodontol,* 31:267–72.

50. Robertson, P. B., Walsh, M., Green, J., Ernster, V., Grady, D., & Hauch, W. (1990). Periodontal effects associated with the use of smokeless tobacco. *J Periodontol,* 61:438–43.

51. Sinusas, K., Coroso, J. G., Sopher, M. D., & Crabtree, B. F. (1992). Smokeless tobacco use and oral pathology in a professional baseball organization. *J Fam Pract,* 34:713–18.

52. Bergstrom, J., Keilani, H., Lundholm, C., & Radestad, U. (2006). Smokeless tobacco (snuff) use and periodontal bone loss. *J Clin Periodontol,* 33:549–54.

53. Fisher, M. A., Taylor, G. W., & Tilashalshi, K. R. (2005). Smokeless tobacco and severe active periodontal disease, NHANES III. *J Dent Res,* 84:705–10.

54. American Academy of Periodontology. (1999). Tobacco use and the periodontal patient. *J Periodontol,* 70:1419–27.

55. Centers for Disease Control and Prevention. (1994). Surveillance for selected tobacco-use behaviors—United States 1900–1994. *MMWR Morb Mortal Wkly Rep,* 43 (SS-3):23.

56. Green, C. R., & Rodgman, A. (1996). The Tobacco Chemists' Research Conference; a half-century of advances in analytical methodology of tobacco and its products. *Recent Adv Tob Sci,* 22:131–304.

57. Hoffmann, D., & Hoffmann, I. (1997). The changing cigarette, 1950–1995. *J Toxicol Environ Health,* 50:307–64.

58. National Cancer Institute, Smoking and Tobacco Control. (1998). *Cigars, health effects and trends* (monograph 9) (NIH Publication No. 98-4302). Bethesda, MD: U.S. Department of Health and Human Services, National Institutes of Health, National Cancer Institute, 73–97.

59. National Toxicology Program. (2000). *9th report on carcinogens* (11th ed.). Bethesda, MD: U.S. Department of Health and Human Sciences, National Institute of Environmental Health Sciences. Retrieved 11/21/06, from http://www.cdc.gov/tobacco/ETS_Toolkit/PublicPlaces/secondhand-smoke.

60. Arbes, S. J., Agustsdottir, H., & Slade, G. D. (2001). Environmental tobacco smoke and periodontal disease in the United States. *Am J Public Health,* 91:253–57.

61. National Cancer Institute, Smoking and Tobacco Control. (2002). *Risks associated with smoking cigarettes with low machine-measured yields of tar and nicotine* (monograph 13) (NIH Publication No. 02-5047). Bethesda, MD: U.S. Department of Health and Human Services, National Institutes of Health, National Cancer Institute, 13–63.

62. Centers for Disease Control and Prevention. (2005). Tobacco use, access, and exposure to tobacco in media among middle and high school students—United States, 2004. *MMWR Morb Mortal Wkly Rep,* 54:297–301.

63. Watson, C. H., Polzin, G. M., Calafat, A. M., & Ashley, D. L. (2003). Determination of the tar, nicotine, and carbon monoxide yields in the smoke of bidi cigarettes. *Nicotine Tob Res,* 5:747–53.

64. Malson, J. L., Lee, E. M., Murty, R., Moolchan, E. T., & Pickworth, W. B. (2003). Clove cigarette smoking: Biochemical, physiological, and subjective effects. *Pharmacol Biochem Behav,* 74:739–45.

65. Asorta, K. (2005). Hooked on hookah? What you don't know can kill you. Tobacco-Related Disease Research Program. University of California. *Burning Issues,* 7 (3):1–11.

66. Shihadeh, A., & Saleh, R. (2005). Polycyclic aromatic hydrocarbons, carbon monoxide, "tar," and nicotine in the mainstream smoke aerosol of the narghile water pipe. *Food Chem Toxicol,* 43:655–61.

67. U.S. Department of Health and Human Services. (1986). *The health consequences of using smokeless tobacco: A report of the Advisory Committee to the Surgeon General* (NIH Publication No. 86-2874). Bethesda, MD: U.S. Department of Health and Human Services, Public Health Service.

68. Hoffman, D., Djordjecic, M. V., Fran, J., Zang, E., Glynn, T., & Connolly, G. N. (1995). Five leading U.S. commercial brands of moist snuff in 1994: Assessment of carcinogenic N-nitrosamines. *J Natl Cancer Inst,* 87:1862–69.

69. Hoffman, D., & Djordjecic, M. V. (1997). Chemical composition and carcinogenicity of smokeless tobacco. *Adv Den Res,* 11:322–29.

70. U.S. Department of Health and Human Services. (2000). *Reducing tobacco use: A report of the Surgeon General.* Atlanta, GA: U.S. Department of Health and Human Services, Centers for Disease Control and Prevention.

71. Centers for Disease Control and Prevention. (1999). Nicotine, pH, and moisture of smokeless tobacco—Florida, January-February. *MMWR Morb Mortal Wkly Rep,* 48:398–401.

72. Going, R. E., Hsu, S. C., Pollack, R. L., & Haugh, L. D. (1980). Sugar and fluoride content of various forms of tobacco. *J Am Dent Assoc,* 100:27–33.

73. Tomar, S. L., & Winn, D. M. (1999). Chew-tobacco use and dental caries among U.S. men. *J Am Dent Assoc,* 130:1601–10.

74. Rubinstein, I., & Pedersen, G. W. (2002). Bacillus species are present in chewing tobacco sold in the United States

and evoke plasma exudation from the oral mucosa. *Clin Diag Lab Immunol,* 9:1057–60.

75. Bowles, W. H., Wilkinson, M. R., Wagner, M. J., & Woody, R. D. (1995). Abrasive particles in tobacco products: A possible factor in dental attrition. *J Am Dent Assoc,* 126:327–31.

76. National Cancer Institute, Centers for Disease Control and Prevention. (September, 2002). Smokeless tobacco fact sheets. Paper presented at the 3rd International Conference on Smokeless Tobacco, Stockholm Center of Public Health, Stockholm, Sweden.

77. International Agency for Research on Cancer (2004). Betel-quid and areca-nut chewing and some areca-nut-derived nitrosamines (Vol. 84). Available at: http://monographs .iarc.fr/ENG/Monographs/vol85/volume85.pdf.

78. Critchley, J. A., & Unal, B. (2003). Health effects associated with smokeless tobacco: A systemic review. *Thorax,* 58:435–43.

79. Fiore, M. C., Bailey, W. C., Cohen, S. J. (2000). *Treating tobacco use and dependence. Clinical practice guideline.* Rockville, MD: US Department of Health and Human Services. Public Health Services.

80. U.S. Department of Health and Human Services. (1988). *Nicotine addiction: The health consequences of smoking: A report of the Surgeon General.* Rockville, MD: Centers for Disease Control and Prevention, National Center for Chronic Disease Prevention and Health Promotion, Office on Smoking and Health.

81. Benowitz, N. L. (1996). Pharmacology of nicotine: Addiction and therapeutics. *Annu Rev Pharmacol Toxicol,* 36:597–613.

82. Benowitz, N. L. (1997). Systemic absorption and effects of nicotine from smokeless tobacco. *Adv Dent Res,* 11:336–40.

83. Perkins, K. A. (1993). Weight gain following smoking cessation. *J Consult Clin Psychol,* 61:768–77.

84. Benwell, M. E. M., Balfour, D. K. J., & Birrell, C. E. (1995). Desensitization of the nicotine-induced mesolimbic dopamine responses during constant infusion with nicotine. *Br J Pharmacol,* 114:454–60.

85. Groman, E., & Fagerstrom, K. (2003). Nicotine dependence: Development, mechanisms, individual differences, and links to possible neurophysiological correlates. *Wein Klim Wochenschr,* 115:155–60.

86. Dodgen, C. E. (2005). *Nicotine dependence: Understanding and applying the most effective treatment interventions.* Washington, DC: American Psychological Association.

87. Henningfield, J. E. (1990, January). Understanding nicotine addiction and physical withdrawal process. *J Am Dent Assoc,* 120, Supplement:2S–6S.

88. American Psychiatric Association. (2000). *Diagnostic criteria from diagnostic statistical manual of mental disorders* (4th ed.). Washington, DC: American Psychiatric Association.

89. Breslau, N., Johnson, E. O., Hiripi, E., & Kessler, R. (2001). Nicotine dependence in the United States. *Arch Gen Psychiatr,* 58:810–16.

90. Tong, E. K., Ong, M. K., Vittinghoff, E., & Perez-Stable, E. J. (2006). Non-daily smokers should be asked and advised to quit. *Am J Prev Med,* 30:23–30.

91. Munafo, M. R., Clark, T. G., Johnstone, E. C., Murphy, M. F. G., & Walton, R. T. (2004). The genetic basis for smoking behavior: A systemic review and meta-analysis. *Nicotine Tob Res,* 6:583–97.

92. Benowitz, N. L., Pomerleau, O. F., Pomerleau, C. S., & Jacob, P. III. (2003). Nicotine metabolite ratio as a predictor of cigarette consumption. *Nicotine Tob Res,* 5:621–24.

93. Bates, C., Jarvis, M., & Connolly, G. (1999). Tobacco additives; cigarette engineering and nicotine addition. London: Action on Smoking and Health (ASH). Retrieved 12/27/06, from http://www.ash.org.uk (ASH Daily News Pages, Product regulation and labelling, Tobacco additives).

94. Kotlyar, M., & Hatsukami, D. K. (2002). Managing nicotine addiction. *J Dent Educ,* 66:1061–73.

95. Centers for Disease Control and Prevention. (2002). Cigarette smoking among adults—United States, 2000. *MMWR Morb Mortal Wkly Rep,* 51:642–45.

96. Tomar, S. L., Husten, C. G., & Manley, M. W. (1996). Do dentists and physicians advise tobacco users to quit? *J Am Dent Assoc,* 127:259–65.

97. George, T. P., & O'Malley, S. S. (2004). Current pharmacological treatments for nicotine dependence. *Trends Pharm Sci,* 25:42–48.

98. Henningfield, J. E., Fant, R. V., Buckhalter, A. R., & Stitzer, M. L. (2005). Pharmacotherapy for nicotine dependence. *CA Cancer J Clin,* 55:281–99.

99. Silagy, C., Stead, L., & Fowler, G. (2006). Nicotine replacement therapy for smoking cessation. (Review). The Cochrane Library, Issue 4:1–109.

100. Cepeda-Benito, A., Reynoso, J. T., & Erath, S. (2004). Meta-analysis of the efficacy of nicotine-replacement therapy for smoking cessation: Differences between men and women. *J Consult Clin Pharm,* 72:712–22.

101. Shiffman, S., Rolf, C. N., Hellebusch, S. J., Gorsline, J., Gorodetzky, C. W., Chiang, Y. K., Schleusener, D. S., Di Marino, M. E. (2001). Real-world efficacy of prescription and over-the-counter nicotine-replacement therapy. *Addiction,* 97:505–16.

102. Pierce, J. P., & Gilpin, E. A. (2002). Impact of over-the-counter sales on effectiveness of pharmaceutical aids for smoking cessation. *J Am Med Assoc,* 288:1260–64.

103. Schneider, N. G., Olmstead, R. E., Franzon, M. A., & Lunell, E. (2001). The nicotine Inhaler; clinical pharmacokinetics and comparison with other nicotine treatments. *Clin Pharmacokinet,* 40:661–84.

104. Le Houezec, J. (2003). Role of nicotine pharmacokinetics in nicotine addiction and nicotine-replacement therapy: A review. *Int J Tuberc Lung Dis,* 7:811–19.

105. Garvey, A. J., Kinnunen, T., Nordstrom, B. L., Utman, C. H., Dohtery, K., Rosner, B., & Vokonas, P. S. (2000). Effects of nicotine gum dose by level of nicotine dependence. *Nicotine Tob Res,* 2:52–63.

106. Shiffman, S., Dresler, C. M., Hajek, P. Gilburt, S. J. A., Targett, D. A., & Strahs, K. R. (2002). Efficacy of a nicotine lozenge for smoking cessation. *Arch Intern Med,* 162:1267–76.

107. Shiffman, S., Gorsline, J., & Gorodetzky, C. W. (2001). Efficacy of the over-the-counter nicotine patch. *Nicotine Tobac Res,* 4:477–83.

108. Bittoun, R. (2006). A combination nicotine-replacement therapy (NRT) algorithm for hard-to-treat smokers. *J Smoking Cessation,* 1:3–6.

109. Heatherton, T. F., Kozlowski, L. T., Frecker, R. C., & Fagerstrom, K. (1991). The Fagerstrom test for nicotine dependence: A revision of the Fagerstrom tolerance questionnaire. *Br J Addict,* 86:1119–27.

110. Heatherton, T. F., Kozlowski, L. T., Frecker, R. C., Rickert, R. C., & Robinson, W. S. (1989). Measuring the heaviness of smoking using self-reported time to first cigarette of the day and the number of cigarettes smoked per day. *Br J Addict,* 84:791–800.

111. Ebbert, J. O., Patten, C. A., & Schroeder, D. R. (2006). The Fagerstrom test for nicotine dependence—smokeless tobacco (FTND-ST). *Addict Behav,* 31:1716–21.

112. Warner, C., & Shoaib, M. (2005). How does bupropion work as a smoking-cessation aid? *Addict Biol,* 10:219–31.

113. Hurt, R. D., Sachs, D. P., Glover, E. D., Offord, K. P., Johnston, J. A., Dale, L. C., Mahayrallah, M. A., Schroeder, D. R., Glover, P. N., Sullivan, C. R., Croghan, I. T., & Sullivan, P. M. (1997). A comparison of sustained-release bupropion and placebo for smoking cessation. *New Engl J Med,* 377:1195–202.

114. Faessel, H. M., Smith, B., Gibbs, M. A., Gobey, J. S., Clark, D. J., & Burstein, A. H. (2006). Single-dose pharmacokinetics of varenicline, a selective receptor partial agonist, in heavy smokers and nonsmokers. *J Clin Pharmacol,* 46:991–98.

115. Gonzales, D., Rennard, S. I., Nides, M., Oncken, C., Azoulay, S., Billing, C. B., Watsky, E. J., Gong, J., Williams, K. E., & Reeves, K. R. (2006). Varenicline, an α 4β2 nicotinic acetylcholine receptor partial agonist, vs. sustained-release bupropion and placebo for smoking cessation. *JAMA,* 296:47–55.

116. Tonstad, S., Tonnesen, P., & Hajek, P. (2006). Effect of maintenance therapy with varenicline on smoking cessation. *JAMA,* 296:64–71.

117. Gordon, J. A., Lichtenstein, E., Severson, H. H., & Andrews, J. A. (2006). Tobacco cessation in dental settings: Research findings and future directions. *Drug Alcohol Rev,* 25:27–37.

118. Dolan, T. A., McGorray, S. P., Grinstead-Skigen, C. L., & Mecklenburg, R. (1997). Tobacco-control activities in U.S. dental practices. *J Am Dent Assoc,* 128:1669–79.

119. Albert, D., Ward, A., Ahluwalia, K., & Sadowsky, D. (2002). Addressing tobacco in managed care: A survey of dentists' knowledge, attitudes, and behaviors. *Am J Public Health,* 92:997–1001.

120. Hu, S., Pallonen, U., McAllister, A. L., Howard, B., Kaminski, R., Stevenson, G., & Servos, T. (2006). Knowing how to help tobacco users; dentists' familiarity and compliance with the clinical practice guidelines. *J Am Dent Assoc,* 137:170–79.

121. Campbell, H. S., Sletten, M., & Petty, T. (1999). Patient perceptions of tobacco-cessation services in dental offices. *J Am Dent Assoc,* 130:219–26.

122. Solenberg, L. I., Boyle, R. G., Davidson, G., Magnan, S. J., & Link Carlson, C. (2001). Patient satisfaction and discussion of smoking cessation during clinical visits. *Mayo Clin Proc,* 78:138–43.

123. Warnakulasuriya, S. (2002). Effectiveness of tobacco counseling in the dental office. *J Dent Educ,* 66:1079–87.

124. Kosden, L. A., Ed. (2003). *ADA guide to dental therapeutics* (3rd ed.). Willard, OH: R.R. Donnelley & Sons, 587–99.

125. Borland, R., Segan, C. J., Livingston, P. M., & Owen, N. (2001). The effectiveness of callback counseling for smoking cessation: A randomized trial. *Addiction,* 96:881–89.

126. Bentz, C. J., Bayley, K. B., Bonin, K. E., Flemming, L., Hollis, J. F., & McAfee, T. (2006). The feasibility of connecting physician offices to a state-level tobacco quit line. *Am J Prev Med,* 30:31–37.

127. Severson, H. H., Andrews, J. A., Lichtenstein, E., Gordon, J. S., & Barckley, M. F. (1998). Using the hygiene visit to deliver a tobacco cessation program: Results of a randomized clinical trial. *J Am Dent Assoc,* 129:993–99.

128. Crews, K. M., Johnson, L., & Nichols, M. (1994). Patient management in a tobacco cessation program in the dental practice. *Compend Contin Educ Dent,* 15:1142–46.

129. Christen, A. G., Jay, S. J., & Christen, J. A. (2003). Tobacco cessation and nicotine replacement therapy for dental practice. *Gen Dent,* 51:525–32.

130. Johnson, N. W. (2004). The role of the dental team in tobacco cessation. *Eur J Dent Educ,* 8 (Suppl 4):18–24.

131. Stafne, E. E., & Bakdash, B. (2004). Tobacco cessation program: Resources to help organize a dental office program. *Northwest Dent,* 31–35.

132. Walsh, M. M, & Ellison, J. A. (2005). Treatment of tobacco use and dependence: The role of the dental professional. *J Dent Educ,* 69:521–37.

Chapter 19

Athletic Mouthguards

Christine N. Nathe

OBJECTIVES

After studying this chapter, the student should be able to:

1. Describe the preventive aspects of athletic mouthguards.
2. Describe the historical aspects of athletic mouthguards.
3. Describe the prevalence of sports-related orofacial and head trauma.
4. List the promotional activities advocating the use of mouthguards.
5. List the sports and activities that should involve the use of athletic mouthguards.
6. Describe the types of athletic mouthguards.
7. Describe the fabrication of custom-made vacuum-formed mouthguards.
8. Describe the dental provider's role in the use of athletic mouthguards.

KEY TERMS

Athletic mouthguard
Dental trauma
Concussions
Repeated mild brain injuries
Cerebral hemorrhages
Incidents of unconsciousness
Jaw fractures
Neck injuries
Condylar-displacement injuries
Study model
Prognathic

INTRODUCTION

Although many orofacial injuries can be prevented during participation in athletic activities, some individuals do not use athletic mouthguards. As a dental provider, it is necessary to promote the use of athletic mouthguards, educate the public on the value of mouth protection during contact sports, and fabricate mouthguards for athletes. In addition, dental providers should promote the use of mouthguards by implementing mouthguard programs in school sports and private athletic organizations.

An **athletic mouthguard** is a removable oral appliance that protects the hard and soft tissues of the oral cavity and brain during contact sports; the appliance is sometimes referred to as a "mouth protector." Mouthguards protect by absorbing energy during an impact, thus decreasing the likelihood of trauma to the oral cavity and brain.

Interestingly, 36% of all unintentional injuries to children and adults occur during sports activities.[1] This issue of prevention is significant considering that 20 million children aged 6 to 16 years are playing out-of-school sports and 25 million youths are participating in competitive sports.[2] Some postulate that coaches and trainers have not been favorably disposed to mouthguard use in organized sports programs.[3,4] These data underscore the need for the promotion of athletic mouthguards by dental providers.

HISTORICAL PERSPECTIVE

Historically, boxers became the first athletes on record to use mouthguards.[5] Marks constructed the first custom-fitted mouthguard in the early 1900s by fabricating a rubber strip that fit securely under the lip and over the outer surfaces of the teeth and gingiva.[6] Interestingly, boxers used to place other materials such as cotton and gutta-percha between lips and teeth for protection.[6]

In 1941 a study revealed that 25% of all football injuries reported among high-school players involved teeth, and in 1950 a study stated that dental injuries were the most common football injury reported by school sports programs.[7] Interestingly, a 1952 photograph of the Notre Dame football team, which appeared in *Life* magazine, visibly educated the public about the extent of orofacial injuries; the caption read "The Football Smile" (Figure 19–1 ■). This smile revealed many individuals with missing teeth and portrayed a natural

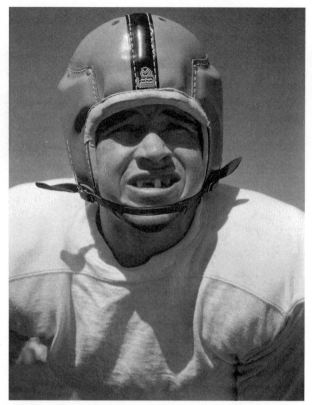

■ **FIGURE 19–1** The "football smile."
(Leonard McCombe/Time & Life Pictures/Getty Images)

correlation between the contact sport and orofacial trauma. However, after a letter was received from the President of Notre Dame, which indicated that at least one of the photographs was actually adjusted to make it look like a player was missing teeth (when he, in fact, had a full dentition), *Life* magazine ran a new photograph of the team. Evidently, it was a common perception that many individuals associated contact sports with dental injuries.

MOUTHGUARD USE

Recommendations have existed for the use of mouthguards dating back to the 1950s when the American Dental Association (ADA) became actively involved in promoting mouthguard use and in determining the extent of oral injuries in football.[8] Then, in 1962, the use of mouthguards was mandated in high school and junior college football by the National Alliance Football Rules Committee. By 1973 the National Collegiate Athletic Association (NCAA) followed suit. The Academy of Sports Dentistry was founded in 1983 to address the prevention of oral and facial injuries during athletic endeavors.[9] Then in the early 1990s, the NCAA expanded the mandated use of mouth protection to include additional sports.[10] The NCAA guidelines on mouthguards are listed in (Table 19–1 ■).

Although the majority of contact sports for youth, high-school, and college athletes mandate the use of mouthguards, there is still controversy over their use. In 2007, Massachusetts coaches complained that the mouthguards inhibited communication on the court and said they were unsanitary, because players would frequently drop them on the floor and have to put them back in their mouths. Subsequently, the Massachusetts Interscholastic Athletic Association voted to remove the mandatory use of the mouthguards.[11]

On the other side of the spectrum, the National Federation of High School Associations' Ice Hockey Rules Committee voted to eliminate a requirement for both boys and girls that a mouthguard be attached to a player's face mask. The committee noted that attached mouthguards make it easier for a player to let the guard dangle and believed their rule change would encourage more players to wear the mouthguards properly.[11]

On a professional level, the National Football League does not require the use of athletic mouthguards.[12] However, professional football players generally are seen on game day with mouthguards in place. In fact, one team from the National Hockey League recently collaborated with Delta Dental of Tennessee to kick off the "Protect Your Fangs" campaign by handing out mouthguards to local youth hockey players to encourage use of mouthguards to prevent injury and maintain oral health.[13]

CONTACT SPORT INJURIES

Many types of orofacial injuries exist, including **dental trauma,** which is injury to the mouth, including teeth, periodontium, soft tissues, and the temporomandibular joint. The U.S. surgeon general's report on oral health identified sporting activities as one of the major causes of craniofacial injuries.[14] Numerous studies have shown a link between athletic activities and dental injuries; furthermore, almost one in six sports-related injuries is to the craniofacial area.[1,14] In fact, approximately 50% of children will sustain traumatic dental injury during childhood.[15] The National Youth Sports Foundation for the Prevention of Athletic Injuries reported that dental injuries are the most common type of injury sustained during participation in sports.[16]

Chipped and avulsed incisor teeth are the most common sports-related orofacial injuries.[17] Mandibular fractures are the most common orofacial fracture, and 31% of all mandibular fractures are sports related; in contrast, 10% of all maxillofacial fractures are sports related.[17,18]

More than 300,000 people suffer traumatic brain injuries while playing sports, most of which are **concussions.**[19] What an athlete experiences during a concussion is actually a temporary trauma-induced alteration in mental status.[20] Many concussions occur without the individual ever losing consciousness, but researchers have determined that **repeated mild brain injuries** occurring over an extended period result in cumulative neurologic and cognitive deficits.[20] In fact, a research study suggests that over 90% of brain concussions resulting in unconsciousness to athletes are a result of a blow or trauma to the jaw.[21]

■ **Table 19–1**   NCAA Guidelines for Mouthguards

1. Properly fitted mouthguards could reduce the potential chipping of tooth enamel surfaces and reduce fractures of teeth, roots, and bones.
2. Properly fitted mouthguards could protect the lip and cheek tissues from being impacted and lacerated against tooth edges.
3. Properly fitted mouthguards could reduce the incidence of fractured jaw caused by a blow delivered to the chin or head.
4. Properly fitted mouthguards could provide protection to toothless spaces; therefore, support is given to the missing dentition of the student athlete.

Source: NCAA Guideline 4C for Mouth Guards. January 1986. Revised August 1999.

MOUTHGUARD PROTECTION AND PREVENTION

Studies have repeatedly revealed the protective value of mouthguards in reducing sports-related injuries to the teeth and soft tissues.[22–24] Mouthguards work by moving soft tissue in the oral cavity away from the teeth and into the upper jaw, preventing laceration and bruising of the lips and cheeks, especially for those individuals who wear orthodontic appliances. In addition, mouthguards act as a simple protectant to the teeth by preventing chipping, fracturing, displacement, and avulsion.

Moreover, the dynamic properties of the mouthguard help absorb the energy associated with the blow the athlete receives. Mouthguards prevent concussions, **cerebral hemorrhages, incidents of unconsciousness, jaw fractures,** and **neck injuries** by helping to avoid situations in which the mandible gets jammed into the maxilla.[25,26] Mouthguards work by providing cushioning between the maxilla and mandible, and by lessening the severity of **condylar-displacement injuries,** which subsequently reduce concussions, as illustrated in (Figure 19–2 ■).

Interestingly, although the majority of studies support the protective value of mouthguards, the Centers for Disease Control and Prevention found insufficient evidence to issue a community-wide recommendation on the effectiveness of mouthguards as a preventive intervention and identified the need for more "high-quality research on their effectiveness."[27]

The ADA has promoted the use of properly fitted mouthguards as the primary means to protect against oral injuries during sports.[28] (Table 19–2 ■) lists activities that require the use of a mouthguard. In particular, some sports are more likely to involve contact that could lead to sports injuries. For that reason, the American Academy of Pediatrics has classified sports according to the degree of contact (Table 19–3 ■). In addition, the American Academy of Pediatric Dentistry recommends the use of properly fitted mouthguards in organized sports.[29] Furthermore, the American Association of Orthodontics and the American Association of Oral and Maxillofacial Surgeons promote April as National Facial Protection Month.[14] The American Dental Hygienists Association supports mandating the use of mouth and head protection for participants during sports activities that involve risk of dental and/or craniofacial injuries.[30]

Interdisciplinary advocacy of mouthguard use was revealed in one study in which 93% of NCAA-certified

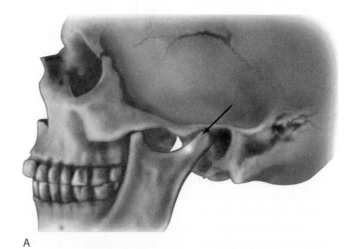

A

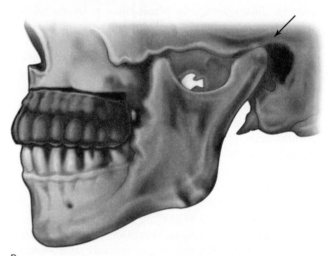

B

■ **FIGURE 19–2** **A.** Note head of condyle and base of the skull without a properly fitted mouthguard. **B.** Note separation in space between the head of the condyle to the base of the skull with a properly fitted mouthguard in place.

athletic trainers reported that athletic mouthguards play a role in prevention.[31] Studies suggest that athletic mouthguards improve the performance of the athletes, by increasing concentration of their efforts on the execution of their sport.[32–34]

Most athletes believe that mouthguards prevent injuries; however, some athletes may not want to wear a mouthguard because they believe that they may not be able to breathe as easily.[35] One study evaluated the oxygen consumption during exercise of athletes wearing mouthguards compared with those not wearing

■ **Table 19–2** *Activities Requiring a Mouthguard*

- Acrobatics
- Basketball
- Bicycling
- Boxing
- Equestrian events
- Extreme sports
- Field events
- Field hockey
- Football
- Gymnastics
- Handball
- Ice hockey
- Inline skating
- Lacrosse
- Martial arts
- Racquetball
- Rugby
- Shot put
- Skateboarding
- Skiing
- Skydiving
- Soccer
- Softball
- Squash
- Surfing
- Volleyball
- Water polo
- Weight lifting
- Wrestling

Source: American Dental Association. (2004). The importance of using mouthguards. *J Am Dent Assoc.* Vol. 135. No. 7. P.1061. Additional information is available at http://www.ada.org.

mouthguards; investigators found no difference in oxygen consumption between the two groups.[36]

TYPES OF MOUTHGUARDS

Three types of mouthguards are commonly available to the athlete: the stock, mouth-formed, and custom-made mouthguard (Table 19–4 ■). The role of any type of mouthguard is to provide protection and prevent orofacial injuries. Although there are inherent differences in types of mouthguards, the mouth-formed mouthguards are used most frequently (90%), but custom-made mouthguards (10%) are most effective at preventing injury.[6]

A stock mouthguard is available in different sizes. It is not custom-made and is not preferred because of the poor fit and excess bulk. Many times athletes will "chew" on this type to make it fit better; athletes also tend to be less compliant with this type of mouthguard because of its fit (Figure 19–3A ■ and B).

A mouth-formed guard, which is generally referred to as a "boil-n-bite" style, can be heated in water and then placed in the mouth. The athlete bites into the guard and an inexact fit is produced. This type of mouthguard can become distorted and does not accommodate an individual athlete's unique oral features. Boil-n-bite mouthguards are the most widely used type (Figure 19–4A ■ and B).

Although there is limited research on the most-effective mouthguard, most dental organizations promote the use of the custom-made mouthguard (Figure 19–5 ■). One study reported no statistical difference between football players wearing boil-n-bite versus custom-made mouthguards in preventing concussions,[24] but another study suggested that custom-made mouthguards were significantly more protective in preventing head and oral injuries than boil-n-bite mouthguards.[37]

In a study comparing the two different types of custom-made mouthguards, it was reported that patients preferred the custom-made, double-layered, heat-and-pressure mouthguard to the custom-made, vacuum-formed mouthguard.[38] Furthermore, Winters suggested that custom-made laminated mouthguards do not break down with use, players do not tend to abuse or alter them, and this type of mouthguard increases separation of teeth, which is desirable to reduce concussions.[39]

Currently, there are two methods of fabricating custom-made mouthguards: vacuum formed and pressure laminated. These types of mouthguard are custom-fabricated and fit precisely on the individual athlete's dentition. Because they are more comfortable and fit better, compliance is increased; therefore, the custom-made mouthguard is more effective at reducing injuries. Both types can be fabricated in the dental office or sent to a laboratory for fabrication. Many dental laboratories fabricate pressure-laminated mouthguards and use the sports team colors on the mouthguard to match the uniforms. Pressure-laminated mouthguards, compared with other mouthguards, seem to maintain minimal and consistent thicknesses in critical areas better. The thicker materials (3–4 mm) are more effective in absorbing impact energy, and the thinner materials show marked deformation at the site of impact.[9] In addition, this type of mouthguard does not need to be replaced unless the athlete has orthodontics or mixed dentition. If cost is an issue, a boil-n-bite mouthguard is recommended.

■ **Table 19–3** American Academy of Pediatrics Classification of Sports

Classification of Sports by Contact		
Contact or Collision	**Limited Contact**	**Noncontact**
Basketball	Baseball	Archery
Boxing*	Bicycling	Badminton
Diving	Cheerleading	Body building
Field hockey	Canoeing or kayaking (white water)	Bowling
Football	Fencing	Canoeing or kayaking (flat water)
Tackle	Field events	Crew or rowing
Ice hockey[†]	High jump	Curling
Lacrosse	Pole vault	Dancing[§]
Martial arts	Floor hockey	Field events
Rodeo	Football	Discus
Rugby	Flag	Javelin
Ski jumping	Gymnastics	Shot put
Soccer	Handball	Golf
Team handball	Horseback riding	Orienteering[||]
Water polo	Racquetball	Power lifting
Wrestling	Skating	Race walking
	Skiing	Riflery
	Cross-country	Rope jumping
	Downhill	Running
	Water	Sailing
	Skateboarding	Scuba diving
	Snowboarding[‡]	Swimming
	Softball	Table tennis
	Squash	Tennis
	Ultimate frisbee	Track
	Volleyball	Weight lifting
	Windsurfing or surfing	

*Participation not recommended by the American Academy of Pediatrics.

[†]The American Academy of Pediatrics recommends limiting the amount of body checking allowed for hockey players 15 years and younger to reduce injuries.[2]

[‡]Snowboarding has been added since previous statement was published.[1]

[§]Dancing has been further classified into ballet, modern, and jazz since previous statement was published.[1]

[||]A race (contest) in which competitors use a map and compass to find their way through unfamiliar territory.

Source: Policy Statement: Medical Conditions Affecting Sports Participation: Committee on Sports Medicine and Fitness. Reproduced with permission from *Pediatrics* Vol. 107 No. 5 May 2001, pp. 1205–1209 by the American Academy of Pediatrics.

FABRICATION OF THE CUSTOM-MADE, VACUUM-FORMED MOUTHGUARD

Although boil-n-bite mouthguards are fabricated easily by placing in hot water and biting into the mouthpiece to leave an "impression," they are not as accurate and do not fit as well as custom-made mouthguards. Custom mouthguards may be fabricated by a dental provider and should fit precisely over the dentition. Fabrication of a mouthguard involves the following general steps:

- Take an alginate impression of the maxillary arch, making sure that the gingival margins and complete anatomy of the arch are impressed. Take care to accurately reproduce the anatomy.

■ **Table 19–4** Types of Mouthguards

Type	Definition
Stock mouthguard	Available in different sizes. Not custom-made. Patients are generally not compliant about wearing this type because of its poor fit and excessive bulk.
Boil-n-bite	A mouth-formed mouthguard. It is heated in water and placed in the mouth. An inexact fit is produced. Many young athletes use this type of mouthguard.
Custom-made mouthguard	A custom-fabricated mouthguard that is made on a study model with the use of a vacuum-forming machine. Can be made in the office or sent to a laboratory. Alginate impression is taken in the dental office. Compliance is increased with this type of mouthguard. This type of mouthguard is the most expensive.

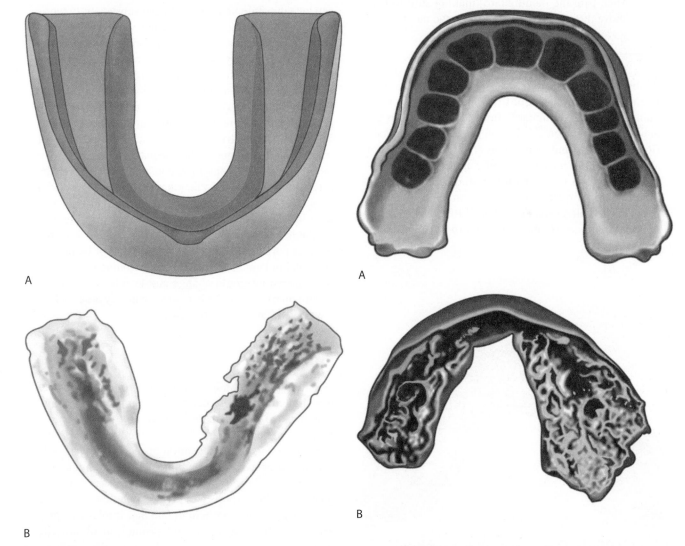

A

A

B

B

■ **FIGURE 19–3** **A.** Stock mouthguard. **B.** Stock mouthguard after several weeks of use.

■ **FIGURE 19–4** **A.** Mouth-formed mouthguard. **B.** Mouth-formed mouthguard after it has been chewed by athlete.

- Pour the dental stone into the accurate alginate impression to form a **study model.** After the model has cooled, spray it with a silicone spray to prevent the thermoplastic mouthguard material from sticking to the model.
- Place the thermoplastic mouthguard material in the frame of the vacuum-forming machine and heat the material. When the material has heated and slumped, lower the frame onto the model and start the machine. Stop the suction after 20 to 30 seconds. Allow the thermoplastic mouthguard material to cool.
- Remove the mouthguard material from the model. Then trim the mouthguard, making sure to trim above the gingival margin to help the mouthguard stay in place during the athletic event.

There are a few special considerations when fabricating athletic mouthguards for certain individuals. If an athlete has a **prognathic** (forward projecting) mandible, the mouthguard should be formed on the mandibular dentition.[40,41] Dental providers should fabricate maxillary and mandibular arch mouthguards for athletes with full fixed orthodontic appliances. [40,41] Silicone putty can be used on the study model during mouthguard fabrication and placed on the orthodontic band area to help prevent undercut.[41] Removable orthodontic appliances should not be worn during athletic events.

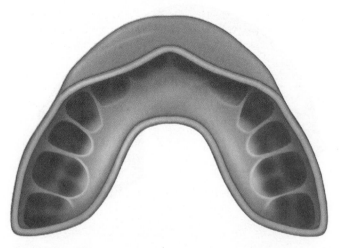

■ **FIGURE 19–5** Custom-made athletic mouthguard.

DENTAL PROVIDER'S ROLE IN MOUTHGUARD USE

Dental providers have the responsibility to educate patients and parents about the necessity of wearing a mouthguard in active sporting events and recreation. Many times, dental hygienists develop unique and close relationships with patients and have the opportunity to promote healthy behaviors frequently and consistently. During conversation with a patient about hobbies and interests is a great time to promote prevention of dental trauma and traumatic brain injury via the use of a mouthguard.

During the dental appointment, the dental provider can take the alginate impression and subsequently fabricate the mouthguard in the office with the use of a vacuum-forming machine. Alternatively, dental providers could send the study model to a laboratory if fabrication is completed off-site. If a boil-n-bite mouthguard is requested by the patient, the dental provider can make recommendations of the size and type, and help the patient locate a store with mouthguards in stock.

The dental hygienist has the responsibility of instructing the patient on the adequate maintenance of a mouthguard. The dental hygienist should suggest the rinsing and brushing of a mouthguard after each use with a soft-bristled, wet toothbrush. Some mouthguards come with brushes. Professional cleaning solutions are also available and specific directions are available with the product purchased. Mouthguards should not be held in hot water or kept in unusually hot environments, because the dimensions could change and lead to distortion.[42] Mouthguards should be kept in a clean, dry area such as a well-ventilated protective case.

SUMMARY

Dental hygienists should be able to promote the use of mouthguards and instruct patients on proper care and maintenance. Mouthguards are used for the prevention of oral trauma and brain injury during recreational and sporting events. The prevention of these traumas could lead to a lifetime of good oral health. Dental hygienists have the responsibility of promoting the use of mouthguards in school sports and private athletic events. The dental hygienists can help create and implement programs for the education and promotion of athletic mouthguards.

REFERENCES

1. Bijur, P. E., Trumbel, A., Harel, Y., Overpeck, M. D., Jones, D., & Scheidt, P. C. (1995). Sports and recreation injuries in US children and adolescents. *Arch Pediatr Adolesc Med,* 149:1009–16.

2. National Youth Sports Foundation. (1994). Fact sheet. Needham, MA: National Youth Sports Foundation.

3. Berg, R., Berkey, D. B., Tang, J. M., Altman, D. S., & Londeree, K. A. (1998). Knowledge and attitudes of Arizona high school coaches regarding oro-facial injuries and mouthguard use among athletes. *J Am Dent Assoc,* 129:1425–35.

4. Kvittem, B., & Roettger, M. (1998). Prospective epidemiological study of oro-facial injuries in high school sports. *J Pub Health Dent,* 58:288–93.

5. (1973). Boxing. In *World Book Encyclopedia* (Vol. 2). Chicago: Field Enterprises Educational Corporation.

6. Mouthguards: history. *Sports Dentistry on Web.* Retrieved 9/13/07 from http://www.sportsdentistry.info/mouthguards.html.

7. Historical backgrounder: Mouthguard development. *Shock Doctor.* Retrieved 7/21/06 from http://www.shockdoc.comm/new/mgHistory.html.

8. Fogan, C. B. (1963). Mouth protection for football players. *J Am Dent Assoc,* 66:3354–55.

9. Academy of Sports Dentistry: About the organization. Retrieved 9/10/07 from http://www.sportsdentistry.org.

10. Kleyman, M. & Vigil, A. (1996, Fall). Use of mouthguards: Review of the literature. *Discloser,* 4–8.

11. Bulletin Board: High school adjusts sports-medicine rules. Retrieved 9/25/07 from http://www.training-conditioning.com.

12. *1999 Official Playing Rules of the National Football League.* Tarrytown, NY: Triumph Books.

13. National Hockey League. (2007, August 29). Predators and Delta Dental launch "Protect Your Fangs." Retrieved 9/25/07 from http://predators.nhl.com/team/app/?service=page&page=NewsPage&articleid=336433.

14. U.S. Department of Health and Human Services. (2000). *Oral health in America: A report of the Surgeon General—Executive summary.* Rockville, MD: U.S. Department of Health and Human Services, National Institute of Dental and Craniofacial Research, National Institutes of Health.

15. Andreasen, J. O. & Andreasen, F. M. (1994). *Textbook and color atlas of traumatic injuries to the teeth* (3rd ed.). St. Louis: Mosby.

16. National Youth Sports Foundation for the Prevention of Athletic Injuries, Inc. Retrieved on 3/24/08 from http://www.sportsdentistry.com/sportsdentistry.html.

17. Emshoff, R., Shoning, H., Rothler, G. Waldhart, E. (1997). Trends in incidence and cause of sports related mandibular fractures. A retrospective analysis. *J Oral Maxillofac Surg,* 55:585–92.

18. Tanaka, N., Hayashi, S., Amagasa, T., & Kohama, G. (1996). Maxillofacial fractures sustained during sports. *J Oral Maxillofac Surg,* 54:715–19.

19. Tyler, J. H., & Nelson, M. E., (2000, May 1). Second Impact Syndrome: Sports Confront Consequenses of Concussions. *USA Today* (magazine).

20. Common Injuries. Maxxgard Custom Fit Laminated Mouthguards. Retrieved on 9/13/07 from http://maxxgard.com/commoninjuries.htm.

21. Stewart, S., & Witzig, J. (1998). New findings of the importance of athletic mouthguards. *VIHJS Newsletter,* 7.

22. Newsome, P. R., Tran, D. C., & Cooke, M. S. (2001). The role of the mouthguard in the prevention of sports-related dental injuries: A review. *Int J Paediatr Dent,* 11:396–404.

23. Onyeaso, C. O. (2004). Secondary school athletes: A study of mouthguards. *J Natl Med Assoc,* 96:240–45.

24. Wisniewski, J. F., Guskiewicz, K., Trope, M., & Sigurdsson, A. (2004). Incidence of cerebral concussions associated with type of mouthguard used in college football. *Dent Traumatol,* 20:143–49.

25. Ranalli, D. (2002). Sports dentistry and dental traumatology. *Dent Traumatol,* 18:231–36.

26. Common Injuries. Maxxgard Custom Fit Laminated Mouthguards. Retrieved on 7/12/06 from http://www.maxxgard.com/commoninjuries.htm.

27. Centers for Disease Control and Prevention. (2001). Promoting oral health: Interventions for preventing dental caries, oral and pharyngeal cancers, and sports-related craniofacial injuries—A report on recommendations of the task force on community preventive services. *MMWR Recomm Rep,* 50(RR-21):1–13.

28. American Dental Association Report. (2006). Using mouthguards to reduce the incidence and severity of sports-related oral injuries. *J Am Dent Assoc,* 37:1712–20.

29. American Academy of Pediatric Dentistry. Policy on prevention of sports-related orofacial injuries. Retrieved 3/23/08 from http://www.aapd.org/pdf/sports.pdf.

30. American Dental Hygienists' Association. (2007). *American Dental Hygienists' Association policy manual, public health policy 7-04.* Chicago: American Dental Hygienists' Association.

31. Hawn, K. L., Visser, M. F., & Sexton, P. J. (2002). Enforcement of mouthguard use and athlete compliance in national collegiate athletic association men's collegiate ice hockey competition. *J Athlet Train,* 37:204–208.

32. Stenger, J. M. (1977). Physiologic Dentistry with Notre Dame athletes. *Basal Facts* 2:8–18.

33. Smith, S. D. (1978). Muscular strength correlated to jaw posture and the temporomandibular joint. *NY State Dental J* 44(7):279–82.

34. Garabee, W. F. (1981). Craniomandibular orthopedics and athletic performance in the long distance runner: A three year study. *Basal Facts* 4(3):77–79.

35. The Academy of Sports Dentistry. (2006). Position statements for properly fitted mouthguard, on athletic mouthguard mandates, and on sports dentistry in the dental school curriculum. Retrieved 3/23/08 from http://www.sportsdentistry-asd.org/position_statement.asp#3.

36. Kececi, A. D., Çetin C., Eroglu E., & Baydar M. L. (2005). Do custom-made mouthguards have negative effects on aerobic performance capacity of athletes? *Dent Traumatol,* 21:276–80.

37. Finch, C., Braham, R., McIntosh, A., McCrory, P., & Wolfe, R. (2005). Should football players wear custom fitted mouthguards? Results from a group randomized controlled trial. *Inj Prev,* 1:242–46.

38. Kenyon, B. J., & Loos, L. G. (2005). Comparing comfort and wearability between Type III single-layered and double-layered EVA mouthguards. *Gen Dent,* 53:261–64.

39. Winters, J. E. (2001, July/September). Role of properly fitted mouthguards in prevention of sport-related concussion. (Commentary). *J Athl Train,* 36:339–41.

40. Johnson, D. C., & Jackson, E. W. (1991). Prevention of intraoral trauma in sports. *Dent Clin North Am,* 35:657–66.

41. Chapman, P. J. (1989). Mouthguards and the role of sporting team dentists. *Aust Dent J,* 34:36–43.

42. Gladwin, M., & Bagby, M. (2009). *Clinical aspects of dental materials* (3rd ed.). Philadelphia: Lippincott Williams & Wilkins. 231.

Chapter 20

Technological Advances in Primary Dental Care

Vicki Gianopoulos

OBJECTIVES

After studying this chapter, the student should be able to:

1. Describe the current status and future of immunizations in oral health care.
2. Describe genetic evolution in oral health care.
3. Describe the current status and future of gene therapy in oral health care.
4. Describe the current status and future of stem cell use in oral health.

KEY TERMS

Immunizations
Immunity
Specific immunity
Passive immunity
Naturally acquired passive immunity
Artificially acquired passive immunity
Active immunity
Naturally acquired active immunity
Artificially acquired active immunity
Human genome project (HGP)
DNA
Genome
Chromosomes
Genes
Proteins
Proteome
Gene polymorphisms
Stem cells

INTRODUCTION

During the past century, society has benefited from tremendous advances in the primary dental sciences, from community water fluoridation to the use of dental sealants in the pit-and-fissure surfaces of teeth, to the utilization of dental hygienists. The proliferation of information technology and the use of computers in dental care delivery will continue to impact the evolution of oral health science and practice (Table 20–1 ■). Dental providers must be equipped to study new innovations and treatment modalities; they also must strive to prevent diseases at their earliest stages. Current technological advances in the science of dental hygiene include the use of stem cells, immunizations, gene therapy, and genetics (Table 20–2 ■).

IMMUNIZATIONS IN ORAL HEALTH

In 1777, a Gloucestershire milkmaid told her physician, Dr. Edward Jenner, that contracting cowpox had been a fortunate event because it conferred protection against smallpox! This bit of folk wisdom led Jenner to research the possibility of preventing smallpox, resulting in the advent of vaccinations. The incentives and rewards for questioning disease and health and, subsequently, for conducting clinical research were never clearer.[1] Since the first live vaccine was introduced by Edward Jenner, live vaccines have been used against a number of viral infections including polio, measles, mumps, rubella, chicken pox, hepatitis A, yellow fever, influenza, and so forth.[2]

■ **Table 20–1**   Primary Preventive Modalities

   I. Toothbrushing
     A. Manual held
     B. Mechanical toothbrush
  II. Dentifrices/Toothpastes
 III. Interdental Adjuncts
     A. Dental floss
     B. Interdental brushes
     C. Wooden interdental cleaners
  IV. Irrigation
   V. Mouthrinses
  VI. Fluoride
 VII. Dental Sealants
VIII. Professional Dental Hygiene Treatment

■ **Table 20–2**   Technological Advances in Primary Preventive Dental Care

   I. Immunizations: Refer to Table 20–3
  II. Genetics and Their Role in Disease
 III. Gene Therapy: Refer to Table 20–4
 IV. Stem Cell Use

Providing specific protection against the most common and damaging pathogens is accomplished by immunizations. Basically, **immunizations** work to prevent diseases from occurring by inducing immunity. **Immunity** means that the body has biological defenses needed to avoid infection or disease.

Specific immunity can be acquired by either passive or active immunization; both modes of immunization can occur by natural or artificial means.[3] Immune cells from an immunized individual may be used to transfer immunity, which is termed **specific immunity. Passive immunity** can be acquired without the immune system being challenged with an antigen. Passive immunity may be acquired naturally or artificially by transfer of serum or gamma-globulins from an immune donor to a nonimmune individual. **Naturally acquired passive immunity** occurs when immunity is transferred from mother to fetus through placental transfer of immunoglobulin G (IgG) or colostral transfer of IgA.[3] **Artificially acquired passive immunity** is often artificially transferred by injection with gamma-globulins from other individuals or gamma-globulin from an immune animal. Passive transfer of immunity with immune globulins or gamma-globulins is practiced in numerous acute situations of infections (diphtheria, tetanus, measles, rabies, etc.) and poisoning (insects, reptiles, botulism), and as a prophylactic measure (hypogammaglobulinemia). In these situations, gamma-globulins of human origin are preferable, although specific antibodies raised in other species are effective and used in some cases (poisoning, diphtheria, tetanus, gas gangrene, botulism).[3]

Active immunity refers to immunity produced by the body following exposure to antigens. **Naturally acquired active immunity** occurs through exposure to different pathogens, which leads to subclinical or clinical infections that result in a protective immune response against these pathogens. In contrast, **artificially acquired active immunity** may be achieved by administering live or dead pathogens or their components. Vaccines used for active immunization consist of live, attenuated, organisms;

killed whole organisms; microbial components; or secreted toxins that have been detoxified[3] (Table 20–3 ■).

Dental Caries

Dental caries is a chronic, infectious disease that may cause severe pain without dental intervention and may result in tooth loss. Worldwide, 5 billion people suffer from tooth decay, and dental cavities affect 60% to 90% of U.S. school children and most adults. In the United States, dental caries remain the most common childhood diseases, five times more common than asthma.[4] How is this disease treated? Use of fluoride in its many forms, use of sugarless products (such as xylitol), sealants, and increased access to dental care are among the approaches that have had a significant impact on the amount of dental disease of the young and economically advantaged. Many of these approaches can be broadly effective. However, economic, behavioral, or cultural barriers to their use have continued the epidemic of dental disease in many populations. Could there be a solution to this disease? There are now studies on vaccinations for the prevention of carious lesions.

Dental caries is a disease caused by a group of organisms called *Streptococcus mutans* (*S. mutans*) and occurs in 3 phases:[5] The first phase involves the initial attachment of the microorganism to the tooth or dental pellicle. This is mediated by an adhesion from *S. mutans* that is known as antigen I/II.[6] The second phase is the accumulation of the bacteria in a biofilm and the production of glucose and glucans by the bacterial enzyme glucosyl transferase (GTFs). The third phase occurs when the multiplication of these bacteria, known as dental plaques, are present with sugars, including sucrose and glucose. This combination produces large amounts of lactic acid, causing enamel dissolution and carious lesion formation.[5] Although other oral microorganisms can be cariogenic, mutans streptococci have unique biochemical features that make them efficient at accumulating and producing carious surfaces; therefore, they are good targets for therapies aimed at the prevention of dental caries. The characteristics that make mutans streptococci particularly efficient at causing dental caries include production of large amounts of lactic acid at a rapid rate and tolerance to extremes of sugar concentration, ionic strength, and pH.[7]

The principle of immunization against dental caries was first introduced by W. H. Bowen who showed that monkeys that were immunized intravenously with *S. mutans* developed little carious disease.[8] Later, studies were done on rats that were immunized subcutaneously in the vicinity of the salivary glands with mutans streptococci, which lead to reductions in the number of mutans streptococci and the extent of dental caries.

In the past decade, several small clinical trials of active immunization with mutans streptococcal antigens have been carried out. Clinical trials have shown increased amounts of salivary secretory IgA specific for the mutans streptococcal antigen that was used for vaccination. In a clinical trial, the vaccine group members were immunized orally with GTF in capsules, and showed substantially reduced reaccumulation of indigenous mutans streptococci for up to 42 days following tooth cleaning and vaccination. Similar delayed reaccumulation was observed after topical application of GTF to the buccal mucosa, which contains minor salivary

■ **Table 20–3** Types of Immunity

Immunity Type	Definition
Specific Immunity	Immunity against a specific antigen or disease
Passive Immunity	Immunity acquired by the transfer of antibodies from another individual, as through injection or placental transfer to a fetus
Naturally Acquired Immunity	Immunity obtained either from the development of antibodies in response to exposure to an antigen, as from vaccination or an attack of an infectious disease, or from the transmission of antibodies, as from mother to fetus through the placenta or the injection of antiserum
Artificially Acquired Immunity	Immunity obtained either from the development of antibodies in response to exposure to an antigen, as from vaccination or an attack of an infectious disease, or from the transmission of antibodies, as from mother to fetus through the placenta or the injection of antiserum

glands and their ducts. In addition, when antigen, either in soluble form or incorporated in liposomes, was administered intranasally or by topical application to the tonsils, the production of antigen-specific salivary IgA was induced. The duration effects on mutans streptococci were short in the young adult populations that were studied. This indicates that immunizations of this population would not affect the accumulation of bacteria on a long-term basis (greater than 42 days).[9] Therefore adults are not the appropriate target population for this vaccine.

Passive-immunization techniques have been studied for dental caries as well. This uses transfer of milk antibody specific for whole mutans streptococci from mother to suckling infant. This has been investigated in animal models and has shown to be protective against dental caries.[5] However, it seems unlikely that this strategy would have significant impact, at least in Western societies, where breast-feeding, if given, usually terminates well before the 'window of infectivity' for mutans streptococci opens.[10]

Although clinical trials have mostly been carried out in young adults (ages 18–23) this is not the target population of choice, primarily because young adults are already infected with mutans streptococci (mainly *S. mutans*). Infants represent the primary target population for caries vaccine. Immunization when infants are about one year old may establish effective immunity against colonization attempts by mutans streptococci.[6, 11]

An ideal vaccine to alleviate dental caries should consist of an antigen that is involved in the molecular pathogenesis of dental caries, should be administered by a route that will reproducibly elicit mucosal antibodies, and should occur when infants are immunocompetent with respect to salivary IgA production and before infection with mutans streptococci occurs.[6] If these features are met, vaccines may be well suited for public health applications, especially in environments that do not lend themselves to regular health care.

Periodontal Diseases

Periodontitis is an oral chronic inflammatory condition that may result in tooth loss attributable to bone and tissue destruction. This disease is associated with pathogenic gram-negative bacteria; *Porphyromonas gingivalis* has been implicated as an important etiologic agent of adult periodontitis.[12,13]

To learn how immunization works, one must have a basic understanding of the method for progression of periodontal disease. It is recognized that the adherence of bacteria to host tissues is a prerequisite for colonization and an important factor in bacterial pathogenesis. An approach to protecting against periodontal diseases is to develop a passive immunization system that blocks two colonization factors of *P. gingivalis* cells involved in its attachment to human host tissues.

One of the colonization factors is the co-aggregation factor, which plays a role in the colonization of *P. gingivalis* in the subgingival area through aggregation with other oral bacteria.[14] *Porphyromonas gingivalis* has the capability of adhering to the surfaces of several gram-positive bacteria such as *Actinomyces viscosus* and streptococci. Therefore, inter-bacterial adherence appears to be an essential step in colonization by *P. gingivalis*. It is well recognized that accumulation of bacteria on the tooth surface follows a sequence, beginning with gram-positive facultative species and shifting over time to gram-negative facultative and anaerobic species. In the earliest stages of dental plaque formation, *P. gingivalis* vesicles aggregate gram-positive bacteria such as *Actinomyces naeslundii,* which was formally named *A. viscosus;* these gram-positive bacteria are also regarded as potential pathogens in periodontal diseases.[15]

Another property of co-aggregation factor is its relationship to pathogenicity, as evidenced by more abscesses being formed by co-aggregates of two strains than those caused by infection with a pure suspension of each microorganism. Furthermore, co-aggregated cells were also more resistant to phagocytosis and killing by neutrophils in vitro and in vivo.[16]

Colonization of *P. gingivalis* at subgingival sites is critical in the pathogenic process of periodontal disease and tissue destruction. Bacterial co-aggregation factors and hemagglutinins likely play major roles in colonization in the subgingival area. Emerging evidence suggests that inhibition of these virulent factors may protect the host against caries and periodontal disease. Recent advances in mucosal immunology and the introduction of novel strategies for inducing mucosal immune responses now raise the possibility that effective and safe vaccines can be constructed. In tests of these vaccines, some successful results were reported in animal experimental models.[16]

No vaccine is absolutely safe, and there is always risk when providing medical intervention in a healthy individual to alleviate future disease. Those who are opposed to immunizations for oral health conditions argue that a vaccination is not justifiable for a condition that is not life threatening. In the future, if dental caries and periodontal disease immunizations prove to have benefits that outweigh risks, this may be the needed solution of prevention to much disease.

GENETICS

Completed in 2003, the **Human Genome Project (HGP)** was a 13-year project coordinated by the U.S. Department of Energy and the National Institutes of Health (Table 20–4 ■). During the early years of the HGP, the Wellcome Trust (U.K.) became a major partner; additional contributions came from Japan, France, Germany, China, and others. Researchers also studied the genetic makeup of several nonhuman organisms, including the common human gut bacterium *Escherichia coli,* the fruit fly, and the laboratory mouse.[17]

An understanding of basic genetics language is needed to discuss the importance of genetics in dentistry. Cells are the fundamental working units of every living system. All the instructions needed to direct their activities are contained within the chemical **DNA** (deoxyribonucleic acid).[17]

DNA from all organisms is made up of the same chemical and physical components. The DNA sequence is the particular side-by-side arrangement of bases along the DNA strand (e.g., ATTCCGGA). This order spells out the exact instructions required to create a particular organism with its own unique traits. The **genome** is an organism's complete set of DNA (Figure 20–1 ■). Genomes vary widely in size: The smallest known genome for a free-living organism (a bacterium) contains about 600,000 DNA base pairs, whereas human and mouse genomes have some 3 billion. Except for mature

■ **Table 20–4**   Human Genome Project Goals and Completion Dates

Area	HGP Goal	Standard Achieved	Date Achieved
Genetic Map	2- to 5-cM resolution map (600–1,500 markers)	1-cM resolution map (3,000 markers)	September 1994
Physical Map	30,000 STSs	52,000 STSs	October 1998
DNA Sequence	95% of gene-containing part of human sequence finished to 99.99% accuracy	99% of gene-containing part of human sequence finished to 99.99% accuracy	April 2003
Capacity and Cost of Finished Sequence	Sequence 500 Mb/year at < $0.25 per finished base	Sequence >1,400 Mb/year at <$0.09 per finished base	November 2002
Human Sequence Variation	100,000 mapped human SNPs	3.7 million mapped human SNPs	February 2003
Gene Identification	Full-length human cDNAs	15,000 full-length human cDNAs	March 2003
Model Organisms	Complete genome sequences of *E. coli, S. cerevisiae, C. elegans, D. melanogaster*	Finished genome sequences of *E. coli, S. cerevisiae, C. elegans, D. melanogaster,* plus whole-genome drafts of several others, including *C. briggsae, D. pseudoobscura,* mouse and rat	April 2003
Functional Analysis	Develop genomic-scale technologies	High-throughput oligonucleotide synthesis	1994
		DNA microarrays	1996
		Eukaryotic, whole-genome knockouts (yeast)	1999
		Scale-up of two-hybrid system for protein-protein interaction	2002

Source: Science 300, 286 (2003) 10.1126/science.1084564. U.S. Genome Project.

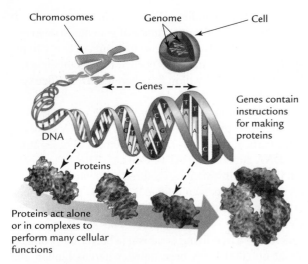

Chromosomes

Genome

Cell

Genes

DNA

Genes contain instructions for making proteins

Proteins

Proteins act alone or in complexes to perform many cellular functions

■ **FIGURE 20–1** Diagram of a Gene. (U.S. Genome Project).

red blood cells, all human cells contain a complete genome.[17]

DNA in the human genome is arranged into 24 distinct **chromosomes**—physically separate molecules that range in length from about 50 million to 250 million base pairs. A few types of major chromosomal abnormalities, including missing or extra copies or gross breaks and rejoinings (translocations), can be detected by microscopic examination. Most changes in DNA, however, are more subtle and require a closer analysis of the DNA molecule to find perhaps single-base differences.[17]

Each chromosome contains many genes, the basic physical and functional units of heredity. **Genes** are specific sequences of bases that encode instructions on how to make proteins. Genes comprise only about 2% of the human genome; the remainder consists of noncoding regions, whose functions may include providing chromosomal structural integrity and regulating where, when, and in what quantity proteins are made. The human genome is estimated to contain 20,000 to 25,000 genes.[17]

Although genes receive a lot of attention, the proteins perform most life functions and even make up the majority of cellular structures. **Proteins** are large, complex molecules made up of smaller subunits called amino acids. Chemical properties that distinguish the 20 different amino acids cause the protein chains to fold up into specific three-dimensional structures that define their particular functions in the cell. The constellation of all proteins in a cell is called its **proteome.** Unlike the relatively unchanging genome, the dynamic proteome

changes from minute to minute in response to tens of thousands of intra- and extracellular environmental signals. A protein's chemistry and behavior are specified by the gene sequence, and by the number and identities of other proteins made in the same cell at the same time and with which the protein associates and reacts[17]

In 1995, the potential impact of gene therapy on dentistry was published; this finding was based on initial studies of gene transfer applications to salivary glands, keratinocytes, and cancer cells.[18] It is now evident that a genetic basis exists for most diseases including periodontal disease and dental caries.[18] In the past 6 years, remarkable progress has been made in the field of gene therapy, including seven areas relevant to dental practice: bone repair, salivary glands, autoimmune disease, pain, DNA vaccinations, keratinocytes, and cancer.[19] Decoding the genome completely depicts the molecular structure, and explains how genes build, maintain, and control all of the biological functions.[19]

Dental Caries

There has been convincing evidence for a number of years that host genetic factors contribute to an individual's susceptibility or resistance to dental caries. This study confirms this evidence and provides additional support for the concept that dental caries is a complex disorder with both environmental and genetic components.[20] This finding has important implications for the practice of dentistry, because it demonstrates that there are additional risk factors for dental caries beyond those that have been traditionally understood. In practice, this finding means that the history of caries in siblings or parents should be evaluated as well as the dietary and oral hygiene behaviors of the individual. It should also be recognized that a genetic susceptibility to caries does not imply that disease is unavoidable, but rather that more intensive preventive interventions are required and that intervention should be started as early as possible.[20]

Periodontal Diseases

Genetic factors that influence an individual's risk for periodontal disease work similarly to environmental factors. The majority of genetic factors are also associated with an exaggerated inflammatory response to periodontal infection. A major genetic factor includes an individual's production of a proinflammatory cytokine interleukin-1B (IL-1B), which is associated with tissue destruction. Interleukin-1B is produced by many cell types, but especially by monocytes in diseased patients.[21] Understanding the human genome and which genes are associated with exaggerated inflammatory response may help dental professionals with the prevention and control of periodontal disease.

In general an individual's genetic background influences his or her susceptibility to many kinds of disease and conditions, including periodontitis. Familial aggregation of a trait or disease can suggest a genetic etiology. However, families also share many aspects of a common environment, including diet, nutrition, and behaviors such as smoking. In addition, certain infectious agents may cluster in families. Thus, familial aggregation may result from shared genes, environmental exposures, and similar socioeconomic influences.[22]

Many aspects of an individual's immune system are inherited and can contribute to a genetic susceptibility to periodontitis.[22] Genetic factors influence inflammatory and immune responses, and periodontitis is largely the result of an exaggerated inflammatory response.

Several studies have investigated genetic polymorphisms for cytokines as potential genetic markers for periodontitis. **Gene polymorphisms,** locations within the genome that vary in sequence between individuals, are very prevalent, affecting at least 1% of the population. The most common form of polymorphism is the single-nucleotide polymorphism, which is a change in a single base pair in the genomic DNA. The rationale for studying single-nucleotide polymorphisms is that they can be used to identify potential markers of susceptibility, severity, and clinical outcome. The results are suggesting that individuals carrying the positive genotype have significantly greater risk for developing periodontitis.[23]

The scientific literature during the decade has seen an increase in the number of reports claiming links for genetic polymorphisms with a variety of medical diseases, particularly chronic immune and inflammatory conditions. However, when studying periodontal diseases the literature reveals that, despite major advances in the awareness of genetic risk factors for periodontal disease (with the exception of periodontitis associated with certain monogenetic conditions), research has not determined a genetic basis for aggressive or chronic periodontitis.[24] Periodontitis is a complex, multifactorial disease and the susceptibility is genetically determined. There is no strong evidence for target genes and gene polymorphisms that play a key role in the susceptibility to and severity of periodontitis. Therefore genetic testing for periodontitis is currently not indicated.[25]

GENE THERAPY

Gene therapy is the insertion of normal DNA directly into cells to correct a genetic defect;[26] the treatment of disease by replacing, altering, or supplementing a gene that is absent or abnormal and whose absence or abnormality is responsible for a disease.[26] Since the advent of gene therapy in dentistry, significant progress has been made to control periodontal disease and reconstruct the dentoalveolar apparatus. However, to date, gene therapy methods have not been developed to control periodontal disease because of its multifactorial origin, complex genetic predisposition, and associated risk.[27]

STEM CELLS IN ORAL HEALTH

Stem cells have the remarkable potential to develop into many different cell types in the body. Serving as a sort of repair system for the body, they can theoretically divide without limit to replenish other cells as long as the person or animal is still alive. When a stem cell divides, each new cell has the potential to either remain a stem cell or become another type of cell with a more specialized function, such as a muscle cell, a red blood cell, or a brain cell.[28] Stem cells have been the subject of heated ethical debates by those opposed to the use of human embryos for study. A new study has revealed a way to turn ordinary human skin cells into what appear to be embryonic stem cells without ever using a human embryo.[29]

Sharks of all species continually shed their teeth and regenerate new teeth, in some cases with up to 50,000 in one lifetime.[30] Humans on the other hand are not as fortunate and frequently rely on the tertiary preventive services of dental providers to replace their teeth with implants or dental prosthetics. Many individuals with missing teeth are faced with the decision of replacing them with implants, bridges, or dental prosthetics. Regeneration of a functional and living tooth is a promising therapeutic strategy for the replacement of a diseased or damaged tooth. Although dental implant therapies have achieved long-term success in the clinic for the recovery of tooth function, the implants require preexisting, high-quality bone structures to support the implants. Regeneration of teeth in individuals without adequate bone support would be a major dental advance.

In 2000, scientists of the National Institute of Health discovered stem cells inside primary teeth. Dr. Shi took a lost primary tooth from his daughter, extracted the pulp and cultured it. Amazingly, some of the tooth cells started to grow.[31]

Recent advances in dental stem cell biotechnology and cell-mediated murine (or rodent) tooth regeneration have encouraged researchers to explore the potential for regenerating living teeth with appropriate functional properties.[32] Murine teeth can be regenerated with the use of many different stem cells to collaboratively form dental structures in vivo. In addition, dentin and pulp tissue and cementum–periodontal complex have been regenerated by human dental pulp stem cells and periodontal ligament stem cells, respectively, when transplanted into immunocompromised mice.[32] However, because of the complexity of human tooth growth and development, the regeneration of a whole tooth structure including enamel, dentin–pulp complex, and periodontal tissues as a functional entity in humans is a promising challenge.[33]

The spatially and temporally organized microenvironment of the tooth bud and its surrounding tissues permits growth and development of the crown and roots, resulting in formation and eruption of the tooth. Root development involves dentin formation, cementum generation, instruction of epithelium, and tooth eruption. From a clinical perspective, the most important part of the tooth is the root, which supports a natural or artificial crown. The crown alone cannot fulfill normal tooth function without a viable root. In contrast, the wide use of synthetic crowns to replace damaged natural crowns has been widely applied in dental clinics with excellent therapeutic outcomes.

Stem cell–mediated root regeneration offers opportunities to regenerate a bio-root and its associated periodontal tissues, which are necessary for maintaining the physiological function of teeth.[34] This cell study reported that tooth regeneration is possible. A new population of stem cells were isolated from the root apical papilla of human teeth (extracted third molars from volunteers ages 18–20 years).[34] Human apical papilla and periodontal ligament stem cells were transplanted to generate a root–periodontal complex capable of supporting a porcelain crown, resulting in normal tooth function.[34] This work integrates a stem cell–mediated strategy for tissue regeneration, engineered materials for structure, and current dental crown technologies. This hybridized tissue-engineering approach led to recovery of tooth strength and appearance.

SUMMARY

Many modalities are used to strive to prevent dental disease; however, many more modalities are being studied. Understanding more about the genetic makeup of an individual will lend information that can help dental providers to understand inherent risk factors and determine the best type of treatment for patients. The information encoded in a patient's genes may be invaluable in treating the patient through prevention of the initiation and the progression of disease. Although the genetic linkage to periodontal disease and the testing for it holds promise, it is more accurate to consider an individual's environmental and genetic factors in an assessment of risk for this disease.

Gene therapy can aid in altering the genetic makeup so that it will be more conducive to health. Research into stem cells will aid in treating diseases and may enhance the practice of tertiary prevention. Finally, immunizations can serve as primary prevention in individuals to prevent diseases from occurring. It is incumbent upon providers to keep up to date in the science of primary dental care, so they can deliver optimum care.

REFERENCES

1. Berg, A. O., Gordon, M. J., and Cherkin, D. C. (1986). Practice-Based Research in Family Medicine. Kansas City: American Academy of Family Physicians.
2. Riedel, S. (2005, 18 January). "Edward Jenner and the History of Smallpox and Vaccination." *Baylor University Medical Center Proceedings.*
3. Ghaffar, A. (2002). Immunization. MBIM 650/720 Medical Microbiology, Lecture 14, University of South Carolina, pp. 2–4.
4. "Dental Vaccine Could Help Billions." (2006, 25 May). *United Press International.* Retrieved May 6, 2008 from http://www.upi.com.
5. (2003, 28 January). "Panel on Caries Vaccine." *National Institute for Dental and Craniofacial Research.*
6. Nash, D. A., & Taubman, M. A. (2006). "The Scientific and Public Health imperative for a vaccine against dental caries." *Science and Society,* 6:255–63.
7. Hamada, S. & Slade, H. D. (1980). Biology, immunology, and cariogenicity to *Streptococcus mutans. Microbiol. Rev.,* 44:331–384.
8. Bowen, W. H. A. (1969). Vaccine against dental caries. A pilot experiment in monkeys (*Macaca irus*). *Br. Dent. J.,* 126, 159–66.
9. Smith, D. J. & Tuabman, M. A. (1987). Oral immunization of humans with *Streptococcus sobrinus* glucosyltransferase. *Infect. Immun.,* 55:2562–69.
10. Russell, M. W., Childers, N. K., Michalek, S. M., Smith, D. J., & Taubman, M. A. (2004). "A Caries Vaccine?" *Caries Research,* 38:230–235.
11. Hajishengallis, G., & Michalek, S. M. (1999). "Caries Vaccine," *Health Mantra,* 1–6.
12. Roberts, F. A., Houston, L. S., Lukehart, S. A., Mancl, L. A., Persson, R. G., & Page, R. C. (2004 February).

"Periodontitis Vaccine Decreases Local Prostaglandin E2 levels in Primate Model," *Infection and Immunity,* 72(2):1166–68.

13. Decarlo, A., Huang, Y., Collyer, A., Langley, D., & Katz, J. (2003 January) "Feasibility of an HA2 Domain-Based Periodontitis Vaccine," *Infection and Immunity,* 71(1): 562–66.

14. Booth, V., Ashley, P., & Lehner, T. (1996 Feb) "Passive Immunization with Monoclonal Antibodies against *Porphyromonas gingivalis* in Patients with Periodontitis," 422–27.

15. Persson, R. G., (2005 October) "Immune Responses and Vaccination against Periodontal Infections." *Journal of Clinical Periodontology,* (32):39–53.

16. Abiko, Y., (2000). "Passive Immunization against Dental Caries and Periodontal Disease: Development of Recombinant and Human Monoclonal Antibodies," *Critical Review in Oral Biology Medicine,* 11(2):140–58.

17. Collins, F. S., Morgan, M., & Patrinos, A. (2003). The Human Genome Project: Lessons from large-scale biology. *Science,* 300:286–90.

18. Baum, B. J., Kok, M., Tran, S. D., & Yamano, S. (2002). The impact of gene therapy on dentistry: A revisiting after six years. *J Am Dent Assoc,* 133:35–44.

19. Yeager, A. L. (2001). Where will the genome lead us? Dentistry in the 21st century. *J Am Dent Assoc,* 132:801–807.

20. Shuler, C. F. (2001). Inherited risks for susceptibility to dental caries. *J Dent Educ,* 65:1038–45.

21. Research, Science and Therapy Committee (2005). Implications of genetic technology for the management of periodontal diseases. *J Periodontol,* 76:850–57.

22. Hodge, P., & Michalowicz, B. (2000). Genetic predisposition to periodontitis in children and young adults. *Periodontology,* 26:113–34.

23. Takashiba, S., & Naruishi, K. (2006). Gene polymorphisms in periodontal health and disease. *Periodontology,* 40:94–106.

24. Kinane, D. F., & Hart, T. C. (2003). Genes and gene polymorphisms associated with periodontal disease. *Critical Reviews in Oral Biology & Medicine,* 14:430–49.

25. Loos, B. G., van der Velden, U., & Laine, M. L. Genetics and periodontitis. *Ned Tijdschr Tandheelkd.* 2008 Feb;115(2):87–92.

26. What Is Gene Therapy? Genetic Home Reference. U.S. National Library of Medicine. Retrieved on May 9, 2008 from http://ghr.nlm.nih.gov/handbook/therapy/genetherapy.

27. Karthikeyan, B. V., & Pradeep, A. R. (2006 Jul 1). Gene therapy in periodontics: A review and future implications. *J Contemp Dent Pract.* 7(3):83–91.

28. Murray, P. E., & Garcia-Godoy, F. (2004). Stem Cells and Development. 13(13):255–62. doi:10.1089/154732804323099181.

29. University of Wisconsin-Madison (2007, November 21). Scientists Guide Human Skin Cells to Embryonic State. *Science Daily.* Retrieved May 9, 2008, from http://www.sciencedaily.com/releases/2007/11/071120092709.htm.

30. Sharks of the Island. Nova online. Retrieved on September 12, 2006 from http://www.pbs.org/wgbh/nova/sharks/world/clickablesans.html.

31. NIH/National Institute of Dental and Craniofacial Research (2003, April 22). Scientists Discover Unique Source of Postnatal Stem Cells in 'Baby' Teeth. *Science Daily.* Retrieved May 9, 2008, from http://www.sciencedaily.com/releases/2003/04/030422075224.htm.

32. Nakara, T., & Yoshiaki, I. D. E. (2007). Tooth regeneration: Implications for the use of bioengineered organs in the first-wave organ replacement. *Human Cell* 20:63–70.

33. Chai Y., & Slavkin H. C. Apr 1, 2003. Prospects for tooth regeneration in the 21st century: A perspective. *Microsc Res Tech.* 60(5):469–79.

34. Sonoyama, W., Liu, Y., Fang, D., Yamaza, T., Seo, B., Zhang C., Liu H., Gronthos, S., Wang, C. Y., Shi, S., & Wang, S. (2006). Mesenchymal Stem Cell-Mediated Functional Tooth Regeneration in Swine. *PloS ONE* 1(1): e79. doi:10.1371/journal.pone.0000079.

Chapter 21

Public Health Programs

Scott L. Tomar

OBJECTIVES

After studying this chapter, the student should be able to:

1. Define public health science and practice.
2. Describe public health approaches.
3. Describe public health activities.
4. Describe dental public health organization and infrastructure.
5. Describe dental health education and promotion programs.

KEY TERMS

Public health
Assessment
Policy development
Assurance
Dental public health
Efficacy
Effectiveness
World Health Organization (WHO)
Pan American Health Organization (PAHO)
World Dental Federation (FDI)
International Federation of Dental
   Hygienists (IFDH)
U.S. Department of Health and Human
   Services (USDHHS)
Administration for Children and Families (ACF)
Health Resources and Services
   Administration (HRSA)
Agency for Healthcare Research
   and Quality (AHRQ)
Centers for Disease Control
   and Prevention (CDC)
Agency for Toxic Substances and Disease
   Registry (ATSDR)
Substance Abuse and Mental Health Services
   Administration (SAMHSA)

KEY TERMS (CONTINUED)
Administration on Aging (AoA)
Food and Drug Administration (FDA)
Centers for Medicare and Medicaid
  Services (CMS)
Indian Health Service (IHS)
National Institutes of Health (NIH)
Office of the Surgeon General
U.S. Public Health Service Commissioned Corps
American Association of Public Health
  Dentistry (AAPHD)
Oral Health Section

American Public Health Association (APHA).
Association of State and Territorial Dental
  Directors (ASTDD).
National Health Interview Survey
Medical Expenditure Panel Survey
Behavioral Risk Factor Surveillance
  System (BRFSS)
National Oral Health Surveillance
  System (NOHSS)
National Governors Association (NGA)
Assurance activities
Health education

INTRODUCTION

Public health is an essential component of developed societies. Many of the major improvements in the health of the American people are the result of public health measures such as ensuring safe food and water, controlling epidemics, and protecting workers from injury. Most people, however, do not give much thought to the public health system until there is a crisis or the system fails. Infectious disease outbreaks, cancer clusters, and the inability of uninsured working people to find affordable health care services are examples of events that draw attention to the infrastructure that protects the health of the public.

PUBLIC HEALTH DEFINED

The Institute of Medicine, in its landmark 1988 report *The Future of Public Health,* defined **public health** as "what we, as a society, do collectively to assure the conditions in which people can be healthy."[1] That 1988 report focused primarily on ways to strengthen the performance of federal, state, and local governmental public health agencies. Recognizing that government alone cannot adequately ensure the public's health, a subsequent Institute of Medicine report, *The Future of the Public's Health in the 21st Century,* expanded the focus to include other sectors of society that are essential partners in the public health system.[2] Those sectors include communities, the health care delivery system, employers and business, the media, and academia.

As former U.S. Surgeon General C. Everett Koop once stated, "Health care is vital to all of us some of the time, but public health is vital to all of us all of the time." Although services such as "safety net" clinics for communities that lack other access to direct health care often fall within the scope of public health agencies, public health is much broader than that. Public health uses organized, interdisciplinary efforts to address the physical, mental, and environmental health concerns of communities and populations. A large part of the mission of public health is achieved through the application of health promotion and disease-prevention technologies and interventions.

The Institute of Medicine identified three core functions that were to be conducted by government public health agencies: assessment, policy development, and assurance.[1]

Assessment involves monitoring of the health of communities and populations at risk to identify health problems and priorities. It includes activities such as public health surveillance, collecting and interpreting data, case finding, and evaluating outcomes of programs and policies.

Policy development is the process by which society makes decisions about problems, chooses goals and strategies to reach them, and allocates resources. Formulation of public policies usually occurs through collaboration between community, private sector, and government leaders.

Assurance involves making certain that all populations have access to appropriate and cost-effective services to reach agreed-upon public health goals. In addition to treatment services for individuals, assurance activities include health promotion and disease-prevention services.

DENTAL PUBLIC HEALTH SCIENCE AND PRACTICE

Dental public health is one of the nine specialties of dentistry recognized by the American Dental Association, and has been defined as the ". . . science and art of preventing and controlling dental diseases and promoting dental health through organized community efforts. It is that form of dental practice which serves the community as a patient rather than the individual. It is concerned with the dental health education of the public, with applied dental research, and with the administration of group dental care programs as well as the prevention and control of dental diseases on a community basis."[3] Although descriptive of what some dental public health practitioners may do, that definition does not fully capture the scope of dental public health practice. In addition to health education and program administration, dental public health is concerned with policy development; advocacy; conduct of research in epidemiology, health services, and disease prevention; and monitoring trends in disease and risk factors in populations. Dental public health is unique in that it straddles two worlds: It is the specialty with dentistry that focuses on public health issues, and it is the segment of the public health infrastructure that is concerned with oral health issues. In reality, personnel who are not board-certified specialists in the field and often are not dentists perform much of what might be considered public health dentistry.

PUBLIC HEALTH APPROACHES

Dental providers traditionally focus primarily on providing care to individual patients on a one-on-one basis. Most U.S. residents seek dental care from dentists in private practice, who diagnose disease, develop a treatment plan, and provide care. It is a model of care that works reasonably well for much of the public, but it has several key deficiencies:

- There are financial, geographic, cultural, attitudinal, and other barriers that restrict access to dental care for a large segment of the public.
- Despite policy statements and recommendations from organizations such as the American Acad-

emy of Pediatric Dentistry,[4] preventive dental visits remain very rare among young children. It remains uncertain whether there is adequate capacity to provide a dental home for all children in the United States by 12 months of age.[5]
- Prevention services often can be delivered in a more cost-effective manner in venues other than private dental offices.
- Dental public health problems often require policy initiatives, community health promotion, and environmental changes that are outside the scope of the individual private-practice dental office.

The difference between a traditional dental approach and a public health approach to dealing with an oral health problem is illustrated by the following example. Typical County Dental Program provides dental services to county residents in a southern U.S. state on a sliding-fee scale, based on household income. It also accepts reimbursement from Medicaid and the State Children's Health Insurance Program (SCHIP). The dental director of Typical County has seen a steady increase in the number of pre-school children experiencing early childhood caries, whose severe disease and young age require treatment in a hospital operating room (OR) under general anesthesia. Typical County Dental Program has just one pediatric dentist on staff. The waiting time for OR cases is now more than 6 months. The dental director reports this problem to the county health director, who then authorizes the dental program to hire two more pediatric dentists. To attract applicants, the director doubles the starting salary for pediatric dentists. As word spreads in the community that the health department has increased the number of dentists who can provide dental care for young children in the OR, private-practice dentists refer young children with early childhood caries who are insured by Medicaid or SCHIP to the Typical County Dental Program. Three years later, the waiting time for pediatric OR cases is still about 6 months.

Progressive County is located in the same state as Typical County. Similar to the Typical County Health Department, the public health dental program has a long waiting list for hospital-based pediatric dental care. The recently hired dental director for the Progressive County Health Department decides to adopt a public health approach to address the problem. First, the director develops an inexpensive surveillance system for dental caries in pre-school children by working with pediatricians and Women, Infants, and Children (WIC) clinics in the county. A simple data collection form is designed and short training sessions are held. For a 2-week period each year, pediatricians and nutritional counselors conduct brief "lift-the-lip" examinations on all 1- to 3-year-olds seen in their facilities. The surveillance data are tabulated, revealing that 35% of the children seen have signs of pre-cavitated or cavitated caries lesions. The dental director forms a community advisory board composed of proponents for children's health and well-being, which uses the data and citizen testimonials to advocate for increased resources from the Progressive County Commission to address dental needs. The county commissioners approve a budget increase for the county dental program. The dental director uses the new funding to implement oral health educational programs for pediatricians, their staff, and WIC counselors, which are aimed at teaching pregnant women and new mothers how to care for their children's teeth. The Progressive County Dental Program also implements a fluoride varnish program in the health department's immunization clinic. Three years later, the prevalence of dental caries among 1- to 3-year-olds has been reduced by 50%, and the demand for OR-based pediatric dental care has been cut in half.

Population versus Individual Approach

The preceding example highlights several key differences between a personal dental care approach and a dental public health approach to controlling oral disease in a population. These are summarized in (Table 21–1 ■). Personal dental care requires an individual to visit a dentist, who then initiates care by taking a dental and medical history and conducting an examination. The dentist

arrives at a diagnosis and develops a treatment plan. After obtaining the patient's informed consent, the dentist renders dental care, collects the fee, and schedules the patient for a follow-up visit.

Dental public health practice follows steps analogous (similar) to those taken by an individual dentist, but the focus is primarily on a population, including those who do not seek care, rather than just one patient in the chair. Through the core public health function of assessment, the dental public health practitioner collects the necessary information to identify community problems, analogous to an individual dentist diagnosing a patient's condition. Similar to a personal dentist's development of a treatment plan, the dental public health practitioner uses the information from the community assessment to develop policies and programs to address the problem. Assurance in a dental public health is analogous to a dentist's provision of care: It involves the delivery of the services to the community.

Reach versus Intensity

Because dental public health is focused on the oral health of communities and populations, and always operates within the constraints of financing and feasibility, the types of services provided involve a balance between what might work best for an individual and what might be possible to deliver to an entire population. Often, programs that reach a wider audience but are less intensive for any one person—and therefore perhaps less effective at an individual level—can produce better population health outcomes than a far more intensive intervention delivered to a much smaller group. For example, intensive smoking-cessation treatments such as group behavior therapy programs are more effective than self-help

■ **Table 21–1** Comparison of the Procedures Used by the Dental Clinician and the Dental Public Health Practitioner

Dental Clinician	*Dental Public Health Practitioner*
Focuses on individual patient	Focuses on community
Conducts examination	Implements public health surveillance
Establishes diagnosis	Conducts analysis
Discusses findings with patient; develops treatment plan	Engages community partners; plans programs; develops policy
Provides treatment	Operates program
Receives payment for services	Obtains financing; conducts cost-effectiveness analysis
Schedules periodic follow-up visits	Conducts program evaluation

alone,[6] but because so few smokers are willing to participate in such programs, they will have almost no measurable effect in reducing the prevalence of smoking in a population. In comparison, less-intensive and relatively inexpensive interventions such as increasing the cost of cigarettes through taxation and changing the environmental norm through workplace smoking restrictions can lead to large reductions in smoking and, consequently, fewer smoking-related deaths.[7] Similar effects are possible with programs for dental-caries prevention. For example, community water fluoridation may have lower effectiveness than professionally applied fluoride varnish for an individual at high risk for caries,[8,9] but water fluoridation may likely prevent much more disease in a population because of its reach.

New drugs, devices, or procedures are frequently tested for how well they work at preventing or treating disease under ideal conditions, which is known as **efficacy.** The prototype for that testing is the double-blinded, randomized, controlled clinical trial, in which subjects' dosages and compliance are tightly monitored, examiners and clinicians are calibrated and tested for reliability, neither subjects nor clinicians know who is receiving the test treatment or the placebo, and subjects are followed over time to measure their outcomes. The extent to which those drugs, devices, or procedures achieve their intended outcomes when deployed in the field for a defined population is known as **effectiveness.** Effectiveness is almost always less than efficacy, because in the real world, circumstances are almost always less than ideal. Public health dwells in the world of effectiveness; it takes technologies established as efficacious in a clinical research setting and applies them to populations.

Balancing Individual Rights and Societal Protection

Public health practice, particularly in the United States, frequently involves a contentious balance between individual rights and the good of society. Motorcycle helmet laws typify this tension: Despite overwhelming epidemiologic evidence that motorcycle helmets reduce fatalities and serious injuries, many motorcycle riders perceive such laws as an infringement on personal liberties.[10] Proponents of motorcycle helmet laws argue that a burden is placed on society when an individual suffers injury or death from preventable motorcycle fatalities.[11] Similar arguments of individual rights versus social good have been made regarding dental public health policies

including, for example, community water fluoridation[12] and school-based dental screening.[13]

DENTAL PUBLIC HEALTH ORGANIZATION AND INFRASTRUCTURE

To be most effective in carrying out the core public health functions regarding oral health, the public health organization must have an adequate dental public health infrastructure. That is, there must be an adequate workforce, a sufficient administrative presence within health agencies and departments, adequate financial resources to implement programs, and the ability to use personnel in an effective and efficient manner. To be most effective, that dental public health workforce should be appropriately trained, represent the diversity of the populations it serves, and be sustainable for the foreseeable future.

Dental public health has a presence internationally and at nearly all levels of government in the United States. The size and scope of these programs vary widely. In addition, there are a number of professional organizations whose primary focus is dental public health.

International Agencies

The **World Health Organization (WHO)** is the directing and coordinating authority for health within the United Nations system. It is responsible for providing leadership on global health matters, shaping the health research agenda, setting norms and standards, articulating evidence-based policy options, providing technical support to countries, and monitoring and assessing health trends. The WHO Global Oral Health Program is one of the technical programs within the agency, located in the Department of Chronic Diseases and Health Promotion. Because oral diseases and conditions share so many common risk factors with major chronic diseases,[14] the WHO Global Oral Health Program focuses largely on modifiable risk behaviors related to diet, nutrition, use of tobacco and excessive consumption of alcohol, and hygiene. The program also stimulates development and implementation of community-oriented demonstration projects for oral health promotion and prevention of oral diseases with focus on disadvantaged and poor population groups in developed and developing countries. The WHO Global Oral Health Program supports countries and regions in their efforts to ensure healthy environments such as access to safe water and sanitation, and encourages national health authorities to implement effective fluoride programs for prevention of dental caries. Such initiatives range from automatic fluoride administration (e.g., water or salt fluoridation) to programs based on the use of affordable fluoridated toothpastes.

The **Pan American Health Organization (PAHO)** is an international public health agency that works to improve health and living standards of the countries of the Americas. It serves as the specialized organization for health of the Inter-American System. It also serves as the Regional Office for the Americas of the WHO and enjoys international recognition as part of the United Nations system. PAHO member states include all 35 countries in the Americas; Puerto Rico is an associate member. France, the Kingdom of the Netherlands, and the United Kingdom of Great Britain and Northern Ireland are participating states, and Portugal and Spain are observer states. The mission of PAHO is to strengthen national and local health systems and improve the health of the peoples of the Americas, in collaboration with ministries of health, other government and international agencies, nongovernmental organizations, universities, social security agencies, community groups, and many others.

Released in 2006, PAHO's proposed 10-Year Regional Plan on Oral Health (see http://www.paho.org/ English/GOV/CE/ce138-14-e.pdf) includes three major goals:

- *Goal 1:* Completion of the unfinished agenda in oral health: "To ensure a minimum level of access to oral health care for all, by addressing gaps in care for the most vulnerable groups."
- *Goal 2:* The integration of oral health care into primary health care services.
- *Goal 3:* Scaling up of proven cost-effective interventions—a multiyear plan for fluoridation programs in the Americas and expansion of oral health coverage with simple technologies.

PAHO has taken an active and visible role in promoting salt fluoridation to prevent dental caries (see http://www .paho.org/English/DD/PUB/SP_615.htm).

The **FDI World Dental Federation** was founded in Paris in 1900 as the Fédération Dentaire Internationale. It is the main organization representing dentists worldwide and organizes a yearly global meeting to bring dentists together to discuss relevant issues. The FDI currently has a membership of more than 150 national dental associations from more than 130 countries, representing nearly 1 million dentists globally. Five standing committees are responsible for addressing the issues of communications and member support, dental practice, education, science, and world dental development and health promotion. The FDI is a non-governmental organization with official relations with the United Nations and the WHO.

One of the missions of the FDI is "to promote optimal oral and general health for all peoples." The FDI plays a role in global dental health issues primarily through advocacy and policy development.

The **International Federation of Dental Hygienists (IFDH)** was officially formed in 1986, although an informal cohort of international dental hygienists called the International Liaison Committee on Dental Hygiene was established in 1973. The IFDH is an international, non-governmental, non-profit organization, free from any political, racial, or religious ties. It unites dental hygiene associations from around the world in their common cause of promoting dental health. The stated purposes of the federation are to (1) represent and advance the profession of dental hygiene; (2) promote professional alliances with its association members as well as with other associations, federations, and organizations whose objectives are similar; (3) promote and coordinate the exchange of knowledge and information about the profession, its education, and its practice; (4) promote access to quality preventive services for oral health care; (5) increase public awareness that oral disease can be prevented through proven regimen; and (6) provide a forum for the understanding and discussion of issues pertaining to dental hygiene.

U.S. Federal Agencies

At the national level, the **U.S. Department of Health and Human Services (USDHHS)** is the department in the executive branch of the federal government that is responsible for the planning and implementation of a wide range of public health programs. The USDHHS includes the Office of the Secretary and 11 agencies, each dealing with different aspects of public health. The **Administration for Children and Families (ACF)** is responsible for numerous programs that provide services and assistance to needy children and families, administers the Temporary Assistance to Needy Families and Head Start programs, provides funds to assist low-income families in paying for child care, and supports state programs for foster care and adoption assistance. The **Health Resources and Services Administration (HRSA)** is the primary federal agency for improving access to health care services for people who are uninsured, isolated, or medically vulnerable. Grantees of this agency provide health care to uninsured people, people living with HIV/AIDS, and pregnant women, mothers, and children. They train health professionals and improve systems of care in rural communities. The HRSA supports training programs and other initiatives to enhance the dental and public health workforces, and funds programs to increase access to oral health care services. The **Agency for Healthcare Research and Quality (AHRQ)** is the lead federal agency charged with improving the quality, safety, efficiency, and effectiveness of health care for all Americans. This agency supports investigator-initiated health services research. The **Centers for Disease Control and Prevention (CDC)** is the lead federal agency for disease-prevention and health-promotion efforts. The CDC administers public health surveillance systems to monitor, investigate, and prevent outbreaks of disease; guards against international disease transmission; maintains national health statistics; provides for immunization services; and conducts and supports research on disease and injury prevention. The CDC's Division of Oral Health supports and disseminates data from national and local oral health surveillance systems, provides technical and financial support to state and local public dental health programs, offers training on water fluoridation engineering, administers the Water Fluoridation Reporting System, and produces guidelines on infection control in dental care settings. The **Agency for Toxic Substances and Disease Registry (ATSDR)** works with states and other federal agencies to prevent exposure to hazardous substances from waste sites. The **Substance Abuse and Mental Health Services Administration (SAMHSA)** focuses on improving the quality and availability of services to prevent and treat substance abuse and mental illness. The **Administration on Aging (AoA)** is one of the nation's largest providers of home- and community-based care for older persons and their caregivers. Its mission is to develop a comprehensive, coordinated, and cost-effective system of long-term care that helps elderly individuals to maintain their dignity in their homes and communities. The AoA also seeks to help society prepare for an aging population. The **Food and Drug Administration (FDA)** ensures the safety of foods and cosmetics, as well as the safety and efficacy of pharmaceuticals, biological products, and medical devices, including those used in personal oral health care and dental public health programs. The **Centers for Medicare and Medicaid Services (CMS)** serves the needs of Medicaid and Medicare beneficiaries. The Medicaid program provides health care benefits to groups of low-income people, some who may have no health insurance or inadequate health insurance. Medicare is a health insurance program for people aged 65 or older, people under age 65 with certain disabilities, and people of all ages with end-stage renal disease. The **Indian Health Service (IHS)** is responsible for providing federal health services to American Indians and Alaska Natives. The provision of health services to members of federally recognized tribes grew out of the special government-to-government relationship between the federal government and Indian tribes. The IHS provides services to approximately 1.5 million American Indians and Alaska Natives who belong to more than 557 federally recognized tribes in 35 states. The **National Institutes of Health (NIH),** the world's premier biomedical research agency, supports research projects nationwide. The National Institute for Dental and Craniofacial Research (NIDCR), one institute within NIH, conducts and supports basic and clinical dental and oral health research.

The **Office of the Surgeon General** is administratively located within the Office of Public Health and Science in the Office of the Secretary, USDHHS. The Office of the Surgeon General oversees the **U.S. Public Health Service Commissioned Corps,** one of the seven uniformed services of the United States. It is a specialized career system designed to attract, develop, and retain health professionals who may be assigned to federal, state, or local agencies, or international organizations. There are approximately 500 dental officers in the U.S. Public Health Service Commissioned Corps. The large majority of Commissioned Corps Dental Officers are assigned to the Indian Health Service, the Bureau of Prisons, or the Department of Homeland Security. There are fewer than 100 dental hygienists in the Commissioned Corps; most are in the Indian Health Service (64%) or the Federal Bureau of Prisons (26%).

State and Local Dental Public Health Programs

Every U.S. state and territory has a health department, although not all state and territorial health departments include an administrative unit focused on oral health. Nearly all state dental public health programs are headed by a state dental director. The size and scope of state dental programs vary widely, although they are typically small. In 2005, state dental public health programs had a median of three full-time employees and two-thirds of programs had annual operating budgets of less than $1 million per year (see http://apps.nccd.cdc.gov/synopses/ NatTrendTableV.asp). Within each state, counties and cities may administer community clinics for oral health treatment through local health departments. These clinics usually serve schools, economically disadvantaged areas, or populations with otherwise limited access to oral health care services.

Professional Organizations in Dental Public Health

There are many national organizations in the United States directly or indirectly involved in dental public health issues. Some of these organizations have dental public health activities as a primary mission, whereas others are focused primarily on other issues such as dental practice, education, or research, but have some involvement in public health issues.

There are three major national dental public health organizations in the United States. The largest of these is the **American Association of Public Health Dentistry (AAPHD),** founded in 1937. The stated mission of AAPHD is "To improve the public's health through oral health research, service, education and policy development." Its vision is "optimal oral health for all."[3] The membership of AAPHD is composed primarily of public health dentists and dental hygienists involved in program administration, education, research, and clinical practice. As of May 2007, AAPHD had 876 members. The second-largest, national, dental public health organization is the **Oral Health Section** of the **American Public Health Association (APHA).** This organization is an association of individuals and organizations working to improve the public's health and to achieve equity in health status for all. It promotes the scientific and professional foundation of public health practice and policy, advocates the conditions for a healthy global society, emphasizes prevention, and seeks to enhance the ability of its members to promote and protect environmental and community health. One of 25 discipline-based sections within APHA, the Oral Health Section, promotes the importance of oral health and increasing the public's access to preventive and treatment services for oral health, and monitors and communicates the oral health needs of the public. As of May 2007, 313 APHA members listed Oral Health Section as their primary section. The other major national organization for dental public

health in the United States is the **Association of State and Territorial Dental Directors (ASTDD).** This national non-profit organization represents the directors and staff of state public health agency programs for oral health. Full membership is limited to one per state, and the member is the state or territorial dental director, except where there is no director of a state oral health program. The ASTDD allows associate membership for persons other than state or territorial dental directors; as of May 2007, ASTDD had 75 associate members.

DENTAL PUBLIC HEALTH ACTIVITIES

The activities of dental public health programs can be organized by the core public health functions: assessment, policy development, and assurance. This section briefly describes the functions of effective dental public health programs, with supporting examples and vignettes to illustrate those activities.

Assessment

As with other public health programs, effective programs for dental public health monitor the health of communities and populations at risk to identify health problems and priorities. Data needed to plan, monitor, and evaluate policies and programs for dental public health come from a number of sources.

Cancer Registries
State-based cancer registries are data systems that collect, manage, and analyze data about cancer cases and cancer deaths. In each state, medical facilities (including hospitals, physicians' offices, therapeutic radiation facilities, freestanding surgical centers, and pathology laboratories) report these data to a central cancer registry. These registries provide the ability to monitor trends in the number of new cases, oral cancer incidence rates (i.e., number of new cases per 100,000 population), oral cancer survival rates, and cancer stage at the time of diagnosis. These statistics are available for the total population within each state as well as by gender, age, and race. Oral cancer incidence rates are available for 47 states and the District of Columbia.[15]

Vital Statistics
Vital statistics include data on birth, death, marriage, and divorce. One vital statistic of interest to dental public health is deaths from oral and pharyngeal cancer. The number of oral and pharyngeal cancer deaths and

mortality rates (i.e., number of deaths from oral cancer per 100,000 population) are available for the nation, all 50 states, and the District of Columbia. Oral and pharyngeal cancer mortality statistics are from CDC's National Vital Statistics System.[15]

Clinical Surveys

The primary current source of national data on the most common oral health conditions is the National Health and Nutrition Examination Survey (NHANES), conducted by NCHS. The survey is unique in that it combines interviews and physical examinations, including oral health examinations conducted by trained dental examiners. The NHANES program began in the early 1960s and was conducted as a series of periodic surveys focusing on different population groups or health topics. In 1999, NHANES became a continuous program. The survey examines a nationally representative sample of about 5,000 persons each year. These persons are located in counties across the country, 15 of which are visited each year. The most recent oral health data from NHANES were released in April 2007 and included data through 2004.[16]

At least 15 state dental programs have conducted statewide clinical surveys within the past 6 years, although none included adults.[17] Most states employed the Basic Screening Survey (BSS), which was developed by the ASTDD.[18] The BSS was developed as a simple training and data collection tool that could be used by screeners with or without dental backgrounds. That approach was taken because non-dental health professionals, such as public health nurses, sometimes have direct access to some population groups, and because some states and communities have few public health dental professionals to assist in screening surveys. The BSS has components for collecting clinical oral health data for pre-school children, school children, and adults.

The primary disadvantages of clinical data collection are the expense and logistic difficulties. Clinical surveys require trained personnel to conduct the examinations; travel to multiple locations; the use of portable or mobile dental equipment; paying attention to infection control; and gaining the cooperation and trust of school officials, parents, and children. Clinical surveys of adults are a particularly difficult and expensive undertaking, which in part explains why there are almost no clinical data on adult oral health at the state or local levels.

Non-Clinical Oral Health Surveys

A good deal of information relevant to planning and monitoring oral health issues can be derived from non-clinical surveys. These surveys involve collection of data via telephone surveys, face-to-face interviews, or self-completed questionnaires, but they do not require clinical examination of participants. These types of surveys are often the most economically and logistically feasible way to reach adults, and valid data on many relevant oral health topics can be covered through self-reported surveys. Some of the major ongoing national surveys of adults that include oral health information are the **National Health Interview Survey,** which collects data on access to dental care as well as behaviors related to oral health such as tobacco use, and the **Medical Expenditure Panel Survey,** which collects information on dental care expenses, use, and insurance. The **Behavioral Risk Factor Surveillance System (BRFSS)** is a state-based ongoing telephone survey on preventive health practices and risk behaviors that are linked to chronic diseases, injuries, and preventable infectious diseases. It includes several oral health variables, including tooth loss, last dental visit, preventive care, and risk factors relevant to oral health. The BRFSS is administered in all states and the District of Columbia.

National Oral Health Surveillance System

Recognizing the need for uniform surveillance for key oral health indicators among the states, the **National Oral Health Surveillance System (NOHSS)** was developed as a collaborative effort between CDC's Division of Oral Health and the ASTDD.[19] The NOHSS is designed to monitor the burden of oral disease, use of the delivery system for oral health care, and the status of community water fluoridation on both a national and state level. It includes nine oral health indicators:

1. **Dental visit:** Adults aged 18+ who have visited a dentist or dental clinic in the past year.
2. **Teeth cleaning:** Adults aged 18+ who have had their teeth cleaned in the past year (among adults with natural teeth who have ever visited a dentist or dental clinic).
3. **Complete tooth loss:** Adults aged 65+ who have lost all of their natural teeth because of tooth decay or gum disease.
4. **Loss of six or more teeth:** Adults aged 65+ who have lost six or more teeth because of tooth decay or gum disease.

5. **Fluoridation status:**   Percentage of people served by public water systems who receive fluoridated water.

6. **Dental sealants:**   Percentage of third-grade students with dental sealants on at least one permanent molar tooth.

7. **Caries experience:**   Percentage of third-grade students with caries experience, including treated and untreated tooth decay.

8. **Untreated tooth decay:**   Percentage of third-grade students with untreated tooth decay.

9. **Cancer of the oral cavity and pharynx:**   Incidence and mortality rates, survival rates, and stage at diagnosis for oral and pharyngeal cancer.

Three of the indicators (nos. 6, 7, and 8) require collection of clinical data, one indicator (no. 9) uses data from the state cancer registry, one indicator (no. 5) is based on monitoring data for water fluoridation collected as part of the Water Fluoridation Reporting System, and the remaining four indicators are based on self-reported data collected by the state BRFSS survey.

Policy Development

Maintain a Strong Oral Health Unit within Health Agencies

An unfortunate reality of state and local dental programs is that they are frequently susceptible to severe budget cuts that threaten their existence. Too often, dental programs and dental care are viewed by legislators and decision makers as nonessential services. As government agencies run by government employees, state programs for dental public health are prohibited from directly lobbying state legislators for continued or enhanced funding. Creative and effective programs, however, are able to build a constituency to advocate on its behalf.

As an example, the Georgia State Oral Health Program faced the threat of elimination with severe budget cuts of state funding for oral health in 1996 and 2000. In response to the threat in 1996, the Georgia Oral Health Coalition (GOHC) was established to build and support state oral health infrastructure. The coalition, composed of interested individuals and organizations, worked diligently in 1996 and 2000 to represent the need for the state's oral health program and necessary dental services. The coalition, along with the Georgia Department of Audits (GDOA) Report, recommended that the state's oral health program remain intact and that the state

expand oral health services. A one-page fact sheet was developed to promote retaining the state dental program; the fact sheet referred to the GDOA report's recommendation to maintain and expand state oral health services, the oral health needs of the state, and the recommendation to maintain the state funding for the oral health program at the present funding level. In addition, consumers, city and county politicians, local boards of health, private dentists, professional health organizations, and advocacy groups sent letters and made calls to the governor and the Department of Human Resources Commissioner. All work was performed by voluntary members and associations. As a result of this effort, the state oral health program was retained and funding reinstated both in 1997 and 2001. The efforts of the GOHC in raising the importance of the state's oral health infrastructure has also led to other benefits including development of a state oral health plan, funding of the school-based Georgia Oral Health Prevention Program, and significant increases in dental Medicaid.

Mobilize Community Partnerships

As discussed above, most state dental programs have few employees and little money, yet are responsible for maintaining and improving the oral health of large populations. Effective programs for dental public health build partnerships and coalitions to help them accomplish their public health goals.

An excellent example of leveraging expertise and assistance is the Maryland Oral Cancer Prevention Coalition. In the early 1990s, cancer registry data showed that Maryland experienced a high oral cancer mortality rate. The Office of Oral Health within the Maryland Department of Health and Mental Hygiene partnered with the University of Maryland Dental School, the National Institute of Dental and Craniofacial Research, the American Cancer Society, the Association of Local and County Dental Health Officers, and others to develop the Maryland Oral Cancer Prevention Coalition. The coalition pooled small grants from each institution to conduct a needs assessment on oral cancer, including (1) an assessment of available funding, educational materials, and interested individuals and agencies; (2) a review of state cancer registry data; (3) the conduct of surveys and focus groups of health care providers to determine their knowledge, attitudes, and practices regarding oral cancer and its early detection; and (4) the conduct of surveys and focus groups of the public regarding prevention and early detection of oral cancer. The coalition's efforts led to publication and dissemination of the survey findings, which it used to secure additional funding and policy changes to prevent oral cancer. The Coalition's efforts provided a template for NIDCR's national request for proposals to develop "State Models for Oral Cancer Prevention and Early Detection" and led to the inclusion of oral cancer as one of seven targeted cancers by the Tobacco Settlement Funds Program in Maryland. Their efforts also led to passage of legislation that established the Maryland Oral Cancer Prevention Initiative.

Develop Policies to Address the Oral Health Needs of the Community: State Oral Health Plans

The past several years have seen many states develop state oral health plans to identify and address oral health concerns through policy and program initiatives. Much of this work has been stimulated by interest in oral health from the **National Governors Association (NGA).** The NGA is the bipartisan organization of the nation's governors through which they influence the development and implementation of national policy, share best practices, and promote visionary leadership on state issues. The NGA Center for Best Practices convened a series of policy academies, throughout 2000 and 2001, to help a selected number of states bolster their ability to serve the oral health needs of low-income children. The objectives of the academies were to (1) help state policy makers develop an oral health action plan that could be realistically implemented in their respective states; (2) learn about innovative solutions that states have used to address critical policy questions and improve program design; and (3) create and reinforce relationships between governors' offices, state legislators, key public program directors, and stakeholders from the private sector. Twenty-one states participated in the academies.

To address the oral health needs of their residents, states are currently undertaking the following policy initiatives:[20]

- *Promoting education and prevention:* Much of the disease experienced by children can be prevented. Several states have launched public awareness campaigns to educate parents and children about proper dental care and to build public support for children's oral health policy initiatives.
- *Increasing coverage and access:* Although many low-income children have dental care coverage

through Medicaid, most receive no preventive dentist visits. Many states are trying to strengthen the safety net by encouraging providers to participate in Medicaid and by including dental benefits in SCHIP.

- *Enhancing the dental workforce:* Many states are trying to attract dentists to chronically underserved areas. States are using loan forgiveness, tax credits, and other incentives, and are trying to enhance dentist training to adequately address pediatric dental care needs.
- *Improving financing and reimbursement:* Many providers refuse to participate in Medicaid because of the low rate at which they are reimbursed. Some states have increased provider reimbursements in Medicaid to attract new dentists as well as to bring back dentists who have stopped participating. As with coverage expansions, this strategy would increase state costs.
- *Improving the quality of data and surveillance:* The lack of reliable state-level data often makes assessing and monitoring the oral health of children a challenge for states. States are working with their public health departments as well as local universities, policy institutes, and the CDC to develop reliable methods to track the prevalence of dental disease.

Assurance in Dental Public Health

Many of the services provided by state and local dental public health programs can be classified as **assurance activities;** that is, these activities are intended to ensure all populations have access to appropriate and cost-effective services to achieve oral health goals. In addition to dental treatment services for individuals, assurance activities include services for oral health promotion and disease prevention.

Community Oral Health Education

Health education has been defined as any combination of learning opportunities designed to aid voluntary adaptations of behavior that are conducive to health.[21] These behaviors may be on the part of individuals, groups, families, institutions, or communities. The etiology of all major dental diseases involves many factors, but individual and community behaviors are major factors involved in the etiology of nearly all of those diseases, including dental caries, most periodontal diseases, and oral cancer. Although it has long been recognized that education alone may not be sufficient to prevent disease, it is an essential part of the process of bringing about desired behavior changes and gaining acceptance as well as use of a preventive measure or program. That is, health education is a necessary, although usually not sufficient, measure for preventing disease in populations.[22]

There are many examples of oral health education programs designed to encourage voluntary adoption of appropriate behavior change. An excellent recent example is the public campaign organized by the Citizen's Watch for Oral Health in Washington State (see http://www.kidsoralhealth.org/index.html). Citizens' Watch for Oral Health is a coalition of labor, business, medical, public health, education, dental, and children's advocacy groups. Through radio public service announcements and print advertisements, which generate media attention, and e-mail communications, public speaking, direct mail, and other communications vehicles, Citizens' Watch for Oral Health seeks to ensure that oral health is viewed as an important health issue, to identify opportunities to prevent oral disease and to advocate for increased prevention, and to engage a powerful constituency to support policies to improve oral health. The campaign resulted in significant increases in Washington residents' knowledge and support for policy solutions such as fluoridation, Medicaid dental care for low-income children, and dental screenings in schools.

The National Spit Tobacco Education Program (NSTEP), developed by Oral Health America, seeks to educate the public about the dangers of using spit (smokeless) tobacco.[23] Through presentations at sporting events, speeches by oral cancer survivors, publications, and educational materials, NSTEP has increased awareness of adverse consequences associated with using those tobacco products.

Community Oral Health Promotion

Health promotion is a broader concept than health education, and classically has been defined as any combination of educational, organizational, economic, and environmental supports for behavior conducive to health.[21] Unlike a strictly educational approach, health promotion seeks to prevent disease even among individuals who have not made personal behavior changes and seeks to remove barriers to adoption of appropriate behaviors. Establishment of smoke-free regulations may

be a prototype of a health promotion approach: This approach involves education of the community about the health risks of exposure to second-hand tobacco smoke, protects non-smokers from exposure to tobacco smoke, changes the environment to de-normalize smoking in workplaces and other public settings, creates additional incentives for smokers to quit, reduces the number of cigarettes smoked per day by those who continue to smoke, and reduces the environmental cues that may lead former smokers to relapse.[24]

Community water fluoridation to prevent dental caries has been described as a health-promotion activity because it alters the living environment of people to improve their health.[25] Instituting and maintaining water fluoridation involves the full range of health promotion activities: education of the public and government leaders, advocation for legislative and policy changes, meeting of engineering and training needs, and addressing of economic issues.

In the United States, most fluoridation laws are enacted and implemented at the local level. The most recent data indicate that 42 of the nation's 50 largest cities are supplied with fluoridated water, and an estimated 67.3% of the U.S. population served by public water systems has access to fluoridated water.[26] The Healthy People 2010 objectives for the nation set a target for at least 75% of the U.S. population served by community water systems to receive optimally fluoridated water by 2010.[27] Although water fluoridation reaches some residents in every state, just 24 of the 50 states provide fluoridated community water to 75% or more of their residents.[26]

Another example of oral health promotion is mouthguard regulations in school-sponsored organized sports. There is compelling evidence that use of mouthguards in sports reduces the risk for dental injuries.[28,29] Education of young people and their parents on the reason for appropriate mouthguard use in sports is essential, but a broader approach to health promotion, which includes regulations that require mouthguards in certain sports, increases use of the devices,[30] creates a cultural norm of wearing them, and ultimately prevents more dental injury than does a strictly voluntary approach.[31]

Linking People to Oral Health Services

One function of dental public health assurance that is most familiar to the public is the provision of dental care services to the public, particularly those unable to access dental services in the private sector. Many state and local health departments provide direct dental services through government-owned fixed or mobile dental clinics. For example, the Duval County (Florida) Health Department Dental Program operates five dental centers in Jacksonville to provide general dental care for children and adults, and operates two mobile dental vans to provide preventive dental care, including sealants, at local elementary schools. Services are primarily funded by the state Medicaid program.

Federally Qualified Health Centers (FQHC) are "safety net" providers such as community health centers, public housing centers, outpatient health programs funded by the Indian Health Service, and programs serving migrants and the homeless. The main purpose of the FQHC program is to enhance the provision of primary care services in underserved urban and rural communities. Health centers are characterized by five essential elements that differentiate them from other providers: (1) They must be located in or serve a high-need community, i.e. "medically underserved areas" or "medically underserved populations"; (2) they must provide comprehensive primary care services as well as supportive services such as translation and transportation services that promote access to health care; (3) their services must be available to all residents of their service areas, with fees adjusted according to patients' ability to pay; (4) they must be governed by a community board with a majority of members being health center patients; and, (5) they must meet other performance and accountability requirements regarding their administrative, clinical, and financial operations. There are more than 1,000 FQHC, which serve 16 million people through 5,000 health center delivery sites in the United States. These centers are supported by federal health center grants, Medicaid, Medicare, private insurance payments, and state/local contributions.[32]

Compared with the general U.S. population, American Indians and Alaskan Natives experience relatively high levels of oral disease and unmet dental care needs.[33-35] As mentioned previously, the IHS is the federal agency responsible for addressing the health needs of more than 1.8 million American Indians and Alaska Natives who belong to more than 557 federally recognized tribes in 35 states. The IHS employs dentists, dental hygienists, and dental assistants either through the uniformed U.S. Public Health Service Commissioned Corps or as civilian employees. In addition, many tribes directly employ their own dental personnel.

One persistent barrier to obtaining regular and periodic preventive dental care is cost, particularly for low-income individuals. Title XIX of the Social Security Act is a federal/state entitlement program that pays for medical assistance for certain individuals and families with low incomes and resources. This program, known as Medicaid, became law in 1965 as a cooperative venture jointly funded by the federal and state governments (including the District of Columbia and the Territories) to assist states in furnishing medical assistance to eligible needy persons. Medicaid is the largest source of funding for medical and health-related services for America's poorest people. Dental services are considered an optional service for the adult population covered by Medicaid. However, dental services are a required service for most Medicaid-eligible individuals under the age of 21, as a required component of the Early and Periodic Screening, Diagnostic and Treatment benefit. Dentists are not required to enroll with their states as providers for Medicaid patients, and in reality relatively few dentists participate in state Medicaid programs.[36] Like Medicaid, the SCHIP is jointly financed by the federal and state governments and administered by the states. The latter program was established in 1997 to help states expand health care coverage to more than 5 million of the nation's uninsured children. Dental services are an optional benefit under SCHIP for all children up to age 19. However, nearly all States have opted to provide coverage for dental services.

Implementing and Supporting Prevention Programs

Assurance in dental public health programs includes prevention activities, arguably the cornerstone of dental public practice. (Table 21–2 ■) lists some of the prevention strategies used in these programs. The details of many of these individual prevention modalities are discussed in Unit Three. Dental public health programs seek to provide these preventive services to whole communities. Many of the programs targeting children use school-based or linked approaches. School-based programs are conducted in schools, and school-linked programs are conducted in schools, private dental practices, and clinic settings outside of schools.

■ **Table 21–2** Community Strategies for Prevention of Key Oral Diseases and Conditions

Dental Caries
- Community-wide health promotion activities, including educational, political, regulatory, and organizational interventions
- Fluoride use
  - Community water fluoridation
  - School water fluoridation
  - Salt fluoridation[a]
  - School-based dietary fluoride tablets
  - School-based fluoride mouthrinse
  - Fluoride varnish
- School-based and school-linked sealant programs
- School-based screening and referral

Periodontal Diseases
- Community-wide health promotion activities, including educational, political, regulatory, and organizational interventions
- School-based personal hygiene, reinforcement of personal oral hygiene habits in Head Start or primary school classrooms
- School-linked screening and referral

Oral and Pharyngeal Cancers
- Community-wide health promotion activities, including educational, political, regulatory, and organizational interventions
- Cancer screening programs

Inherited Disorders
- Early detection programs

Trauma
- Community-wide health promotion activities, including educational, political, regulatory, and organizational interventions
- Mouth protector fittings for entire team

[a]Salt fluoridation is not currently used in the United States, but is used in several European and South American countries.
Source: U.S. Department of Health and Human Services. (2000). *Oral health in America: A report of the Surgeon General.* Bethesda, MD: U.S. Department of Health and Human Services, National Institutes of Health, National Institute of Dental and Craniofacial Research, 156.

SUMMARY

Dental public health uses organized, interdisciplinary efforts to address the oral health concerns of communities and populations. A large part of the mission of dental public health is achieved through the application of health-promotion and disease-prevention technologies and interventions. Dental public health is also concerned with policy development; advocacy; conduct of research in epidemiology, health services, and disease prevention; and monitoring trends in disease and risk factors in populations. Public health frequently involves achieving a balance between individual versus population approaches to controlling disease, between individual rights and societal good, and between intensity versus reach.

The activities of dental public health programs can be classified into one of the three core functions of public health organizations: assessment, policy development, and assurance. These activities occur at all levels of jurisdiction although perhaps with varying distribution, with international and national organizations and agencies generally more involved with assessment and policy development, and local agencies more heavily involved in assurance activities.

Meeting the future oral health needs of the public in an era of rapidly growing health care costs, an increasingly diverse population, and growing public expectations for good oral health for a lifetime will require effective and efficient approaches to reaching all members of society. The traditional approach to managing oral disease will become increasingly expensive and unacceptable. The demand for better methods of monitoring the oral status of populations, preventing disease, and ensuring access to necessary services will continue to increase. The dental public health model will remain the most equitable and cost-effective approach to maintaining and improving the nation's oral health.

REFERENCES

1. Institute of Medicine. (1998). *The future of public health.* Washington, DC: National Academies Press.
2. Institute of Medicine. (2002). *The future of the public's health in the 21st century.* Washington, DC: National Academies Press.
3. American Dental Association, Council on Access, Prevention and Interprofessional Relations. (1976). *Definitions of recognized dental specialties: Dental public health.* Retrieved June 1, 2007, from http://www.ada.org/prof/ed/specialties/definitions.asp.
4. American Academy of Pediatric Dentistry. (2006). Policy on the dental home. In *American Academy of Pediatric Dentistry reference manual 2005–2006.* Chicago: American Academy of Pediatric Dentistry, 22–23.
5. Jones, K., & Tomar, S. L. (2005). Estimated impact of competing policy recommendations for age of first dental visit. *Pediatrics,* 115:906–14.
6. Stead, L. F., & Lancaster, T. (2005). Group behaviour therapy programmes for smoking cessation. *Cochrane Database Syst Rev,* Issue 2. Art. No.: CD001007.
7. Burns, D. M. (2000). Smoking cessation: Recent indicators of what's working at a population level. In National Cancer Institute. *Population based smoking cessation: Proceedings of a conference on what works to influence cessation in the general population* (NIH Publication No. 00-4892). (Smoking and Tobacco Monograph No. 12). Bethesda, MD: U.S. Department of Health and Human Services, National Institutes of Health, National Cancer Institute, 1–24.
8. Truman, B. I., Gooch, B. F., Sulemana, I., Gift, H. C., Horowitz, A. M., Evans, C. A., Griffin, S. O., & Carande-Kulis, V. G. (2002). Task Force on Community Preventive Services. Reviews of evidence on interventions to prevent dental caries, oral and pharyngeal cancers, and sports-related craniofacial injuries. *Am J Prev Med,* 23 (1 Suppl):21–54.
9. Marinho, V. C. C., Higgins, J. P. T., Logan, S., & Sheiham, A. (2002). Fluoride varnishes for preventing dental caries in children and adolescents. *Cochrane Database Syst Rev,* Issue 1. Art. No.: CD002279.
10. Jones, M. M., & Bayer, R. (2007). Paternalism and its discontents: Motorcycle helmet laws, libertarian values, and public health. *Am J Public Health,* 97:208–17.
11. Baker, S. P. (1980). On lobbies, liberty, and the public good. *Am J Public Health,* 70:573–75.
12. Martin, B. (1991). *Scientific knowledge in controversy: The social dynamics of the fluoridation debate.* Albany, NY: State University of New York Press.
13. Tickle, M., Milsom, K. M., Buchanan, K., & Blinkhorn, A. S. (2006). Dental screening in schools: The views of parents,

teachers and school nurses. *Br Dent J,* 201:769–73; discussion 767.
14. Sheiham, A., & Watt, R. G. (2000). The common risk factor approach: A rational basis for promoting oral health. *Community Dent Oral Epidemiol,* 28:399–406.
15. U.S. Cancer Statistics Working Group. (2006). *United States cancer statistics: 2003 incidence and mortality.* Atlanta, GA: U.S. Department of Health and Human Services, Centers for Disease Control and Prevention and National Cancer Institute.
16. Dye, B. A., Tan, S., Smith, V., Lewis, B. G., Barker, L. K., Thornton-Evans, G., Eke, P. I., Beltrán-Aguilar, E. D., Horowitz, A. M., & Li, C. H. (2007). *Trends in oral health status: United States, 1988–1994 and 1999–2004* (DHHS Publication No. (PHS) 2007-1698). (Vital Health Stat 11(248)). Hyattsville, MD: U.S. Department of Health and Human Services, Centers for Disease Control and Prevention, National Center for Health Statistics.
17. Association of State and Territorial Dental Directors. (2007). *State & territorial dental public health activities: A collection of descriptive summaries. Acquiring oral health data.* Retrieved June 1, 2007, from http://www.astdd.org/index.php?template=sactnav_temp.php&topic=Acquiring%20Oral%20Health%20Data.
18. Association of State and Territorial Dental Directors. (2003). *Basic screening surveys: An approach to monitoring community oral health.* Columbus, OH: Association of State and Territorial Dental Directors.
19. Centers for Disease Control and Prevention. (2006). *National Oral Health Surveillance System.* Retrieved June 1, 2007, from http://www.cdc.gov/nohss/.
20. National Governors Association (NGA) Center for Best Practices, Health Policies Studies Division. (2002). *Issue brief: State efforts to improve children's oral health.* Washington, DC: NGA Center for Best Practices.
21. Green, L. W., & Johnson, K. W. (1983). Health education and health promotion. In Mechanic, D., Ed. *Handbook of health, healthcare, and the health professions.* New York: Wiley, 744–65.
22. Frazier, P. J., & Horowitz, A. M. (1990). Oral health education and promotion in maternal and child health: A position paper. *J Public Health Dent,* 50 (6 Spec No.):390–95.
23. Oral Health America. (2006). *National Spit Tobacco Education Program. Smokeless does not mean harmless.* Retrieved June 1, 2007, from http://www.nstep.org/index.htm.
24. Centers for Disease Control and Prevention. (2002). *Reducing tobacco use: A report of the Surgeon General.* Atlanta, GA: U.S. Department of Health and Human Services, Centers for Disease Control and Prevention, National Center for Chronic Disease Prevention and Health Promotion, Office on Smoking and Health.

25. Kressin, N. R., & De Souza, M. B. Oral health education and health promotion. In Gluck, G. M., & Morganstein, W. M., Eds. *Jong's community dental health* (5th ed.). St. Louis: Mosby, 277–328.

26. American Dental Association. (2005). *Fluoridation facts.* Chicago: American Dental Association.

27. U.S. Department of Health and Human Services. (2000). *Healthy people 2010* (Vols. I–II) (2nd ed.). (With understanding and improving health and objectives for improving health). Washington, DC: U.S. Government Printing Office.

28. American Dental Association Council on Access, Prevention and Interprofessional Relations and Council on Scientific Affairs. (2006). Using mouthguards to reduce the incidence and severity of sports-related oral injuries. *J Am Dent Assoc,* 137:1712–20; quiz 1731.

29. Knapik, J. J., Marshall, S. W., Lee, R. B., Darakjy, S. S., Jones, S. B., Mitchener, T. A., delaCruz, G. G., & Jones, B. H. (2007). Mouthguards in sport activities: history, physical properties and injury prevention effectiveness. *Sports Med,* 37:117–44.

30. Ranalli, D. N., & Lancaster, D. M. (1995). Attitudes of college football coaches regarding NCAA mouthguard regulations and player compliance. *J Public Health Dent,* 55:139–42.

31. Quarrie, K. L., Gianotti, S. M., Chalmers, D. J., & Hopkins, W. G. (2005). An evaluation of mouthguard requirements and dental injuries in New Zealand rugby union. *Br J Sports Med,* 39:650–51.

32. National Association of Community Health Centers, I. (2007). *About NACHC.* Retrieved June 11, 2007, from http://www.nachc.com/about/.

33. Niendorff, W. J., & Jones, C. M. (2000). Prevalence and severity of dental caries among American Indians and Alaska Natives. *J Public Health Dent,* 60 (Suppl 1): 243–49.

34. Broderick, E. B., & Niendorff, W. J. (2000). Estimating dental treatment needs among American Indians and Alaska Natives. *J Public Health Dent,* 60 (Suppl 1):250–55.

35. Zuckerman, S., Haley, J., Roubideaux, Y., & Lillie-Blanton, M. (2004). Health service access, use, and insurance coverage among American Indians/Alaska Natives and Whites: What role does the Indian Health Service play? *Am J Public Health,* 94:53–59.

36. U.S. General Accounting Office. (2000). *Oral health: Factors contributing to low use of dental services by low-income populations* (GAO Publication No. GAO/HEHS-00-149). Washington, DC: U.S. General Accounting Office.

Chapter 22

Pregnancy and Infancy

Sharon G. Peterson

OBJECTIVES

After reading this chapter, the student should be able to:

1. Describe and define this target population.
2. Describe common oral conditions and diseases of pregnant and infant patients.
3. Describe specific preventive strategies to use with pregnant and infant patients.
4. Describe the role of the dental provider in treating pregnant and infant patients.

KEY TERMS

Target population
Early childhood caries
Pregnancy gingivitis
Preterm birth
Low birth weight

INTRODUCTION TO TARGET POPULATIONS AND PREVENTIVE STRATEGIES

Target population is a term used to represent a certain segment of the population that consists of groups of individuals with similarities of some sort, whether it be age, race, educational background, life situation, and/or health conditions. The term is broad and can represent 3-year-old children, a group of youths involved in a local church group, or even elderly in an assisted-living community. Basically, age can be a representative factor of a target group, but the group members usually have other commonalties as well. An example would be that, although the children in the group are 3 years old, they may also share other characteristics in that they attend the same Head Start program, live in the same geographic area, come from families in similar income sectors, have one parent, and live with extended families. In addition, many of the children have the same ethnic background. So, although we know that these children are 3 years old, many factors are helpful when planning a dental hygiene in-service for this group. This chapter and the chapters that follow will discuss target populations, cultural diversity, and barriers to dental care that may be encountered.

INTRODUCTION TO PREGNANCY AND INFANCY

Pregnancy and infancy present significant risk for oral disease. Current trends show that the medical and dental disciplines are merging interests and expertise to improve access to oral health care services so as to deter the detrimental effects of dental decay, gingival inflammation, and periodontal destruction. These disease processes span the life of the individual and can be diminished or inhibited with well-constructed prevention programs.

The dental profession possesses the knowledge and technology to assist parents in raising children free of dental disease. In fact, the goal of dental care is to help infants and toddlers avoid the pain and devastation that accompanies **early childhood caries** (ECC); provide them with a pleasant, nonthreatening introduction to dental care; and establish and reinforce the foundation of preventive oral habits. The inclusion of oral health in anticipatory guidance during well-child care visits ensures that the child's oral health needs can be addressed in infancy. Recommendations indicate that the first dental risk assessment should occur as early as 6 months of age, and the establishment of a dental home should occur by approximately 1 year of age.[1]

As health professionals, dental care providers must identify the potential for the development of disease and institute effective measures for preventing initiation of the disease; it is then a sound and logical practice to intervene before onset of the disease, rather than treat the effects of the disease. Pediatricians recommend that the infant be evaluated five times during the first year and three times during the second year of life. Although these visits are aimed at evaluating development, prevention, or early detection of disease, physicians should not be expected to provide a thorough oral evaluation or proper preventive oral health counseling. It is the dental professionals that must be proactive and assume the responsibility.

POPULATION CHARACTERISTICS
Pregnant Women

In the short period after the diagnosis of pregnancy, an expectant mother is exposed to a barrage of information applicable to her health and that of her unborn child. Dental health information should be included in this routine. At the time of the oral health consultation, a dentist or dental hygienist should be the source of the essential information.

Women are particularly susceptible to periodontal disease, because female hormones affect the periodontal structures. The increased risk of **pregnancy gingivitis** appears to be primarily the result of resistance changes that occur during pregnancy in the connective tissues composing the structure of the periodontium. If the pregnant mother does not have well-established oral self-care, she may not be aware of these changes. Predominant manifestations are gingival enlargement, increased erythema, tissue sensitivity, and spontaneous bleeding. These manifestations of periodontal diseases can deter the mother from effective oral care.

It is a common misunderstanding that bleeding is a sign of injury. With an increase in gingival inflammation, including bleeding, the pregnant mother often avoids flossing to reduce the incidence of bleeding. In addition, toothbrushing can be problematic if the mother is experiencing morning sickness. The placement or movement of the toothbrush in the posterior of the oral cavity may trigger an overactive gag reflex that is common in morning sickness. The increased acidity in the oral cavity as a result of frequent vomiting can irritate the mucosa and gingiva, as well as increase the probability of demineralized tooth structures. Chronic avoidance of dental care during pregnancy is common; therefore, maintenance of oral health care should be a primary focus of oral health consultation from both the medical and dental professions.

Research studies have consistently reported that oral disease has an effect on systemic diseases such as cardiovascular disease, stroke, endocarditis, and bacterial pneumonia. A relationship has been drawn between the incidence of periodontitis and low-birth-weight, preterm babies. Researchers assert that the litany of inflammatory factors, as a result of the periodontitis process, are not limited to the oral environment.[2] Li, Kolltveit, Tronstad, and Olsen have identified three mechanisms in which oral infections can affect or manifest in a secondary site: "metastatic spread of infection from the oral cavity as a result of transient bacteremia, metastatic injury from the effects of circulating oral microbial toxins, and metastatic inflammation caused by immunological injury induced by oral microorganisms."[3] One or all of these processes probably exist in the mother with periodontitis; however, the concept of injury, as a result of circulating endotoxins that cross the placental barrier, has been the most likely focus of the research.

Infection in the chorion and amniotic apparatus supports an association between **preterm birth** (PTB) or **low birth weight** (LBW) and infection during pregnancy.[4] In an abbreviated explanation, the presence of amniotic inflammatory factors promotes production of cytokines, which release prostaglandins. These prostaglandins, once they have reached a threshold level, appear to facilitate the onset of preterm labor through cervical dilation. In some cases, in which periodontal disease is not the primary cause of premature delivery, it has been identified as a contributing factor to low-birth-weight babies.

Infants

Significant progress has been made toward determining factors that contribute to poor birth outcomes. Rates for mothers receiving prenatal care have increased, tobacco use among pregnant women has decreased, and improvements have been made in neonatal intensive care units. But despite these improvements, PTB and LBW have not shown a corresponding decline. A pioneer in studying the association between pregnancy and periodontal disease, Offenbacher and other researchers were the first to suggest the presence of maternal periodontal disease as a possible factor in delivery of a preterm/low-birth-weight infant. In a case-control study of 124 pregnant women,

they observed that women who delivered an infant weighing less than 2500 grams or at less than 37 weeks' gestation had significantly worse periodontal disease than control women.[5]

PTB and LBW have been shown to be the two most significant predictors of infant health and survival. In fact, LBW is a major worldwide public health problem; these infants confront a significant survival disadvantage that accounts for almost half of the nation's infant mortality. In addition, LBW babies also can suffer from a number of medical disorders such as cerebral palsy, blindness, respiratory conditions, cardiovascular malformations, and other developmental disabilities. Compared with term infants, PTB infants are nearly 7 times more likely to die before their first birthdays. Both PTB and LBW infants account for a large proportion of maternal and neonatal mortality and morbidity.[6]

Oral health counseling should come early, because the first trimester of pregnancy is a critical time. All organ systems are forming during this period. Tooth buds begin formation at the fourth to fifth weeks of gestation, followed by the initial mineralization of bones and teeth from the ninth to twelfth weeks. Stress experienced by the unborn child at this time can produce dento-oral deformities. For example, a cleft lip or palate results when the maxillae fail to unite between the fourth to sixth weeks. These changes can result from a variety of etiologic factors affecting the mother, such as genetics, stress of an injury, severe virus infection, alcohol toxicity, or smoking. An excessive stress to the fetus at any critical time in development can result in a temporary, but often irreparable, arrest in cellular growth.

COMMON ORAL MANIFESTATIONS
Pregnant Women

A study of 903 pregnant women conducted at the University of North Carolina showed a significant increase in women with periodontal disease who exhibited four or more sites with attachment loss measuring greater than or equal to 2 mm. A significant association between maternal periodontal disease, race, smoking, and insurance status was also found. Results showed that pregnant black women were more likely than white women to have periodontal disease.[7]

The effect of periodontal interventions on pregnancy outcome was assessed in a prospective study designed to examine the relationship between periodontal disease and preterm LBW infants in a cohort of young, minority, pregnant, and postpartum women. Of 164 women for whom birth outcome data were available, 74 were subjected to oral prophylaxis during pregnancy, and 90 received no periodontal treatment. The preterm/LBW rate was lower among women who received periodontal treatment compared with those who did not (13.5% versus 18.9%).[8]

Research conducted to estimate whether maternal periodontal disease was predictive of preterm (less than 37 weeks) or very preterm (less than 32 weeks) births showed "the incidence of preterm birth was 11.2% among periodontally healthy women, compared with 28.6% in women with moderate-severe periodontal disease and antepartum moderate-severe periodontal disease was associated with an increased incidence of spontaneous preterm births. The unadjusted rate of very preterm delivery was 6.4% among women with periodontal disease progression, significantly higher than the 1.8% rate among women without disease progression."[9]

Jeffcoat et al. examined the relationship between maternal periodontal disease and spontaneous PTB among 1,313 pregnant women; they found that moderate-severe maternal periodontal disease identified early in pregnancy was associated with an increased risk for spontaneous preterm birth, independent of other traditional risk factors.[10] Clearly periodontal health has an impact on the overall health of the child and warrants the earliest intervention. All health care providers should establish routines of oral health counseling and referral for dental care in early pregnancy. In a study conducted in Washington state, 54% of the pregnant women reported that they had not been counseled on how to care for their teeth and gums, and the overall frequency of pregnant women not receiving dental care during pregnancy was relatively high.[11]

A pregnant woman is often at considerable risk of caries development. The mother's teeth do not lose calcium as postulated in a number of myths; instead, the risk of dental caries probably increases because of changes in eating habits. For example, the sucking of hard candy to reduce nausea, dietary cravings, and frequent between-meal snacks of refined carbohydrates can raise the caries potential of the dental plaque. In addition, the mother often experiences nausea or "morning sickness," causing vomiting with a regurgitation of stomach acid, which may cause erosion and demineralization of the lingual surfaces of the teeth. Many times, only a toothbrush or a sudsy dentifrice is needed to trigger a gag reflex.

Avoidance of aberrant eating habits and snacking, exercise of sugar discipline, and use of xylitol products can greatly minimize the possibility of caries development. There are few reports available that indicate a decrease in caries prevalence of children born to mothers taking a fluoride supplement.[12] Primary teeth could benefit from prenatal exposure to dietary fluoride supplements taken by the mother: however, recent studies do not support maternal prenatal fluoride supplementation.[13] A study of prenatal and postnatal fluoride supplements compared to postnatal fluoride supplementation only was conducted to determine the existing amount of fluoride in enamel and dentin of deciduous teeth. The researchers concluded that "fluoride exposure during the prenatal period offered no additional measurable fluoride uptake by dental tissues beyond that attributable to postnatal fluoride alone.[14] The expectant mother should be provided with appropriate treatment and recall appointments during the period of pregnancy. Professionally applied topical fluorides and systemic fluoride supplementation can benefit the mother's oral health in conjunction with additional daily self-care with fluoride dentifrices and mouthrinses. These measures will both prevent demineralization of the mother's teeth and facilitate remineralization in the event of the development of an incipient lesion.

Infants

Dental caries can and does occur in infants and toddlers well before 3 years of age. Early infant caries has been observed in children as young as 12 months of age.[15–21]

One of the first major hazards to the child's primary dentition is ECCs. This condition has also been referred to as "nursing caries," nursing bottle caries, nursing bottle mouth, baby-bottle syndrome, baby-bottle tooth decay, and bottle-mouth caries. The caries pattern of this condition is highlighted by rampant dental caries initially involving the maxillary primary incisors and progressing to the first primary molars in later stages[18–26] (Figure 22–1 ■). The decay is caused by continual, prolonged exposure of the primary teeth to milk, infant formula, fruit juices, soft drinks, or other sugar/carbohydrate–containing fluids placed in the nursing bottle or sipping ("sippy") cup.

Once teeth erupt, the practice of offering a child a bottle filled with cariogenic fluid as a pacifier or at naptime or bedtime should be discouraged. Once teeth erupt and plaque accumulates, the ingestion of sugar-containing fluids during bedtime or naptime places the child at

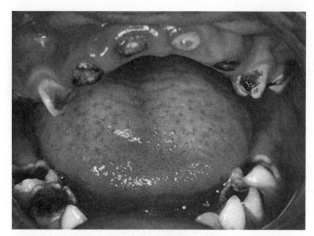

■ **FIGURE 22–1**   Early childhood caries.
(Courtesy of Dr. Lezley McIlveen, Department of Dentistry,
Children's National Medical Center, Washington, DC.)

considerable risk for dental caries, because salivary flow decreases during sleep and the fluid pools around the teeth, creating a highly acidic environment. The pooling of the oral fluids occurs around the maxillary anterior teeth.[19] Not all primary teeth are equally attacked. During sucking of the nipple of either the bottle or the breast, the tongue overlies the lower incisors, which directs the sweetened liquid against the maxillary incisors and to the back of the palate. The mandibular incisors often are either completely intact or only slightly affected, whereas the maxillary incisors bear the brunt of the repeated acid attacks. The other primary teeth are involved to various degrees, depending on the suckling habits of the infant.

The caries attack begins with the appearance of white areas of demineralization around the gingival third of the teeth (Figure 22–1). With time, these incipient lesions begin to turn brown as active caries progresses. Eventually, the carious lesions that ring the cervical areas of the teeth can result in entire crowns being lost, either by fracture of the undermined enamel or by the continuous action of the caries. In either event, only the exposed root is left in the alveolous (Figure 22–1).

A child should not be put to sleep with a bottle or no-spill sippy training cup. Frequent prolonged bottle feedings or use of a sippy cup containing beverages high in sugar (e.g., fruit drinks, soda, or fruit juice), milk, or formula during the day or at night should be avoided.[18] If a bottle is to be used as a pacifier, it should be filled with water only.[23]

Early childhood caries can also occur in some breast-fed children who are nursed every time the infant indicates a desire for feeding (demand feeding, with ten more nursing events over a 24-hour period).[24] However, frequent bottle feeding at night, breast-feeding upon demand, and extended and repetitive use of a no-spill training cup are associated with, but not consistently implicated in, ECC.[25]

The loss of teeth resulting from ECC can have far-reaching effects on the child's eventual face growth.[14] In addition, premature loss of primary molars predisposes children to malocclusion (improper alignment of the jaws and teeth).[27] The loss of tooth function, the ability to chew, or facial variance may result in low self-esteem for both the parent and child.

On occasion, there will be a pattern of multiple, severe caries in a toddler without a substantiated history of early nursing patterns that placed the infant at an increased risk. The caries process is certainly multifactorial and, at times, a definite cause may not be identifiable. Nevertheless, sound primary preventive strategies early on will provide the appropriate environment for the prevention of dental caries.

Evidence suggests that dental caries is an infectious disease process initiated via the transmission of *Streptococcus mutans* from parents to their infants.[28–32] The specific plaque hypothesis suggests microbial specificity in dental caries, and longitudinal evidence supports the role of *S. mutans* in caries initiation.[33,34] The following characteristics of *S. mutans* are important relative to dental caries in children.

- Permanent *S. mutans* colonization of the oral cavity in infants can occur before the primary teeth erupt.[17]
- Sucrose facilitates the adherence of *S. mutans* to the tooth surface.[35,36,37]
- The source of infection of the infant with *S. mutans* is from within the family, most likely the mother.[14–18,38]
- Initial acquisition of infant caries takes place during the "window of infectivity."[38–40]

Transmission of *S. mutans* to the infant most likely occurs in the first year of life, during a specific time period, identified as the window of infectivity, between 6 and 30 months of age. Furthermore, there is higher risk between 18 and 30 months of age.[24,25] If the infant has a high-sucrose diet in the presence of *S. mutans,* the conditions are favorable for the initiation of caries. The early establishment of oral hygiene measures and the adoption of a low-cariogenic diet and low-risk feeding patterns should begin in infancy.

With the above bulleted points as a backdrop, it is possible to develop guidelines that minimize the possibility of transmittal of cariogenic flora from members of the family who will be most closely associated with the child. The most important goal is to reduce the bacterial challenge to the point that the potential for transmission of *S. mutans* is minimal. For the mother especially, this goal will require continual maintenance of a high level of oral hygiene. Preferably, such a program should commence no later than the sixth month of pregnancy and continue throughout the time of the eruption of the child's teeth and onward until a mature, stable, nonpathogenic plaque has been established (i.e., very low *S. mutans* count) on the child's erupted primary teeth.[41] Such a program includes appropriately spaced professional visits for prophylaxis, bacterial counts, and monitoring of oral health. For the mother, the manual and chemical plaque control procedures may include, in addition to the toothbrush, irrigation devices and use of such anti-plaque rinses as chlorhexidine, which can specifically target *S. mutans*. For the child, the most important procedure from time of birth would be a restriction of cariogenic foods and attention to oral hygiene as discussed later in this chapter. Recent studies have validated the use of xylitol products to suppress proliferation of *S. mutans* in both the mother and child.[42,43] The long-term use of xylitol by the mother can prevent caries in the offspring by inhibiting bacterial transference from mother to child and has been found to be very cost-effective.[44,45]

PREVENTIVE STRATEGIES

Preventive strategies for pregnant women and infants need to be initiated in a multifaceted approach that bridges oral health stakeholders. Cross-profession training in the oral disease process and prevention strategies ensures a diverse workforce who can better serve those at risk. The First Five Oral Health training program in the state of California, instituted by the First Five Commission, recognizes the need for cross-profession training. This program is a statewide oral health project to provide various levels of training to oral health and other health providers about the prevention and treatment of dental disease for children aged zero to 5 years. The project's goals are to educate 30,000 dental professionals and 10,000 medical professionals, and to deliver intensive

training to 14,000 dental professionals and more than 3,500 medical professionals statewide. This program also provides education on the prevention of ECC to parents and caretakers of young children, including those with disabilities and other special needs.[46]

Pregnant Women

It is important to provide oral health counseling throughout the pregnancy. The counseling should include dental hygiene and dental care as needed, which, hopefully, would include at least one to two visits to the dental provider. Therefore, oral health counseling and assessment of existing oral conditions should be conducted in the medical office during obstetrical visits, because the mother would be seen more frequently (typically monthly) by her obstetrical doctor. This approach would provide the mother with the most comprehensive prevention efforts during the scope of her pregnancy.

Proper nutrition during pregnancy is essential. Although nutritional deficiencies in the mother usually must be severe to affect the unborn child, a daily balanced diet provides the necessary proteins, fats, carbohydrates, vitamins, and minerals. The American Dietetic Association's position regarding pregnancy is that the key components of a health-promoting lifestyle during pregnancy include appropriate weight gain; consumption of a variety of foods in accordance with the Food Guide Pyramid; appropriate and timely vitamin and mineral supplementation; avoidance of alcohol, tobacco, and other harmful substances; and safe handling of food.[47]

All obstetric services should develop a positive referral system to ensure that expectant mothers receive an early dental examination, preventive oral health counseling for themselves and the future child, as well as necessary treatment. The referral may be to a private practice, a hospital dental service, or to a public health facility.

The mother-to-be should be encouraged to seek a flexible dental program, if available, in which prevention, monitoring, and therapy are commensurate with the severity of the dental condition. Many women who become pregnant are already long overdue for treatment; to postpone needed care for 9 more months could cause severe oral problems, leading to the potential premature or LBW baby. During pregnancy, it would be ideal to see the mother twice during her pregnancy for preventive care and oral health counseling. To accomplish this goal, the mother would need to be seen in the first trimester and the last trimester.

With pregnancy, modification in treatment necessitates alteration of the dental chair incline to accommodate comfort. It is recommended that the mother not be reclined completely in the last trimester because of the potential decrease in blood flow and increased pressure on the fetus. It is common for the mother to experience increased difficulty in breathing while reclining because of the pressure directed toward the diaphragm. With additional pressure directed toward the bladder, treatment may need to be presented in stages with frequent breaks. Dental radiographs for emergencies may be necessary but should be avoided whenever possible during the first trimester. If radiographs are necessary, careful gonadal and abdominal shielding is required as with all dental patients. According to the Food and Drug Administration (FDA), dental radiographs may be prescribed for pregnant patients as long as there is careful adherence to the FDA selection criteria guidelines.[48,49] Dental disease left untreated during pregnancy can lead to problems for both the mother and the fetus, and dental radiographs may be required for proper diagnosis and management.[50]

All therapeutic or restorative dental treatment should be completed by the end of the second trimester, because the position of the baby by the third trimester affects the woman's posture, making long dental appointments quite uncomfortable. Once the treatment is completed, the attending dentist should supply feedback to the obstetrician, indicating completion of the primary, secondary, and tertiary preventive dentistry treatment plans. The collaboration of medical and dental providers can ensure that both the mother and child are being given the greatest opportunity for optimal oral health. Further collaborations in research can draw together financial resources and create cohesive treatment protocols for early intervention programs.

The New York State Health Department has developed the publication *Oral Health Care During Pregnancy and Early Childhood Practice Guidelines*, established to focus on the oral health needs of pregnant women. These recommendations have been developed to assist health care professionals to educate women about oral health and to improve the overall health of women and children. These guidelines will enable health care professionals to work together as a team to improve the care delivered to mothers and children. This improved integration of care is expected to have significant health benefits.[51] An invaluable element of the guide is succinct recommendations for (1) prenatal care providers, (2) oral health professionals, and (3) child health professionals. The guidelines provide supplemental information to be made available to pregnant women on dietary habits, pediatric health and dental care, as well as resources for health professionals on referral for oral care, guidelines for prescribing dental radiographs, anticipatory guidance, and effective prevention programs. This proactive guide demonstrates the national trend to recognize overarching goals of medicine and dentistry.

The Prenatal Education and Treatment project, funded by the Osteopathic Heritage Foundation, is a current program that was initiated by the Columbus Children's Hospital Dental Clinic to incorporate oral health into prenatal health. The program formed a partnership with three local prenatal clinics where low-income pregnant women receive their prenatal care. Risk assessment, dental screening, and education are conducted by a hygienist during prenatal visits as part of overall prenatal care. Case-management activities are incorporated to assist with transportation and establishment of a dental home for those needing treatment (as well as an infant dental home). Follow-up dental services, including comprehensive dental care, are provided at Columbus Children's Hospital Dental Clinic. In addition, the project educates non-dental health professionals about the importance of oral health during pregnancy.[52]

This emphasis on excellent maternal oral health is required for three reasons: (1) to reduce the possibility of onset and/or progression of caries and periodontal disease throughout the pregnancy; (2) to provide a greater possibility of better care for the expected child as a result of the mother's personal involvement with dental treatment, prevention, and counseling; (3) to reduce the number of cariogenic organisms in the mother's mouth.

Infants

Because health professionals can identify the potential for the development of disease and have effective measures available for preventing the initiation of disease, it is a sound and logical practice to intervene before the onset of disease whenever possible, rather than to wait and treat the effects of the disease. Examples of primary prevention exist in pediatric medicine with well-baby evaluations and immunization programs. Pediatricians recommend that the infant be evaluated five times during the first year and three times during the second year of life (Table 22–1 ■). Although these visits are aimed at evaluating development and prevention or early detection of disease, physicians are not adequately trained to provide a thorough dental evaluation or proper preventive dental health counseling. The dental profession must be proactive and assume this responsibility.

■ **Table 22-1** Infant and Toddler Oral Health Anticipatory Guidance Schedule

Age	Appropriate Guidance
Prenatal	Importance of good oral health for mother
	Signs of disease
	Preventing disease
1 month	Function of baby teeth
	Importance of baby teeth
	How decay occurs
3 months	Appropriate bottle use
	Appropriate breast feeding
	Comforting tips
6 months	Characteristics of early childhood caries
	Causes of early childhood caries
	Effects of early childhood caries
	Prevention of early childhood caries
9 months	Importance of cleaning baby teeth
	How to clean baby teeth
	Teach
	"Lift the Lip"
12 months	Switching from breast or bottle to cup
	Importance of regular dental care
	Resources for dental care
18 months	Healthy eating
24 months	Establish that healthy behaviors have been implemented
	Screen for early childhood caries

Source: Nevada State Health Division. Used with permission.

Because of events such as ECC, there is a growing desire by parents of infants and toddlers to receive an early dental evaluation for their children and obtain information on the prevention of dental diseases in their children. According to parents, the major reasons they seek early dental evaluations are:

- Desire for information on preventing tooth decay for their child.
- Desire to avoid unpleasant experiences that the parents had suffered.
- Desire to learn their role in their child's oral health.
- Recommendation by their pediatrician or family physician.

The education process can probably best start with the obstetrician and pediatrician explaining to the expectant or new parents the consequences of continued intake of sugary fluids. The physician can further aid in reducing the problem by prescribing bottle formulas that contain the least sugar. For instance, there is a considerable range in the amount of sugar found in the various commercially available baby foods. Finally, the dental profession should emphasize the need for high-school and community dental education programs to alert would-be parents of their responsibilities in dental care for their infant.

The First Smiles Program in Vancouver, Washington, provides oral hygiene information, fluoride varnish applications, nutrition counseling, and dental referrals to interested clients of the Special Supplemental Nutrition Program for Women, Infants and Children (WIC) at the Clark County Health Department. The First Smiles Program began in 1995 to address the high incidence of decay in Head Start children. The program primarily operates from Medicaid reimbursement. This program is unique because it partners a dental hygienist and WIC staff to improve the oral health of the clients they serve. A nutritionist from WIC provides dietary risk assessment, and the dental hygienist provides dental screenings, fluoride varnish applications, and individualized oral health education. Frequency of return treatment for these children is based on the presence or absence of white spot lesions. Dental hygiene students from Clark

Community College are also used to provide oral health education and dental cleanings at the health department to pregnant women enrolled in WIC. The goal of the First Smiles Program is to prevent or reduce ECC in high-risk children. The program promotes xylitol in their dietary counseling and instructs clients on the benefits of xylitol. The program publishes a patient brochure on how xylitol prevents decay and how to use xylitol gum. [53]

Early Dental Care

The newborn should become accustomed to oral care early. After feeding, the ridges where the teeth will later appear and the palate should be gently wiped with gauze or a soft washcloth. This removes leftover food, and establishes a routine for the mother to clean inside the child's mouth. Children need directly supervised oral hygiene care throughout childhood. It was traditionally recommended that a child should visit the dental office no later than 2 1/2 years of age. Ideally, the child's first dental visit should occur at 6 months of age and no later than 1 year of age.[1] The purpose of this initial visit is to permit an evaluation of the mouth and jaws for proper formation and alignment of structures. A second objective is to allow the child to become familiar with the dental office and its personnel under pleasant circumstances to forestall future apprehension.

Infant Oral Health Education

According to the United Nations' Convention on "The Rights of the Child," articles 2 and 24, all children should have the same rights and have the right to health and medical service. Early childhood caries is a lifestyle disease with biologic, behavioral, and social determinants. An early screening of all children at around 1 year of age is an excellent opportunity for early detection of risk factors and risk indicators that may increase the possibilities for its prevention. The caries risk evaluation should form the base for appropriate recommendations of preventive measures.[54]

The American Academy of Pediatric Dentistry states: "Infant dental care begins with dental health counseling for the newborn, which should include a dental office visit for preventive oral health counseling no later than 12 months of age. However, for those children who are delayed in erupting teeth, the first visit may be postponed, but should occur within 6 months following the eruption of the first tooth."[13]

A federal program called Early and Periodic Screening, Diagnosis, and Treatment (EPSDT), which mandates that medical and dental services be provided to children from low-income families, adopted the policy that children in the EPSDT program receive a dental screening by 12 months of age. A survey of 54 dental school departments of pediatric dentistry showed that 86% teach students to see infants at 12 months of age or younger.[55]

One study evaluated a promotion program for oral health in which "health visitors" met with mothers of 8-month-old babies to address some of the risk factors associated with nursing caries. The program significantly improved the mothers' recall of advice given by health visitors that encouraged the use of a feeder cup, brushing of their babies' teeth with fluoride toothpaste, and restriction of sugary foods and drinks. Significant improvements were also found in recall of advice regarding the use of sugar-free medicine and registration of babies with a dentist. The program also encouraged a higher proportion of the mothers to bring their children to clinics for a hearing check.[56]

The advantages of the infant oral health approach are:

- Identifying and modifying detrimental feeding habits, thus reducing potential risk of caries.
- Assisting parents in establishing for their children dietary and snack patterns that have a low risk of caries.
- Explaining and demonstrating tooth-cleaning procedures for infants and toddlers.
- Determining fluoride status and recommending an optimum fluoride program.
- Introducing dentistry to the child in a pleasant, non-threatening manner.
- Preparing parents for upcoming dental events for their child (anticipatory guidance).

A Protocol For Early Preventive Intervention

The interview The interview process and counseling session should be thorough and specific, yet concise. The attention span of the infant is limited: Once the child becomes bored and seeks attention from the parent(s), their attentiveness to your discussion will be limited at best. Experience shows that the interview and preventive counseling are best accomplished before the examination of the infant for the following reasons:

- Specific parental concerns can be identified and addressed during the examination.
- Should the infant fuss during the examination (normal behavior), the parent(s) usually direct their attention toward the child during the ensuing discussion, not toward the dentist.

• The child can be kept busy with toys or other distractions before the examination in a nonthreatening environment, and the parent(s) will be better able to direct their attention toward the dentist.

The interview should begin with a discussion of the parents' reason for seeking care. Historical information gathered at the initial interview will assist the practitioner in developing the most appropriate and individualized preventive program for the family. Categories of helpful information are discussed in the following paragraphs.

1. *Growth and Development.* An abnormal pattern of development may be discovered or suspected, prompting a referral for further evaluation. Also, the date of the eruption of the first tooth will provide a baseline for determining patterns of dental development and assist in answering future questions from parents regarding their child's dental development.

2. *Feeding History.* Knowledge of the feeding patterns during infancy is critical (1) to assist the dentist in assessing the child's risk for developing ECC by discovering potentially harmful feeding habits, and (2) to help form a basis for recommendations regarding proper feeding practices that minimize the potential for dental disease.

3. *Medical History.* A complete medical history is important. Knowledge of any systemic conditions that may adversely affect dental health will assist in developing appropriate preventive strategies. For example, long-term, frequent intake of sucrose-based medications may require additional recommendations for tooth cleaning to offset the increased caries risk from the sucrose intake.

4. *Preventive Assessment.* Information regarding dental development, dental health attitudes, and current oral hygiene practices will serve as a starting point for counseling parents about an appropriate preventive program for their child. A history of tooth decay in the family ("soft teeth") will provide insight into the environmental influences as well as parental attitudes about dental health and serve to guide the dentist's discussion regarding preventive strategies.

5. *Fluoride Supplementation.* It is important to know if the child has access to fluoride in drinking water. It is not sufficient to establish that a family lives in a fluoridated community. On occasion, the family may drink bottled water, which contains an unknown quantity of fluoride. On the other hand, a family drinking well water may or may not be receiving systemic fluoride depending on the concentration of fluoride in the water. Before any fluoride supplements are prescribed, the water should be tested for fluoride concentration; then, supplements should be prescribed accordingly. Some families live in rural settings with well water, but the child spends the majority of the day in a location with fluoridated water such as a day care facility or school. Therefore, an accurate assessment of all potential sources of fluoride intake should be explored before making any recommendations regarding fluoride supplementation.

If the daily intake of fluoride is insufficient, parents should be informed that small daily dosages are beneficial to a child's teeth. Table 22–2 ■ will aid in determining the amount of fluoride supplementation needed. Initially, supplementation is best accomplished by the use of fluoride drops. Around the age of 3 years, the drops can be replaced by fluoride tablets, which are swallowed. Later, as the child gains skill in chewing the tablet, the fluoride-laden saliva can be swished around the mouth and then swallowed to provide a topical application as well as systemic benefits. The practice of using a tablet a day should continue until the child is at least 12 years old, although many believe that fluoride supplementation should be considered as long as the individual—child or adult—has a fluoride-deficient intake.

6. *Oral Hygiene.* An assessment of current tooth-cleaning activities is important to establish the parents' role in oral hygiene for their child. Many parents think

■ **Table 22–2**   Fluoride Supplementation Depends on the Fluoride Content of the Drinking Water

Age	*< 0.3 ppm*	*0.3–0.6 ppm*	*> 0.6 ppm*
Birth–6 mos.	0	0	0
6 mos.–3 yrs.	0.25	0	0
3 yrs.–6 yrs.	0.5	0.25	0
6 yrs.–16 yrs.	1.0	0.5	0

that allowing an infant or toddler to brush their own teeth is adequate. If the infant's teeth are being brushed, it is important to establish how, when, and by whom, and to inquire whether the parents experience any difficulties during the process.

In one study, almost half of the parents interviewed had started toothbrushing programs for their infants at 12 months and 75% had done so by 18 months.[57] With such infant and toddler toothbrushing programs, only a small amount, approximately the size of a pea, of a fluoridated dentifrice should be used to avoid the possibility of the child ingesting an excess of fluoride. Around the age of 6 years, daily fluoride mouthrinses may be initiated as part of the total lifelong program for oral health.

The following are a recommended set of interview questions to ask pregnant women and new mothers within the first 30 months of the child's life:[58]

- Do you have any problems with your teeth?
- Does your family have any inherited problems/ diseases affecting the teeth?
- Do you know the fluoride status of your drinking water?
- Are you brushing and flossing regularly?
- As your child grows up, do you think you can help your child prevent tooth decay? What kinds of things do you want to do to protect your child's teeth?

Counseling   On the basis of the information gathered to this point, the practitioner is ready to provide recommendations on how parents can play an active role in preventing dental disease in their child by assuming responsibility for the child's oral hygiene and diet.

Parents should be educated regarding the following tooth-cleaning recommendations:

- A parent, other adult, or older sibling must assume total responsibility for tooth cleaning in infants and young children. Many children are unable to perform adequate plaque removal until they are 6 to 8 years of age.
- Tooth cleaning should be done in a comfortable location and pleasant environment. Positioning will be demonstrated during the examination.
- A dentifrice is not necessary for infants. In many cases, it may be a source for objection because of the taste and foaming action.

- If a dentifrice is used, only a pea-sized amount should be placed on the brush to avoid ingestion of excess fluoride.
- Tooth cleaning should be accomplished with a small, soft-bristled toothbrush.
- Tooth cleaning should be accomplished at least once daily.
- The evening tooth cleaning may be easier to accomplish after the infant's last feeding instead of waiting until just before bedtime, because a tired infant can frequently be fussy during the procedure.

Parents have control, for the most part, over their child's diet during the early years. The exceptions include time spent with babysitters and in day care settings. Parents can have some influence in those situations, however, if they make their wishes known. The following information should be shared with parents.

- Infants should be weaned from the bottle around 12 months of age.
- The bottle should not be used as a pacifier nor given during bedtime or naptime.
- Only water, formula, or milk should be offered in the bottle.
- Frequent, prolonged episodes of breast-feeding could be a caries risk.
- Sleeping with the child and allowing nursing through the night should be avoided.
- Infants and young children generally will eat more frequently than three times daily.
- Between-meal snacks should consist of foods that have a low cariogenic potential.
- Total amount of cariogenic foods is not the issue; rather, the frequency of ingestion and retentiveness of the food are the factors that contribute to the caries risk.

The examination   Once the interview and counseling aspects of the visit are completed, the dentist is ready to proceed with the examination of the infant or toddler. The dental chair and overhead light are neither required nor very useful for examining children this young. Because one of the prime objectives is to provide a dental examination in a pleasant, nonthreatening manner, the procedure is best accomplished in the knee-to-knee position for children under 3 years of age. This position provides a stable, yet comfortable, environment that incorporates the security of parental involvement, which may produce a calming effect on infants and toddlers who lack the cognitive ability to cooperate. Should the child offer resistance, the dentist can easily and gently stabilize the child's mouth and head, which is cradled in the dentist's lap, while the parent holds the child's hands and, if needed, stabilizes the child's legs by cradling them with the elbows. Many of the infants and toddlers accept the examination procedures in this position without resistance. It is important in those instances in which the children resist or cry that the parents be assured that the behavior is normal (and expected) for the child's age and should not be considered "bad" or "uncooperative."

The examination should begin with a soft touch, with the extraoral head and neck conditions evaluated first, allowing the child to become accustomed to the dentist's actions. The examination of the oral cavity should begin by using the fingers to palpate the oral structures before introducing the dental instruments. Illumination can be provided with a penlight or flashlight held by the dental assistant. Access and stabilization of the mouth can be obtained by placing a finger on the gum pad distal to the most posterior tooth in a maxillary quadrant. After inspection of the oral soft and hard tissues, a dental cleaning (plaque removal) is accomplished with a soft-bristled, moist, child-sized toothbrush. Rarely will a rubber cup and polishing paste be required for stain removal. The tooth-cleaning process is discussed and demonstrated as you remove the plaque. At this point, it is very important that the child be repositioned with the head cradled in the parent's lap and the parent given the opportunity to practice the tooth-cleaning process with the dentist's supervision and guidance. This approch will help some parents get over their reluctance to clean their child's teeth, especially when the child resists. Occasionally, some infants and toddlers exhibit tight contacts between the anterior as well as the posterior teeth, which accumulate considerable plaque. The parent can be shown how to clean these areas using dental floss in a holder with relative ease. The parents are advised that they need to perform tooth cleaning for their child at least once per day, but preferably after each meal. The most critical time to clean the teeth is after the last meal or snack of the day. It is emphasized that toothpaste is not required and is usually objectionable to the infant. If it is used, only a minimal quantity should be placed on the brush.

It should also be emphasized early that, when the child is becoming accustomed to the routine of having a parent brush the teeth, the tooth cleaning should not become an unpleasant struggle for those infants and toddlers who initially resist the procedure. On those occasions when the child struggles considerably, the procedure should not be abandoned. Rather, less attention can be placed on performing thorough plaque removal, while maintaining a consistent effort to establish a routine with the child. A more thorough tooth cleaning can be performed another day when the child is more cooperative. Parents can be reminded of other routines that are accomplished despite the child's objections, such as washing the child's hair. If the tooth-cleaning routine is established during the first 12 months of age, strong objections and resistance to the procedure during the "terrible twos" can usually be avoided.

Concluding the appointment   The appointment is concluded by addressing the following areas:

- Provide the parents with a summary of your clinical findings.
- Make appropriate recommendations that are based on the clinical findings.
- Solicit and answer any remaining questions that the parents may have.
- Reinforce the parents' role and responsibilities in their child's oral health care.
- Establish an optimal fluoride program (pending any water analysis).
- Distribute educational pamphlets/brochures as desired.
- Provide anticipatory guidance information.
- Establish an appropriate recall schedule.

Anticipatory guidance   Anticipatory guidance is a process for preparing the parents for upcoming developmental changes and concerns that may arise before the next scheduled dental visit so as to minimize the negative effects that may arise. Wherever possible, information on preventive oral health should be provided to expectant parents during prenatal education programs.

Establishing a recall schedule   The recall appointment may be scheduled for 3, 6, or 12 months depending on the child's potential risk for developing dental disease, which is based on clinical findings, stage of dental development, and feeding or diet patterns. Examples for determining appropriate recall schedules are listed in (Table 22–3 ■).

■ **Table 22–3** Clinical Findings According to Child's Age and Expected Feeding or Diet Patterns and Dental Development Characteristics

	Clinical Findings	*Feeding or Diet Patterns*	*Dental Development*
3 months	Enamel decalcification Considerable plaque build-up Amelogenesis imperfecta Dentinogenesis imperfecta	Bottle used at bedtime or naptime Bottle used as a pacifier Bottle used past 12 months of age Frequent cariogenic diet or snacks	Stage of dental development has minimal influence on decision for a 3-month recall
6 months	Posterior proximal contacts No previous tooth cleaning Primary dentition crowding Moderate plaque build-up	Relatively cariogenic diet or frequent snacking on cariogenic foods	Second primary molar eruption is anticipated within 6 months
12 months	Generalized spacing present Good oral hygiene exhibited Shallow occlusal anatomy	Good dietary habits exhibiting a low cariogenic potential	Second primary molar eruption anticipated within 12 months

SUMMARY

The potential exists today for dental health professionals to assist parents in raising caries-free children. The knowledge and technology are available, and the request for this service is growing. The dental professional has the opportunity to accept this role with enthusiasm and continue to be a leader among the health professions in disease prevention. Dental providers must not ignore the oral health needs of infants and toddlers under 3 years of age. They must, instead, take advantage of their knowledge and technology to begin disease prevention efforts with children as infants and to educate parents-to-be and new parents about their important role in the oral health of their children. By doing so, dental providers can provide a pleasant and logical introduction to dentistry and promote the profession in a most positive way.

REFERENCES

1. New York State Department of Health. (2006, August). *Oral health care during pregnancy and early childhood practice guidelines.* Albany, NY: New York State Department of Health, 6–9, 15. Also available at: http://www.health.state.ny.us/publications/0824.pdf.

2. Thoden van Velzen, S. K., Abraham-Inpijn, L., & Moorer, W. R. (1984). Plaque and systemic disease: A reappraisal of the focal infection concept. *J Clin Periodontol,* 11:209–20.

3. Li, X., Kolltveit, K. M., Tronstad, L., & Olsen, I. (2000, October). Systemic diseases caused by oral infection. *Clin Micrbiol Rev,* 13(4):547–58.

4. Offenbacher, S., Beck, J. D., Lieff, S., & Slade, G. (1998). Role of periodontitis in systemic health: Spontaneous preterm birth. *J Dent Educ,* 62:852–58.

5. Offenbacher, S., Katz, V., Fertik, G., Collins, J., Boyd, D., Maynor, G., McKaig, R., & Beck, J. (1996). Periodontal infection as a possible risk factor for preterm low birth weight. *J Periodontol,* 67:1103–13.

6. ACOG Practice Bulletin. (2001). Assessment of risk factors for preterm birth. Clinical management guidelines for obstetrician-gynecologists. Number 31, October 2001. *Obstet Gynecol,* 98(4):709–16.

7. Jared, H. L., Lieff, S., Wilder, R. S., & Offenbacher, S. (1999, March). Periondontal disease and low birthweight: A critical link. *Access,* 13:32–37.

8. Lieff, S., Boggess, K. A., Murtha, A. P., Jared, H., Madianos, P. N., Moss, K., Beck, J., & Offenbacher, S. (2004). The oral conditions and pregnancy study: Periodontal status of a cohort of pregnant women. *J Periodontol,* 75(1):116–26.

9. Offenbacher S., Boggess, K. A., Murtha, A. P., Jared, H. L., Lieff, S., McKaig, R. G., Mauriello, S. M., Moss, K. L., & Beck, J. D. (2006, January). Progressive periodontal disease and risk of very preterm delivery. *Obstet Gynecol.* 107(1):29–36.

10. Jeffcoat, M. K., Geurs, N. C., Reddy, M. S., Cliver, S. P., Goldenerg, R. L., & Hauth, J. C. (2001). Periodontal infection and preterm birth: Results of a prospective study. *J Am Dent Assoc,* 132:875–80.

11. Lydon-Rochelle, M. T., Krakowiak, P., Hujoel, P. P., & Peters, R. M. (2004). Dental care use and self-reported dental problems in relation to pregnancy. *Am J Public Health,* 94(5):765–71.

12. Casamassimo, P. S. (2001, July). Maternal oral health. *Dent Clin North Am,* 45(3):469-78, v-vi.

13. Moss, S. J. (1988). The year 2000 health objectives for the nation. *Pediatr Dent,* 10:228–33.

14. Sa Roriz Fonteles, C., Zero, D. T., Moss, M. E., & Fu, J. (2005, Nov-Dec). Fluoride concentrations in enamel and dentin of primary teeth after pre- and postnatal fluoride exposure. *Caries Res* 39 (6): 505–508.

15. Dimitrova, M. M., Kukleva, M. P., & Kondeva, V. K. (2000). A study of caries polarization in 1-, 2- and 3-year-old children. *Folia Med* (Plovdiv), 42:55–59.

16. Dimitrova, M. M., Kukleva, M. P., & Kondeva, V. K. (2000). Specificity of caries attack in early childhood. *Folia Med* (Plovdiv), 42:50–54.

17. Dimitrova, M. M., Kukleva, M. P., & Kondeva, V. K. (2000). Early childhood caries—incidence and need for treatment. *Folia Med* (Plovdiv), 42:46–49.

18. Behrendt, A., Sziegoleit, F., Muler-Lessmann, V., Ipek-Ozdemir, G., & Wetzel, W. E. (2001). Nursing-bottle syndrome caused by prolonged drinking from vessels with bill-shaped extensions. *ASDC J Dent Child,* 68:47–50.

19. Petti, S., Cairella, G., & Tarsitani, G. (2000). Rampant early childhood dental decay: An example from Italy. *J Public Health Dent,* 60:159–66.

20. Faye, M., Ba, A. A., Yam, A. A., Ba, I. (2006). Caries patterns and diet in early childhood caries. *Dakar Med.* 51(2):72–77.

21. Psoter, W. J., Pendrys, D. G., Morse, D. E., Zhang, H., Mayne, S. T. (2006 Winter). Associations of ethnicity/race and socioeconomic status with early childhood caries patterns. *J Public Health Dent.* 66(1):23–29.

22. Dini, E. L., Holt, R. D., & Bedi, R. (2000). Caries and its association with infant feeding and oral health-related behaviours in 3-4-year-old Brazilian children. *Community Dent Oral Epidemiol,* 28:241–48.

23. National Maternal and Child Oral Health Resource Center. (2006). Open wide: Oral health training for health professionals. Retrieved 3/07 from http://www.mchoralhealth.org/OpenWide/index.htm.

24. Valaitis, R., Hesch, R., Passarelli, C., Sheehan, D., & Sinton, J. (2000). A systematic review of the relationship between breastfeeding and early childhood caries. *Can J Public Health,* 91:411–17.

25. Mouradian, W. E., Huebner, C. E., Ramos-Gomez, F., Slavkin, H. C. (2007 May). Beyond access: The role of family and community in children's oral health. *J Dent Educ.* 71(5):619–31.

26. U.S. Department of Health and Human Services. (2000). Healthy people 2010 (Vol. II) (2nd ed.). Washington, DC: U.S. Department of Health and Human Services. Also available at: http://www.healthypeople.gov/Document/HTML/Volume2/21Oral.htm.

27. Herbert, F. L., Lenchner, V., & Pinkham, J. R. (1994). In Starkey, P. A., Ed. *The answer book.* Chicago: American Society of Dentistry for Children.

28. Thorild, I., Lindau-Jonson, B., & Twetman, S. (2002). Prevalence of salivary *Streptococcus mutans* in mothers and in their preschool children. *Int J Paediatr Dent,* 12:2–7.

29. Li, Y., Wang, W., & Caufield, P. W. (2000). The fidelity of mutans streptococci transmission and caries status correlate with breast-feeding experience among Chinese families. *Caries Res,* 34:123–32.

30. Ercan, E., Dülgergil, C. T., Yildirim, I., Dalli, M. (2007, August). Prevention of maternal bacterial transmission on children's dental-caries-development: 4-year results of a pilot study in a rural-child population. *Arch Oral Biol.* 52(8):748–52.

31. Berkowitz, R. (2006). Mutans streptococci: Acquisition and transmission. *Pediatr Dent,* 28(2):106–109.

32. Lindquist, B., & Emilson, C. (2004) Colonization of Streptococcus mutans and Streptococcus sobrinus genotypes and caries development in children to mothers harboring both species. *Caries Res,* 38(2):95–103.

33. Li, S., Liu, T. J., Xiao, X. R., Ye, W. W. (2004, November). Acquisition of Mutans streptococci by children of 3-4 years with possible source of the pathogen from their mothers. *Sichuan Da Xue Xue Bao Yi Xue Ban.* 35(6):818–20.

34. Tanzer, J. M., Livingston, J., & Thompson, A. M. (2001). The microbiology of primary dental caries in humans. *J Dent Educ,* 65:1028–37.

35. Ooshima, T., Matsumura, M., Hoshino, T., Kawabata, S., Sobue, S., & Fujiwara, T. (2001). Contributions of three glycosyltransferases to sucrose-dependent adherence of *Streptococcus mutans. J Dent Res,* 80:1672–77.

36. Sheiham, A. (2001). Dietary effects on dental diseases. *Public Health Nutr,* 4:569–91.

37. Shemesh, M., Tam, A., Steinberg, D. (2007, November). Expression of biofilm-associated genes of Streptococcus mutans in response to glucose and sucrose. *J Med Microbiol.* 56(Pt 11):1528–35.

38. Caufield, P. W., Dasanayake, A. P., Li, Y., Pan, Y., Hsu, J., & Hardin, J. M. (2000). Natural history of Streptococcus sanguinis in the oral cavity of infants: Evidence for a discrete window of infectivity. *Infect Immun,* 68:4018–23.

39. Carletto, K. F., Cornejo, L., & Gimenez, M., (2005). Early acquisition of Streptococcus mutans for children. *Acta Odontol Latinoam,* 18(2):69–74.

40. Brambilla, E., Felloni, A., Gagliani, M., Malerba, A., García-Godoy, F., & Strohmenger, L. (1998). Caries prevention during pregnancy. Results of a 30-month study. *J Am Dent Assoc,* 129:871–77.

41. Russell, S. L., & Mayberry, L. J. (2008 Jan-Feb). Pregnancy and oral health: A review and recommendations to reduce gaps in practice and research. *MCN Am J Matern Child Nurs.* 33(1):32–37.

42. Caglar, E., Kavaloglu, S. C., Kuscu, O. O., Sandalli, N., Holgerson, P. L., & Twetman, S. (2007, December). Effect

of chewing gums containing xylitol or probiotic bacteria on salivary mutans streptococci and lactobacilli. *Clin Oral Investig.* 11(4):425–29. Epub 2007 June 16.

43. Haresaku, S., Hanioka, T., Tsutsui, A., Yamamoto, M., Chou, T., & Gunjishima, Y. (2007). Long-term effect of xylitol gum use on mutans streptococci in adults. *Caries Res.* 2007; 41(3):198–203.

44. Soderling, E., Isokangas, P., Pienihakkinen, K., Tenovuo, J., & Alanen, P. (2001). Influence of maternal xylitol consumption on mother-child transmission of mutans streptococci: 6-year follow-up. *Caries Res,* 35(3):173–77.

45. Thorild, I., Lindau, B., & Twetman, S. (2003). Effect of maternal use of chewing gums containing xylitol, chlorhexidine or fluoride on mutans streptococci colonization in the mothers' infant children. *Oral Health Prev Dent,* 1(1):53–57.

46. First Five Training Program. Healthy teeth begin at birth. Retrieved 3/28/08 from http://www.first5oralhealth.org/downloads/brochure_May_25_2005.pdf.

47. Kaiser, L. L., & Allen, L. American Dietetics Association. (2002). Nutrition and lifestyle for a healthy pregnancy outcome. (Position paper on Nutrition and Pregnancy). *J Am Diet Assoc,* 102:1470–90.

48. National Council for Radiation Protection & Measurements. (2003). *Radiation protection in dentistry.* Bethesda, MD: National Council for Radiation Protection & Measurements.

49. U.S. Department of Health and Human Services, Public Health Service, Food and Drug Administration; and American Dental Association, Council on Dental Benefit Programs, Council on Scientific Affairs. (2004). The selection of patients for dental radiographic examinations. (Rev. ed.). Retrieved from http://www.ada.org/prof/resources/topics/radiography.

50. Little, J. W., Falace, D. A., Miller, C. S., & Rhodus, N. L. (2002). *Dental management of the medically compromised patient.* (6th ed.). St. Louis: Mosby, 306.

51. New York State Department of Health. (2006, August). *Oral health care during pregnancy and early childhood practice guidelines.* Albany, NY: New York State Department of Health, 31–38. Also available at: http://www.health.state.ny.us/publications/0824.pdf.

52. Homa, A., & Casamassimo, P. S. (2007, Nov). Access to dental care during pregnancy: An innovative approach. *APHA 135th Annual Meeting and Expo. Poster Abstract.,* Program Information: http://apha.confex.com/apha/135am/techprogram/paper_147787.htm.

53. First Smiles Program. (1995). "Xylitol Gum." Vancouver, WA: Clark County Public Health. Retrieved 3/26/08 from http://www.co.clark.wa.us/health/oralhealth/documents/xylitol-eng-1.pdf.

54. Twetman, S., Garcia-Godoy, F., & Goepferd, S. J. (2000). Infant oral health. *Dent Clin North Am,* 44:487–505.

55. McWhorter, A. G., Seale, N. S., & King, S. A. (2001). Infant oral health education in U.S. dental school curricula. *Pediatr Dent,* 23:407–409.

56. Hamilton, F. A., Davis, K. E., & Blinkhorn, A. S. (1999). An oral health promotion programme for nursing caries. *Int J Paediatr Dent,* 9:195–200.

57. Davies, G. M., Duxbury, J. T., Boothman, N. J., Davies, R. M., & Blinkhorn, A. S. (2005, June). A staged intervention dental health promotion programme to reduce early childhood caries. *Community Dent Health.* 22(2):118–22.

58. Holt, K., & Barzel, R. (2006). Health professional's guide to pediatric oral health management. National Maternal and Child Oral Health Resource Center (OHRC). Retrieved 3/3/07 from http://www.mchoralhealth.org/PediatricOH/mod2_2_2.htm.

Chapter 23

Pediatrics

Tamara L. Donald

OBJECTIVES

After reading this chapter, the student should be able to:

1. Describe and define this pediatric population.
2. Describe common oral conditions and diseases of pediatric patients.
3. Describe specific preventive strategies to use with pediatric patients.
4. Describe the role of the dental provider in treating pediatric patients.

KEY TERMS

Early childhood
School-aged
Adolescence
Cognitive development
Social learning theory
Classical conditioning
Operant conditioning
Psychosocial development
Easy child
Difficult child
Slow-to-warm-up child
Early childhood caries
Behavior management
Communication
Tell-show-do technique
Voice control
Positive reinforcement
Distraction

INTRODUCTION

Oral health is essential in children's overall health, functional capacity, and social welfare.[1] Dental care is an indispensable health service for children, because dental caries and untreated dental disease can have significant consequences for a child's health and well-being. Children can experience pain, infection, dysfunction, poor appearance, and low self-esteem as well as drastic alterations to their ability to eat, communicate, sleep, and play.[1–3] Furthermore, dental caries and untreated dental disease provide a reservoir of infection for systemic spread and have been associated with low social functioning and failure to thrive.[4,5]

For a child, dental experiences are a unique psychological and behavioral experience, which can cause distinct challenges to the delivery of treatment. These challenges place unique demands on dental providers.[6] The highest level of technical skill and knowledge is used when treating a child patient. To ensure effective treatment, dental professionals need familiarity with the developmental norms of different ages and an understanding of the underlying dynamics of childhood. As this requirement indicates, treating children is different.

One reason we have not made more progress in eradicating common oral diseases in childhood may be a narrow interpretation of their needs, which fails to consider the broader social, developmental, and environmental context of children's lives.[5]

POPULATION CHARACTERISTICS

Dental care has been identified as the most prevalent unmet health need in U.S. children.[4] Millions of children continue to suffer needlessly from preventable oral diseases as a result of extensive disparities existing in oral health and access to care.[1,2,4,7] Furthermore, dental caries remains the preeminent oral disease of childhood.[1,2,7,8]

The vast majority of children are affected by dental caries to some degree by the time they reach adulthood.[8] Children from lower-income households and ethnic minority families are disproportionately affected by dental caries, because prevalence and severity of childhood dental caries are linked to socioeconomic status across all age groups.[1,2,5,7] Consequently, this group of children experiences 80% of all dental caries.[1,4]

American children experience an estimated 52 million hours lost from school in addition to problems with schoolwork completion and deterioration of school performance because of dental problems.[2,3,5] Children also experience costly emergency room visits, and hospital-based medical and surgical treatments because of pain or dental problems.[1,5] Moreover, children with poor oral health may be subjected to acute or chronic pain; the impact of pain on children varies depending on the child's developmental level.[9]

Many changes have evolved since the years when dental care for children was predominately secondary and tertiary care.[7,8,10] Today, however, pediatric dental care is prevention-oriented. By limiting children's experience of dental pain and infection, their capacity to function well, grow normally, and engage in normal activities will be enhanced.[1] Accordingly, dental professionals possess the potential to reduce oral disease in children and establish a healthy functioning dentition through the use of preventive dental services.

In childhood, changes occur rapidly, particularly changes in children's abilities to think, reason, understand, and consequently make thoughtful decisions about their behavior. The rapidity and power of such changes make knowledge imperative for anyone wishing to understand the health care needs of any child at any given age.[11]

Each period of development is characterized by specific, sequentially developing skills and traits. Dental providers must consider the ability or readiness of a child to perform a given task and assess the child's capacity for understanding information and cooperating with care.[5,12] It is critical that dental providers be competent in approaching children during different stages of development to build a trusting relationship.[13] Although adult patients require a one-to-one relationship involving the dental provider and patient, children necessitate a one-to-two relationship consisting of the dental provider, child patient, and parent.[12] Consequently, every time a child presents for treatment, parental concerns must be considered as well.[14]

This section will focus on the pediatric patient, involving the **early childhood** (2–5 years), **school-aged** (6–11 years), and **adolescence** (12–19 years) stages of development. Although each stage illustrates the behavior trends for each age group, the information is given as a guide to anticipated abilities and behaviors in children, because each child has an individual pattern of growth.

Child Development

Children are not little adults; they are dynamic beings who are in a state of constant development.[15,16] Children encounter diverse challenges and specific needs in each developmental stage, which require fulfillment so they can progress to the next stage. Therefore, to better understand children's behavior and respond to their age-related needs, dental providers must have a philosophical appreciation of child development, and they must recognize that the major changes taking place in the various stages of growth and development are important considerations that impact preventive care and treatment.[6]

Child development theories can provide a framework for understanding many issues related to children, such as behaviors, their own understanding of their illness process and treatments, their interaction with peers and family members, and their ability to cope in others settings.[17] This understanding can help guide the dental professionals in planning, implementing, and evaluating patient care while fostering the healthy development of children.

Piaget's Cognitive Developmental Theory

Jean Piaget theorized that children actively construct their understanding of the world and go through four stages of **cognitive development** (Table 23–1 ■): sensorimotor (birth to 2 years of age), preoperational (2 to 7 years of age), concrete operational (7 to 11 years of age), and formal operational (11 years of age through adulthood).[13,18,19] The stages occur in a fixed sequence in which the accomplishments of one stage provide the foundation for the next stage, and the transition from one stage to another is gradual, not abrupt; children often show aspects of two stages while going through these transitions.[20]

Piaget's stages of cognitive development provide additional aspects of development to consider when treating the child patient: their intellectual capabilities and their level of understanding.[13] This cognitive development is crucial to a child's ability to understand the relationships between behavior and health, and to make decisions about their own health behavior. A child's understanding may affect how they interpret and comply with treatment. Children's increasing cognitive sophistication leads them toward a greater ability to engage in self-protective behavior and to assume responsibility for preventing problems and promoting health. A child's age may influence the psychological and behavioral responses to illness and treatment.[11]

Social Learning Theory

Albert Bandura studied how learning through observation (modeling and imitation) affects behavior and thought. He contended that many behaviors or responses are

■ **Table 23–1**   Piaget's Four Stages of Cognitive Development

Age Range	Stage of Development	Primary Points of Development
Birth–2 years	Sensorimotor stage	The infant constructs an understanding of the world by coordinating sensory experiences with physical actions. An infant progresses from reflexive, instinctual action at birth to the beginning of symbolic thought toward the end of the stage.
2–7 years	Preoperational stage	The child begins to represent the world with words and images. These words and images reflect increased symbolic thinking and go beyond the connection of sensory information and physical action.
7–11 years	Concrete operational stage	The child can now reason logically about concrete events and classify objects into different sets.
11 years–adulthood	Formal operational stage	The adolescent reasons in more abstract, idealistic, and logical ways.

Source: Modified from Santrock, 2004;[18] Beauman, 2001;[13] Child Development Institute, 1998–2005;[15] and Microsoft Corporation, 2005.[19]

acquired through observational learning.[20] Bandura's **social learning theory** emphasizes reciprocal interactions among the person, behavior, and environment.[19] It maintains that children can learn through observations of others or from vicarious experience through others.[21] An example would be a child watching another child patient cry or scream during dental treatment. The very act of observing a negative reaction to dental treatment could cause the observing child to become fearful of dental treatment. Essentially, by observing the person's experience, that particular experience also becomes the child's.[21]

Pavlov's Classical Conditioning

Ivan Pavlov's theory was based on the principle of **classical conditioning,** in which a neutral stimulus acquires the ability to produce a response originally produced by another stimulus, that is, learning by association. It occurs when a person makes a mental association between two events or stimuli, and a simple encounter with the first stimulus produces a response once associated only with the second stimulus.[19] For instance, many children have developed a dental phobia after having painful dental procedures. These children fear a dental drill, along with a wide range of stimuli associated with it—the waiting room, the dental chair, the dental operatory. In the conditioning of fear, a conditioned stimulus, such as the dental drill, is associated with an aversive stimulus, such as the pain that can happen in the course of a dental procedure, in a new or unfamiliar environment. After one such pairing (dental drill and pain), children can develop a long-lasting fear of the conditioned stimulus and of the context.

Skinner's Operant Conditioning

B. F. Skinner's theory says the consequences of a behavior produce changes in the probability of the behavior's occurrence, a process of trial and error known as **operant conditioning.**[18,22] Skinner claimed that the inner mental events such as thoughts, feelings, or perceptions are themselves behaviors and, like any other behaviors, are shaped and determined by environmental forces.[20] Reinforcement is a key concept in operant conditioning; this concept may be defined as any event that follows a response and strengthens or increases the probability of the response being repeated.[20] Positive reinforcement (toys, stickers, hand shakes, verbal praise) increases the probability that behavior will be repeated, and a negative reinforcement (punishment, omission, avoidance) decreases the probability that the behavior will be repeated.[19,22]

Just as individuals engage in behaviors to get positive reinforcement, they also engage in behaviors to avoid or escape unpleasant conditions. Therefore, it is important to reinforce only desired behavior, and it is equally important to avoid reinforcing behavior that is not desired.[22] For instance, halting treatment because of behavioral resistance by a child (negative reinforcement) is likely to reinforce undesirable behavior for subsequent visits, because the child has now established that the previous response (behavioral resistance) successfully ended the perceived unpleasant condition (treatment).

Erikson's Psychosocial Theory

Erikson's theory describes **psychosocial development** as a series of eight stages (Table 23–2 ■). Each stage consists of a unique developmental task that confronts individuals with a crisis that must be resolved.[18] Erikson's first five stages are related to the child patient. These stages and their associated psychosocial crises are trust versus mistrust (birth to 1 year of age); autonomy versus shame and doubt (1 to 3 years of age); initiative versus guilt (3 to 6 years of age); industry versus inferiority (7 to 12 years of age); and identity versus identity confusion (adolescence to early adulthood).[13,18,23]

Erikson's stages of psychosocial development provide a framework for approaching children at different ages and stages with consideration for their emotional needs. Psychosocial development refers to the changes in a child's relationships with other people, especially their ability to function as an autonomous individual. Enhancements in psychosocial development influence a child's behavior with regard to health promotion and prevention, their psychological response to illness, and the ability to assume personal responsibility for their health.[13,23]

Early Childhood Development: 2 to 5 Years of Age

Physical

Physical growth during early childhood is characterized by a steady rate of change. Children typically grow about 3 inches in height and approximately 4.5 pounds annually, with a broad range of variation for normal height and weight. During this time, children become taller, slimmer, heavier, and less top-heavy. Also, their gross motor skills (Table 23–3 ■) continue to increase dramatically as the child masters the standing posture, walking becomes

■ **Table 23-2** Erickson's Psychosocial Developmental Stages

Stage of Development and Basic Conflict	Age Range	Important Events and Primary Points of Development
Trust versus mistrust (hope)	Birth–1 year	A sense of trust requires infants' basic physical needs to be met and a loving, nurturing, relationship to be formed with parents or caregiver. If requirements are not met, infants will develop insecurity and mistrust. Trust in infancy allows a lifelong expectation that the world will be a good and pleasant place to live.
Autonomy versus shame and doubt (will)	1–3 years	Infants begin to discover that their behavior is their own. Their energies are centered on developing physical skills, controlling body functions, and making decisions. They develop an ability to do things for themselves and assert their sense of autonomy. They realize their *will*. "Well-parented" children emerge from this stage sure of themselves, elated, and proud of their newly found control. If children are restrained too much or punished too harshly, they may develop shame and doubt.
Initiative versus guilt (purpose)	3–6 years	Children develop a vigorous curiosity, foster a strong imagination, and use fantasy and play to broaden their skills. They use active, purposeful behavior to cope with the challenges of the widening social world. They are asked to assume responsibility for their bodies, their behavior, and their possessions, which develops their sense of initiative. Uncomfortable guilt feelings may arise if a child's curiosity or sense of initiative is restricted.
Industry versus inferiority (competence)	7–12 years	Children are mastering knowledge and intellectual skill. They learn to compete and cooperate with others. They are enthusiastic about learning and want real achievement to be industrious. They can be reasoned with and can understand explanations. These "school-aged" children must deal with demands to learn new skills or experience feelings of defeat, failure, incompetence, or inferiority.
Identity versus identity confusion (fidelity)	Adolescence	Adolescents experiment with various roles, trying to find out who they are, what they are all about, and where they are going in life. They are confronted with many new adult responsibilities and statuses. They seek someone to inspire or lead them. They establish sexual identity, and gradually develop socially agreeable and desirable ideals. Adolescents will face identity confusion if self-certainty is not achieved.

Source: Modified from Santrock, 2004;[18] Beauman, 2001;[13] and Child Development Institute, 1998–2005.[15]

instinctive, and reaching and throwing are refined. Furthermore, their fine motor skills (Table 23–4 ■) improve substantially from sophistication of reaching, grasping, and manipulating small objects. Moreover, there is an increase in brain maturation, which contributes to improved cognitive abilities.[18]

Cognitive

Early in this period of intellectual growth, children constantly ask questions because of their curiosity and exploration of surroundings and perceived objects. They can recall specific past experiences; however, if they are not given appropriate cues and prompts, the information may

■ **Table 23–3** Gross Motor Skills in Early Childhood

Age	Examples of Gross Motor Skills
2 years	Running Kicking a ball Picking up an object without falling down
3 years	Walking up stairs by alternating feet Pedaling a tricycle Throwing a ball forward Jumping in place
4 years	Performing a standing broad jump Catching a large ball Hopping on one foot
5 years	Skipping smoothly Balancing on one foot

Source: Modified from Dworkin, 1988.[32]

■ **Table 23–4** Fine Motor Skills of Early Childhood

Age	Examples of Fine Motor Skills
2 years	Turning pages of a book Eating well with a spoon Holding a glass securely Building a tower of six blocks
3 years	Scribbling with a crayon Building a tower of nine to ten blocks Using a fork Pouring from a pitcher
4 years	Buttoning clothing Lacing shoes Cutting with scissors
5 years	Brushing teeth Combing hair Washing face

Source: Modified from Dworkin, 1988.[32]

be unreliable and incomplete, because they can remember only the features of an experience that capture their attention instead of the relevant dimensions. Furthermore, there is an increase in children's attention span and vocabulary, as well as dramatic enhancements in language development during this time.

Socioemotional

Children become more proficient at talking about their own emotions as well as the emotions of others during early childhood. The amount of terms used to describe emotion increases as they learn more about the causes and consequences of feelings—along with the understanding that a single event can generate different emotions in different people.[18] Children's rich imagination leads to magical thinking and pretend play, causing them to interpret what they are told quite literally. It is this vivid fantasy that aids children in emotional development by allowing them to experiment with strong feelings, work through areas of tension, and assume aspects of identification of those around them.[24] During this period, children struggle to ascertain autonomy and independence as well as to establish self-identity, self-awareness, and a capacity for self-monitoring.[25] Their emotional attachments to parents and other caregivers, however, still remain a vital source of emotional well-being, because the strongest fears at this time are those of separation from parents and self-injury.[25] Children also begin to experience self-referential emotions such as pride, guilt, shame, and embarrassment in addition to developing an awareness of gender and a sense of gender-specific behavior.[19] Moreover, early childhood is a time when cooperative play and group play are possible because of the greater development of impulse control. Children will actively seek social contact with their peers, although there are wide ranges of how aggressively they will pursue such contacts, depending on the child's temperament, or behavioral style.[25]

School-Aged Development: 6 to 11 Years of Age

Physical

Children grow more slowly and gradually during the school-aged period. They gain 2 to 3 inches in height and about 5 pounds in weight each year. Body proportions change: They become slimmer as "baby fat" begins to decrease, and muscle mass and strength steadily increase.[18] Motor development becomes much smoother and more coordinated because of improved myelination of the central nervous system, enabling children to use their hands more dexterously for fine motor skills such as handwriting, producing arts and crafts, and playing instruments. In addition, they can perform gross motor skills such as running, climbing, skipping rope, swimming, bicycle riding, batting a ball, and skating. These skills allow them to participate in organized sports. School-aged children gain greater control over their bodies and experience energetic physical health during this period; however, they are far from having physical maturity and possess a need to be active.[18]

Cognitive

During this period of development, children's cognitive skills are well suited to begin a formal education by attending school; therefore, the stage is called "school-aged." These children can concentrate better and longer than before, and their capacity for thought and reasoning significantly increases with more systematic and selective learning that is applied with increasing ease to a variety of contexts.[19] Also, school-aged children gain improved verbal reasoning and use of symbolic and graphic representations through a refined use of language and advances in reading, vocabulary, grammatical skills, science, and mathematics.[25] They begin to master and appreciate their intellect by becoming more consciously aware of their mental processes and are capable of attaining cognitive skills to accomplish goals. By the end of this stage, children have the intellectual skills to function competently in the adult world; however, abstract and hypothetical issues remain difficult to understand, because this stage is characterized by concrete operational thinking.[18,19]

Socioemotional

The emotional development of school-aged children is a period when the child learns about the outside world and becomes increasingly independent of his parents.[25] The child develops a conscience or a sense of responsibility about matters of importance to the child. These are the years when closely-knit groups are formed, such as clubs and gangs, to fulfill the child's need for peer acceptance. During this period, the child is introduced to the culture of society through the public or private school. These years are important for learning how to get along with other people and to abide by the rules of society. During this time, children link achievement with self-concept and are constantly measuring themselves and their achievements against others.[24] They have an increased understanding of complex emotions such as pride and shame, as well as the ability to detect that more than one emotion can be experienced in particular situations and the capability to consider the circumstances that led up to the emotional reaction. In addition, school-aged children improve their ability to suppress and conceal emotions, and they use self-initiated strategies to redirect emotions.

This period is marked by children's quest for social involvement and social acceptance.[24] Doing the "in thing" becomes extremely important, and most school-aged children pursue gender-stereotyped activities with same-gender friendship groupings. Their success in maintaining a positive sense of self during the many changing friendships depends on the resilience of their coping and social skills, which encompass a good sense of humor, an ability to make others feel wanted, a willingness to share, a positive mood, creativity, leadership, and negotiation abilities. Finally, children with positive peer relations tend to give and receive positive attention, conform to classroom rules, and perform well academically; they also initiate social contact in a positive manner and develop pleasant social interchanges with others.

Adolescent Development: 12 to 19 Years of Age

Physical

The most important marker of the beginning of adolescence is puberty. During this time, accelerated growth in height and weight occurs, as well as a process of "filling out" that is largely under the influence of the sex hormones and gives the appearance of sexual characteristics and ability to reproduce.[25] Throughout this sexual maturation, major changes occur in the distribution of body fat and musculature, genitals enlarge, breasts develop, and skin becomes oily.

Cognitive

Adolescents move toward the stage of cognitive development known as formal operational thinking. In this stage, they develop critical thinking, conceptual thinking, and introspection through their increased speed, automaticity, and capacity of information processing; they also have more breadth of content knowledge in a variety of domains, increased ability to construct new combinations of knowledge, and a greater range and more spontaneous use of strategies or procedures for applying or obtaining knowledge.[18] And they have the cognitive ability to develop hypotheses followed by deduction or conclusion for solving problems. Furthermore, adolescents are capable of making competent decisions as well as moral judgments.

At this time, adolescents can apply a set of solutions to a specific problem, as well as contemplate the effect of all possible variables. Furthermore, having reached this stage, the adolescent can now think in abstract terms and deal with hypothetical situations. Consideration is now given to the *possible* and *what might be*.[25] They begin to ask and answer the question, "what if . . ." Adolescents begin to think about things that cannot be seen, heard, or touched, such as faith, trust, beliefs, and spirituality as they journey toward self-reflection and self-identity.[26,27]

Socioemotional

Adolescence is the period of transition from childhood to adulthood; the transition is accompanied by a series of baffling and sometimes highly disturbing emotional and social problems attributable to the structural and physiologic changes occurring as a process of physical alterations and sexual maturation.[25] Personal appearance becomes a source of great conflict because of an adolescents' heightened interest in body image and agonizing self-consciousness. Furthermore, adolescents develop a need to separate from parents and establish their own identities as individuals, which requires the support of a peer group for the safe psychological shelter in which to grow outside the family.[25] Separation from the family need not be physical, although it often is, but refers to confidence in the adolescent's decision making and an ability to perform socially on an equal basis with peers.[25] Moreover, there is a dramatic increase in the emotional importance and intimacy of close friends given that peers are looked to as role models for dress, music, entertainment, and life style; nonetheless, adolescents need reassurance, support, and physical affections from their parents.

Children's Development and Behavior

Temperament

Temperament is an individual's behavioral style and characteristic way of emotionally responding.[18] It is the foundation for the child's distinct personality given that personality is determined by the interaction of temperament traits with the environment.[24,28] Temperamental characteristics influence all aspects of development and behavior. The three basic types, or clusters, of temperament are (1) easy child, (2) difficult child, and (3) slow-to-warm-up child.[18,24,25,28] The **easy child** is characterized by regularity, easy adaptability, and a positive mood in the approach to new situations. The **difficult child** demonstrates considerable irregularity, many negative mood expressions, slow adaptability, and frequently reacts negatively to new situations. Lastly, the **slow-to-warm-up child** has a low activity level and mild reactions, is somewhat negative, and shows low adaptability.

Parents

Parents influence how children think, socialize, and become self-aware.[19] Consequently, parents play an important role in the dental experience of their children, because they decide the importance they will place on the dental health of their child and the role they will take in supervising oral hygiene, scheduling regular dental appointments, and monitoring the child's diet.[29] Furthermore, children look to the parents for information on appropriate and inappropriate behavior in a strange situation.[30] The level of anxiety experienced by children is often a reflection of parental fears; parental anxiety (mostly maternal) correlates with a child's mood, cooperativity, anxiety, and anxious behavior during treatment.[12,14,29,31] Thus, a child's behavior during the dental appointment is affected significantly by the parents.

Economics

Children from low-income families can experience greater domestic turmoil, nutritional deficiencies, child abuse or neglect, as well as a lack of role models and an intellectually stimulating environment.[32] Furthermore, children who identify with their poor families are vulnerable to feelings of shame, anxiety, anger, or psychological impotence that can portray as a chronic mental stress.[33] Consequently, these children have an inability to coordinate behavior with identified authority, which causes a more compromised ability to work well with adults, particularly adults who are authoritative and seek compliance. Moreover, they may harbor rejection and resentment of the dental professional during an appointment.[29]

The abilities of children from low-income families to learn and communicate are adversely affected. For example, when children grow up in impoverished circumstances, and when their parents do not use a large number of vocabulary words in communicating with them, their vocabulary development suffers; they also acquire language more slowly, retain immature pronunciations longer, and speak in shorter sentences.[18,25,29] Thus, it is suggested that a clinician speak slower, repeat information more often than usual, and use visual aids when communicating with low-income children.[29]

Culture

Child development is powerfully influenced by the cultural context in which it occurs. Culture is the complex internal psychological structures that determine values, sense of self and others, as well as expected patterns of behavior. It establishes ideas about health and illness, personal responsibility in health and disease, and nature of healing, which influence the experience of a health care encounter as well as dental hygiene treatment.[24]

Setting

Protective equipment such as goggles and a facemask can elicit anxiety if worn during the initial contact with the child patient. Also, wearing plain white clothing or a white coat can elicit fear from a small number of child patients.[34] Furthermore, if the dental professional shows insecurity around children, child patients may demonstrate increased behavioral problems compared with their reaction to experienced clinicians.[29] It is reported that providers who express greater confidence perform more effectively and experience less uncooperative behavior from children.[35]

COMMON ORAL MANIFESTATIONS

The more common oral conditions of early childhood are dental caries, oral mucosal infections, accidental and intentional dental and oral trauma, developmental disturbances associated with teething or tooth formation, and developmental clefts of the lip and/or palate. In addition, parents frequently request information on additional concerns including sucking habits, tooth alignment, timing and order of tooth eruption, and tooth coloration. Of these conditions, dental caries is the preeminent concern because of its tremendous prevalence and consequences.[1]

Early Childhood Caries

Dental caries among very young children is referred to as **early childhood caries** (ECC). This condition is defined as the presence of one or more decayed, missing, or filled tooth surfaces in any primary tooth in a young child. This unique pattern of dental caries affects the smooth surfaces of primary maxillary incisors and occlusal fissures of the first molar teeth.

PREVENTIVE STRATEGIES

Children exhibit a broad range of physical, cognitive, and socioemotional development as well as diverse behavioral characteristics; therefore, maintaining the child's compliance in the dental environment may require behavior-management techniques. **Behavior management** can be described as a continuum of interaction with a child/parent directed toward communication and education. Its goal is to ease fear and anxiety while promoting an understanding of the need for good dental health and the process by which it is achieved.[36]

Cooperative behavioral management with children and families can assist in promoting optimal dental care, because a number of specific dental and dental hygiene procedures can cause anxiety or discomfort.[37]

Tables 23–5 ■ through 23–7 ■ outline implications of dental treatments for the three developmental stages. The following behavior-management techniques are communication based; therefore, no specific consent or documentation is necessary before use.

■ **Table 23–5** Implications for Dental Treatment during Early Childhood

- Develop rapport with child and parent as a foundation for cooperation and trust.
- Regard the parent as a partner in the child's oral health care.
- Talk to children in short sentences using simple words without double meanings; do not use metaphors, because children interpret language literally.
- Maintain a calm, slow, reassuring voice that is not intimidating to the child.
- Explain all procedures in simple, concrete terms.
- Clarify what the child's role is during treatment, and set acceptable rules for behavior.
- Demonstrate the use of equipment, and involve the child in the dental care as much as possible.
- Use substitution words (e.g., refer to the suction as a "straw;" describe the handpiece as a "tooth tickler;" portray x-rays as using a "camera" to take "pictures" of the teeth).
- Give simple instructions and directions one at a time.
- Make use of gestures and facial expressions.
- Use a confident manner and positive voice when inviting children to sit in the dental chair independently.
- Consider allowing the child to sit on their parents' lap, depending on parental attachment.
- Allow the child to explore the environment through smell, taste, touch, sight, and sound (e.g., smelling the fluoride, hearing the compressed air, handling a mirror, tasting prophylactic paste).
- Do not lie to children about pain; describe to the child exactly what the procedure will feel like.
- Avoid logic because the child lacks reasoning skills during this stage.
- Allow children to make choices whenever possible, and give them a means to interrupt treatment, such as raising a hand to signal discomfort.
- Answer questions and encourage curiosity.
- Avoid over directing the very cooperative child.
- Be aware that negativism (saying "no") may be the child's only way of control and that temper tantrums are a possibility.
- Teach parent and child appropriate oral hygiene care according to the child's needs.
- Offer suggestions and/or recommendations to parents concerning risk factors and their assisting the child with oral hygiene activities.
- Ignore inappropriate behaviors while praising appropriate behaviors and cooperation.
- Reward good behavior with a tangible gift (e.g., toothbrush, sticker, toy).

Communication

Communication is the most fundamental form of behavior management. It is the foundation for cooperation and trust, as well as the basis for establishing a relationship with the child that may allow for successful completion of dental procedures, and at the same time, help the child develop a positive attitude toward dental health.[36]

Communication is the process by which a person sends a message to another person with the intention of evoking a response; the objective of communication is understanding.[37,38] Communication can be applied with both cooperative and uncooperative pediatric patients; many different approaches are required to communicate with the variety of children who enter the dental operatory, because they need communication, teaching, and guidance in the new environment.[39]

Communicating with children takes skill, thoughtfulness, and practice.[40] In addition, working with and educating children successfully require the dental professional to analyze the child's developmental level and comprehension skills so as to communicate according to age, behavior, and the context of the interaction.[22,36–38,40] The intellectual development of children sets absolute limits on what can be communicated with young patients; a greater understanding of their developmental stage—their cognitive and personality development, their fears and desires, their individual backgrounds—will enable the dental professional to communicate more successfully in terms the children will understand.[38] Consequently, if a dental professional uses language the patient cannot understand, the child loses attention and cooperation, decreasing the chances that goals will be achieved.[37]

A child's essential link to parents emphasizes the need for effective communication with parents. Moreover, parents' behavior and attitudes can have a key effect on their children's behavior during treatment. Anything that can be done to improve communication with parents

■ **Table 23–6**   Implications for Dental Treatment for School-Aged Children

- Develop rapport with child as a foundation for cooperation and trust.
- Talk with children about their friends, school, and outside interests.
- Direct questions toward the child first, ensuring that the child is your patient.
- Develop rapport with the parents, and consider them partners in the child's oral health care.
- Dispel myths that children may have learned from other children and/or adults about dental visits.[6]
- Clarify what the child's role is during treatment, and set acceptable rules for behavior.
- Encourage questions and give straight answers.
- Explain procedures using simple vocabulary.
- Regularly ask children to repeat (in their own words) what has just been said or explained to them to ensure understanding.
- Describe the operation of equipment and reasons for its use.
- Give clear explanations of what the patient will experience in terms of pain or discomfort; do not lie to or mislead the child.
- Help these patients retain control by including them in decision making, soliciting their help, giving them the opportunity to make choices involving their care when possible, and providing them a means to interrupt treatment, such as raising a hand to signal discomfort.
- Introduce children to routine care of their teeth and gums, including regular brushing, flossing, and reductions in sugar consumption (e.g., candy, sodas).
- Teach parents to monitor their child's oral hygiene activities, and offer suggestions to parents who struggle with their children regarding these issues.
- Be positive and supportive to the child, thus avoiding judgment and embarrassment.
- Be aware that children in this stage can have temper tantrums that are difficult to control and their behavior can be unpredictable: from cooperative to obstructive to withdrawn to enthusiastic.
- Distinguish between emotional crying (pain, fear) and crying used to control the environment (tantrums); handle emotional crying with patience and empathy; tantrums require behavior-management techniques.
- Understand that praise becomes a stronger reinforcer and that "rewards" used for appropriate behaviors can become less tangible.

■ **Table 23–7**   Implications for Dental Treatment of the Adolescent

- Develop rapport with the adolescent as a foundation for cooperation and trust.
- Talk with the adolescent about friends, school, interests, and hobbies.
- Allow sufficient time for patients of this age to adjust before asking demanding questions, because they are at first distrustful of authority.[6]
- Reassure the adolescent about confidentiality and privacy issues.
- Set reasonable limits and standards for cooperation and behavior.
- Help these patients retain control by including them in decision making, soliciting their help, giving them the opportunity to make choices involving their care when possible, and providing them a means to interrupt treatment, such as raising a hand to signal discomfort.
- Allow self-expression and avoid being judgmental.
- Listen, be attentive, and attempt to understand the adolescent while making sure to respond in consistent standard English.[43]
- Be supportive and be a good role model and resource.
- Set goals for oral hygiene activities and future recall appointments.
- Appeal to the impact of their oral health on social interactions (e.g., plaque and oral bacteria can cause bad breath).
- Dispel myths of idealized media images of dental health (e.g., extremely white teeth).
- Understand that adolescents can exhibit arrogant and disrespectful attitudes.
- Treat all questions seriously and provide full explanations.
- Discuss oral health in terms of disease and infections; give explanations and consequences, especially physical consequences.
- Give clear explanations of what the patient will experience in terms of pain or discomfort; do not lie to or mislead the patient.
- Include dietary habits, tobacco, alcohol, and drug use in health education messages.
- Strive for a positive dental hygiene experience, allowing the adolescent to gain more self-esteem.

will likely lead to better dental experiences for the parent and child, because more-informed parents will likely be more relaxed and, therefore, may influence their child in a more positive way.[36]

Tell-Show-Do

The **tell-show-do technique** is a basic and straightforward strategy used to help introduce a new experience in conjunction with helping to minimize fear of the unknown.[34] This method of behavior shaping involves the following concepts:

- *Tell:* Verbal explanations of procedures in phrases appropriate to the developmental level of the patient.
- *Show:* Demonstrations for the patient of the visual, auditory, olfactory, and tactile aspects of the procedures in a carefully defined, nonthreatening setting.
- *Do:* Completion of the procedure, without deviating from the explanation and demonstration.

The tell-show-do method is indicated for all patients to teach them important aspects of the dental visit, to gain positive behavior at the subsequent appointments, and to shape the patient's response to procedures through desensitization; this method grants the patient the ability to learn new and more pleasant associations with anxiety-provoking stimuli.[22,36]

Voice Control

Voice control is a controlled alteration of voice volume, tone, or pace to influence and direct the patient's behavior to gain the patient's attention and compliance, avert negative or avoidance behavior, and establish appropriate adult–child roles.[36] It has been reported that the contingent and specific use of firm commands, at points where children were beginning to lose control and drift away from communication, led to much more control, compliance, and good behavior during dental treatment; this tactic also led to the patient's better sense of self-worth after treatment.[41]

Positive Reinforcement

Positive reinforcement refers to the presentation of a stimulus immediately after desirable patient behavior that results in an increase in the frequency of the behavior.[41]

Social reinforcers can be the most influential consequences for increasing the occurrence of adaptive behaviors. They include verbal reinforcers (e.g., "good job keeping your mouth open"), appropriate physical demonstrations (e.g., patting the child's shoulder, shaking the child's hand), or through nonverbal gestures (e.g., smile, thumbs-up). Tangible reinforcers (e.g., toys, stickers) can also be used to reinforce desired behaviors; however, access to these "rewards" should occur only after the appropriate behavior in order for the behavior to remain effective.[36,42]

Distraction

Distraction is the technique of diverting the patient's attention (e.g., listening to music with earphones) from what may be perceived as an unpleasant procedure by decreasing children's perceptions and expectations of unpleasantness, thus preventing negative behavior.[36]

SUMMARY

For all children, oral health is an essential component of overall health, and dental care is an essential health service. Dental professionals need to understand several dimensions of a child's psychological development to relate effectively to and guide the child patient. The dental professional needs to know what emotional and social behaviors to expect from children in different age groups. The dental professional also must be able to communicate on a level consistent with the child's view of the world. In addition, knowledge is needed about how children learn so that the dental professional can teach the child desirable behavior. The definitive achievement of oral health care for children is the prevention of oral disease.

REFERENCES

1. Edelstein, B. L. (2002). Dental care considerations for young children. *Spec Care Dent,* 22 (3 Suppl):11S–25S.
2. U.S. Department of Health and Human Services. (2000). *Oral health in America: A report of the Surgeon General—Executive summary.* Rockville, MD: U.S. Department of Health and Human Services, National Institute of Dental and Craniofacial Research, National Institute of Health.
3. Kanellis, M. J. (2000). The impact of poor oral health on children's ability to function. *J Southeastern Soc Pediatr Dent,* 6 (2):12–13.

4. Mouradian, W. E., Wehr, E., & Crall, J. J. (2000). Disparities in children's oral health and access to dental care. *JAMA,* 284:2625–31.

5. Mouradian, W. E. (2001). The face of a child: Children's oral health and dental education. *J Dent Educ,* 65: 821–31.

6. Windmer, R. (2002). Implications of child development on the practice of oral care. *Compend Contin Educ Dent,* 23 (3 Supp 2):4–9.

7. Crall, J. J. (2002). Children's oral health services: Organization and financing considerations. *Ambul Pediatr,* 2 (2 Suppl):148–53.

8. Edelstein, B. L. (2002). Disparities in oral health and access to care: Findings of national surveys. *Ambul Pediatr,* 2 (2 Suppl):141–47.

9. Schechter, N. (2000). The impact of acute and chronic dental pain on child development. *J Southeastern Soc Pediatr Dent,* 6 (2):16–17.

10. American Dental Education Association. (2003). Improving the oral health status of all Americans: Roles and responsibilities of academic dental institutions. The Report of the ADEA President's Commission. Washington, DC: American Dental Education Association, ADEA Center for Educational Policy and Research. *J Am Dent Assoc,* 67:563–83.

11. Maddux, J. E., Roberts, M. C., Sledden, E. A., & Wright, L. (1986). Developmental Issues in child health psychology. *Am Psychol,* 41:25–34.

12. McDonald, R. E., Avery, D. R., & Dean, J. A. (2004). *Dentistry for the child and adolescent* (8th ed.). St. Louis: Mosby, chapter 3, pp. 35–49.

13. Beauman, S. S. (2001). Didactic components of a comprehensive pediatric competency program. *J Infus Nurs,* 24:367–74.

14. Mallin, K., & Lazarus, M. C. (2005). Treating children is different. *Dermatol Clin,* 23:171–80.

15. Child Development Institute. *Stages of intellectual development in children and teenagers.* Retrieved 1/7/06 from http://www.childdevelopmentinfo.comdevelopment/ piaget/shtml. Copyright © 1998–2005 by Child Development Institute.

16. Price, S. (1994). The special needs of children. *J Adv Nurs,* 20:227–32.

17. Revell, G. M., & Liptalk, G. S. (1991). Understanding the child with special health care needs: A developmental perspective. *J Pediatr Nurs,* 6:258–67.

18. Santrock, J. W. (2004). *Life-span development* (9th ed.). Boston: McGraw-Hill Higher Education, chapters 1–13. pp. 1–435 (actual pages info found pp. 18–20, 42–52, 73, 161–166, 183–185, 194–201, 210–214, 235–238, 276–277, 331, 339, 372–376, 399)

19. Thompson, R. A. (2005). Child development. Microsoft® Encarta® Encyclopedia 2005 1993–2004, Microsoft Corporation, Redmond, WA.

20. Wood, S. E., Wood, E. G., & Boyd, D. (2006). *Mastering the world of psychology* (2nd ed.). Boston: Pearson Education, 136–67.

21. Do, C. (2004). Applying the social learning theory to children with dental anxiety. *J Contemp Dent Pract,* 5:126–35.

22. Baghdadi, Z. D. (2001). Principles and application of learning theory in child patient management. *Quintessence Int,* 32:134–41.

23. George, J. M., & McIver, F. T. (1983). Three theories of psychological development: Implications for children's dentistry. *J Dent Educ,* 47:112–13.

24. Dixon, S. D., & Stein, M. T. (2000). *Encounters with children: Pediatric behavior and development* (3rd ed.). St. Louis: Mosby, 14–22, 304–305, 349, 377.

25. Lowrey, G. H. (1986). *Growth and development of children* (8th ed.). Chicago-London: Year Book Medical Publishers, Chapters 6, 9. (chapter 6 pp. 143–219, chapter 9 pp. 323–343) (actual pages used pp. 158–160, 170–173, 199–210, 343–357).

26. Huebner, A. (2000, March). *Adolescent growth and development* (Family and Child Development, Publication 350-850). Virginia Cooperative Extension, Virginia Polytechnic Institute and State University; Virginia State University; U.S. Department of Agriculture. Retrieved 4/25/06, from http://www.ext.vt.edu/pubs/family/ 350-850/350-850.html.

27. Barnett, R. V. (2005). *Helping teens answer the question "Who am I": Cognitive development in adolescents* (Document FCS2241). Family Youth and Community Sciences Department, Florida Cooperative Extension Service, Institute of Food and Agricultural Sciences, University of Florida. Retrieved 4/25/06, from http://www.edis.ifas.ufl .edu/FY769.

28. Child Development Institute. *Temperament and your child's personality.* Retrieved 1/7/06 from http://www .childdevelopmentinfo.comdevelopment/temperament_ and_your_child.html. Copyright © 1998–2005 by Child Development Institute.

29. Pinkham, J. R. (1995). Personality development: Managing behavior of the cooperative preschool child. *Dent Clin North Am,* 39:771–87.

30. Newton, J. T., & Harrison, V. (2005). The cognitive and social development of the child. *Dent Update,* 32:33–34, 37–38.

31. Kagan, J. (1999). The role of parents in children's psychological development. *Pediatrics* 104:164–67.

32. Dworkin, P. H. (1988). The preschool child: Developmental themes and clinical issues. *Curr Probl Pediatr,* 18:73–134.

33. Fayle, S. A., & Tabmassebi, J. F. (2003). Pediatric dentistry in the new millennium: 2. Behaviour management—Helping children to accept dentistry. *Dent Update,* 30:294—98.

34. Musselman, R. J. (1991). Considerations in behavior management of the pediatric dental patient: Helping children cope with dental treatment. *Pediatr Clin North Am,* 38:1309–23.

35. Wurster, C. A., Wenstein, P., & Cohen, A. J. (1979). Communication patterns in pedodontics. *Percept Mot Skills,* 48:159–66.

36. American Academy of Pediatric Dentistry. (2004). Reference manual, 2004–2005: Clinical guideline on behavior management. *Pediatr Dent,* 26:89–94.

37. Darby, M. L., & Walsh, M. M. *Dental hygiene theory and practice.* Philadelphia: W.B. Saunders, 75–101.

38. Chambers, D. W. (1976). Communicating with the young dental patient. *J Am Dent Assoc,* 93:793–99.

39. Feigal, Robert J. (2001). Guiding and managing the child dental patient: A fresh look at old pedagogy. *J Dent Educ,* 65:1369–77.

40. Deering, C. G. & Cody, D. J. (2002). Communicating with children and adolescents. *Am J Nurs,* 102 (3):34–41.

41. Greenbaum, P. E., Turner, C., Cook, E. W., & Melamed, B. G. (1990). Dentists's voice control: Effects on children's disruptive and affective behavior. *Health Psychol,* 9:546–58.

42. MacDonald, E. K. (2003). Principles of behavioral assessment and management. *Pediatr Clin North Am,* 50:801–16.

Chapter 24

Adult Dental Care

Maria Perno Goldie

OBJECTIVES

After reading this chapter, the student should be able to:

1. Describe and define this target population.
2. Describe common oral conditions and diseases of adult patients.
3. Describe specific preventive strategies to use with adult patients.
4. Describe the role of the dental provider in treating adult patients

KEY TERMS

Oral health
Adolescence
Hormonal changes
Hormonal imbalances
Oral contraceptives
Pregnancy granulomas
Osteoporosis
Menopause
Periomylosis
Floating amalgams
Pregnancy gingivitis
Iatrogenic disease

INTRODUCTION

Oral diseases continue to be among the most prevalent problems in our society, despite the importance of oral health to personal overall health and well-being. **Oral health** is defined as being without oral cancer, dental caries, periodontal diseases, or other forms of oral problems.[1] The general level of oral health has improved steadily in recent decades. The baby boomer generation will be the first in which the majority will maintain their natural teeth over their entire lifetime, having benefited from water fluoridation and fluoride toothpastes. Over the past 10 years, the number of adults missing all their natural teeth has declined from 31% to 25% for those aged 60 years and older, and from 9% to 5% for those adults between 40 and 59 years. However, 5% means a surprising one of twenty middle-aged adults are missing all their teeth. More than 40% of poor adults (20 years and older) have at least one untreated decayed tooth compared with 16% of nonpoor adults.[2] Dental caries and periodontal diseases are preventable and controllable. Dental caries can be prevented by a combination of fluoride, dental sealants, and other new technologies. Periodontal diseases can be prevented mainly by personal and professional control of plaque biofilm.

POPULATION CHARACTERISTICS

Humans go through a variety of life stages, from birth to old age. Changes usually begin at puberty when the adult life cycle begins. The following sections illustrate the characteristics of specific age groups of adults.

Adolescence to Young Adulthood: 13–20 Years of Age

Adolescence is a period of transition from the dependence of childhood to the independence of adulthood. It can be identified in terms of sexual maturity, identity development, and a period of social transition into adulthood. Puberty and associated physical changes may occur between the ages of 9 and 17 years. The pituitary gland is responsible for the control of the production of estrogens, from the ovaries in females, and androgens, from the testes in males. These hormones, responsible for the development of sex organs, continue to cause profound physical and emotional influences during this life stage. Physically, both males and females experience accelerated growth, height, weight, and muscle mass. Because of the pattern of growth spurts, adolescents may appear clumsy and awkward. Lack of physical coordination may become an issue and may affect self-esteem. Dermatological changes are often evident in this life stage and may cause immense concern in teens.

Early Adulthood: 21–39 Years of Age

The transition from adolescence to adulthood is marked by independent choices, a sense of identity, and psychological and social adjustments that ready one for marriage, parenthood, and career choice. Although this is a period in which individuals are generally in good health (i.e., peak bone mass, stabilized hormones), chronic disease that may appear later in life may be affected by lifestyle choices made during this time. During this life stage, many females may take oral contraceptives. Individuals also may marry and start families, so oral care of expectant mothers and unborn children becomes a relevant issue.

Mature Adulthood: 40–60 Years of Age

As the middle years of adulthood approach, many people are established, have definite lifestyles, and have found their role within the societal structure. This is also a time of reflection and slowing of the pace of their life. An important trend seen in this age group is the increasing role as a caregiver. Individuals may now have to care for aging parents, adult children who have returned home, or grandchildren.[3] Hair begins to gray and thin, weight gain is more apparent, and physical inabilities due to arthritis or other conditions may surface. Lifestyle choices, such as lack of exercise, poor nutrition, increased stress, tobacco use, obesity, and alcohol abuse, may have consequences not seen before. Risk for disease increases, orally and systemically. Numerous physiologic changes occur during this life stage that have an effect on oral health. Conversely, many oral conditions may affect other aspects of physiologic health. A patient's understanding of the impact of oral health on overall health is extremely important. Initially the link of periodontal diseases to systemic diseases was thought to be unidirectional, but growing evidence shows that the relationship may be bidirectional.

As women approach midlife, hormonal imbalances become evident in the cessation of menstruation and presentation of various symptoms indicative of the changing hormone levels during perimenopause and menopause. Some females choose hormone replacement therapy or estrogen replacement therapy to control symptoms such as vaginal dryness, hot flashes, and increased urinary frequency. However, since the release of the results of the Women's Health Initiative Study, fewer women are taking oral hormones because of their potential deleterious effects.[4] These effects include, but are not limited to, increased risk of breast cancer, heart disease, and stroke.[4] Having lower levels of circulating sex hormones causes systemic and oral symptoms.

COMMON ORAL MANIFESTATIONS

Systemic conditions that affect oral health include **hormonal changes** and **imbalances.** Oral disease can affect a patient's life in many ways. Certain oral conditions may undermine self-image and self-esteem, discourage social interaction, and be noteworthy chronic stressors.[3] Some conditions may also lead to or contribute to other health issues, such as heart disease, diabetes, and low-birth-weight babies, and interference with vital functions, such as food selection, chewing, and swallowing.

The strong connection between oral health and a person's overall well-being emphasizes the importance of the dental hygienist's interaction with patients on many psychosocial–behavioral levels: attitude, health beliefs, motivating factors, living situation, and previous dental experiences. Just as physical–physiologic factors demonstrate some crossover, psychosocial–behavioral factors may, in turn, affect diagnosis and therapy. For example, a psychiatric disorder influences oral health (e.g., bulimia, which causes tooth destruction through regurgitation, or depression, which can impair oral hygiene), or fear of dental procedures impairs communication or otherwise interferes with the provision of care.

Dental Caries

Dental caries is still as prevalent as ever.[5] Dental caries affects not only children; it is also a problem among adults (Table 24–1 ■; Figures 24–1 ■ and 24–2 ■). Recurrent caries and root caries are prevalent among adults and the

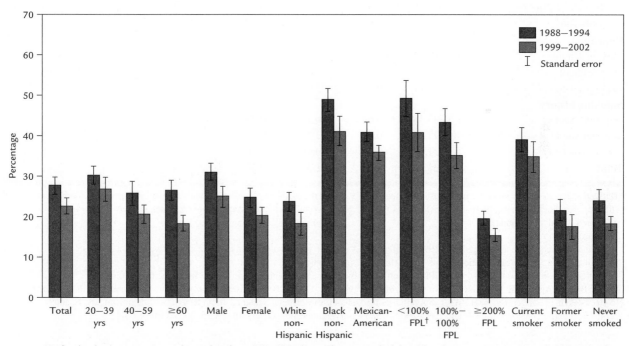

*Defined as having one or more decayed surfaces (DS>0) in the tooth crowns of adults with at least one permanent tooth (dentate). All estimates are adjusted by age (10-year groups) and sex to the U.S. 2000 standard population, except sex, which is adjusted only by age.
†Percentage of the Federal Poverty Level (FPL), which varies by income and number of persons living in the household.

■ **FIGURE 24–1**   Prevalence of untreated dental decay[a] among dentate adults aged 20 years and older, by selected characteristics—United States, National Health and Nutrition Examination Survey, 1988–1994 and 1999–2002. (Beltrán-Aguilar ED, Barker LK, Canto MT, Dye BA, Gooch BF, Griffin SO, Hyman J, Jaramillo F, Kingman A, Nowjack-Raymer R, Selwitz RH, Wu T. Surveillance for Dental Caries, Dental Sealants, Tooth Retention, Edentulism, and Enamel Fluorosis—United States, 1988–1994 and 1999–2002. *MMWR Surveillance Summaries*, August 26, 2005/54(03); 1–44.)

■ **Table 24-1** Prevalence of Coronal Caries in Permanent Teeth among Dentate Adults* Aged 20 Years or Older, by Selected Characteristics—United States, National Health and Nutrition Examination Survey, 1988–1994 and 1999–2002

Characteristic	1988–1994		1999–2002		Difference in %[¶]	% Change[¶]
	%[†]	SE[§]	%	SE		
Age group (yrs)						
20–39	93.11	0.52	86.76	0.85	−6.35	−6.82
40–59	96.25	0.43	95.07	0.44	−1.18	−1.23
≥ 60	94.58	0.53	93.10	0.56	−1.48	−1.56
Sex						
Male	93.83	0.45	90.34	0.64	−3.49	−3.72
Female	95.41	0.27	92.27	0.51	−3.14	−3.29
Race/Ethnicity**						
White, non-Hispanic	96.37	0.28	93.32	0.38	−3.05	−3.17
Black, non-Hispanic	88.35	0.68	84.61	0.85	−3.74	−4.24
Mexican-American	87.29	0.70	83.50	1.62	−3.79	−4.34
Poverty status?[††]						
<100% FPL	86.89	1.17	86.65	1.28	−0.24	−0.28
100%–199% FPL	92.75	0.73	89.06	0.93	−3.69	−3.98
≥ 200% FPL	96.27	0.28	93.17	0.47	−3.10	−3.22
Education						
<High school	89.65	0.59	84.53	1.11	−5.12	−5.71
High school	96.01	0.33	92.63	0.85	−3.38	−3.52
>High school	96.11	0.37	93.16	0.39	−2.95	−3.07
Smoking history						
Current smoker	93.45	0.64	90.19	0.85	−3.26	−3.49
Former smoker	95.15	0.71	92.47	0.93	−2.68	−2.82
Never smoked	94.66	0.42	90.96	0.46	−3.70	−3.91
Total	94.62	0.27	91.30	0.36	− 3.32	− 3.51

*Defined as having one or more decayed or filled surfaces (DFS > 0) in the tooth crowns of adults with at least one permanent tooth (dentate). All estimates are adjusted by age (10-year groups) and sex to the U.S. 2000 standard population, except sex, which is adjusted only by age.
[†] Weighted prevalence estimates.
[§] Standard error.
[¶] Between the two surveys and using 1988–1994 as reference. A positive value indicates an increase, a negative value a decrease.
**Calculated using "other race/ethnicity" and "other Hispanic" in the denominator.
[††]Percentage of the Federal Poverty Level (FPL), which varies by income and number of persons living in the household.
Source: Beltrán-Aguilar, E. D., Barker, L. K., Canto, M. T., Dye, B. A., Gooch, B. F., Griffin, S. O., Hyman, J., Jaramillo, F., Kingman, A., Nowjack-Raymer, R., Selwitz, R. H., Wu T. Surveillance for Dental Caries, Dental Sealants, Tooth Retention, Edentulism, and Enamel Fluorosis—United States, 1988–1994 and 1999–2002. *MMWR Surveillance Summaries*, August 26, 2005/54(03): 1–44.

elderly. Again, the segment of the general population most prone to caries is also the most vulnerable: In the adult population it is the poor, ethnic minorities, and those with certain medical conditions or disabilities. Ongoing investigation is needed to identify the most effective health education messages for the prevention of caries, particu-larly for the vulnerable populations. New methods to diagnose, control, and prevent caries throughout the life-span may be on the horizon, as more is understood about the molecular consequences of the interaction between host and microbes, and about the genomic makeup of bacteria implicated in dental caries.

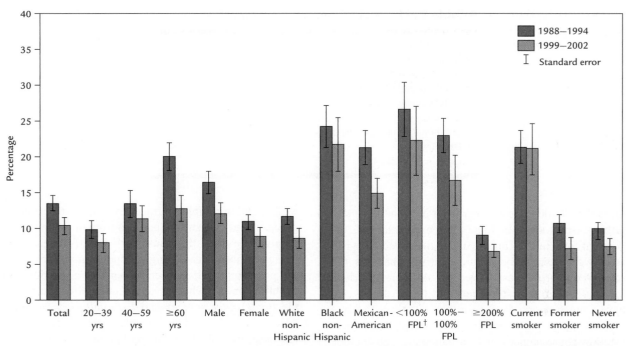

*Defined as having one or more untreated decayed surfaces in the tooth roots of adults with at least one permanent tooth (dentate). All estimates are adjusted by age (10-year groups) and sex to the U.S. 2000 standard population, except sex, which is adjusted only by age.
†Percentage of the Federal Poverty Level (FPL), which varies by income and number of persons living in the household.

■ **FIGURE 24-2**   Prevalence of untreated root caries[a] in dentate adults aged 20 years and older, by selected characteristics—United States, National Health and Nutrition Examination Survey, 1988–1994 and 1999–2002.
(Beltrán-Aguilar ED, Barker LK, Canto MT, Dye BA, Gooch BF, Griffin SO, Hyman J, Jaramillo F, Kingman A, owjack-Raymer R, Selwitz RH, Wu T. Surveillance for Dental Caries, Dental Sealants, Tooth Retention, Edentulism, and Enamel Fluorosis—United States, 1988–1994 and 1999–2002. *MMWR Surveillance Summaries*, August 26, 2005/54(03); 1–44.)

Periodontal Diseases

Periodontal diseases are a result of infections caused by bacteria in the biofilm that forms on the teeth and in the periodontal pocket.[6] The mildest form, gingivitis, is the only reversible stage. Gingivitis may lead to periodontitis, a more severe form of the disease that can destroy the periodontal ligament and surrounding bone and, in some cases, lead to the loss of teeth. Almost half of U.S. adults aged 35 to 44 years have gingivitis and about one fourth have periodontitis.[7] Severe periodontal diseases affect 14% of adults aged 45 to 54 years and 23% of those aged 65 to 74 years.[7] Tobacco use is a major risk factor for the development and progression of periodontal diseases.[8] There also is significant substantiation that diabetes, particularly if poorly controlled, increases the risk for periodontal disease (Table 24–2 ■).

Treatment of periodontal diseases includes surgical as well as nonsurgical methods, and advances in regeneration of tissues have increased through the years. Specific treatment for periodontal disease will be determined by a number of factors, including age, overall health, and medical history; extent of the disease; tolerance for specific medications, procedures, or therapies; expectations for the course of the disease and treatment outcomes; and patient opinion or preference. Treatment may include any or a combination of the following: scaling and root planing; pharmaceuticals; or surgery, including pocket reduction, regeneration procedures, soft tissue grafts, crown lengthening, or dental implants. As with all diseases, prevention is the best way to manage this problem.

Oral and Pharyngeal Cancer

Oral and pharyngeal cancer is the sixth most common cancer in the developed world.[9] Each year, an estimated 28,900 Americans are diagnosed with this disease and

■ **Table 24-2** Risk Factors for Periodontal Diseases

- Genetics
- Lifestyle choices
- A diet low in nutrients
- Smoking and use of smokeless tobacco
- Autoimmune and systemic diseases
- Diabetes
- Hormonal changes in the body
- Bruxism
- Certain medications

more than 7,400 die each year from it.[10] The most disturbing aspect about oral and pharyngeal cancer is the survival rate. In the United States, the 5-year survival rate is approximately 50%, a statistic that has not improved over the past 20 years.[11] African American men suffer the highest incidence of these cancers and have a much poorer 5-year survival rate than do white men, regardless of diagnostic stage.[12] Despite the devastating consequences of oral cancer, which include impaired ability to chew, swallow, and speak, and often disfigurement from extensive surgery to remove parts of the face and oral structures, only 14% of U.S. adults report receiving oral cancer examinations that can detect early disease. Reconstruction and management of the oral cancer survivor come at a high price, both economically and socially. More efforts are needed to increase public and professional knowledge about oral cancer and its prevention. A critical need involves developing biomarkers and diagnostic tests that can be used to improve cancer diagnosis and more accurately predict the course of the disease. There also is a pressing need to develop more-effective, individualized treatments that spare healthy tissues and improve quality of life.

Women's Oral Health

Women taking oral contraceptives and pregnant women experience significant hormonal changes. The woman who uses **oral contraceptives** (OCs) will experience hormonal imbalances similar to those in pregnancy. The hormones contained in OCs act to inhibit the release of the ovum from the ovary, thereby preventing fertilization. These hormonal changes can result in oral manifestations such as hormonal gingivitis, an important topic for oral care education. The relative proportion of the *Bacteroides* species, implicated in periodontitis, is increased 55-fold in pregnant women and 16-fold in

women taking oral contraceptives over the control group.[13] We see a shift in bacteria from those that cause gingivitis to those that cause periodontitis when circulating sex hormones are high. Both hormones, estrogen and progesterone, have been shown to be a substitute for naphthoquinone, which is an essential growth factor for the *Bacteroides* species and *Prevotella intermedia*.[13] Also, the bacteria and the lipopolysaccharide elicit a host response, including production of cytokines and proinflammatory mediators, which contribute to the negative tissue response.[14] Synthesis of prostaglandins (mediators of inflammation) is high during pregnancy, and it is suggested that progesterone functions as an immunosuppressant in the gingival tissues of pregnant women.[15] This effect can be observed clinically as an exaggerated appearance of inflammation. Progesterone-induced inhibition of collagenase, superimposed on vascular changes, is stated as the cause of **pregnancy granulomas.** These combined effects result in the accumulation of collagen within the connective tissue, sometimes causing these tumor-like growths.[16]

Young adults who needed orthodontic treatment during adolescence, but did not receive treatment, may have that orthodontic treatment performed at this time. Patients of this age are beginning to realize the importance of their teeth from an esthetic standpoint and as an important element of their general health. The esthetic appearance of their teeth is indeed important to their overall oral health.

The oral health of patients in this group increases in complexity as they age. They also begin to experience the onset of various chronic conditions. These conditions, or often the therapies used to treat them, may have significant effect on the oral tissues. For example, the onset of diabetes in someone with previously excellent plaque control may result in significant bleeding. The bleeding may frighten the patient, and the clinician should consider this in treatment planning and observation.

During this time frame, most women experience perimenopause and menopause. With the accompanying decline of estrogen, women are more susceptible to reduced bone density, called **osteoporosis,** which also may affect the dental alveolar structure.[17,18] Loss of dental alveolar bone that often may accompany osteoporosis is usually completely unexpected by the patient. The effect of reduced estrogen levels on bone density must be considered a potential contributing factor in the onset of periodontal disease.[19]

Cosmetic options to restore a more youthful smile range from cosmetic whitening with a peroxide-based product to more significant procedures, including veneers, replacement of amalgam restorations with composite materials, and porcelain crowns. The patient may be more likely to feel comfortable discussing these topics with the dental hygienist, at least initially, before consultation with the dentist.

The female patient approaching middle age is faced with hormonal changes inevitably brought about with the onset of **menopause.** These changes often present as alterations in emotions, because the hormonal changes may cause mood swings, depression, anxiety, and a general feeling of malaise.[20] Clinicians must be alert to these changes, in addition to the potential physiologic ones mentioned earlier, and approach the patient in a calm and courteous manner.

These transitional years are filled with psychologic milestones that the clinician must consider in the determination of treatment plans and provision of treatment. Awareness of and sensitivity to the major life changes people face may make a tremendous difference in the relationship that develops between patient and clinician. This relationship may be rewarding and enriching to both parties.

PREVENTIVE STRATEGIES

Adolescence to Young Adulthood: 13–20 Years of Age

Dental providers may experience some difficulty when trying to relay oral health messages to individuals in this age group. The importance of good oral hygiene and plaque biofilm control must be stressed to minimize caries and periodontal disease. Contributing to periodontal diseases in this age group are the abundant sex hormones circulating in the bloodstream.[21] Females are particularly sensitive, because they have high levels of circulating estrogen and progesterone. Oral tissue has many receptors for these hormones and will most likely be affected as these hormones accumulate in the tissue. Effects include increased vascularity, decreased cell-mediated immunity, increased subgingival bacteria, increased gingival swelling, increased redness, bleeding on probing, increased vascular effects/edema, and increased number of *Prevotella intermedia.*[22] Increased efficacy and frequency of self care are vital during this life phase.

An oral condition that becomes evident and has greater importance during adolescence is malocclusion.[23] Malocclusion is a condition or variation from proper alignment of the teeth and jaw; minor alignment problems have very little impact on patient health.[24] Conversely, some malocclusions can be esthetically displeasing, may affect chewing and speaking, and may necessitate treatment to maintain health and function. This is also a life stage when orthodontic treatment is considered; risk factors, potential benefits, and costs should also be taken into account. A noteworthy psychologic advantage often realized with orthodontic treatment is an enhanced self-image, which may have a positive effect on an adolescent's life.

Eating disorders are more prevalent in this stage of life.[25] Purging behavior of those with eating disorders may result in **periomylosis,** in which the enamel of teeth is dissolved by the acid produced by repeated vomiting.[26] The teeth may have a dull, chalky enamel surface. Often the lingual/palatal surfaces appear eroded, and restorations appeared raised from the tooth (**"floating amalgams"**). An oral examination indicating disordered eating should result in a frank discussion with the patient and a referral to the appropriate health care professional. This particular psychologic problem should be approached from a medical–dental team perspective. The psychiatrist or other mental health professional should be aware of and involved in the progress or deterioration of the patient's oral health as it relates to the patient's recovery from this eating disorder.[27]

Early Adulthood: 21–39 Years of Age

The dental hygienist can expect to educate pregnant women about their oral health before and after conception, and the impact that certain lifestyle choices can have on the oral health of the baby. Dispelling myths such as "you lose one tooth for every child you have" is another aspect in the education of the patient in this life stage. An expectant woman should not fear damage to her teeth during pregnancy if she maintains adequate care and gets the necessary vitamins and minerals for both herself and her unborn child. Explaining the relationship between gingivitis during pregnancy and its effects on fetal development (e.g., preterm low birth weight) can significantly elevate the importance of oral self-care during this phase of adult life.[28] **Pregnancy gingivitis** is present in over 30% of pregnant women.[29] Clinically, the gingival tissues appear bright red and edematous at the marginal gingiva and interdental papilla, with an increased tendency to bleed. This is a period of great receptivity to medical–dental knowledge, because expectant parents generally seek and appreciate information regarding health changes during this very important period of their life.

The current focus on wellness may be a powerful motivational strategy for patients and may provide dental providers with opportunities for patient education about oral health. Health promotion theory indicates that people are often more willing to comply with health instruction if a visually pleasing advantage is realized versus only a health improvement.[30] An example may be tobacco cessation. Although a significant health benefit exists when one ceases use of tobacco products, it may be the lack of stain on the teeth or fewer facial wrinkles that are the true motivators behind the change in behavior. Knowledge of health promotion theory allows the dental hygienist to present information about oral self-care or treatment options to patients in terms that are relevant to their needs and desires—and beyond expected health benefits.

Mature Adulthood: 40–60 Years of Age

As the U.S. population ages, life expectancy is increasing. Life expectancy has increased from 47.3 years of age in 1900 to 77.8 years of age in 2004.[31] This increase is accompanied by an expectation of a good quality of life. Oral problems have a negative effect on quality of life, because a problem with the oral cavity can affect the ability to eat, digest food, and communicate. Diet, nutrition, sleep, psychologic status, and social interaction are all affected by impaired oral health. Oral health and disease also have a significant impact on general health and disease.

To understand an individual patient's attitudes, one must evaluate the cultural, psychologic, educational, social, economic, dietary, and chronologically specific cohort experiences that may have influenced that patient's life.[32] Oral health status is affected by these same factors and is the sum of an individual's life experiences

with oral health care, as well as with caries, periodontal disease, and **iatrogenic disease** (disease caused inadvertently by a medical provider, a medical treatment, or a diagnostic procedure).

A comprehensive approach to the provision of preventive services, counseling, education, and disease screening for average-risk, asymptomatic adults includes regular assessments of health risks. Individuals with chronic disorders or who are members of high-risk populations may need further interventions. Screening and counseling includes risk stratification and health assessment; tobacco use screening; hypertension screening via blood pressure measurement; problem-drinking screening; osteoporosis screening via bone mineral density testing; and of course oral health screening for periodontal disease, dental caries, xerostomia, oral cancer, and other diseases and conditions.[33]

About 25% of adults 60 years old and older no longer have any natural teeth.[34] Periodontal disease or dental caries are the most frequent causes of tooth loss. Older Americans continue to experience dental decay, and older adults may have new tooth decay at higher rates than children.[34]

Severity of periodontal disease increases with age. At all ages men are more likely than women to have more severe disease. In addition, at all life stages, people at the lowest socioeconomic level have the most severe periodontal disease.

Root caries is a common problem among the elderly. It afflicts a large percentage of geriatric patients and is difficult to manage. The dental provider should conduct a detailed history and clinical examination, including a check of salivary flow, medication history for hyposalivatory medications, and the possibility of a high sugar intake (sucking candies; consuming sweetened tea or coffee, soft drinks, candy, gum, ice cream).[35] The etiology of root caries includes dietary habits, microbial plaque biofilm, and decreased salivary flow.[36] To rule out xerostomia as an etiologic factor, a salivary volume study can be performed, as well as a buffering capacity test.[35]

Root lesions are often very difficult to restore because of their location, problems with moisture control, and proximity to the pulp; therefore, they are prone to high recurrence rates. Prevention is the best treatment. As a primary, secondary, or tertiary intervention, chewing gum can be used as an adjunct to preventive therapy, because it has been shown to increase pH of the plaque and saliva, thereby assisting in neutralization of plaque acid formation.[37] Xylitol-containing gum stimulates saliva, inhibits bacterial plaque biofilm, and is a five-carbon sugar alcohol that cariogenic bacteria cannot metabolize for energy production.[38] Antimicrobial agents are effective against the infective process of caries: Chlorhexidine is extensively used as a mouthrinse to reduce the bacterial load intraorally.[39]

Fluoride is the primary preventive measure, because it has an antimicrobial effect on the bacteria that cause dental caries and supports remineralization of tooth structure.[40] Fluoride can be delivered to a patient in different forms including rinses, pastes, gels, varnishes, lozenges, tablets, and drinking water. Low-dose fluoride (1000 to 11,100 ppm) in a dentifrice has been reported to reduce caries by maintaining a low concentration of salivary fluoride available for remineralization with daily uses.[41] Mouthrinses (0.05% sodium fluoride) available for purchase over the counter are also retained in the saliva and dental plaque and, when used daily or weekly, help to prevent dental caries. Prescription-strength fluoride is available at a higher potency (5000 ppm dentifrice or 2.0% sodium fluoride rinse) for added caries protection. The effectiveness of all at-home products depends on patient compliance.

Professionally applied topical fluoride in the form of acidulated phosphate fluoride (1.23%) provides a long-term, low-fluoride-release source of calcium fluoride. This agent can slowly release fluoride and maintain the salivary fluoride level. Varnishes offer a high concentration (5% sodium fluoride at 22,600 ppm) of fluoride that adheres to the tooth structure, is applied professionally, and creates a film of calcium fluoride, which is then released in a timed manner.

Products containing calcium phosphates are now available. These products support remineralization by increasing calcium and phosphate in saliva, thus changing the pH balance toward remineralization. NovaMin is a synthetic mineral composed of calcium, sodium, phosphorous, and silica, which binds to the tooth surface and releases rapid, continuous deposition of a natural crystalline hydroxyl carbonate.[42] Recaldent contains casein phosphopeptide, a milk-derived peptide, that is bound to amorphous calcium phosphate. Casein phosphopeptide binds the compound to the tooth structure, and amorphous calcium phosphate is released during acidic challenges.[43] Studies have shown this compound to be effective in remineralizing caries lesions and interfering with the adhesion of some bacteria to the tooth surface.[44]

Enabling individuals to maintain good oral hygiene is an important preventive strategy for reducing gingival inflammation, particularly for dependent older people and others who may have difficulty maintaining adequate self-care. Aids such as power toothbrushes are a useful approach for individuals with decreased dexterity and visual acuity. Dietary modification suitable to the oral condition is another health promotion strategy among the elderly.

In summary, fluoridated water and use of fluoride toothpaste provide protection against dental decay at all ages. Practicing effective oral hygiene will reduce dental plaque biofilm and can help prevent periodontal disease and dental caries. Regular professional visits to the dental provider are vital, even if a person has no natural teeth and wears dentures. Professional care helps to maintain the overall health of the teeth and mouth, and provides for early detection of precancerous or cancerous lesions. Tobacco-cessation counseling is vital to reduce general health risks posed by tobacco use. Smokers have 7 times the risk of developing periodontal disease compared with non-smokers. The Smoking Cessation Leadership Center is an excellent resource.[45] Tobacco used in any form increases the risk for periodontal disease, oral and throat cancers, and oral fungal infection, namely oral candidiasis.[46] Spit tobacco containing sugar also increases the risk of dental caries.[47] Limiting alcoholic beverages reduces the risk for oral and throat cancers, because alcohol and tobacco used together are the primary risk factors for these cancers. Oral care before cancer chemotherapy or radiation to the head or neck is important, because these therapies can damage or destroy oral tissues and result in severe irritation of the oral tissues, mouth ulcers, loss of salivary function, rampant tooth decay, and destruction of bone. Caregivers should reinforce the daily oral hygiene routines of elders who are unable to perform these activities independently.

Individuals taking bisphosphonates for cancer or osteoporosis must be evaluated thoroughly. The development of bisphosphonate-related osteonecrotic lesions of the jaw is a clinical problem in which spontaneous exposure of alveolar bone occurs or, much worse, the patient presenting for routine dental extractions or periodontal curettage develops an area of necrotic bone that does not respond to conservative treatment or surgical management. The burden now falls on dental providers to consider the ramifications of bisphosphonate therapy in the patient population carefully before undertaking what may seem to be routine dental care.[48] If osteonecrosis is suspected, panoramic and tomographic imaging may be performed; however, radiographic changes are not evident until there is significant bone involvement. A thorough history and intraoral clinical examination is the most effective way to establish the diagnosis.

SUMMARY

The challenge to enhance public knowledge of oral health care remains for health care professionals in the private and public sectors, for developers of school programs, and for the news media. These groups can join forces to develop and implement a variety of relevant, culturally sensitive, and effective approaches for the appropriate use of fluorides and dental sealants, control of gingival conditions, and increasing awareness of the value of community water fluoridation, specifically for adults in their roles as eligible voters or parents.

Barriers to oral health care include availability, accessibility, affordability, and acceptability. Additional barriers include the functional and medical status of the individual, previous patterns of use of dental treatment, lack of knowledge, and fear.

We must be aware that the time is fast approaching when the demand for oral health care, especially geriatric care, will far exceed the number of dentists currently willing and able to provide such care. Alternative providers, such as dental hygienists, are a viable option to increase access to preventive and therapeutic care.

REFERENCES

1. Barker, B. D., & Gift, H. C. (1990). Oral health problems in the second fifty. In *The second fifty years: promoting health and preventing disability,* Berg, R. L., & Cassells, J. S., Eds. Washington, DC: National Academy Press, 119–135.
2. United States Department of Health and Human Services, Centers for Disease Control and Prevention. Oral health for adults. Retrieved 12/06 from http://www.cdc.gov/OralHealth/publications/factsheets/adult.htm. Posted December 2006. Viewed March 24, 2008.
3. U.S. Department of Health and Human Services. (2002). *Oral health in America: A report of the surgeon general.* Rockville, MD: U.S. Department of Health and Human Services, National Institute of Dental and Craniofacial Research, National Institutes of Health. Also available at: http://profiles.nlm.nih.gov/NN/B/B/J/V/_/nnbbjv.pdf.
4. The Writing Group for the WHI Investigators. (2002). Risks and benefits of estrogen plus progestin in healthy post-menopausal women: Principal results of the Women's Health Initiative randomized controlled trial. *JAMA* 288(3):321–33.
5. Hopcraft, M. S., & Morgan, M. V. (2006). Pattern of dental caries experience on tooth surfaces in an adult population. *Community Dent Oral Epidemiol,* 34(3):174–83.
6. NIDCR/CDC Dental, Oral and Craniofacial Data Resource Center. Oral health, U.S. 2002 annual report. Retrieved from http://drc.hhs.gov/report/3_0.HTM. Accessed March 24, 2008.
7. Brown, L. J., & Löe, H. (2000). Prevalence, extent, severity and progression of periodontal disease. *Periodontology,* 2(1):57–71.
8. Johnson, G. K., & Slach, N. A. (2001). Impact of tobacco use on periodontal status. *J Dent Educ,* 65(4):313–21.
9. Horowitz, A., Drury, T. F., Goodman, H. S., & Yellowitz, J. A. (2000, April). Oral pharyngeal cancer prevention and early detection—Dentists' opinions and practices. *J Am Dent Assoc,* 131(4):453–62.
10. National Institute of Dental and Craniofacial Research. *NIDCR strategic plan. The burden of oral diseases.* Bethesda, MD: U.S. Department of Health and Human Services, National Institute of Dental and Craniofacial Research, National Institutes of Health. Also available at: http://www2.nidcr.nih.gov/about/strat-plan/burden.asp#4. Accessed March 24, 2008.
11. Swango, P. A. (1996). Cancer of the oral cavity and pharynx in the United States: An epidemiologic review. *J Public Health Dent,* 56(6):309–18.
12. National Cancer Institute. (1999). *SEER cancer statistics review, 1973–1996.* Bethesda, MD: National Cancer Institute.
13. Sooriyamoorthy, M. & Gower, D. B. (1989, April). Hormonal influences on gingival tissue: Relationship to periodontal disease. *J Clin Periodontol,* 16(4):201.
14. Roberts, F. A., & Darveau, R. P. (2000). Beneficial bacteria of the periodontium. *Periodontology,* 30(1):40–50.
15. Majerus, P. W. (1998, January 29). Prostaglandins: Critical roles in pregnancy and colon cancer. *Curr Biol,* 8(3):R87–R89.
16. Amar, S, Chung, K. M. (1994) Influence of hormonal variation on the periodontium in women. Periodontology 2000 6 (1) , 79–87 doi:10.1111/j.1600-0757.1994.tb00028.x.
17. Willing, M., Sowers, M., Aron, D., Clark, M. K., Burns, T., Bunten, C., Crutchfield, M., D'Agostino, D., & Jannausch, M. (1998, April). Bone mineral density and its change in white women: Estrogen and vitamin D receptor genotypes and their interaction. *J Bone Miner Res,* 13:695–705.
18. Anbinder, A. L., Prado, M., Spalding, M., Balducci, I., Carvalho, Y. R., & da Rocha, R. F. (2006). Estrogen deficiency and periodontal condition in rats: A radiographic and macroscopic study. *Braz Dent J,* 17(3):201–207.
19. Yoshihara, A., Seida, Y., Hanada, N., & Miyazaki, H. (2004). A longitudinal study of the relationship between periodontal disease and bone mineral density in community-dwelling older adults. *J Clin Periodontol,* 31(8):680–84.

20. Halbreich, U., & Kahn, L. S. (2001). Role of estrogen in the aetiology and treatment of mood disorders. Review article. *CNS Drugs,* 15(10):797–817.

21. Mariotti, A. (1994). Sex steroid hormones and cell dynamics in the periodontium. *Critical Rev Oral Biol Med,* 5(1):27–53. Also available at: http://crobm.iadrjournals .org/cgi/reprint/5/1/27.pdf.

22. Machtei, E. E. (2004). The effect of menstrual cycle on periodontal health. *J Periodontol,* 75(3):408–12.

23. Feldmann, I., Lundström, F., & Peck, S. (1999). Occlusal changes from adolescence to adulthood in untreated patients with Class II Division 1 deepbite malocclusion. *Angle Orthodont,* 69(1):33–38.

24. Siegel, M. A. (2002). A matter of class: Interpreting subdivision in a malocclusion. *Am J Orthod Dentofacial Orthop,* 122(6):582–86.

25. Sheiham, A., Steele, J. G., Marcenes, W., Tsakos, G., Finch, S., & Walls, A. W. (2001). Prevalence of impacts of dental and oral disorders and their effects on eating among older people: A national survey in Great Britain. *Community Dent Oral Epidemiol,* 29(3):195–203.

26. Little, J. W. (2002). Eating disorders: Dental implications. *Oral Surg Oral Med Oral Pathol Oral Radiol Endod,* 93(2):138–43.

27. Fairburn, C., & Harrison, P. (2003, Feb.) Eating disorders. *Lancet,* 361(9355):407–16.

28. Pirie, M., Cooke, I., Linden, G., & Irwin, C. (2007). Dental manifestations of pregnancy. *Obstetrician Gynaecologist,* 9:1:21–26.

29. New York State Department of Health. (2006, August). Oral health care during pregnancy and early childhood practice guidelines. Retrieved from http://www.health .state.ny.us/publications/0824.pdf.

30. Earp, J. A. & Ennett, S. T. (1991). Conceptual models for health education research and practice. *Health Educ Res,* 6(2):163–71.

31. National Center for Health Statistics. (2006). *Health, United States, 2006 with chartbook on trends in the health of Americans.* Hyattsville, MD: National Center for Health Statistics.

32. John, J., Mani, S. A., & Azizah, Y. (2004). Oral health care in the elderly population in Malaysia—A review. *Med J Malaysia,* 59(3), 433–39.

33. Institute for Clinical Systems Improvement (ICSI). (2006, October). *Preventive services for adults.* Bloomington, MN: Institute for Clinical Systems Improvement, 1–48.

34. Centers for Disease Control and Prevention. CDC fact sheet. Oral health for older Americans. Retrieved 3/24/08 from http://www.cdc.gov/OralHealth/factsheets/ adult-older.htm. Modified November 21, 2006.

35. Faine, M. P., Allender, M. S., Baab, D., Persson, R., & Lamont, R. J. (1992). Dietary and salivary factors associated with root caries. *Spec Care Dent,* 12:177–82.

36. Cohen, G., Negron, R. J., & Bockler, M. A clinical approach to the treatment and management of rampant root caries. Retrieved 3/24/08 from http://www.cumc .columbia.edu/news/dental/cdr96/cohen.html.

37. Park, K. K., Schemehorn, B. R., Bolton, J. W., & Stookey, J. K. (1990). Effect of sorbitol gum chewing on plaque pH response after ingesting snacks containing predominantly sucrose or starch. *Am J Dent,* 3:185–91.

38. Anderson, M. H., Bratthall, D., Einwag, J., Eldertom, R. J., Ernst, C.-P., Levin, R. P., Tynelius-Bratthall, G., & Willershausen-Zonnchen, B. (1994). *Professional prevention in dentistry.* Baltimore, MD: Williams & Wilkins.

39. Santos, S., Herrera, D., López, E., O'Connor, A., González, I., & Sanz, M. (2004). A randomized clinical trial on the short-term clinical and microbiological effects of the adjunctive use of a 0.05% chlorhexidine mouth rinse for patients in supportive periodontal care. *J Clin Periodontol,* 31(1):45–51.

40. Rozier, R. G. (2001). Effectiveness of methods used by dental professionals for the primary prevention of dental caries. *J Dent Educ,* 65(10):1063–1072.

41. Wolfgang, H. A. (2006). Effect of fluoride tooth pastes on enamel demineralization. *BMC Oral Health,* 6:8.

42. Retrieved 5/21/08 from http://novamin.com/tooth-remineralization-technology.html.

43. Aimutis, W. R. (2004, April). Bioactive Properties of Milk Proteins with Particular Focus on Anticariogenesis. Supplement: The Emerging Role of Dairy Proteins and Bioactive Peptides in Nutrition and Health. The American Society for Nutritional Sciences *J. Nutr.* 134:989S–995S.

44. Reynolds, E. C. (1997). Remineralization of enamel subsurface lesions by casein phosphopeptide-stabilized calcium phosphate solutions. *J Dent Res,* 76:1587–95.

45. Retrieved 5/21/08 from http://smokingcessationleadership .ucsf.edu/.

46. Barbour, S. E., Nakashima, K., Zhang, J. B., Tangada, S., Hahn, C. L., Schenkein, H. A. & Tew, J. G. (1997). Tobacco and smoking: Environmental factors that modify the host response (immune system) and have an impact on periodontal health. *Crit Rev Oral Biol Med,* 8:437–60.

47. Tomar, S. L. & Winn, D. (1999). Chewing tobabcco use and dental caries among U.S. men. *J Am Dent Assoc,* 130(11):1601–10.

48. Salmassy, D. (2007, July). Fosamax: Bad to the bone? *Mod Hyg,* 3:7.

Chapter 25

Geriatrics

Charles D. Tatlock

OBJECTIVES

After reading this chapter, the student should be able to:

1. Describe and define this target population.
2. Describe common oral conditions and diseases of geriatric patients.
3. Describe specific preventive strategies to use with geriatric patients.
4. Describe the role of the dental provider in treating geriatric patients.

KEY TERMS

Elderly
Old
Very old
Functionally independent
Frail elderly
Kyphosis
Functional status
Dementia
Functional dentition
Long-term care

INTRODUCTION

"One of the undeniable facts about living is that every day we are getting older."[1] The good news is that people in the United States are living longer and healthier lives than ever before. Despite this fact, the current "Baby Boomer" generation—the cohort representing those born between the years 1946 and 1964—demonstrates a strong and consuming desire to stem the tide of the aging process. These efforts notwithstanding, projections by the U.S. Census Bureau predict that in 30 years, one of every five Americans will be 65 or older. In addition, the present geriatric population is one of the fastest growing segments of our society.

A number of significant changes occur during aging. Fortunately, most of these normal changes do not cause oral diseases.[2,3] Instead, it is the cumulative effects of both oral and systemic diseases that result in the prevalence of oral disease among the elderly. It is interesting to note that increasing numbers of "well elderly" are able to retain their natural teeth and enjoy normal oral function throughout old age. The current Baby Boomer generation is becoming increasingly aware of the fact that oral health is important, both in terms of one's general health status and the effects of oral health on physical appearances and the development of positive self-concepts.[4]

With regard to the twenty-first century, older adults by the year 2040 are expected to account for approximately 21% of the population in the United States, a significant increase from 4% in 1900 and 12% in 1990. The 85-and-older age group is the most rapidly growing segment in the U.S. population. Projections by the U.S. Census Bureau suggest that this population could grow from about 4 million in 2000 to 19 million by 2050.[5]

POPULATION CHARACTERISTICS

The U.S. older population grew rapidly for most of the twentieth century, from 3.1 million in 1900 to 35 million in 2000. In addition, the number of centenarians, people at least 100 years old, has increased in the last decade from about 37,000 in 1990 to over 50,000 in 2000. About 80% of centenarians are women (Figure 25–1 ■). Except during the 1990s, the growth of the older population has outpaced that of the total population. This growth rate has prompted social observers to describe the older population as being on the threshold of a boom.[5]

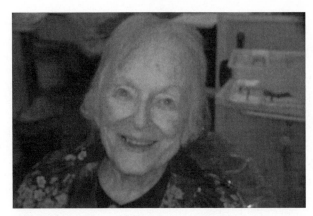

■ **FIGURE 25–1** Heloise A. Arnold, RDH and Centenarian. A graduate from the first school of dental hygiene, Fones School of Dental Hygiene in Bridgeport, Connecticut.
(Charles D. Tatlock, DDS, MPH, University of New Mexico, Albuquerque, NM)

The Baby Boomer cohorts' impact on the country's age structure will continue into the first half of the twenty-first century. By 2020 the Baby Boomer cohorts will be aged 56 to 74 years (Figure 25–2 ■), and by 2030, one fifth of the American population will be 65 or older. The size of the older population is projected to double over the next 30 years, growing to 70 million by 2030. Also note that in Figure 25–2 the U.S. Census Bureau projects that the population aged 85 and older could grow from about 4 million in 2000 to 19 million by 2050. After 2030 the Baby Boomers will become the oldest old, and the country's age structure is expected to change (Figures 25–3 ■ through 25–6 ■).[5]

This age structure is unprecedented in American history. Currently, Baby Boomers include over 76 million people, of whom 25% have a college education. In addition, they are the first generation to have benefited from widespread community water fluoridation and fluoride in toothpaste. As a result, many will reach older adulthood with their dentition virtually intact.[6]

In response to this changing U.S. and world demographic, the World Health Organization (WHO) issued a document in 2002 titled *Active Ageing: A Policy Framework*,[7] which outlines essential approaches toward healthy aging. As a way for people to enjoy longevity and sustain health-related quality of life with age, this document emphasizes the importance of minimizing risk factors that contribute to chronic disease and functional decline while maximizing protective factors against such problems.

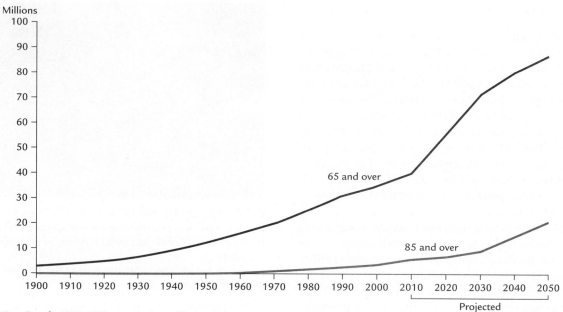

Note: Data for 2010–2050 are projections of the population.
Reference population: These data refer to the resident population.

■ **FIGURE 25–2** Number of People Age 65 and Over, by Age Group, Selected Years 1900–2000 and Projected 2010–2050
(*Source:* U.S. Census Bureau, Decennial Census and Projections.)

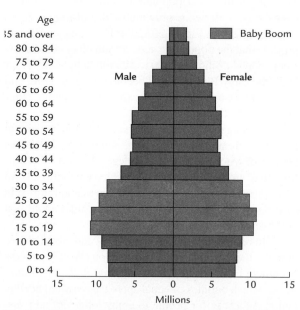

Note: The reference population for these data is the resident population.

■ **FIGURE 25–3** Population by Age and Sex: 1980
(*Source:* U.S.Bureau of the Census, 1983, Table 44. For full citation, see references at end of chapter.)

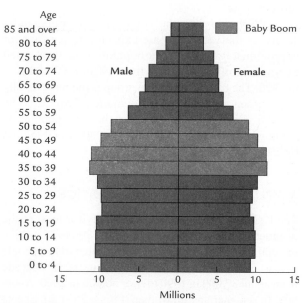

Note: The reference population for these data is the resident population.

■ **FIGURE 25–4** Population by Age and Sex: 2000
(*Source:* U.S. Census Bureau, 2001, Table PCT12. For full citation, see references at end of chapter.)

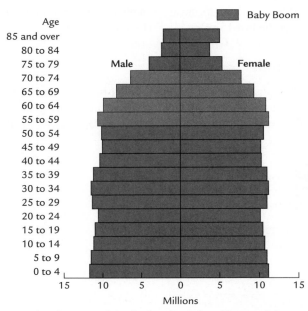

Note: The reference population for these data is the resident population.

■ **FIGURE 25–5** Population by Age and Sex: 2020 (Source: U.S. Census Bureau, 2004. For full citation, see references at end of chapter.)

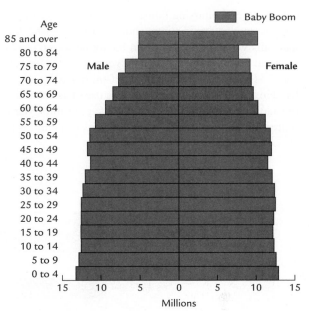

Note: The reference population for these data is the resident population.

■ **FIGURE 25–6** Population by Age and Sex: 2040 (Source: U.S. Census Bureau, 2004. For full citation, see references at end of chapter.)

It is important to recognize that *oral health* is an identified component of "active aging" and is included in the WHO policy proposals. In many ways, this is a visionary statement. Whereas it generally has been agreed that good oral health care should begin at birth, relatively few have argued and advocated for oral health among the elderly. Slowly, and thanks in part to advocacy by former U.S. Surgeons General, a national realization is emerging that oral health is important to overall health for people of all ages.

The WHO defines the population between 65 and 75 years as "**elderly.**" The term "**old**" is used for individuals between 76 and 90 years and "**very old**" for those over age 90. Elderly and old individuals are often very different with respect to their physiologic function, burden of illness, and any associated disability.[8] In essence, when we are describing the geriatric population, we are dealing with a very heterogeneous group.

Frail Elderly

Ettinger and Beck[9] developed a functional definition of the elderly based upon an older person's ability to seek

dental services. The categorization that they developed can be divided into three groups:[10]

- The functionally independent older adult
- The frail older adult
- The functionally dependent older adult

According to this description, the vast majority of older adults, 70%, are able to get to the dentist and are categorized as **functionally independent.** About 14% of community-dwelling elderly fall under the **frail elderly** category. These are persons with chronic conditions contributing to major limitations in mobility. About 5% of community-dwelling elderly are homebound or functionally dependent. Another group of functionally dependent older adults are those who are institutionalized in nursing homes.[10]

Living arrangements of America's older adults are closely linked to income, health status, and the availability of caregivers. Older persons who live alone are more likely to be in poverty and experience health problems, compared with older persons who live with a spouse or a relative. In 1997, 1.6 million elderly, less than 5% of the elderly, lived in nursing homes.[1] The percentage of the population who live in nursing homes also increased dramatically with age, ranging from 1% for persons 65 to 74 years, to 5% for persons 75 to 84 years, to 19% for persons 85+ years.[1] In 2000, over a half-million older adults lived in assisted-living facilities. The use of assisted-living facilities, board and care homes, continuing-care retirement communities, and other types of facilities in addition to long-term care in a nursing home has grown over the last 15 years.[1,11–17] (Figure 25–7 ■).

Health

The most common illnesses found in older American adults are arthritis, hypertension, impaired hearing, heart disease, and impaired vision (Table 25–1 ■). Nearly 90% of

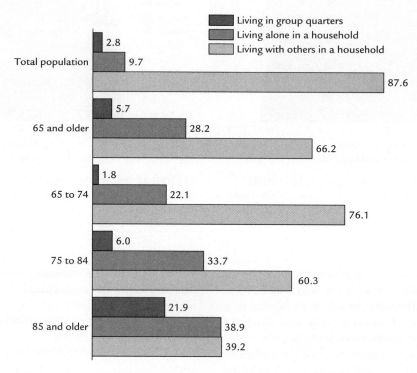

■ **FIGURE 25–7** Living Arrangements: 2000 (Percent distribution. Data based on sample. For information on confidentiality protection, sampling error, nonsampling error, and definitions, see *www.census.gov/prod/cen2000/doc/sf4.pdf*)

(*Source:* U.S. Census Bureau, Census 2000 special tabulation.)

■ **Table 25–1**   Top Five Chronic Conditions among Community-Dwelling Seniors by Gender

Men	*Women*
1. Arthritis	1. Arthritis
2. Hearing impairments	2. Hypertension
3. Heart condition	3. Heart condition
4. Hypertension	4. Hearing Impairments
5. Deformities: orthopedic impairments	5. Cataracts

Source: From: U.S. Bureau of the Census, Statistical Abstract of the United States, 1996. (118th Edition), Washington, DC, 1998.

all older adults have a chronic illness. At present, 30% of the individuals over age 65 have three or more chronic illnesses and account for more than 33% of the costs for health care in the United States.[9] Yet, almost 71% of noninstitutionalized older adults describe their general health to be excellent, very good, or good, compared with others their age.[4]

The leading causes of death in adults over the age of 65, which account for approximately 75% of all the deaths, are heart disease, cancer, stroke, and Alzheimer's disease or dementing illnesses.[4,9] Cardiovascular disease remains the leading cause of death in older adults but has experienced a significant reduction since 1940 (since then a marked reduction in cardiovascular deaths for all age groups has occurred). The 85-years-and-older group has had the least reduction, which was 20%.[9,18]

Cancer (lung, breast, prostate, and colon) is the second most-common cause of death in older adults. Since 1940, a 20% increase has occurred in cancer deaths for persons 55 years of age and older. Statistics show that 37% of men and 22% of women aged 60 to 79 years will develop invasive cancer. The risk for invasive cancer from birth to death is 50% in men and 30% in women. The most marked increase has been in cancer of the lung in both men and women.[9,19]

The third leading cause of death in older adults is cerebrovascular disease (stroke). The incidence has been decreasing since 1960.[20,21] Approximately 10 stroke patients exist per 1000 population in the United States. Prevalence rises in men from 14.6 per 1,000 adults at 45 to 64 years to 77.5 per 1,000 for men ages 75 and older, and from 15.9 to 79.6 in the respective age groups in women.[9,22,23]

In light of the above information, a dramatic increase is expected in the number of older adults in this country and in the proportion with significant chronic illnesses. These older adults will need dental care at an increasing level in years to come. Oral health professionals must be aware of the special management needed to treat this group of patients.[9] For example, drug dosages and duration of treatment may have to be modified, certain drugs may have to be avoided, antibiotic prophylaxis may have to be administered, and special precautions may have to be made before surgery to avoid excessive bleeding.[9,20]

Physiologic Changes

Physiologic changes associated with aging can impact every system in the body and have an effect on the way dental care is delivered. Overall, changes occur for all people, tissues, and organs; but these changes occur with differing rates and individual variability. However, many of the deficits traditionally attributed to aging are actually signs of pathologic processes.[4]

The major results of the aging process are (1) a reduced physiologic reserve of many body functions (i.e., heart, lungs, kidney); (2) an impaired homeostasis mechanism by which bodily activities are kept adjusted (i.e., fluid balance, temperature control, and blood pressure control); (3) an impaired immunologic system, as well as a related increased incidence of neoplastic and age-related autoimmune conditions.[4,24]

Bone remains metabolically active throughout life. Age-related bone loss is extremely common, reflecting an imbalance between bone resorption by osteoclasts and bone formation by osteoblasts. *Osteoporosis,* a common problem in the elderly, is an age-related disorder characterized by a decrease in bone mass and by an increased susceptibility to bone fractures. Clinically, advanced osteoporosis can present with chronic back pain, from mechanical strain caused by **kyphosis** or vertebral compression fractures.[4] Kyphosis is the condition that generally results in the stooping posture and rounded-shoulder appearance of the affected elder.

Recent studies indicate that changes in alveolar bone as a result of osteoporosis may contribute to the progression of periodontal disease.[4,25] Also, a significant decrease in bone mass of the mandible may lead to fragility and increased resorption, risk of fracture, and failure of osseointegration of dental implants. Prevention, rather than treatment, is the key to the management of osteoporosis. Exercise, vitamins, a balanced diet, dietary calcium, and estrogen play a role in the treatment and prevention of osteoporosis.[4]

It is incumbent upon the dental team to be aware and adaptable to the commonly seen age-related changes in their patients. Modifications of office design and patient management techniques will facilitate and enhance the practices of those providing oral health care to a growing older population who inevitably will be seeking dental care.

Functional Status

According to geriatricians, functional status is a critical indicator of health and well-being in the older person. Furthermore, it is one of the most challenging issues in health care of older adults. **Functional status** is often used as a way to describe an individual's health status rather than the presence of specific diseases.[4] As an overarching concept, it describes a more complete picture that includes impairments in physical and cognitive functioning, and also helps predict mortality, institutionalization, and the type and amount of health care services needed. Identifying a person's functional status requires a comprehensive health assessment, including an assessment of the individual's functional abilities, health status, physical, psychological, and oral health status.[4]

Cognitive Changes

Recent studies of the aging brain demonstrate that major cognitive declines do not occur in the absence of disease, trauma, or stress. These studies suggest that developmental transitions, life events, and environmental changes may interfere with older adults' ability to concentrate and to think clearly.[4] Research has indicated that a person's intellect does not decline as an outcome of aging, but rather as a result of many conditions including poor nutrition, vitamin deficiencies, disease, and hormonal changes.[26] An older person usually takes longer than a younger adult to learn the same information, but when given sufficient time, the end result is similar for both individuals. In general, more time is needed for an older person to encode, that is, to retrieve or to recall the information. In later life, mental health is measured by the capacity to cope effectively with relationships and environment and by the satisfaction experienced in doing so.[4]

Because of the multiplicity of factors that relate to the treatment of the elderly, it is important to evaluate the ability of the patient to communicate and to understand, consent to, and participate in the treatment. The practitioner must determine, either through an interview or professional services, the capacity of the individual to respond to treatment.[4]

Dementia is the loss of established intellectual activity that interferes with occupational and social function. It includes impairment of memory, language, perception, calculation, abstract thinking, judgment, and executive function.[9] The most common type of dementia in the elderly is senile dementia of the Alzheimer's type (SDAT), accounting for over 50% of all dementias seen in the elderly.[4] The second most common cause of dementia in the elderly is multi-infarct dementia, or vascular dementia, accounting for 15% to 25% of cases.[27] Both of these types of dementia are irreversible. Between 10% and 20% of the cases of dementia are classified as reversible.[9,21] The reversible dementias may be associated with the following medical diseases: hepatic encephalopathy, acid–base disturbances, hypoglycemia, thyroid disease, uremia, AIDS, trauma, syphilis, multiple sclerosis, and stroke.[9]

Alzheimer's disease is discussed here briefly, because it is the most common type of dementia seen in elders. Senile dementia of the Alzheimer's type (SDAT) is a progressive, degenerative, dementing illness that attacks the brain and leads to the loss of memory, intellectual capacity, and ability to think, and to changes in behavior. Approximately 10% of older adults over age 65 years and 45% over age 85 years have SDAT. In the early stages of the disease, the individual generally maintains good social skills and is often able to "disguise" the presence of the disease. At this stage, the disease is often very difficult to assess and is generally denied by family members.[4]

The cause of SDAT is not known; however, several possibilities are under investigation, including genetics, nutrition, environment, and infectious agents.[9] Currently there is no cure for SDAT. A relatively new drug, tacrine (Cognex) has shown short-term benefit; tacrine has a high rate of toxicity though.[21,28] Another new drug, donepezil (Aricept), has shown about the same level of benefit as tacrine but without the high rate of toxicity.[29] Velnacrine, a metabolite of tacrine, also has been used to treat SDAT with limited results.[30]

Despite treatment, the disease progresses over a period of from 2 to 20 years and presents as a complex picture of overlapping symptoms that reflect a continuous decline in memory, ability to think, and behavior control. Cognitive skills and competency in life skills decline. There is loss of memory, language, intellectual prowess, concentration, and emotionality, as well as altered spatial motor performance. Both verbal and nonverbal communication is affected.[4]

Alzheimer's patients are managed best by an understanding and empathetic approach. The oral health professional should keep the patient's attention and explain what is going to happen before doing it. The provider should communicate using short words and sentences, and should repeat instructions and explanations. Nonverbal communication can be very helpful. Facial motion and body posture of the dental professional should show support, willingness to care, and cues that the patient is understood. Positive nonverbal communication includes direct eye contact, smiling, touching of the arm, patting of the hand, and so on.[9] Patients with SDAT should be placed on an aggressive preventive dentistry program including 3-month recall, oral examination, prophylaxis, fluoride gel application, oral hygiene instruction, and adjustment of prosthesis.[31]

COMMON ORAL MANIFESTATIONS

It is essential to recognize that no broad, generalized declining changes in oral health occur simply with age. Healthy older people can expect to keep their teeth throughout their lifetime. However, in the presence of one or more medical conditions and/or their treatments, oral functions may be altered, which can then impact the patients' general and oral health status.[4]

During the past 50 years, one of the major changes in patterns of oral disease in the United States has been a steady decrease in the rate of edentulism. It is likely that, for the first time in recorded history, there are now more older adults with natural teeth than without teeth.[4] In 1986, almost 30% of those 65 to 74 years were edentulous, whereas in 2024 it is predicted that only 10% of this group will be edentulous.[32] This decline in edentulism appears to be the result of water fluoridation, increased public awareness of preventive approaches, improved access to services, and a decrease in early tooth loss.[4,33]

Consequently, older adults today retain more teeth than did earlier generations. And they often maintain so-called **functional dentition,** defined as the presence of at least 20 natural teeth, many of which may be heavily restored with fillings, crowns, and bridges.[8]

Although the prevalence of edentulism increases in the noninstitutionalized older age groups, these rates have steadily decreased over time.[34] At the same time that more teeth are being retained, this decline in tooth loss results in more natural teeth at risk for caries (coronal, recurrent, and root) and periodontal diseases. As these trends continue, more restorative and preventive services will need to be performed in future dental practices.[4]

Recent reports have found that the prevalence of coronal caries is decreasing for children and young adults of middle to high socioeconomic status. Although dental caries has not traditionally been perceived as a problem for the elderly, decay rates have been found to be higher in some adult groups than in children. As long as teeth are present, individuals remain at risk of dental caries.[4,34] Unfortunately, many older adults do not place a priority on oral health care; they think the only reason to see a dentist is to relieve pain and discomfort. This effect, coupled with a reduced sensory ability, means many older adults tend to seek care only when their decay is in a late stage.[4] Root caries is common and frequently occurs in this age group. Root caries has been found in 65% of the males and 53% of the females in the 1985–86 National Institute of Dental Research study.[35] With the use of new preventive approaches and restorative materials, the dilemma associated with restoring root-carious lesions is expected to diminish in the future.[4]

Contrary to many long-held views, periodontal disease is not an age-related disease. Although the prevalence of periodontal disease appears to increase with age, this increase is likely due to the long-standing cumulative nature of the disease, with its onset earlier in adulthood. It is estimated that 90% of adults aged 65+ years need periodontal treatment, with 15% needing complex treatment.[36] With new diagnostic methods complementing traditional clinical techniques, earlier identification of periodontal disease and risk factors will be possible, as well as early treatment to help reduce disease progression and its subsequent loss of teeth.[4]

Like most cancers, oral cancer occurs primarily in the older age segments of the population, with the majority of cases diagnosed after age 65 and more than 95% occurring after age 40.[37] The key issue related to oral cancer problems is the need for early and effective diagnosis. Although the primary risk factors for the development of oral squamous cell carcinoma, the most-common form of oral cancer, have traditionally included alcohol abuse and use of tobacco products, these risk factors do not have to be present for a lesion to develop.[38] Thus, it is of vital importance for the oral health care professional to provide oral cancer examinations to all patients on a regular (at least annual) basis. Early diagnosis of oral cancer greatly improves the prognosis of the disease. Many factors influence the timing at which oral cancers are diagnosed, such as lack of access to care and patient delay in seeking treatment.[39] Therefore, oral health professionals must provide, when appropriate, routine comprehensive intra- and extraoral examinations of their patient populations.[4]

Through frequent recall visits and regular professional examinations, adults will be able to better maintain their dentition throughout their life. Prevention of oral disease is the critical component for oral health maintenance. In addition to promoting and monitoring basic oral hygiene practices, the practitioner needs to be aware of the changing physical, psychologic, socioeconomic, and medication status of their older adult patients.[4] In addition, the practitioner needs to be ready and willing to intervene, to make necessary modifications to treatment, and to make referrals to community resources. Older adults and their caregivers need to be educated and have their education reinforced so as to enhance their knowledge of oral care protocols.

Long-Term Care

Long-term care refers to health, social, and residential services provided to chronically disabled persons over an extended time.[4,14] Population studies in the United States suggest that persons 65 years and older have a 40% chance of spending some time in a long-term care facility before they die. Of those who enter nursing homes, 55% will spend at least 1 year there, and over 20% will spend more than 5 years there. Two of the most-common symptoms that lead to nursing home placement are incontinence and behavioral problems such as wandering or disruptive actions often associated with dementia and Alzheimer's disease.[4,15]

This population has been characterized as having high levels of edentulism, coronal and root caries, poor oral hygiene, periodontal diseases, and soft tissue lesions.[4,16,17] Residents of long-term care facilities could have their oral health needs met on-site in light of new technological advances in portable and mobile dental equipment. With an increasing number of oral health professionals willing to provide mobile services, comprehensive oral health programs would become feasible and logical activities in this setting.

Surgeon General's Report

The U.S. Surgeon General's report, *Oral Health in America,* emphasizes the fact that oral health is integral to general health and describes the disparities in the availability of dental care, especially for very young and very old populations.[40] The report uses the phrase "silent epidemic" to characterize the disparity between the epidemic of oral disease and the silence from those who need care. This report highlights many reasons that dental care is of particular importance for frail older adults:[1]

- Oral diseases are cumulative and become more complex over time. The older adult population has high rates of oral diseases. This is complicated further by the fact that many senior adults lose their dental insurance when they retire. Medicare does not reimburse for routine dental services, and many states do not have Medicaid dental coverage for the frail elderly.[1]
- Oral problems have a negative effect on quality of life. Oral–facial pain and tooth loss can greatly reduce the quality of life and restrict major functions. Problems with the teeth and mouth can affect the ability to eat and communicate. Individuals with facial disfigurements due to oral diseases often experience loss of self-esteem, anxiety, depression, and social stigma. Diet, nutrition, sleep, psychological status, and social interaction are all affected by impaired oral health.[1]
- Dental disease has a significant impact on general health. The oral cavity can be a portal of entry for microbial infections that affect the whole body. Oral diseases give rise to pathogens, which can be blood-borne[41] or aspirated into the lungs,[42] bringing about severe, even life-threatening, consequences. Recent research findings have linked possible associations between chronic oral infections and diabetes, heart and lung disease, and stroke.[1]

Older adults suffer from the cumulative effects of oral diseases over their lifetime. This results in extensive oral disease.[43] Berkey, Berg, Ettinger, and Meskin, in a comprehensive review of oral health studies of institutionalized elderly published between 1970 and 1989, described the compromised oral health status of nursing home residents. Up to 70% of residents had unmet oral needs, exhibiting high rates of edentulism (complete tooth loss), dental caries (decay), poor oral hygiene, periodontal disease (diseases of the supporting structures of the teeth), and soft tissue lesions.[16]

Over 30% of community-dwelling elderly in 1997 were edentulous, with the rate rising to 43% of those older than 85 years.[1] Approximately one third of community-dwelling elderly have untreated coronal or root caries and other oral health problems including periodontal disease, attrition, unreplaced missing teeth, abrasion and erosion, broken or failing older dental restorations, dry mouth, mucosal diseases, oral cancer, and alveolar ridge atrophy.[1] The homebound often face insurmountable barriers to dental access. Among the elderly receiving home health services noted in one study, the majority reported their oral health was "fair" or "poor," and nearly 80% reported a perceived dental care need. In addition, only 26% reported having been to the dentist within the past 2 years, whereas 40% reported not having been to the dentist in more than 10 years.[17]

A major impact of systemic diseases on the oral health of older adults is caused by the side effects of medications. With increasing age and associated chronic disease, the elderly are prescribed an ever-expanding variety of medications. Besides the desired therapeutic outcome, adverse side effects may alter the integrity of the oral mucosa. Problems such as xerostomia (dry mouth), bleeding disorders of the tissues, lichenoid reactions (oral tissue changes), tissue overgrowth, and hypersensitivity reactions may occur as a result of drug therapy.[44]

The dental treatment needs of the elderly differ from those of younger adults, and newer cohorts of elderly have significantly different needs than older cohorts. Shay reports that in 1957, 70% of adults aged 75 years were fully edentulous, whereas today the number has dropped to less than 40%. This finding means that, 40 years ago, most dental treatment for older adults involved making and repairing full dentures. Today the picture has changed dramatically, with far more natural teeth present, and significantly different attitudes toward oral health and dental care among newer cohorts of the elderly. The elderly now receive a full range of dental services from examinations and preventive services to complex restorative and periodontal services.[45]

Aging has an impact on oral tissues just as it has on other tissues throughout the body. As teeth age, the enamel, dentin, and pulp undergo progressive changes. The enamel becomes less hydrated (drier). In addition, the thickness of the enamel decreases as enamel is lost from abrasion and attrition. Dentin changes more profoundly over a lifetime. The dentin volume expands into the pulp chamber as secondary dentin forms in response to decay and mastication. Many dentinal tubules narrow and others close altogether, forming sclerotic dentin. These changes make the older tooth more brittle, less resilient, less soluble, less permeable, and darker in color.[1] The pulp chamber, where the blood vessels and nerves of the teeth are located, also undergoes significant changes. The volume of the chamber declines as secondary dentin is deposited. The blood vessels and nerves in the pulp decline with a loss of myelinated nerve fibers and a gain of dystrophic calcium.[46]

PREVENTIVE STRATEGIES

It has been said that the greatest failure in modern dentistry is the failure to treat. At the same time that dentistry is able to provide implants, esthetic veneers, and other "high-tech" treatments that would have been unimaginable only a few years ago, large segments of the population, including the frail elderly, lack access to necessary basic care.[1]

A major question is whether older adults today, as well as baby boomers who will be entering their seventies within the next decade, will demand dental care as part of their overall well-being. The current cohort of elders varies widely in its use of dental services, from regular preventive users to nonusers who report that they have not been to a dentist in more than 20 years. In 1999, 53.5% of older adults reported that they had visited a dentist, the lowest rate of any age group beyond 18 years of age.[47]

Perhaps one should not expect current cohorts of older adults—born before 1940—to value oral health and dental esthetics in the same way younger generations do. Several researchers have reported significant differences between younger and older adults in oral health status and utilization patterns.[48] In studies in which age groups are compared, significant differences generally emerge, with older adults more likely to report not seeking dental care within the most recent 5 or more years. Utilization appears to peak in middle age, then declines dramatically by age 65; 1999 National Health Interview Survey (NHIS) data revealed that only 53.5% of adults aged 65 and older had seen a dentist in the past year, compared with 67% of those aged 35 to 54 years. More than a quarter (28%) of the older group had not been to a dentist in more than 10 years. Nevertheless, utilization rates for all groups increased between 1989 and 1999, with the greatest increase among the oldest age group, from 43.2% to 53.5%.[48,49]

Senior-Friendly Dental Practice

Many frail older adults can be seen at a regular dental office, provided that they are mobile and the office is accessible and senior-friendly. In some instances, modifications are needed to accommodate the frail older adult. Erickson developed the list of essentials for the senior-friendly office.[50]

Health Promotion

Health promotion has become an important means of improving older adults' behaviors in a variety of areas, including exercise, weight loss, management of diabetes, and hypertension.[51] Unfortunately, it has received less attention in dentistry except for some early efforts 20 or more years ago. With the rapid advances in materials and methods for home-based oral hygiene as well as in the materials and techniques in dental practice, it is important to educate the general population on an ongoing basis. Even those who make semiannual dental visits generally do not receive oral health education. Many patients would welcome such efforts, as illustrated by the findings of Abrams and colleagues that 73% of adults younger than 55 years and 62% of those 55 and older indicated a desire for educational programs in their dentist's office.[52] For those who do not seek regular dental care, this information is even more critical and should be provided in alternative settings such as senior centers, assisted-living facilities, and adult day health centers, as well as non-traditional settings such as faith community centers and malls. Advocates of oral health care for current and future cohorts of elders can adopt many of the techniques used by the medical community to assist patients with chronic systemic diseases. The dental care community must find creative ways to reach out to underserved segments of older adults.[51]

Although one expects to observe an increase in dentures among the elderly, a question remains as to whether the non-edentulous elderly receive an array of dental care similar to other adults.[51] Examinations and preventive care on a continuing and regular basis over the life span are essential for good oral health and for reducing the incidence of periodontal disease and requirements for dentures.

In other words, this population represents those for whom the broader range of dental services is appropriate. The diminished use of preventive services (cleaning and examinations) currently experienced by the older adult population, however, does suggest a special effort may be needed to encourage older adults to use preventive dentistry and to develop assurances that improved access to dental care will be extended to all ages in the life span.[51]

Public Policy

Although preventive dentistry has increased in the United States in recent years, the gains have been most dramatic among the younger cohorts. Programs to encourage and support access to dental care for the elderly are needed to reduce the age-based utilization gap and to improve the oral health of elders.

What can health care policy makers do to ensure that there are enough trained health professionals for America's future? As the dental needs of frail elderly adults discussed in this chapter become more apparent, some recommendations have been set forward. Table 25–2 ■ delineates action steps proposed by Helgeson and colleagues, which are among the most concise and far-reaching recommendations that the author has encountered regarding the issue of increased access to oral health care for the geriatric population.[1]

■ **Table 25–2**   Policy Strategies to Change Perceptions toward Oral Health Care for Elders

Work to Change Perceptions Regarding Oral Health and Disease So that Oral Health Becomes an Accepted Component of General Health
Include oral health services in all health promotion, disease prevention, and care delivery programs. Develop training programs for non-dental health professionals to emphasize how they can and should work to enhance oral health.

Accelerate the Building of the Science and Evidence Base and Apply Science Effectively to Improve Oral Health
Survey dental needs among older adults living in a variety of settings, including senior housing, board and care homes, assisted living facilities, nursing homes, and other long-term care facilities.

Build an Effective Oral Health Infrastructure that Meets the Needs of All Americans
Develop community-based dental care delivery systems at regional and state levels to reduce gaps in prevention and care for low-income older adults, nursing home residents, and elderly people with disabilities.

Remove Known Barriers between People and Oral Health Services
Increase the number of dental professionals who are trained to provide mobile, on-site dental care for frail elderly adults and other groups with special dental access needs.
Provide oral health benefits in all public health programs, especially those for elderly adults.

Use Public-Private Partnerships to Improve the Oral Health of Those Who Still Suffer Disproportionately from Oral Diseases
Increase the number of dental, medical, and nursing programs with active partnerships or cooperative working agreements with public and private community-based organizations that serve people with special access needs, such as frail elderly adults.

Source: From Helgeson, M. et.al., (2001). Frail Elderly Adults. Dental Care Considerations of Disadvantaged and Special Care Populations. Proceedings of the Conference Held April 18–19, 2001, in Baltimore, Maryland. U. S. Department of Health and Human Services, Health Resources and Services Administration. Rockville, Md.

Dental Providers

The role of the oral health professional will focus more on the diagnosis and treatment of oral diseases and disorders and the use of new modalities. As diseases of the hard tissues are resolved, more emphasis will be placed on the diagnosis and treatment of soft tissue lesions. With new and improved diagnostic skills, the older adult, the group identified as having the highest risk of oral cancer, may no longer require the extensive and often disfiguring surgical remedies currently being administered. These projected oral health outcomes justify that preventive oral health approaches need to be maintained throughout the lifespan.[4]

To provide optimal care to the aging population, one must remain current on oral medicine, pharmacotherapeutics, and changing technologies. Oral health care professionals must address how this aging population will manage in a variety of dental settings, and at a minimum, have accessible, senior-friendly offices, medical history forms printed in large type, as well as easy-to-read signs, health literature, and appointment cards.[4]

Oral health is important to overall health for people of all ages. There is definitive research that shows the connections between poor oral health and systemic diseases, such as diabetes, cardiovascular disease, and respiratory disease, particularly among older adults. Oral cancers are known to be more prevalent in people over the age of 50.[9]

New research is pointing to potential connections between oral health and other systemic conditions.[53] Researchers are still learning about the links between oral health and general health, but in itself, oral disease can cause pain, tooth loss, and bad breath. Seniors living in long-term care facilities, as well as some seniors being cared for in their home, are at particular risk of complications from poor oral health because of frailty, poor health, and increased dependence on others for personal care. In many cases, oral health problems in residents of long-term care facilities go undetected until there are acute symptoms, such as pain or infection.

The changing marital and family composition that is occurring in the United States is likely to change the types of familial support that are available to people at older ages. The future older population is likely to be better educated than the current older population, especially when Baby Boomers start reaching age 65. Their increased levels of education may accompany better health, higher incomes, and more wealth, and consequently higher standards of living in retirement. Research on genetic, biologic, and physiologic aspects of aging is likely to change the future for the older population. In the medical and public health arenas, research to understand chronic diseases, such as diabetes and Alzheimer disease, may produce significant improvements for treatment and prevention.[53]

SUMMARY

The oral health professional of today and of the future will be called on to treat an ever-increasing number of older adults. The future elderly will differ from the cohort seen today. The future elderly will have more teeth, visit the dental professional more often, and have a higher level of education, better finances and a dramatically different perspective on needs. They are, and will continue to be, a heterogeneous mix of individuals with various levels of functional, socioeconomic, and oral health status. Advances in materials and technology, combined with the changing patterns of oral diseases, will continue to have dramatic effects on the practice of dentistry.[4]

The social and economic implications of the aging of the Baby Boom generation will be a significant concern for policy makers, the public health and private sectors, and individuals. The size and longevity of this group will trigger debate about possible modifications to Social Security, Medicaid, Medicare, and disability and retirement benefits, among other issues.[5] And to think this was the generation that once vowed never to trust anyone over 30.[54]

This chapter has underscored the notion that oral health is important to overall health for people of all ages. And ideally, this important component of health care should continue past retirement into the twilight years. Proper dental care must now be understood as a lifetime commitment. As we learn more about the link between oral and systemic health, and as more people keep their natural teeth into old age, it is critical to help older adults learn and practice preventive oral health care.

REFERENCES

1. Helgeson, M., Smith, B. J., Johnsen, M., & Ebert, C. (2001). Frail elderly adults. In Health Resources and Services Administration. Proceedings of a conference on Dental Care Considerations of Disadvantaged and Special Care Populations. Rockville, MD: U.S. Department of Health and Human Services, Health Resources and Services Administration. (U. S. Government Printing Office: 2001, 491-191/43013.

2. Baum, B. J., & Ship, J. A. (1991). Oral disorders. In Beck, J., Ed. *Geriatrics review syllabus—A core curriculum in geriatric medicine.* New York: American Geriatrics Society, 332–36.

3. Beck, J. D. (1984). Epidemiology of dental diseases in the elderly. *Gerodontology,* 3:5–15.

4. Yellowitz, J. A., & Strayer, M. S. (2004). Geriatric dental care. In Harris, N. O., & Garcia-Godoy, F., Eds. *Primary preventive dentistry.* (6th ed.). Upper Saddle River, NJ: Prentice Hall, 589–604.

5. U.S. Census Bureau. (2005). 65+ *in the United State: 2005.* U.S. Census Bureau. Washington, DC; www.census.gov/prod/2005pubs.

6. Niessen, L. C., & Gibson, G. (2000). Aging and oral health for the 21st century. *Gen Dent,* 48(5): 544–49.

7. Report of the World Health Organization. (2002). Active ageing: A policy framework. *Aging Male,* 5(1):1–37.

8. Alian, A. Y., McNally, M. E., Fure, S., & Birkhed, D. (2006). Assessment of caries risk in elderly patients using the Cariogram model. *J Can Dent Assoc,* 72(5):459–63.

9. Little, J. W., Falace, D. A., Miller, C. S., & Rhodus, N. L. (2002). Dental management of older adults. In *Dental management of the medically compromised patient.* St. Louis: Mosby, 526–40.

10. Ettinger, R. L, & Beck, J. D. (1984). Geriatric dental curriculum and the needs of the elderly. *Spec Care Dent,* 4:207–13.

11. Leon, J., & Lai, R. T. (1990). *Functional status of non-institutionalized elderly: Estimates of ADL and IADL difficulties* (DHHS Publication No. (PHS) 90-3462). Rockville, Md: U.S. Department of Health and Human Services, Agency for the Health Care Policy and Research.

12. U.S. Census Bureau. (2004). We the people: Aging in the United States. Retrieved 12/1/06 from http//www.census.gov/prod/2001pubs/c2kbr01-10.pdf.

13. U.S. Department of Health and Human Services. (2006, April 11). Advance Data From Vital and Health Statistics (Number 370). Rockville, MD: U.S. Department of Health and Human Services.

14. Doty, P., Liu, K., & Weiner, J. (1985). Special report. An overview of long-term care. *Health Care Financ Rev,* 6:69–78.

15. Ouslander, J. G., Osterweil, D., & Morley, J. E. (1997). *Medical care in the nursing home* (2nd ed.). New York: McGraw-Hill.

16. Berkey, D. B., Berg, R. G., Ettinger, R. L, & Meskin, L. H. (1991). Research review of oral health status and service use among institutionalized older adults in the United States and Canada. *Spec Care Dent,* 11:131–36.

17. Strayer, M. S, & Ibrahim, M. (1991). Dental management needs of homebound and nursing home patients. *Community Dent Oral Epidemiol,* 19:176–77.

18. Fein Leib, M., & Zarate, A. D. (1992). Reconsidering age adjustment procedures: Workshop proceedings, National Center for Health Statistics. *Vital Health Stat,* 4(29):5–17.

19. Landis, S. H., (1998). Cancer statistics. *CA Cancer J Clin,* 48:6–29.

20. Ferri, F. F., Fretwell, M. D., Wachtel, T. J. (1997). *Practical guide to the care of the geriatric patient,* (2nd ed.). St. Louis: Mosby.

21. Katz, M. S., & Gerety, M. B. (1998). Gerontology and geriatric medicine. In Stein, J. H., Ed. *Internal medicine.* St. Louis: Mosby, 2282–93.

22. Kannel, W. B., Thom, T. J. (1990). Incidence, prevalence, and mortality of cardiovascular diseases. In Hurst, J. W., Ed. *The heart, arteries, and veins.* New York: McGraw-Hill.

23. Adams, P. F., & Benson, V. (1990). Current estimates from the National Health Interview Survey 1989. In *Vital and health statistics* (Series 10). Atlanta, GA: Center for Disease Control and Prevention, National Center for Health Statistics.

24. Medalie, J. (1986). The practice of geriatrics. In Calkins, E., Davis, P. J., & Ford, A. B., Eds. *An approach to common problems in the elderly.* Philadelphia: W.B. Saunders. 378–402.

25. Rose, L. F., Steinberg, B. J., & Minsk, L. (2000). The relationship between periodontal disease and systemic conditions. *Compend Continu Educ Dent,* 21(10A): 870–77.

26. Jarvik, L. (1988). Aging of the brain. How can we prevent it? *Gerontology,* 28:739–47.

27. White, L., Cartwright, W. S., Cornoni-Huntley, J., & Brock, D. B. (1986). Geriatric epidemiology. *Annu Rev Gerontol Geriatr,* 6:215–311.

28. Thornburg, J. E. (1994). Gerontological pharmacology. In Brody, T. M., Larner, J., & Minneman, K. P., Eds. *Human pharmacology: molecular to clinical.* St. Louis: Mosby, 855–60.

29. Scharre, D. W., & Cummings, J. L. (1998). Dementia. In Yoshikawa, T. T., Cobbs, E. L., & Brummel-Smith, K., Eds. *Practical ambulatory geriatrics.* St. Louis: Mosby. 333–45.

30. Antunono, P. G. (1995). Effectiveness and safety of velnacrine for the treatment of Alzheimer's disease: A double-blind placebo-controlled study. *Arch Intern Med,* 155:1766–73.

31. Friedlander, A. H., & Jarvik, L. F. (1987). The dental management of the patient with dementia. *Oral Surg,* 64:549–53.

32. Weintraub, J. A., & Burt, B. A. (1985). Oral health status in the United States: Tooth loss in the United States. *J Dent Educ,* 49:368–78.

33. Bloom, B., Gift, H. C., & Jack, S. S. (1992). Dental services and oral health, National Health Interview Survey, 1989. In *Vital health and statistics* (Series 10). Atlanta, GA: Centers for Disease Control and Prevention, National Center for Health Statistics.

34. Papas, A., Joshi, A., & Giunta, J. (1992). Prevalence and intraoral distribution of coronal and root caries in middle-aged and older adults. *Caries Res,* 26:459–65.

35. National Institutes of Health. (1987). *Oral health of United States adults: National findings* (NIH Publication No. 87-2868). Washington, DC: National Institutes of Health, National Institute of Dental Research.

36. Berg, R. L., & Cassells, J. S. (1990). Oral health problems in the 'Second Fifty.' In *The second fifty years: Promoting health and preventing disability.* Washington, DC: National Academy Press.

37. Berkey, D. B., Berg, R. G., Ettinger, R. L., & Meskin, L. H. (1991). Research review of oral health status and service use among institutionalized older adults in the United States and Canada. *Spec Care Dent,* 11:131–36.

38. Greer, R. O. (1993). Recent clinical and molecular biological advances in diagnosis and treatment of oral cancer. In *Scientific frontiers in clinical dentistry, an update.* Washington, DC: National Institutes of Health, National Institute of Dental Research.

39. Sadowsky, D. C., Kunzel, C., & Phelan, J. (1988). Dentists' knowledge, case-finding behavior and confirmed diagnosis of oral cancer. *J Cancer Educ,* 3:127–34.

40. Satcher, D. (2000). Oral health in America: A report of the Surgeon General. Rockville, MD: U.S. Department of Health and Human Services, National Institutes of Health, National Institute of Dental and Craniofacial Research.

41. Mulligan, R., & Navazesh, M. (1992). Relationship between oral conditions and systemic diseases in the elderly. *J Dent Res,* 71 (Spec Iss):316. Abstract1681.

42. Bartlett, J. G. (1994). Pneumonia. In Hazzard, W. R., Bierman, E. L., Blass, J. P., Eds., Editor emeritus, Reubin Andres, *Principles of geriatric medicine and gerontology* (3rd ed.). New York: McGraw-Hill, 332–36.

43. Beck, J. D., & Hunt, R. J. (1985). Oral health status in the United States: Problems of special patients. *J Dent Educ,* 49(6):407–25.

44. Ettinger, R. L, Watkins, C., & Cowen, H. (2000). Reflections on changes in geriatric dentistry. *J Dent Educ,* 64:715–22.

45. Shay, K. (2000). Restorative considerations in the dental treatment of the older patient. *Gen Dent,* 48(5):550–53.

46. Burke, F. M., & Samarawickrama, D. Y. D. (1995). Progressive changes in the pulpo-dentinal complex and their clinical consequences. *Gerodontology,* 12:57.

47. Wall, T. P., & Brown, L. J. (2003). Recent trends in dental visits and private dental insurance, 1989 and 1999. *J Am Dent Assoc,* 134:621–27.

48. Ettinger, R. L. (1992). Attitudes and values concerning oral health utilization of services among the elderly. *Int Dent J,* 42:373–84.

49. Manski, R. J., Goodman, H. S., Reid, B. C., & Macek, M. D. (2004). Dental insurance visits and expenditures among older adults, 1995–1997. *MMWR CDC Surveill Summ,* 48:51–88.

50. Erickson, L. (2000). The senior friendly office. *Gen Dent,* 48(5):562.

51. Kiyak, H. A., & Reichmuth, M. (2005). Barriers and enablers of older adults' use of dental services. *J Dent Educ,* 69(9):975–86.

52. Abrams, R. A., Ayers, C. S., & Lloyd, P. M. (1992). Attitudes of older versus younger adults toward dentistry and dentists. *Med Care,* 12:67–70.

53. Crozier, S. (2006). Elder care. Resolution addresses oral health news of 'vulnerable' older adults. *ADA News,* 37(20):24.

54. Vorenberg, S. (2007, January 1). Going out with a Boom: A generation faces its mortality. *The Albuquerque Tribune,* p. 1. Also available at: http://www.abqtrib.com.

Chapter 26

Medically Compromised Populations

Elaine Sanchez Dils

OBJECTIVES

After reading this chapter, the student should be able to:

1. Describe and define this target population.
2. Describe common oral conditions and diseases of medically compromised patients.
3. Describe specific preventive strategies to use with medically compromised patients.
4. Describe the role of the dental provider in treating medically compromised patients.

KEY TERMS

Arthritis
Bulimia nervosa
Cancer
Trismus
Cardiac arrhythmias
Tachycardia
Bradycardia
Congestive heart failure
Depressive disorders
Major depression
Dysthymia
Bipolar disorder
Diabetes mellitus
Type 1 diabetes
Gestational diabetes
Epilepsy
Hemophilia
Human immunodeficiency virus
Acquired immune deficiency syndrome
Acquired immunodeficiency syndrome
Oral hairy leukoplakia
Kaposi sarcoma
Linear gingival erythema

KEY TERMS (CONTINUED)
Necrotizing ulcerative periodontitis
Hypertension
Lichenoid reaction
Solid organ/tissue transplant
Hematopoietic cell transplantation
Bone marrow transplant
Chronic obstructive pulmonary disease
Asthma
Kidney or renal disease and failure
Substance abuse
Psychoactive

Alcoholism
Petechiae
Ecchymoses
Marijuana
Oral papillomas
Cocaine
Methamphetamine
Hyperthyroidism
Thyrotoxicosis
Hypothyroidism
Osteoporosis
Lingual thyroid

INTRODUCTION

The dental practitioner encounters patients with various types of medical conditions. It is important for each professional to understand what oral changes may occur as a result of an altered medical state. Furthermore, in an attempt to provide the patient with proper methods of preventive care, the dental professional should be aware of approaches unique to each patient and their condition. This chapter will briefly address the characteristics of several conditions, their oral manifestations, and preventive strategies for each category.

ARTHRITIS

Population Characteristics and Common Oral Manifestations

Arthritis literally means joint inflammation.[1–3] The word is used to describe more than 100 rheumatic diseases and conditions. These diseases and conditions affect joints, the surrounding tissues of the joints, and other related connective tissues. Generally, arthritic states are characterized by pain, stiffness, aching, and swelling of the affected areas.[2,4] Arthritis can have a gradual or sudden onset.[2] The most common forms of arthritic diseases are rheumatoid arthritis, osteoarthritis, systemic lupus erythematosus, Lyme disease, and Sjögren's syndrome.[5,6] According to the Centers for Disease Control and Prevention, in 2002, 43 million American adults were living

with some type of arthritis, and an estimated 67 million will be diagnosed with arthritis by 2030.[4]

Strategies to Prevent Oral Manifestations

Rheumatoid arthritis is generally seen as a systemic inflammation of the joints, whereas osteoarthritis is typically isolated to a few select joints. In both conditions, the dental practitioner should be aware of the possible effects to the temporomandibular joint (TMJ). If the TMJ is involved, the dental professional should consider several factors including decreased jaw function, possible need for a soft-food diet, and any medication the patient is taking to manage discomfort.[7] Dental practitioners need to consider the use of either heat or cold therapy to relax and soothe the joint during and after treatment. The dental provider also needs to assess the possible benefits of an oral appliance to decrease pressure exerted on the TMJ.

Patients with an arthritic condition need individualized treatment plans. These plans need to consider the possible need for shorter visits. Another consideration when assessing appointment length are visits with enough time to allow the patient to walk around as needed, adjust any physical supports, or change position frequently while in the dental chair. Plans for personalized oral hygiene instruction should also be addressed. The patient with an arthritic condition may not have the strength, movement, or dexterity to perform typical self-care regimens.

BULIMIA

Population Characteristics and Common Oral Manifestations

Bulimia nervosa is an eating disorder characterized by a person having recurrent episodes of overeating otherwise known as binge eating. These episodes are generally associated with a feeling of loss of control. The individuals then use some means to "get rid" of the food such as vomiting or excessive exercise, or using diuretics, laxatives, and enemas to prevent weight gain.[8]

Bulimia has been associated with both depression and overachieving behaviors.[5,9] These conditions can be effectively treated by antidepressant medication, cognitive-behavior therapy, and interpersonal therapy.

Strategies to Prevent Oral Manifestations

When a patient with bulimia is in the dental chair, the practitioner must pay special attention to the condition of the teeth. The teeth can be damaged by the repeated insult of acid from purging, as well as from high-carbohydrate foods taken in during a binging episode. Both factors will increase the likelihood of multiple caries. A person with evidence of this damage should be placed on a self-care fluoride regimen in addition to professionally applied fluoride. Also, the dental provider should highly stress the oral hygiene instruction to clear the mouth of anything that may increase caries and periodontal rates. Lastly, the dental provider should refer these individuals for further medical consultations.

CANCER

Population Characteristics and Common Oral Manifestations

There are multiple types of cancer, each type having its own unique characteristics. This section will discuss cancer in very general terms, attempting to address concerns the dental provider may encounter. **Cancer** is characterized by an out-of-control growth of abnormal cells. These cells have the ability to outlive normal cells. The development of these abnormal cells is due to damage to DNA. The proliferation of the abnormal cells allows them to spread relatively easily from the organ of origin to other sites throughout the body.[10] The dental professional should start with a thorough

health history of their patients at each visit, followed by an oral cancer screening.

When cancer is diagnosed, it is categorized by a stage (see Chapter 5). The stage I, II, III, or IV is based on the size of the tumor and how far it has spread. In stage I, the cancer remains in the original organ. In stage II, the cancer is in a regional area, having spread to nearby structures. In stage III, the cells have moved even farther away from the site of origin. If the cancer has been diagnosed as stage IV, the cancer can be found throughout the body. Depending on the type and stage of the cancer, various treatments can be recommended. The most common treatments are surgical removal of the affected tissues, radiation therapy, chemotherapy, and biologic therapies.[11]

As a result of both the cancer itself and the treatments, the patient may experience several dental manifestations. These manifestations include mucositis, xerostomia, ulcers, increased susceptibility to infection, and poor healing, to name a few.[5]

Strategies to Prevent Oral Manifestations

If the patient has encountered any of the manifestations of cancer, the dental professional should consider placing the patient on an antimicrobial mouthrinse to decrease the numbers of oral pathogens present. This measure will help the patient's body fight off any possible infection, hopefully averting any need for additional healing. Saliva substitutes should also be recommended to keep the oral cavity moist. These products will increase general comfort as well as reduce the propensity toward caries and periodontal disease.

If the patient is suffering with ulcers of the oral cavity, a rinse with diphenhydramine can be used to decrease oral pain. Patients may also experience oral burning sensations. These sensations can be reduced by a rinse with sodium bicarbonate and water. Candidiasis is also prevalent in individuals undergoing cancer treatments. An antifungal agent can be prescribed to eliminate this condition. Mouth exercises and tongue depressors may assist in opening the mouth; they can be recommended for the patient who is suffering from **trismus** (involuntary contraction of the muscles used in chewing). With all of these potential culprits damaging the oral cavity, the one component of the individual treatment plan that would be most beneficial for patients with cancer is to place them on self-care fluoride treatments.

Having soft, custom-fit trays for daily application of a fluoride gel can help protect the teeth.

Patient education is another important area in which a dental professional can help to fight cancer. Information about risk factors can be easily included during patient education. Some of the most common risk factors are tobacco use, unprotected sun exposure, poor diet, infectious diseases, chemicals, and radiation exposure.[12]

CARDIAC ARRHYTHMIAS

Population Characteristics and Common Oral Manifestations

Cardiac arrhythmias occur when electrical impulses in the heart do not function properly.[13] This condition can be any change from a normal sequence of electrical impulses.[14] A proper heartbeat needs a rhythmic coordination of impulses. A lack of this rhythmic coordination can result in many types of ailments. The most common are an inadequate circulation of the blood supply, damage to or death of the heart tissues, coronary artery disease, cardiomyopathy, and valvular heart disease.[15] There are two types of cardiac arrhythmias: tachycardia and bradycardia. **Tachycardia** is an abnormally rapid heartbeat, whereas **bradycardia** is an atypically slow heart beat for an individual.[16]

A cardiac arrhythmia may not have any signs or symptoms. Some things to look for are a fluttering feeling, racing or slow pulse rate, chest pain, shortness of breath, and lightheadedness with dizziness and possible fainting. Although there are not any specific oral manifestations of a cardiac arrhythmia, the *medications* used to treat an arrhythmia can induce some manifestations. Drug-induced xerostomia and ulcerations can be seen.

Strategies to Prevent Oral Manifestations

Patients with these conditions should use saliva substitutes and stimulants, and self-care fluoride treatments are recommended. If oral signs of the condition are causing pain, a diphenhydramine rinse may be helpful. In addition to maintaining a low-stress environment, use of a local anesthetic with epinephrine should be considered. Excessive amounts of epinephrine, however, could cause a life-threatening arrhythmia.

CONGESTIVE HEART FAILURE

Population Characteristics and Common Oral Manifestations

Congestive heart failure (CHF) is a life-threatening condition in which the heart can no longer pump enough blood to the rest of the body. When the organs do not receive enough blood, they are not getting adequate oxygen or nutrients. This deficiency results in damage to the organs, which in turn reduces their function. The most common causes of CHF are hypertension and coronary heart disease.[17] Congestive heart failure can also result after a heart attack from the scar tissue that was produced, coronary artery disease, heart valve disease, and any additional heart defects.[18]

The symptoms associated with CHF are weight gain; swelling of the feet, ankles, and abdomen; and pronounced neck veins. In addition, a person experiencing CHF may have shortness of breath, general weakness, and decreased urine production.[17]

Strategies to Prevent Oral Manifestations

Patients with well-controlled CHF can have routine dental treatment. However, the dental professional should remember that these patients are more susceptible to infections. Stressing the importance of good oral hygiene is imperative. These patients will also most likely be on medications related to the causative factors of CHF. These medications can cause xerostomia. Saliva substitutes and stimulants can help relieve the dry mouth. If the patient is taking digitalis, the amount of epinephrine used should be carefully determined. Digitalis also exacerbates the gag reflex. In addition, dental appointments should be short and stress free.

DEPRESSION

Population Characteristics and Common Oral Manifestations

Depressive disorders are illnesses involving the body, mood, and thoughts. The three most common types of depressive disorders are major depression, dysthymia, and bipolar disorder.[19] **Major depression** is characterized by a feeling of sadness or hopelessness most of the day, decreased energy, change in weight, difficulty concentrating, and either insomnia or hypersomnia.

These symptoms must last longer than 2 weeks to be classified as depression. **Dysthymia** has similar symptoms, but they are less severe and last longer than 2 years. **Bipolar disorder** is manifested as episodes of mania, a euphoric high, mixed with episodes of major depression. The causes of depression are not totally clear. Depression is thought to be tied to low self-esteem, an inherited trait, or some major physical change that leads to a brain–mental change.[19]

Strategies to Prevent Oral Manifestations

All of these types of depression can have effects on the dental patient. Patients may experience drug-induced xerostomia, which could be helped with saliva substitutes and stimulants. In addition, patients experiencing depressive states could have little or no interest in maintaining proper oral hygiene. Providing proper oral hygiene education and referring patients to other medical professionals could help reduce the frequency or severity of these depressive episodes. Patients experiencing a manic phase could do damage to their oral tissues by aggressively cleaning their mouths. Reinforcing the proper techniques and proper dental adjuncts could prevent these injuries.

DIABETES

Population Characteristics and Common Oral Manifestations

Diabetes mellitus is a group of metabolic diseases in which the body does not produce or properly use insulin.[20,21] Insulin is a hormone produced by the pancreas that helps convert sugars, starches, and other food into energy.[20,22] Approximately 7% of the U.S. population has been diagnosed with diabetes. It is also named as the sixth leading cause of death in the United States.[22]

There are three basic types of diabetes: type 1, type 2, and gestational diabetes. **Type 1 diabetes** occurs when the body fails to produce insulin.[20] This type most commonly presents in childhood or adolescence, but can occur at any age and requires daily insulin injections. Individuals with type 1 diabetes tend to be slender in stature, have thick saliva, and are prone to other autoimmune diseases.

Individuals with type 2 diabetes produce insulin, but their bodies are unable to properly use the insulin. This diabetic state has a gradual onset. Eighty-five percent of these patients are obese or have increased abdominal fat. Most frequently, type 2 diabetes occurs in adults, but recently it is being seen more often in overweight, underactive children.[20]

Gestational diabetes is a temporary condition that occurs in women during pregnancy. Although this condition is reversible, it does predispose the individual to developing type 2 diabetes.

Strategies to Prevent Oral Manifestations

With any type of uncontrolled diabetes, oral complications increase: Both candidiasis and angular cheilitis are seen. The increased glucose levels provide a favorable environment for fungal organisms. Treatment with a topical antifungal medication can help alleviate these conditions. An altered immune response is the primary culprit behind an increase in caries and periodontal disease. The goal of the dental professional is to educate patients on the oral effects of diabetes and ensure that patients are managing their diabetic condition appropriately. Patients who experience ulcerations, numbness, burning, or pain of the oral tissues can try to reduce these symptoms with a sodium bicarbonate and water rinse or a diphenhydramine rinse.

EPILEPSY

Population Characteristics and Common Oral Manifestations

Epilepsy is a disorder of the brain in which cells create abnormal electricity that causes a seizure.[23] Seizures can manifest in several different ways. In addition to the well-known jerky movements, a seizure can be a loss of consciousness, a period of confusion, a staring spell, or muscle spasms.[23,24,25] Seizures can occur with several different illnesses including stress, sleep deprivation, fever, alcohol or drug withdrawal, and syncope (fainting).[5,25] There are two basic types of seizures: a partial and a generalized seizure. A partial seizure involves only one part of the brain, whereas a generalized seizure engages most or all of the brain.[26] Not all seizures are considered epilepsy. A true diagnosis of epilepsy indicates that the individual has recurrent seizures.[24,25]

Strategies to Prevent Oral Manifestations

Phenytoin-induced gingival hyperplasia is the major oral complication associated with epilepsy. This gingival overgrowth can be reduced and controlled with thorough oral hygiene. In addition, any overhanging restorations and calculus must be removed in an attempt to control the overgrowth. If these relatively mild treatments do not work, surgical reduction of the gingival tissues might be necessary.

A dental provider must stress the importance of regular examinations for the patient with epilepsy. Early identification of any oral injury may prevent severe discomfort later. Grand mal seizures are severe epilepsy seizures that are initially tonic (prolonged contraction of muscles occurs), but become clonic (alternating contractions and partial relaxations of muscles occur) and usually result in loss of consciousness. With this type of seizure, fractured teeth and injuries to the lips and tongue may occur.[27]

HEMOPHILIA

Population Characteristics and Common Oral Manifestations

Hemophilia is a disorder of the body's blood-clotting system. The body has difficulty changing blood from a liquid to a solid state to stop bleeding.[28,29] Hemophilia may be considered if a patient answers positively to having unexplained bleeding or bruising, blood in the urine or stool, large, deep bruises, or prolonged bleeding from a cut. Further medical evaluation should also take place if an individual has spontaneous nosebleeds or tightness in their joints.[30]

Strategies to Prevent Oral Manifestations

When a hemophiliac presents for dental care, the most important thing to stress is the need for impeccable oral hygiene. The patient cannot risk unnecessary infection.[31]

Patients with mild-to-moderate hemophilia can typically be treated in a traditional dental setting. Those with severe cases should have their dental treatment in a hospital setting.[29,32] If a person with hemophilia is scheduled for multiple extractions, it is important that a splint is made to cover and protect the extraction sites. In mild and moderate hemophiliac patients, pressure packs can be used alongside a product containing thrombin to control bleeding.

HIV AND AIDS

Population Characteristics and Common Oral Manifestations

Human immunodeficiency virus (HIV) is a virus that infects and attacks human cells, primarily the CD4 cells. HIV causes decreased and disordered immunity that progresses over time. As the CD4 cell count drops over time, the patient becomes more susceptible to opportunistic infections. When HIV advances, it develops into **acquired immune deficiency syndrome** or **acquired immunodeficiency syndrome** (AIDS). Treatments are available for HIV and AIDS, but they only control the disease; there is no cure. Both conditions are eventually fatal.

HIV is transmitted several ways. The virus can be acquired through sexual contact, including anal, vaginal, and oral sexual encounters, with an HIV-positive person. In addition, a mother can infect her child with HIV in utero (in the uterus), during birth, and through breast-feeding. This type of transmission is preventable with medications; therefore, all pregnant women should be tested. HIV is also transferred in blood-to-blood contacts. This type of transference is very pertinent to the dental professional, because contaminated instruments and needle sticks are a method of transmitting blood. Although small amounts of the virus are detectable in saliva, there is very little concern about it being a primary infective factor.[33]

Many oral manifestations are associated with HIV and AIDS. Table 26–1 ■ lists various categories of oral conditions. The development of oral candidiasis

■ **Table 26–1**   HIV Oral Manifestations

Mucosal	Hyperplastic	Ulcers	Gingival Disease	Other
Candidiasis	Papillomavirus warts	Aphthous ulcers	Linear erythema	Caries
Oral hairy leukoplakia	Kaposi sarcoma	Herpes simplex	Gingivitis	Xerostomia
Hyperpigmentation	Bacillary angiomatosis	Varicella-zoster	Necrotizing periodontal	Lymphadenopathy
	Other malignancies	Cytomegalovirus	disease	Parotid disease
	and fungi			

suggests an immune dysfunction of some type. In the HIV-positive patient, it is usually indicative of a lower CD4 count. Candidiasis can have a range of presentations in the mouth (Figures 26–1 ■ through 26–3 ■). The three most commonly seen types of oral candidiasis are angular cheilitis, erythematous candidiasis, and psuedomembranous candidiasis.[34–36] They can be treated with several antifungal drugs.

Additional common findings are **oral hairy leukoplakia** (OHL) (Figure 26–4 ■), which is caused by the Epstein-Barr virus; herpes simplex virus; and major apthous-like ulcers.[35,36] Although OHL is rarely treated, the herpes virus (Figure 26–5 ■) can be treated with an antiviral drug such as acyclovir (Zovirax),

famciclovir (Famvir), or valacyclovir (Valtrex).[37] Major aphthous-like ulcers (Figure 26–6 ■) tend to respond well to both systemic or topical corticosteroid therapy. **Kaposi sarcoma** is also widely seen[35] (Figure 26–7 ■). It typically presents on the skin first, then intraorally. As a lesion becomes more severe and internally located, the body corresponds with a decreasing CD4 count. Kaposi sarcoma can be treated with an antiretroviral therapy and chemotherapy or radiation for refractory cases.

Periodontal involvement in the HIV-positive patient can advance rapidly compared with the general population. This advancement is thought to be associated with the immunocompromised state. Two specific

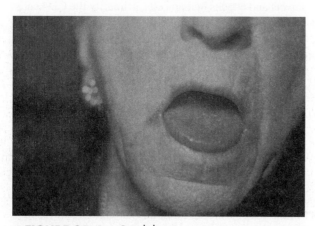

■ **FIGURE 26–1** Candidiasis.
(Centers for Disease Control and Prevention, CDC)

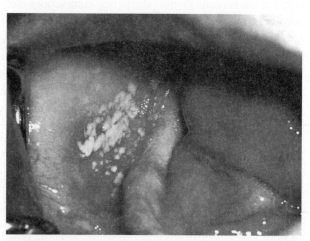

■ **FIGURE 26–3** Acute oral pseudomembranous candidiasis of an HIV-positive patient.
(Centers for Disease Control and Prevention, CDC)

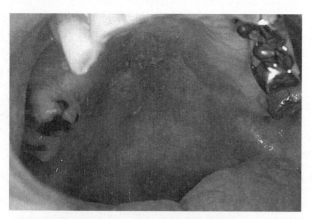

■ **FIGURE 26–2** Erythematous candidiasis.
(Centers for Disease Control and Prevention, CDC)

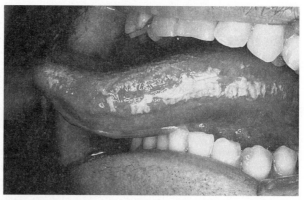

■ **FIGURE 26–4** Oral hairy leukoplakia of an HIV-positive patient.
(Centers for Disease Control and Prevention, CDC)

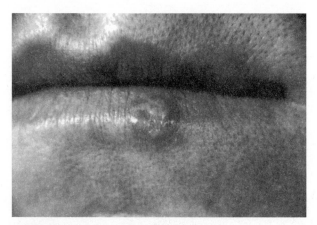

■ FIGURE 26–5 Herpes simplex lesion.
(Centers for Disease Control and Prevention, CDC)

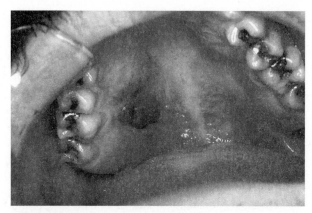

■ FIGURE 26–7 Kaposi sarcoma.
(Centers for Disease Control and Prevention, CDC)

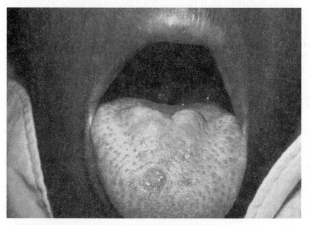

■ FIGURE 26–6 Aphthous stomatitis.
(Centers for Disease Control and Prevention, CDC)

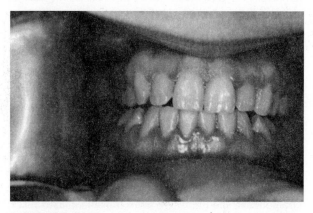

■ FIGURE 26–8 Acute necrotizing ulcerative gingivitis.
(Centers for Disease Control and Prevention, CDC)

states more frequently seen in the HIV patient are **linear gingival erythema** and **necrotizing ulcerative periodontitis** (NUP) (Figure 26–8 ■). Both states can be prevented and treated with debridement of the plaque and calculus followed by a regimen of chlorhexidine 0.12% rinses for several weeks. In addition, the patient experiencing NUP will most likely need systemic antibiotic therapy.[34]

Strategies to Prevent Oral Manifestations

The HIV and AIDS patient will benefit the most from prevention and control of the microbial buildup in the oral cavity. Adequate professional care and self-knowledge of how to maintain a plaque- and calculus-free environment

will limit these patients from getting secondary oral infections. HIV/AIDS patients must seek regular dental examinations and treatments, because most common lesions are easily detected.

HYPERTENSION

Population Characteristics and Common Oral Manifestations

Blood pressure is determined by the amount of blood the heart pumps and the amount of resistance to blood flow in the arteries. As the heart pumps more blood and the arteries narrow, the blood pressure increases. High blood pressure is called **hypertension.**[38] Typically, there are no signs or symptoms associated with hypertension.[39]

Strategies to Prevent Oral Manifestations

Although there are no direct oral manifestations of hypertension, several of the medications to treat this condition can affect the oral cavity.[40] Some antihypertensive drugs, especially diuretics, can cause a dry mouth. This irritation can be helped by salivary stimulators and substitutes. Several different medications to treat high blood pressure can give the patient a **lichenoid reaction** characterized by the eruption of shiny, violet-colored, flat-topped elevations of mucosal tissue. Angiotensin-converting enzyme inhibitors have been known to delay healing times and increase gingival bleeding. Calcium antagonists, another class of drugs used for treatment of hypertension, have been shown to cause an increase in gingival hyperplasia.[5]

ORGAN TRANSPLANTS

Population Characteristics and Common Oral Manifestations

The first type of organ transplantation is a **solid organ/tissue transplant,** and the second type is a **hematopoietic cell transplantation,** also known as a **bone marrow transplant.** Solid organ/tissue transplants include the heart, lungs, kidneys, livers, intestines, pancreas, skin, eye components, and limbs.[41] When a transplant takes place, the greatest risk of failure is the recipient's body rejecting the tissue. This rejection is where most of the dental considerations begin. The immunosuppressive drugs that are administered to a patient are typically the cause of many oral manifestations.

Excessive immunosuppression can lead to mucositis, herpes infections, ulcerations, candidiasis, and alveolar bone loss. Gingival overgrowth has also been indicated with immunosuppression and poor oral hygiene.[42,43]

Strategies to Prevent Oral Manifestations

Patients with an organ transplant need to ensure their periodontal health is stable by undergoing a professional dental hygiene evaluation. Periodontal health will limit the body's ability to rapidly progress the periodontal disease. Keeping the oral cavity as plaque free as possible will continue to maintain the healthy environment.

PULMONARY DISEASE

Population Characteristics and Common Oral Manifestations

Chronic obstructive pulmonary disease (COPD) is a generic term used to describe damage to the lungs that makes it difficult to breathe.[44] The two most common diseases named under the classification of COPD are bronchitis and emphysema. Although these diseases have considerations during dental treatment, there are no specific oral manifestations found as a direct result of the disease. However, the typical causative factor leading to the development of COPD is cigarette smoking.[45] The oral manifestations and preventive strategies related to smoking are discussed later in this section.

Asthma is a disease of the respiratory system in which the airway constricts, becomes inflamed, or is lined with excessive amounts of mucus. Several different stimuli including allergens, respiratory infections, exercise, and certain drugs can trigger an asthma attack.

Asthma itself does not cause oral disease; however, some of the asthma treatments can. Beta$_2$-agonist inhalers decrease salivary flow and plaque pH levels. These conditions are related to an increase in the number of caries and the prevalence of gingivitis. Asthmatics tend to have a greater-than-average amount of acid reflux. This reflux gives way to an increase in enamel erosion.

Inhaled steroids are common treatments for asthma and COPD.[46] These steroids decrease the normal immune function in the oral cavity. This change is associated with increased cases of candidiasis.

Strategies to Prevent Oral Manifestations

Those individuals with caries and erosion can benefit from self-care fluoride regimens. All of the above-mentioned oral conditions will benefit from thorough oral hygiene, which should be planned and taught by the dental professional.

Candidiasis can be treated with an antifungal medication; however, there are preventive measures patients can take to reduce the outbreak of the *Candida* species. Patients who rinse with water after using their inhalers can reduce the incidence of candidiasis. Also, using inhalers with a "space" chamber will reduce the likelihood of developing candidiasis.[47]

RENAL DISEASE/FAILURE

Population Characteristics and Common Oral Manifestations

The kidneys' function is to excrete wastes, concentrate urine, and regulate electrolytes.[48] In **kidney or renal disease and failure,** the kidneys quit effectively removing metabolic end products from the blood, and fail to regulate the fluid level, electrolyte balance, and pH balance of the extracellular fluid. Systemic symptoms of kidney failure are weight loss, fatigue, decreased urine production, easy bruising, yellowing of the skin, and a decreased sensation in the extremities. The only treatments for renal failure or end-stage kidney disease are dialysis or kidney transplantation.[49,50]

A very common oral manifestation of someone in chronic renal failure is pallor (paleness) of the oral mucosa, which is due to the lowering of the number of red blood cells present.[51] Patients also may complain of a metallic taste in their mouths. This taste alteration is caused by a high concentration of urea in the saliva.[51] The higher concentration of urea does, however, inhibit the growth of lactobacilli, which in turn decreases the caries rate.[52] Xerostomia and candidal infections are also prevalent. A lack of vitamin C gives the gingiva an abnormal red appearance; the gingiva is also spongy and bleeds easily.[53,54,55] In addition to these oral manifestations, evidence of chronic renal failure is seen in radiographs. A loss of the lamina dura, demineralized bone, and radiolucent jaw lesions may be present.[56,57]

Strategies to Prevent Oral Manifestations

The first step for the dental professional is prescribing individualized oral hygiene for the patients. With increased susceptibility for infection, the number of oral pathogens must be controlled. Moreover, the general comfort of the patient must be considered. Conditions such as xerostomia and ulcerations can cause discomfort that can be controlled by saliva substitutes, fluoride treatments, or diphenhydramine rinses. If the patient has candidiasis, an antifungal agent can be prescribed.

SUBSTANCE ABUSE DISORDERS

Substance abuse refers to the overindulgence in and dependence on a **psychoactive** (substance that affects the mind or behavior), leading to effects that are detrimental to the individual's physical health or mental health, or the welfare of others.[58] Although several types of substances can be abused, this section will focus on a few frequently encountered substances with associated oral manifestations. For all of these substance abuse disorders, the most important strategy for a dental provider is to encourage these patients to obtain the proper help required to control and eventually stop the habitual cycle of the abuse.

Population Characteristics of Alcohol Abuse and Common Oral Manifestations

Alcoholism is defined as a primary, chronic disease characterized by impaired control of overdrinking, preoccupation with the drug alcohol, use of alcohol despite adverse consequences, and distortions in thinking.[59] In the United States, approximately 75,000 deaths per year are caused by excessive alcohol use.[60] Over time, abusive alcohol consumption can lead to many physical problems. These problems include, but are not limited to, strokes, cardiovascular issues, depression, liver diseases, and gastrointestinal problems, as well as social troubles.[61–70]

Direct oral manifestations of alcohol abuse are xerostomia, **petechiae** (localized hemorrhaging of skin or mucosal surfaces characterized by small reddish/purplish spots), **ecchymoses** (escape of blood into tissues from ruptured blood vessels), and increased gingival bleeding. Tooth erosion is also evident, predominately from vomiting that may follow episodes of binge drinking.[71] An overall neglect of the body leads to poor oral hygiene, increasing the risk of dental caries and periodontal disease.[72] Increases in stress levels add to bruxism and allow for opportunistic infections such as candidiasis to develop.[73] It is 10 to 15 times more likely for a chronic alcoholic to develop oral squamous cell carcinomas.[74]

Population Characteristics of Tobacco Use and Common Oral Manifestations

Cigarette smoking is the most popular means of tobacco use; however, smokeless tobacco products such as snuff and chewing tobacco are also very popular. Cigars and pipes are other ways to smoke tobacco without inhaling the smoke into the lungs. Nicotine, a highly addictive chemical in tobacco, is absorbed through mucous membranes. As the nicotine enters the blood stream, the body releases adrenaline, which stimulates a release of blood glucose, and an increase of blood pressure, respiration, and heart rates.[75] The National Center for Health Statistics reports that, in 2004, approximately 21% of the U.S. population smoked cigarettes.[76]

Oral effects such as oral cancer, leukoplakia, nicotine stomatitis, and hairy tongue may result from tobacco use. Tobacco users have a 4 times greater chance than people who do not use tobacco to develop oral cancer.[77] Leukoplakia, which can become cancerous, develops from tobacco contacting the oral mucosa for long periods of time.[78] Nicotine stomatitis is a precancerous mucosal change of the hard palate. It is caused by the heat of smoking tobacco, as opposed to the chemicals in the tobacco.[79] Hairy tongue is a result of the elongation of the filiform papillae of the tongue. It is thought that the tobacco causes the epithelial cells of the tongue to stop shedding.[77] Patients who use tobacco are also seen to have a greater incidence of periodontitis and a higher caries rate.[80,81] Contributing to these conditions and to xerostomia is a decrease of salivary production.[81]

Population Characteristics of Marijuana Use and Common Oral Manifestations

Marijuana is a mix of flowers, stems, seeds, and leaves of the hemp plant *Cannabis sativa*. It is usually smoked either as a cigarette or through a pipe. THC (delta-9-tetrahydrocannabinol) is the addictive chemical in marijuana. A high is experienced by users from the binding of certain nerve cells to THC.[82] In 2004, it was found that approximately 14.6 million Americans used marijuana at least once a month.[83] Many terms are used to name marijuana including pot, herb, weed, grass, ganja, and hash.

In general, marijuana abusers have poorer oral health than nonusers, with an increased risk of caries and periodontal diseases.[84] Xerostomia is a major effect of marijuana, which can also increase the risk of caries and periodontitis.[85] Marijuana smoke acts as a carcinogen and is associated with dysplastic changes and premalignant lesions in oral mucosas.[86] Users are prone to oral infections, such as benign epithelial tumors that project from the surrounding oral mucosa, called **oral papillomas,** which are most likely due to the immunosuppressive effects of marijuana.[85,87] These effects may also be the link to the increased prevalence of candidiasis.[88]

Population Characteristics of Cocaine Abuse and Common Oral Manifestations

Cocaine is a highly addictive stimulant of the central nervous system. It is an alkaloid ester extracted from the leaves of plants.[89] There are two basic forms of cocaine: hydrochloride salt and freebase, which is also called "crack cocaine." Hydrochloride salt, the powdered form of cocaine, is dissolved in water and can be taken intravenously or intranasally. *Freebase* refers to a compound that has not been neutralized by an acid to make the salt. This drug is smoked.[90] There are several street names for cocaine including blow, nose candy, snowball, tornado, wicky stick, and Perico.[91]

Cocaine interferes with the reabsorption process of dopamine. The buildup of dopamine causes continuous stimulation of the receiving neurons. This stimulation is associated with feelings of euphoria.[92,93]

Topically applied cocaine can be locally destructive to the oral mucosa and dentition. Ulceration, necrosis, and rapid recession are seen. In addition, erosion of both enamel and dentin is seen.[94] These oral manifestations can be attributed to addicts checking the purity of the cocaine on these areas of the mouth.[95] When crack cocaine is smoked, the crack pipe directs extremely hot smoke to the midline of the hard palate. The heat can lead to ulcerations or, in extreme cases, perforation of the hard palate.[96,97] Necrotic ulcers of the tongue and epiglottis are also related to smoking freebase cocaine.[97] Candidiasis may be seen as a result of the weakened immune system. Craving of sweets during cocaine use leads to an increased caries rate. Prolonged periods of stimulation of the central nervous system leads to long periods of bruxism, giving way to severe tooth wear.[95] Aggressive toothbrushing while on a cocaine high has been implicated as the cause of both cervical and tooth abrasion and gingival lacerations.[94]

Population Characteristics of Methamphetamine Abuse and Common Oral Manifestations

Methamphetamine is a potent stimulant that releases high levels of dopamine, norepinephrine, and serotonin. This drug also blocks the reuptake of these same substances. Similar to cocaine, the dopamine stimulates brain cells, which in turn enhance mood and body movements.[98] Cocaine has been found to increase dopamine units by 350, and methamphetamine increases it by 1250 units compared with base levels of dopamine.[99] Excessive norepinephrine may be responsible for the alertness and lack of fatigue felt by methamphetamine users. The extra serotonin is thought to cause cognitive impairment and eventual depression.[100]

Methamphetamine is an odorless, white, crystalline powder that has a bitter taste. This powder dissolves in water or alcohol. The drug can be taken orally or intranasally, smoked, or injected. Methamphetamine is known on the streets by names such as speed and chalk. Methamphetamine hydrochloride is the form that can be smoked. Because it presents in crystals that resemble ice, methamphetamine hydrochloride is referred to as ice, crystal, glass, and tina.[101] Crank is the less pure form of methamphetamine.

The most common and related oral manifestation of methamphetamine use is rampant caries. This rapid decay process begins between the teeth and moves around the teeth at the cervical junction[102] (Figure 26–9 ■). One cause of this destructive process is said to be the caustic substances used in the production of methamphetamine. Methamphetamines have also been implicated in slowing salivary production, an extreme desire for sugary soda consumption, and a lack of desire for good oral hygiene. It is thought that smokers have worse dental effects, because the chemicals are brought in direct contact with the oral cavity, causing sores and infections. Injectors of methamphetamine do not experience the same severe tooth decay; however, they do experience more severe clenching and grinding. The increased bruxism is attributed to the more powerful effects of the injected drug.[103]

Strategies to Prevent Oral Manifestations

As previously stated, the most important role of the dental provider is to educate patients to not engage in these types of damaging activities. If a patient however is a

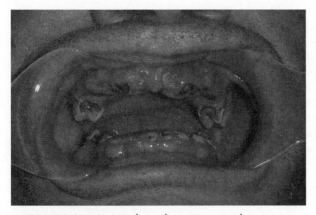

■ **FIGURE 26–9**   Methamphetamine mouth.
(Charles D. Tatlock, DDS, MPH, Associate Professor, University of New Mexico, Albuquerque, NM)

substance abuser, the dental professional should help to direct patients to a safe environment to receive the necessary care to get clean and sober.

Encouraging these patients to seek consistent dental visits is of top priority. These visits will allow the patients to be taught appropriate, individualized self-care regimens. Proper self-care will allow patients to keep the oral environment less conducive to the bacteria that cause caries and periodontal diseases. In addition, the patients need regular screenings for oral cancer. Early detection increases the likelihood of successful treatment of an oral cancer lesion. If the patient has xerostomia, the patient should be directed to consider the integration of saliva substitutes and stimulants into the daily dental routines. Topical fluoride treatment could help with this problem as well as help to prevent caries. An antifungal medication may be prescribed to lessen the insult of the *Candida* species if present in the patient's mouth. If the patient is feeling discomfort from ulcerative lesions, a diphenhydramine rinse may be beneficial. If attrition from clenching and grinding is present, a mouthguard can be recommended to stop the progression of the tooth wear.

THYROID DYSFUNCTION

Population Characteristics and Common Oral Manifestations

The thyroid gland is an endocrine gland that secretes three hormones: thyroxine, triiodothyronine, and calcitonin. Thyroxine, also know as T4, contains four iodine molecules, and is produced only by the thyroid. Triiodothyronine, referred to as T3, is a variation of T4 and contains three iodine molecules.[104] These hormones are transported through the blood by binding to plasma proteins and are regulated by the hypothalamic–pituitary–thyroid axis.[104] There are two basic types of thyroid dysfunction: hypothyroidism and hyperthyroidism. **Hyperthyroidism,** also known as **thyrotoxicosis,** is an overactivity of the thyroid gland, which causes high levels of T4 or T3 in the blood.[104,105] This excessive level of hormone results in an acceleration of vital body functions, leading to higher physical and mental activity.[105–107] **Hypothyroidism,** by contrast, is the underactivity of the thyroid gland. This subnormal secretion of the T4 hormone causes the body's normal functioning rate to slow, causing a decrease in overall mental and physical activity.[104,105,107,108] The patient with hyperthyroidism will have an increase in their rates of dental caries and periodontal disease. Contributing to this is **osteoporosis** of the alveolar ridges,[109,110] which is characterized by decreased bone mass resulting from decreased bone density and enlargement of bone spaces. The bone is more porous and susceptible to fracture.

Hypothyroidism has very different oral manifestations. These patients will frequently have an enlarged tongue and delayed eruption of their teeth. Delayed wound healing contributes to the poor periodontal health seen in these individuals.[109]

Strategies to Prevent Oral Manifestations

Demonstrating proper plaque control and then evaluating the patients' plaque-control technique will help increase the patients' ability to control the progression of oral diseases related to thyroid dysfunction. In addition, these patients will experience early loss of their primary dentition, followed by accelerated eruption of their permanent teeth. Excessive tissue on the lateral posterior tongue, called a **lingual thyroid,** may also be seen. Patients also commonly complain of a burning sensation in their mouths.[109] These patients could benefit from rinsing with sodium bicarbonate and water.

SUMMARY

Patients with medical conditions will be present every day in the dental practice. Dental providers need to help their patients find a means to prevent and care for oral conditions that may be associated with medical states. Each medical circumstance has unique oral manifestations. Being knowledgeable about these characteristics and associated preventive strategies will be beneficial to both the practitioner and the patients. Table 26–2 ■ gives a synopsis of several medical conditions and their characteristics, associated oral manifestations, and preventive strategies.

■ **Table 26–2** Synopsis of Medical Conditions, Their Oral Manifestations, and Preventive Strategies

Condition	*Characteristics*	*Oral Manifestations*	*Preventive Strategies*
Alcohol abuse	Excessive consumption of ethanol	Oral cancer Poor oral hygiene Xerostomia Petechiae Ecchymoses Increased bleeding Candidiasis Tooth erosion	Individualized oral hygiene instruction Saliva stimulants and substitutes Self-care fluoride treatments Antifungal agent Diphenhydramine rinse
Arthritis	Group of diseases that damage joints	Poor oral hygiene TMJ issues	Individualized oral hygiene instruction Short appointment times Oral appliance Alternative positioning during appointments
Asthma	Abnormal function of the lungs	Candidiasis Increased caries Increase gingivitis	Antifungal agent Diphenhydramine rinse
Bulimia	Binge eating followed by purging	Tooth erosion Increased caries and periodontitis Tooth sensitivity	Individualized oral hygiene instruction Self-care fluoride treatments
Cancer	Out-of-control growth of abnormal cells	Mucositis Candidiasis Xerostomia Loss of taste Trismus Cervical caries Sensitive teeth Excessive/spontaneous bleeding Poor healing Increased susceptibility to infection	Antifungal agent Individualized oral hygiene instruction Saliva stimulants and substitutes Self-care fluoride treatments Antimicrobial rinse Mouth exercises Tongue depressors to open mouth

■ **Table 26–2**   (Continued)

Condition	Characteristics	Oral Manifestations	Preventive Strategies
Cardiac arrhythmias	Abnormal heartbeat or rate	Xerostomia Ulceration Petechiae	Diphenhydramine rinse Saliva stimulants and substitutes Self-care fluoride treatments

Cocaine use	Use of addictive stimulant
	  drug
		Ulceration of mucosa
		Palatal perforation
		Necrosis of gingiva
		Bruxism
		Cervical tooth abrasion
		Tooth erosion
			Individualized oral hygiene
			  instruction
			Mouthguard
			Diphenhydramine rinse

Congestive heart
failure
	Inability of heart to pump
	  enough blood to the
	  body's other organs
		Infection
		Bleeding
		Petechiae
		Ecchymoses
		Xerostomia
			Saliva stimulants and
			  substitutes
			Self-care fluoride treatments

Depression	Illness of mind, body, and
	  thoughts
		Poor oral hygiene
		Xerostomia
		Damage to tissues due
		to "over" cleaning
			Saliva stimulants and
			  substitutes
			Self-care fluoride treatments

Diabetes	Metabolic disorder
	  resulting in abnormal
	  blood glucose levels
		Impaired healing
		Increased susceptibility to infections
		Candidiasis
		Accelerated periodontal disease
		Xerostomia
		Ulcerations
		Numbness/burning/pain of oral tissues
			Antifungal agent
			Diphenhydramine rinse
			Sodium bicarbonate
			  and water rinse
			Saliva stimulants and
			  substitutes
			Self-care fluoride treatments

Epilepsy	Neurologic disorder
	  causing seizures
		Gingival hyperplasia
		Fractured teeth
		Injury to lips and tongue
			Individualized oral hygiene
			  instruction
			Surgical reduction of gingival

Hemophilia	Bleeding disorder	Spontaneous bleeding Prolonged bleeding Hematomas	Individualized oral hygiene instruction
HIV/AIDS	Immune system failure	Candidiasis Kaposi sarcoma Hairy leukoplakia Linear gingival erythema NUG/NUP	Antifungal agent Individualized oral hygiene instruction Antibiotics Corticosteroid therapy

Hypertension	Elevation of blood
	  pressure
		Xerostomia
		Ulceration
		Lichenoid reactions
		Decreased healing
		Increased bleeding
		Gingival hyperplasia
			Diphenhydramine rinse
			Saliva stimulants and
			  substitutes
			Self-care fluoride treatments

Hyperthyroidism	Excessive release
	  of thyroid hormone
		Progressive periodontal disease
		Extensive caries
		Tumors on tongue
		Osteoporosis of alveolar ridge
		Premature loss of teeth
		Early eruption patterns
		Burning sensation
			Sodium bicarbonate
			  and water rinse
			Individualized oral hygiene
			  instruction

(Continued)

■ **Table 26–2** (Continued)

Condition	Characteristics	Oral Manifestations	Preventive Strategies
Hypothyroidism	Thyroid failure	Increased tongue size Delayed eruption of teeth Delayed wound healing	Individualized oral hygiene instruction
Liver disease	Inflammation of the liver	Bleeding, lichenoid eruptions	Individualized oral hygiene instruction

Marijuana use	Smoking of plant
	    Cannabis sativa
		Xerostomia
		Oral cancer
		Poor oral hygiene
		Candidiasis
		Increased gingivitis and periodontitis
			Individualized oral hygiene
			    instruction
			Antifungal agent
			Saliva stimulants
			    and substitutes

Methamphetamine
use
	Use of addictive
	    stimulant drug
		Poor oral hygiene
		Xerostomia
		Rampant decay
			Individualized oral hygiene
			    instruction
			Saliva stimulants
			    and substitutes
			Self-care fluoride treatments

Organ transplants	Solid organ/tissue or
	    hematopoietic cell
	    transplantation
		Candidiasis
		Herpes (simplex and zoster)
		Hairy leukoplakia
		Kaposi sarcoma
		Aphthous stomatitis
		Spontaneous bleeding
		Increased infection
		Ulceration
		Petechiae
		Ecchymoses
		Gingival hyperplasia
		Salivary gland dysfunction
		Xerostomia
			Individualized oral hygiene
			    instruction
			Antifungal agent
			Saliva stimulants
			    and substitutes

Renal disease	Complete or near
	    failure of the kidneys
		Mucosal pallor
		Xerostomia
		Metallic taste
		Ammonia breath
		Stomatitis
		Loss of lamina dura
		Bone radiolucencies
		Increased bleeding
		Ulcerations
		Candidiasis
			Antifungal agent
			Diphenhydramine rinse
			Saliva stimulants
			    and substitutes
			Self-care fluoride treatments
			Individualized oral hygiene
			    instruction

Tobacco use	Use of plants in the
	    genus *Nicotiana*
		Oral cancer
		Leukoplakia
		Xerostomia
		Alveolar bone damage
		Gingival damage
		Hairy tongue
		Nicotine stomatitis
		Increased caries
			Saliva stimulants
			    and substitutes
			Self-care fluoride treatments

REFERENCES

1. What is arthritis? Retrieved 1/8/07 from www.arthritis. org. Adapted from: The Arthritis Foundation Guide to Good Living with Rheumatoid Arthritis. Posted 6/9/2007.

2. Centers for Disease Control and Prevention, National Center for Chronic Disease Prevention and Health Promotion. (2007, May 24). Arthritis overview. Retrieved 11/22/06 from http://www.cdc.gov/arthritis/arthritis/index.htm.

3. Abramson, S. B., & Yazici, Y. (2006). Biologics in development for rheumatoid arthritis: Relevance to osteoarthritis. *Adv Drug Deliv Rev,* 58:212–25.

4. U.S. Department of Health and Human Services, Centers for Disease Control and Prevention. (2007, May 24). *Chronic disease—Arthritis—At a glance.* Retrieved 12/15/07 from http://www.cdc.gov/nccdphp/publications/aag/arthritis.htm.

5. Little, J., Falace, D., Miller, C., & Rhodus, N. (2002). *Dental management of the medically compromised patient* (6th ed.). St. Louis: Mosby.

6. Mahalik, J., Shigaki, C. L., Baldwin, D., & Johnstone, B. (2006). A review of employability and worksite interventions for persons with rheumatoid arthritis and osteoarthritis. *Work,* 26:303–11.

7. Ardic, F., Gokharman, D., Atsu, S., Guner, S., Yilmaz, M., & Yorgancioglu, R. (2006). The comprehensive evaluation of temporomandibular disorders seen in rheumatoid arthritis. *Aust Dent J,* 51:23–28.

8. Reba, L., Thornton, L., Tozzi, F, Klump, K. L., Brandt, H., Crawford, S., Crow, S., Fichter, M. M., Halmi, K. A., Johnson, C., Kaplan, A. S., Keel, P., LaVia, M., Mitchell, J., Strober, M., Woodside, D. B., Rotono, A., Berrettini, W. H., Kaye, W. H., & Bulik, C. M. (2005). Relationships between features associated with vomiting in purging-type eating disorders. *Int J Eat Disord,* 38:287–94.

9. Johnson, C. D., Koh, S. H., Shynett, B., Koh, J., & Johnson, C. (2006). An uncommon dental presentation during pregnancy resulting from multiple eating disorders: Pica and bulimia: Case report. *Gen Dent,* 54:198–200.

10. American Cancer Society. (2006, February 6). Cancer reference information: What is cancer? Retrieved 11/22/06 from http://www.cancer.org/docroot/CRI/content/CRI_2_4_1x_What_Is_Cancer.asp?sitearea.

11. American Cancer Society (n.d.) *Cancer reference information: How is cancer treated?* Retrieved 11/22/06 from http://www.cancer.org/docroot/CRI/content/CRI_2_4_4x_How_Is_Cancer_Treated.asp?

12. American Cancer Society. *Cancer reference information: What are the risk factors for cancer?* Retrieved 3/27/08 from http://www.cancer.org/docroot/CRI/content/CRI_2_4_2x_What_are_the_risk_factors_for_cancer_72.asp?sitearea=.

13. Mayo Clinic Staff. (2005, February). *Heart arrhythmias introduction.* Retrieved 2/16/08 from http://mayoclinic.com/health/heart-arrhythmias/DS00290.

14. American Heart Association. What are arrhythmias? Retrieved 3/27/08 from http://www.americanheart.org/presenter.jhtml?identifier=4469.

15. Mayo Clinic Staff. (2005, February). *Heart arrhythmias causes.* Retrieved 2/16/08 from http://mayoclinic.com/health/heart-arrhythmias/DS00290.

16. Brasel, K. J., Guse, C., Gentilello, L. M., & Nirula, R. (2007). Heart rate: Is it truly a vital sign? *J Trauma,* 62:812–17.

17. Gandelman, G. (2006, July). Heart failure. In *MedlinePlus Medical Encyclopedia.* Retrieved 11/22/06 from http://www.nlm.nih.gov/medlineplus/ency/article/000158.htm.

18. American Heart Association. (n.d.). *Congestive heart failure.* Retrieved 11/22/06 from http://www.americanheart.org/presenter.jhtml?identifier=4585.

19. National Institutes of Health Depression. Retrieved 3/20/08 from http://www.nimh.nih.gov/health/topics/depression/index.shtml.

20. American Diabetes Association. (n.d.). *All about diabetes.* Retrieved 11/22/06 from http://www.diabetes.org/utils/printthispage.jsp?PageID=ALLABOUTDIABETES_233165.

21. American Diabetes Association. (2004). *American Diabetes Association: Clinical practice recommendations 2004. Report of the expert committee on the diagnosis and classification of diabetes mellitus.* Alexandria, VA: American Diabetes Association.

22. Centers for Disease Control and Prevention, National Center for Chronic Disease Prevention and Health Promotion. (2006, June 27). CDC's diabetes program. What is diabetes? Retrieved 11/22/06 from http://www.cdc.gov/diabetes/faq/basics.htm.

23. American Academy of Family Physicians. (1994, September). *Epilepsy.* Retrieved 11/22/06 from http://familydoctor.org/214.xml?printxml.

24. Mayo Clinic Staff. (2005, April). *Epilepsy.* Retrieved 11/22/06 from http://www.mayoclinic.com/health/epilepsy/DS00342.

25. Kohrman, M. H. (2007). What is epilepsy? Clinical perspectives in the diagnosis and treatment. *J Clin Neurophysiol,* 24:87–95.

26. Mayo Clinic Staff. (2005, April). *Epilepsy signs and symptoms.* Retrieved 11/22/06 from http://www.mayoclinic.com/health/epilepsy/DS00342/DSECTION=2.

27. Aragon, C. E., & Burneo, J. G. (2007). Understanding the patient with epilepsy and seizures in the dental practice. *J Can Dent Assoc,* 73:71–76.

28. Mayo Clinic Staff. (2005, May). *Hemophilia.* Retrieved 11/22/06 from http://www.mayoclinic.com/health/hemophilia/DS00218.

29. Israels, S., Schwetz, N., Boyar, R., & McNicol, A. (2006). Bleeding disorders: Characterization, dental considerations and management. *J Can Dent Assoc,* 72:827.

30. Mayo Clinic Staff. (2005, May). *Hemophilia signs and symptoms.* Retrieved 11/22/06 from http://www.mayoclinic.com/health/hemophilia/DS00218/DSECTION=2.

31. Hoots, W. K., & Nugent, D. J. (2006). Evidence for the benefits of prophylaxis in the management of hemophilia A. *Thromb Haemost,* 96:433–40.

32. Correa, M. E., Annicchino-Bizzacchi, J. M., Jorge, J., Paes de Almeida, O., Ozelo, M. C., Aranha, F. J., & Lourdes Barjas-Castro, M. (2006). Clinical impact of oral health indexes in dental extraction of hemophilic patients. *J Oral Maxillofac Surg,* 64:785–88.

33. Centers for Disease Control and Prevention. (1999, July). HIV and Its Transmission. Bethesda, MD: U.S. Department of Health and Human Services, Centers for Disease Control and Prevention.

34. Reznik, D. (2005, December–2006, January). Oral manifestations of HIV disease. *Perspective,* 13 (5) pages 143–148.

35. Baccaglini, L., Atkinson, J. C., Patton, L. L., Glick M., Ficarra, G., & Peterson, D. E. (2007). Management of oral lesions in HIV-positive patients. *Oral Surg Oral Med Oral Pathol Oral Radiol Endod,* 103 (Suppl):S50.e1–23.

36. Sroussi, H. Y., Villines, D., Epstein, J., Alves, M. C., & Alves, M. E. (2007). Oral lesions in HIV-positive dental patients—One more argument for tobacco smoking cessation. *Oral Dis,* 13:324–28.

37. Emmert, D. (2000, March). *Treatment of common cutaneous herpes simplex virus infections. Am Fam Physician* 2000; 61:1697–704,1705–706,1708.

38. Mayo Clinic Staff. (2006, September). *High blood pressure (hypertension).* Retrieved 3/27/08 from http://mayoclinic.com/health/high-blood-pressure/DS00100.

39. Mayo Clinic Staff. (2006, September). *High blood pressure (hypertension)—Signs and symptoms.* Retrieved 3/27/08 from http://mayoclinic.com/health/high-blood-pressure/DS00100.

40. Gibson, R. M., & Meechan, J. G. (2007). The effects of antihypertensive medication on dental treatment. *Dent Update,* 34:70–72, 75–76. 78.

41. Sollecito, T. Transplantation medicine. (2003). *Burket's Oral Medicine Diagnosis and Treatment.* Tenth Ed.: Chapter 19, p.503–24. Lewiston, NY: BC Decker Inc.

42. Ellis, J. S., Seymour, R. A., Taylor, J. J., & Thomason, J. M. (2004). Prevalence of gingival overgrowth in transplant patients immunosuppressed with tacrolimus. *J Clin Periodontol,* 32:2.

43. Oliveira Costa, F., Ferreira, S. D., Lages, E. J., Costa, J. E., Oliveira, A. M., & Cota, L. O. (2007). Demographic, pharmacologic, and periodontal variables for gingival overgrowth in subjects medicated with cyclosporine in the absence of calcium channel blockers. *J Periodontol,* 78:254–61.

44. Fehrenbach, C. Chronic obstructive pulmonary disease. (2002, November 20–26). *Nurs Stand,* 17 (10):45–51.

45. Mannino, D. M., Gagnon, R. C., Petty, T. L., & Lydick, E. (2000). Obstructive lung disease and low lung function in adults in the United States: Data from the National Health and Nutrition Examination Survey 1988–1994. *Arch Intern Med,* 160:1683–89.

46. Antoniu, S. A., Mihaescu, T., & Donner, C. F. (2007). Inhaled therapy for stable chronic obstructive pulmonary disease. *Expert Opin Tharmacother,* 8:777–85.

47. Casiglia, J., & Mirowski, G. (2006, October 5). *Oral manifestations of systemic diseases.* Retrieved 11/22/06 from http://www.emedicine.com/derm/topic887.htm#section~author_information.

48. U.S. National Library of Medicine, National Institutes of Health. End-stage kidney disease. In *MedlinePlus Medical Encyclopedia.* Retrieved 11/22/06 from http://www.nlm.nih.gov/medlineplus/ency/article/000500.htm.

49. National Institute of Diabetes and Digestive and Kidney Diseases, National Institutes of Health. (2006 December). *Treatment methods for kidney failure: Hemodialysis.* Retrieved 11/22/06 from http://kidney.niddk.nih.gov/kudiseases/pubs/hemodialysis/.

50. Sharma, D. C., & Pradeep, A. R. (2007, January). End stage renal disease and its dental management. *NY State Dent J,* 73 (1):43–47.

51. DeRossi, S. S., & Glick, M. (1996). Dental considerations for the patient with chronic renal disease receiving hemodialysis. *J Am Dent Assoc,* 127:211–19.

52. Brescia, M. J., Cimino, J. E., & Appel, K. (1966). Chronic hemodialysis using veni-puncture in a surgically created arteriovenous fistula. *N Engl J Med,* 275:1089–92.

53. Kerr, A. R. (2001). Update on renal disease for the dental practitioner. *Oral Surg Oral Med Oral Path,* 92:9–16.

54. Spielman, A. L., Bivona, P., & Rifkin, B. R. (1996). Halitosis. A common oral problem. *NY State Dent J,* 62(10):36–42.

55. Eigner, T. L., Jastak, J. T., & Bennet, W. M. (1986). Achieving oral health in patients with renal failure and renal transplants. *J Am Dent Assoc,* 113:612–16.

56. Gavalda, C., Bagan, J., Scully, C., Silvestre, F., Milian, M., & Jimenez, Y. (1999). Renal hemodialysis patients: Oral, salivary, dental and periodontal findings in 105 adult cases. *Oral Dis,* 5:299–302.

57. Syrjanen, S., & Lampainen, E. (1983). Mandibular changes in panoramic radiographs in patients with end-stage renal disease. *Dentomaxillofac Radiol,* 12:51–56.

58. Anderson, K. N., Anderson, L. E., & Glanze, W. D. (1998). *Mosby's medical, nursing, and allied health dictionary* (5th ed.). St. Louis: C.V. Mosby.

59. The Joint Committee of the National Council on Alcoholism and Drug Dependence and the American Society of Addictive Medicine to Study the Definition and Criteria for the Diagnosis of Alcoholism. (1992). The definition of alcoholism. *JAMA,* 268(8):1012–14.

60. Stahre, M. A., Brewer, R. D., Naimi, T. S., & Miller, J. W. (2004). Alcohol-attributable deaths and years of potential life lost—United States, 2001. *MMWR Morb Mortal Wkly Rep,* 53:866–70.

61. Corrao, G., Rubbiati, L., Zambon, A., & Arico, S. (2002). Alcohol-attributable and alcohol-preventable mortality in Italy. *Eur J Public Health,* 12:214–23.

62. Corrao, G., Bagnardi, V., Zambon, A., & La Vecchia, C. (2004). A meta-analysis of alcohol consumption and the risk of 15 diseases. *Prev Med,* 38:613–19.

63. Rehm, J., Gmel, G., Sepos, C. T., & Trevisan, M. (2003). Alcohol-related morbidity and mortality. *Alcohol Res Health,* 27:39–51.

64. Castandeda, R., Sussman, N., Westreich, L., Levy, R., & O'Malley, M. (1996). A review of the effects of moderate alcohol intake on the treatment of anxiety and mood disorders. *J Clin Psychiatr,* 57:207–12.

65. Kochanek, K. E., Murphy, S. C., Anderson, R. N., & Scott, C. (2004). Deaths: Final data for 2002 (National Vital Statistics Reports 53(5)). Hyattsville, MD: National Center for Health Statistics.

66. Schiff, E. R. (1997). Hepatitis C and alcohol. *Hepatology,* 26 (Suppl 1):39S–42S.

67. Lesher. S. D. H., & Lee. Y. T. M. (1989). Acute pancreatitis in a military hospital. *Military Med,* 154:559–64.

68. Kelly, J. P., Kaufman, D. W., Koff, R. S., Laslow, A., Wiholm, B. E., & Shapiro, S. (1995). Alcohol consumption and the risk of major upper gastrointestinal bleeding. *Am J Gastroenterol,* 90:1058–64.

69. Booth, B. M., & Feng, W. (2002). The impact of drinking and drinking consequences on short-term employment outcomes in at-risk drinkers in six southern states. *J Behav Health Serv Res,* 29:157–66.

70. Leonard, K. E., & Rothbard, J. C. (1999). Alcohol and the marriage effect. *J Stud Alcohol Suppl* 13:139–46.

71. Olshan, A. F., Weissler, M. C., Watson, M. A., & Bell, D. A. (2001). Risk of head and neck cancer and the alcohol dehydrogenase 3genotype. *Carcinogenesis,* 22:57–61.

72. Genco, R. J. (1999). Current view of risk factors for periodontal disease. *J Periodontol,* 67 (Suppl):1041–49.

73. Wynder, E. L., & Bross, I. J. (1998). Etiological factors in mouth cancer: An approach to its prevention. *BMJ,* 1:389–95.

74. Holbrook, T. L., & Barrett-Conner, E. (1998). A prospective study of alcohol consumption and bone density. *BMJ,* 306:1506–509.

75. National Institute on Drug Abuse. (2006). Tobacco addiction. Research Report Series. Bethesda, MD: U.S. Department of Health and Human Services, National Institutes of Health, National Institute on Drug Abuse. Rockville, MD. NIDA Research Report - Tobacco Addiction: NIH Publication No. 06-4342, Printed 1998, Reprinted 2001, Revised 2006.

76. National Center for Health Statistics. (2006). Health, United States, 2006 with chartbook on trends in the health of Americans (Library of Congress Catalog No. 76-641496). Hyattsville, MD: National Center for Health Statistics.

77. Walsh, P., & Epstein, J. (2000). The oral effects of smokeless tobacco. Retrieved 3/27/08 from http://www.cda-adc.ca/jcda/vol-66/issue-1/22.html.

78. Bergstrom, J., Keilani, H., Lundholm, C., & Radestad, U. (2006). Smokeless tobacco (snuff) use and periodontal bone loss. *J Clin Periodontol,* 33;549–54.

79. Academy of General Dentistry. (1996). How many teeth are in that cigarette pack? Retrieved 11/06 from http://www.agd.org.

80. Rao, L. P., Das, S. R., Mathews, A., Naik, B. R., Chacko, E., & Pandey, M. (2004). Mandibular invasion in oral squamous cell carcinoma. *Int J Oral Maxillofac Surg,* 33:454–57.

81. Frije, J., & Kumar, J. V. (2001, March). Prevention of cancers of oral cavity and pharynx in New York State. *NY State Dent J,* 67 (3):26–30.

82. National Institute on Drug Abuse. (2006, April). NIDA InfoFacts: Marijuana. Bethesda, MD: U.S. Department of Health and Human Services, National Institutes of Health.

83. Office of Applied Studies. (2004). Results from the 2004 National Survey on Drug Use and Health: National findings (DHHS Publication No. SMA 05-4061). (Office of Applied Studies NSDUH Series H-27). Rockville, MD: Office of Applied Studies.

84. Darling, M. R., & Arendorf, T. M. (1992). Effects of cannabis smoking on oral health. *Int Dent J,* 42:19–22.

85. Darling, M. R., & Arendorf, T. M. (1993). Effects of cannabis smoking on oral soft tissues. *Community Dent Oral Epidemiol,* 21:78–81.

86. Hashibe, M., Ford, D., & Zhang, A. (2002). Marijuana smoking and head and neck cancer. *J Clin Pharmacol,* 42:103S–107S.

87. Cho, C. M., Hirsch, R., & Johnstone, S. (2005). General and oral health implications of cannabis use. *Aust Dent J,* 50:70–74.

88. Darling, M. R., Arendorf, T. M., & Coldrey, N. A. (1990). Effects of cannabis smoking on oral candidal carriage. *J Oral Pathol Med,* 19:319–21.

89. Seyer, B., Grist, W., & Muller, S. (2002). Aggressive destructive midfacial lesion from cocaine abuse. *Oral Surg Oral Med Oral Pathol Oral Radiol Endod,* 94:465–70.

90. National Institute on Drug Abuse. (2006). *Cocaine abuse and addiction.* (Research Report Series). Rockville, MD: U.S. Department of Health and Human Services, National Institutes of Health, National Institute on Drug Abuse.

91. U.S. Department of Justice, U.S. Drug Enforcement Administration. (2006 August). *Cocaine.* Retrieved 10/07 from http://www.dea.gov/concern/cocaine.html.

92. National Institute on Drug Abuse. (2006, April). *NIDA InfoFacts: Crack and cocaine.* U.S. Department of Health and Human Services, National Institutes of Health, National Institute on Drug Abuse.

93. Swan, N. (2005). Brain scans open window to view cocaine's effects on the brain. U.S. Department of Health and Human Services, National Institutes of Health, National Institute on Drug Abuse. Available from http://www.nida.nih.gov/NIDA_Notes/NNVol13N2/Brain.html.

94. Villa, P. D. (1999). Midfacial complications of prolonged cocaine snort. *J Can Dent Assoc,* 65:218–23.

95. Darby, M. L. & Walsh, M. (2003). *Dental hygiene theory and practice.* St. Louis: Elsevier Saunders.

96. Smith, J., Kacker, A., & Anand, V. K. (2002). Midline nasal and hard palate destruction in cocaine abusers and cocaine's role in rhinologic practice. *Ear Nose Throat J,* 81(3):172–77.

97. Ibsen, O. A. C., & Phelan, J. A. (2000). *Oral pathology for the dental hygienist.* St Louis: Saunders.

98. Chang, L., Ernst, T., Speck, O., & Grob, C. (2005). Addictive effects of HIV and chronic methamphetamine use on brain metabolite abnormalities. *Am J Psychiatr,* 162:361–69.

99. Richards, J., & Brofeldt. B. (2000). Patterns of tooth wear associated with methamphetamine use. *J Periodontol,* 71:1271–74.

100. Stein, W. (2005, September–October). Rotten times are here again. *Northwest Dent,* 84(5):10.

101. National Institute on Drug Abuse. (2006, April). *NIDA InfoFacts: Methamphetamine.* U.S. Department of Health and Human Services, National Institutes of Health, National Institute on Drug Abuse.

102. Curtis, E. (2006). Meth mouth: A review of methamphetamine abuse and its oral manifestations. *Gen Den,* 54:125–29.

103. Saini, T., Edwards, P., Kimmes, N., Carroll, L. R., Shaner, J. W., & Dowd, F. J. (2005). Etiology of xerostomia and dental caries among methamphetamine abusers. *Oral Health Prev Dent,* 3:189–95.

104. Streff, M., & Pachucki-Hyde, L. (1996). Management of the patient with thyroid disease. *Nurs Clin North Am,* 31:779–96.

105. Thyroid gland disorders. In *Merck manual of medical information: Second home edition.* Whitehouse Station, NJ: Merck Research Laboratories, Chapter 163.

106. Mayo Clinic Staff. (2006). Hypterthyroidism. Retrieved 3/27/08 from http://mayoclinic.com/health/hyperthyroidism/DS00344.

107. Greene, C. (2005). Thyroid gland. World Book Online References Center. World Book, Inc. Retrieved 4/1/08 from http://www.worldbookonline.com/wb/Login?ed=wb.

108. U.S. National Library of Medicine, National Institutes of Health. Hypothyroidism. In *MedlinePlus medical encyclopedia.* Retrieved 11/22/06 from http://www.nlm.nih.gov/medlineplus/ency/article/000353.htm.

109. Silverton, S. (2003). Endocrine disease. In Greensberg, M., & Glick, M., Eds. *Burket's oral medicine diagnosis and treatment* (19th ed.). Ontario: BC Decker Inc, 578–91.

110. Sun, L., Davies, T. F., Blair, H. C., Abe, E., & Zaidi, M. (2006). TSH and bone loss. *Ann NY Acad Sci,* 1068:309–18.

Chapter 27

Populations with Developmental Disabilities

Elaine Sanchez Dils

OBJECTIVES

After reading this chapter, the student should be able to:

1. Describe and define this target population.
2. Describe common oral conditions and diseases of patients with developmental disabilities.
3. Describe specific preventive strategies to use with patients with developmental disabilities.
4. Describe the role of the dental provider in treating patients with developmental disabilities.

KEY TERMS

Developmental disability
Mental retardation
Perseveration
Pica
Autism
Cerebral palsy
Macroglossia

INTRODUCTION

Typically, a **developmental disability** is defined as a severe, chronic disability attributable to mental or physical impairment that manifests before the age of 22 years. This disability is likely to continue indefinitely, resulting in functional limitations and a need for planned care and treatment.[1,2] Approximately 4.5 million individuals in the United States have a developmental disability.[3]

The U.S. Surgeon General, in his 2001 conference and report, *Closing the Gap: A National Blueprint for Improving the Health of Individuals with Mental Retardation*, discussed the failure of the health care system to provide reasonable access to quality medical and dental care for persons with mental retardation.[4] One of the goals of the report was to increase the number of health care providers with appropriate training to treat persons with developmental disabilities. One of the results of recognizing this problem has been action taken by the Commission on Dental Accreditation (CODA). As of 2004, CODA requires that students who graduate from an accredited dental or dental hygiene school "must be competent in assessing the treatment needs of patients with special needs."[5] Dental professionals need an understanding of the limits and conditions that could possibly affect patients who have these disabilities. Although all patients must be considered on an individual basis, a basic knowledge of developmental disabilities will help the dental practitioner understand the disability, anticipate some of the challenges that might be encountered, and understand how to effectively treat and prevent diseases in this population.

Populations with developmental disabilities can have varying degrees of functional level. In a dental setting, patients considered to be high-functioning would be able to respond to the dental provider. For example, this level of function would be moving the head when prompted, relaxing the lips and tongue, and having radiographs taken without assistance. In contrast, patients considered to be low-functioning would need the dental team to manipulate all functions for them. These patients may not respond to basic commands or have a conscious swallowing ability.

Many different conditions and diagnoses can be considered a developmental disability. Developmental disabilities include bipolar disorder, fetal alcohol syndrome, microcephaly, multiple sclerosis, Prader-Willi syndrome, schizophrenia, spina bifida, traumatic brain injuries, deafness, and blindness. The four most frequently seen and studied conditions are mental retardation, autism, cerebral palsy, and Down syndrome.

MENTAL RETARDATION
Population Characteristics and Common Oral Manifestations

To be diagnosed with **mental retardation,** a person must meet three criteria.[6] First, the person must have a general learning deficiency. Next, impairments in communication, self-care, or mobility are exhibited. Finally, the first two criteria must be recognized during the developmental years, that is, 18 years or younger. It has been found that approximately 12 of every 1,000 births result in a child with mental retardation.[7] Although mental retardation is frequently found to correspond with other disabilities, it can be a stand-alone diagnosis.[8,9]

There are several causes of mental retardation. Chromosomal variations or defective genes are genetic causes. Physical, or brain, damage can also be the causative factor. This damage can occur at the prenatal, neonatal, or postnatal stage.[6] Prenatal harm is typically caused by maternal influences such as malnutrition, exposure to excessive radiation, alcohol use, and drug use. In addition, infections in the mother such as rubella and syphilis can also be the culprit. Premature birth, insufficient oxygen, or a birth injury may also cause mental retardation. Infections such as meningitis, toxins like lead, a brain tumor, or a traumatic brain injury could lead to mental retardation in the postnatal stage.

In addition to the above-mentioned origins, mental retardation can also be categorized into a variety of causative groups: cultural or familial, multifactor, psychosocial, and diagnosis unknown.[6] A person whose parents have significantly limited intelligence, are indifferent to the child, or have rejected the child may be the cause for mental retardation. Sensory deprivation can also be implicated as a root of mental retardation.

The intellectual characteristics of individuals with mental retardation vary widely.[6] These persons learn visual and auditory discrimination slowly, and they have difficulty with abstract terminology and verbal cues. In addition, they may experience short-term memory deficiencies and difficulty predicting outcomes. These individuals also are easily distracted and may have perseveration habits.[9] **Perseveration** means that the patient may have uncontrollable repetition of a particular response, such as a word, phrase, or gesture, despite the absence or cessation of a stimulus.

A person with mental retardation has several oral manifestations. An increase in the prevalence of periodontal diseases related to medications the patient takes, malocclusion, and poor oral hygiene are seen. Although the *number of untreated caries* is much higher in populations with mental retardation, the *caries rate* is comparable to that of the general population. Missing permanent teeth, delayed eruption, and enamel hypoplasia are more prevalent in these individuals. Increases in damaging oral habits are diagnosed such as bruxism, mouth breathing, tongue thrusting, biting lips, and **pica** (an appetite for substances not fit as food or of no nutritional value).[9]

Preventive Strategies

The most important strategy for preventive dental care in this population is addressed with either the individual or the caregivers. Stressing the need for regular maintenance appointments is the critical first step. Developing individualized treatment plans that incorporate the individual's abilities and the role of the caregiver is important. Also ensuring sufficient use of preventive aids such as fluorides will help with their oral health needs.

AUTISM
Population Characteristics and Common Oral Manifestations

The symptoms and severity vary widely in people diagnosed with autism. **Autism** impairs communication, and social, behavioral, and intellectual functioning.[10,11] For every 1,000 births in the United States, 3.4 babies will be diagnosed with autism.[12] A person with autism may appear aloof, distant, or detached and does not respond to common verbal or social cues as expected. In addition, hyperactivity and the tendency to become frustrated quickly are commonly seen. The continuous, meaningless repetition of words, phrases, or movements (perseveration) may be noted.[10]

Rates of periodontal diseases and caries in persons with autism correspond to those of the general population. As with all persons, a softer food diet high in sugar without proper dental self-care will increase the likelihood of caries and periodontal disease. An increase in damaging oral habits such as bruxism, biting of ones' lips, and pica may also be found in patients with autism. These habits may be self-coping mechanisms, exploration, or one of many repetitive behaviors seen in individuals with autism.

Preventive Strategies

When the dental provider is providing oral hygiene instruction, the patient's learning level should be assessed to ensure the instruction is being delivered at the appropriate level.[10] This approach will help the individual understand the importance of and need for proper self-care. The autistic person can be sensitive to changes; therefore, consistency and structure in dental appointments and instruction are also very important. If the patient can tolerate a mouthguard, its use should be considered for patients who have problems with self-injurious behavior or bruxism (see Chapter 19).

CEREBRAL PALSY
Population Characteristics and Common Oral Manifestations

Cerebral palsy (CP) is a nonprogressive, neuromuscular disorder caused by damage to the immature brain. Cerebral palsy does not refer to a specific disease; rather, it is an injury to the motor portion of the brain. This injury can be associated with uncontrolled body movements, seizures, balance problems, sensory dysfunction, and mental retardation.[13–16]

The causes of CP are again seen at the prenatal, neonatal, and postnatal stages.[14,16] Specifically, CP is seen in 3.1 of 1,000 births.[7] Maternal diabetes, hypertension, or infections, such as herpes, can be implicated. Rh factor incompatibility, excess radiation, and drugs taken by the mother are also seen in the development of CP. Oxygen deprivation, birth injury, and prolonged or difficult labor contribute to CP that develops during the prenatal and neonatal stages. Postnatally, trauma, brain tumors, infections, such as encephalitis and meningitis, and toxins, such as lead and hydrocarbons, contribute to the number of people with CP.

Cerebral palsy is classified by the severity (mild, moderate, or severe), the area of brain involved, and the resultant disorder.[16] The types of CP seen are spasticity, athetosis, ataxia, tremors, rigidity, and mixed.[15,16] Approximately 50% to 70% of people with CP also have mental retardation. The remaining persons have normal or superior intelligence.[16]

Roughly 30% of CP patients have epilepsy.[16] Most patients with CP have visual, hearing, and speech defects.[14,16] Their speech can be slow because of an inability to control muscles involved in speech and mastication. A swallowing dysfunction can also lead to frequent drooling. Constant involuntary movements can make eating difficult.[15,17] An inadequate cough reflex may increase choking, coughing, and aspiration.[16]

Preventive Strategies

Periodontal diseases and caries are both more widespread in this population.[15,16] Enamel hypoplasia, mouth breathing, and food retention in the mouth all contribute to the increased rates of periodontal disease and caries.[13,14] In addition, physical constraints of the patient with CP can make proper oral hygiene difficult. For these reasons, a unique, individualized dental care plan that can be performed by the patient or caregiver, if necessary, must be developed. A wide-handled, powered toothbrush may assist these patients (Figure 27–1 ■). A manual toothbrush with an enlarged handle, elastic cuff, or small strap attached to the brush may help patients who do not have a high level of fine muscle control.[18] The toothbrush modifications shown in Figure 27–1 through 27–4 ■ may be used with manual toothbrushes. A regimen of daily fluoride treatments along with individualized, personal, and caregiver-directed plaque control measures, such as the use of a floss threader (Figure 27–5 ■), can help reduce the incidence of these diseases.

Because of the number of individuals with CP who also have epilepsy, several cases of gingival hyperplasia may be seen.[16,19] In cases with excessive growth of gingival tissue, gingival reduction may be considered a treatment option. An increase in the number of class II malocclusions is found in patients with CP.[15–17] The malocclusion is due to skeletal problems, not just tooth misalignment or the common habit of tongue thrusting.[16] The increased rate of temporomandibular joint disorder corresponds with a higher rate of bruxism.[15–17] Severe bruxism can cause wear of tooth facets, tooth fractures, and possibly pulpal exposure of teeth. The loss of the vertical dimension of the posterior teeth, seen in bruxism, is thought to be a large contributing factor to temporo-

mandibular joint problems. If reasonable for the individual, orthodontics may be considered. Patients with cerebral palsy also tend to have hyperactive bite and gag

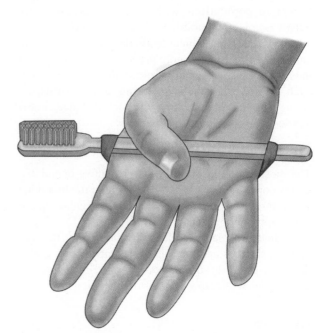

■ **FIGURE 27–2**   Toothbrush attached to hand with rubber band.

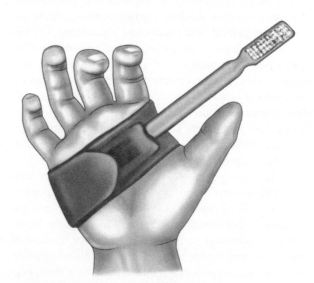

■ **FIGURE 27–3**   Toothbrush attached to hand with Velcro.

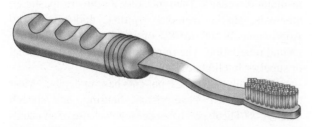

■ **FIGURE 27–1**   A wide-handled, grip toothbrush.

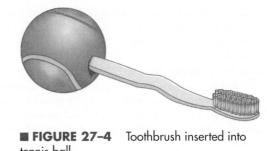

■ **FIGURE 27–4** Toothbrush inserted into tennis ball.

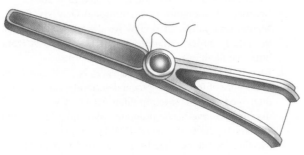

■ **FIGURE 27–5** Dental floss holder.

reflexes.[15] In these cases a mouthguard may help reduce the effects of the prolonged bruxing and clenching.

DOWN SYNDROME

Population Characteristics and Common Oral Manifestations

Down syndrome occurs in 1 of every 733 births in the United States; the person affected is found to have an extra twenty-first chromosome.[20–23,24,25] Nearly all patients with Down syndrome have some level of mental retardation. These individuals have specific orofacial characteristics: a nose with a flat, broad bridge; low-set ears; slanted, almond-shaped eyes; lack of a supraorbital ridge, which contributes to the broad, short head; and, frequently, absent or reduced maxillary sinuses.[23,25–26]

About 40% of persons with Down syndrome have mitral valve prolapse.[18,22–27] As a result of the absent or reduced maxillary sinus, many of these patients suffer from sleep apnea.[27] An increase in upper respiratory tract infections is due to an impaired immune system.[23–27] Signs of Alzheimer's disease and dementia begin around the age of 35 years.[23,25] Generalized

ligament laxity also is seen frequently.[25] Speech, hearing, and vision problems are common as well. These patients tend to be below average height, obese, and sexually underdeveloped.[23,25]

Preventive Strategies

Patients with Down syndrome have severe, early onset of periodontal disease attributable to a decreased immune response with ligament laxity.[18,19,21] Proper oral hygiene performed at an early age by both the patient and caregivers is imperative. A lower rate of decay is seen in the patient with Down syndrome compared with the general population.[19] This characteristic is attributed to the delayed eruption of the teeth and open proximal contacts. Underdevelopment of the midface gives way to a large number of class III malocclusions.[18,19,21] **Macroglossia** (enlarged tongue) and a fissured, protruding tongue are evident as a result of the forward position of the mandible and slightly opened mouth.[18,19]

Use of fluoride treatments and saliva substitutes may decrease xerostomia for the patient contending with this syndrome. Variable tooth morphology and short roots may also be seen. An increase in bruxism is also common among patients with Down syndrome.[21] Although no definitive preventive measure can be taken with the anatomic development, educating the patient and caregiver(s) on known oral issues and management strategies is best.

SUMMARY

Although several developmentally disabled patients are able to brush their own teeth and can often do so with support and encouragement from dental personnel, it is very important to intimately involve the patient's primary caregiver in oral hygiene instruction. Personalized techniques can be demonstrated and explained to suit each patient's needs. For some patients with developmental disabilities, dental professionals and caregivers may need to alter their methods of performing oral examinations or dental prophylaxis. Some examples of alternative positioning can be seen in Figure 27–6 ■ and Figure 27–7 ■.

Individuals with developmental disabilities face many challenges unique to their condition. To provide care that reflects the unique needs of these individuals, the dental team must understand the underlying condition.

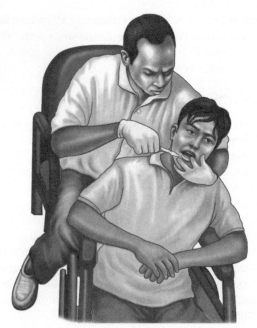

■ **FIGURE 27–6**   Sitting behind patient in wheelchair.

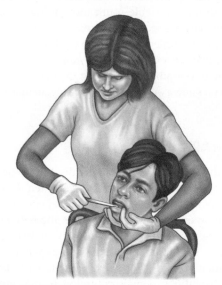

■ **FIGURE 27–7**   Standing behind patient in chair.

REFERENCES

1. Calderone, J. (1996). *Memorandum: Functional definitions.* Albuquerque, NM: New Mexico Department of Health.
2. National Institute of Health. *Oral health care for people with developmental disabilities.* Bethesda, MD: National Institutes of Health, National Oral Health Information Clearinghouse.
3. Administration for Families and Children, Administration on Developmental Disabilities. *Fact sheet.* (n.d.) Retrieved 10/16/06 from http://www.acf.hhs.gov/programs/add/.
4. U.S. Public Health Service. (2001). *Closing the gap: A national blueprint for improving the health of individuals with mental retardation. Report of the Surgeon General's conference on health disparities and mental retardation.* Washington, DC: U.S. Government Printing Office.
5. Commission on Dental Accreditation. Accreditation Standards For Dental Education Programs. Standard 2-26. American Dental Association. Adopted July, 2004.
6. Southern Association of Institutional Dentists. (n.d.). Mental retardation: A review for dental professionals. Self-study course, module 1. Retrieved 4/1/08 from http://saiddent.org/modules/9_module1.pdf.
7. Bhasin, T. K., Brocksen, S., Avchen, R. N., & Braun, K. V. Prevalence of four developmental disabilities among children aged 8 years—Metropolitan Atlanta developmental disabilities surveillance program 1996 and 2000. Posted January 18, 2006. Retrieved 4/1/08 from www.cdc.gov.
8. Merriam Webster Online Dictionary. (n.d.). Mental retardation. Retrieved 5/06 from http://www.merriam-webster.com/dictionary/Mental%20retardation.
9. U.S. Department of Health and Human Services. (2004, May). *Practical oral care for people with mental retardation* (NIH Publication No. 04-5194). Rockville, MD: U.S. Department of Health and Human Services, National Institute of Dental and Craniofacial Research, National Institutes of Health.
10. U.S. Department of Health and Human Services. (2004, May). *Practical oral care for people with autism* (NIH Publication No. 04-5190). Rockville, MD: U.S. Department of Health and Human Services, National Institute of Dental and Craniofacial Research, National Institutes of Health.
11. Merriam Webster Online Dictionary. (n.d.). Autism. Retrieved 5/06 from http://www.merriam-webster.com/dictionary/autism.
12. National Institute of Mental Health. Autism spectrum disorders (pervasive developmental disorders). (n.d.) Retrieved 4/1/08 from http://www.nimh.nih.gov.
13. Merriam Webster Online Dictionary. (n.d.). Cerebral palsy. Retrieved 5/06 from http://www.merriam-webster.com/dictionary/cerebral%20palsy.
14. Aswal, S., Russman, B. S., Blasco, P. A., Miller, G., Sandler, A., Shevell, M., & Stevenson, R. *Practice parameter: Diagnostic assessment of the child with cerebral palsy: Report of the Quality Standards Subcommittee of the American Academy of Neurology and the Practice Committee of the Child Neurology Society.* 2004 Mar 23; 62(6):851–63.
15. U.S. Department of Health and Human Services. (2004, May). *Practical oral care for people with cerebral palsy* (NIH Publication No. 04-5190). Rockville, MD: U.S.

Department of Health and Human Services, National Institute of Dental and Craniofacial Research, National Institutes of Health.

16. Southern Association of Institutional Dentists. (n.d.). Cerebral palsy: A review for dental professionals. Self-study course, module 4. Retrieved 4/1/08 from http://saiddent.org/modules/12_module4.pdf.

17. Scheutz, F., & Langeback, J. (1995). Dental care of infectious patients in Denmark. *Community Dent Oral Epidemiol,* 23:226–31.

18. Bhowate, R., & Dubey, A. (2005). Dentofacial changes and oral health status in mentally challenged children. *J Indian Soc Pedodont Prev Dent,* 23:71–73.

19. Fenton, S., Hood, H., Holder, M., May, P., & Mouradian, W. (2003, Dec.) The American Academy of Developmental Medicine and Dentistry: Eliminating health disparities for individuals with mental retardation and other developmental disabilities. *J Dent Edu,* 67(12):1337–44.

20. National Down Syndrome Society. Information topics. Retrieved 10/16/06 from http://www.ndss.org.

21. Merriam Webster Online Dictionary. Down syndrome. Retrieved 5/06 from http://www.merriam-webster.com/dictionary/down%20syndrome.

22. Saenz, R. (1999, Jan 15). Primary care of infants and young children with Down syndrome. *Am Fam Physician,* 59(2):381–90, 392, 395–96.

23. Southern Association of Institutional Dentists. (n.d.). Down syndrome: A review for dental professionals. Self-study course, module 3. Retrieved 4/1/08 from http://saiddent.org/modules/11_module3.pdf.

26. U.S. Department of Health and Human Services. (2004, May). *Practical oral care for people with Down syndrome* (NIH Publication No. 04-5193). Rockville, MD: U.S. Department of Health and Human Services, National Institute of Dental and Craniofacial Research, National Institutes of Health.

27. Steffens-Picher, E. (n.d.) Treating the patient with Down syndrome (Continuing Education Course). Retrieved 5/06 from http://www.dentalcare.com/soap/conteduc/index.htm.

24. Waldman, H. B., & Perlman, S. (2002, Jan). Preparing to meet the dental needs of individuals with disabilities. *J Dent Educ,* 66(1):82–85.

25. Chung, E., Sung, E., & Sakurai, K. (2004, May). Dental management of the Down and Eisenmenger syndrome patient. *J Contemp Dent Pract,* 15;5(2):70–80.

Glossary

A

Abutment teeth: The teeth to which the two ends of a bridge are attached.

Acidogenesis: Acid production.

Aciduric: The ability to thrive in a relatively acidic environment.

Acquired pellicle: The coating of saliva origin that forms on exposed tooth surfaces.

Actinic cheilitis: A precancerous condition on the lip that is due to prolonged exposure to the sun. Sometimes referred to as "farmer's lips" or "sailor's lips."

Active immunity: The production of antibodies against a specific agent by the immune system that can be acquired in two ways, by contracting an infectious disease or by receiving a vaccination.

Adhesion: The surface appendage of a bacterium that allows the microbe to attach to receptor sites on the tooth or on other bacteria in the plaque.

Aerobic bacteria: Bacteria that require oxygen for survival.

Ageusia: The loss of taste functions of the tongue, particularly the inability to detect sweetness, sourness, bitterness and saltiness.

Alimentary tract: The mucous membrane-lined tube of the digestive system through which food passes, in which digestion takes place, and from which wastes are eliminated.

Alternative restorative technique (ART): The excavation of cavitated carious lesions with hand instruments and restoration of the cavities and associate pits an fissures with a glass ionomer or dental sealant material.

Alveolar crest fibers: The periodontal fibers that attach to the cementum just apical to the cementoenamel junction, run downward, and insert into the alveolar bone.

Alveolar fracture: A fracture of the alveolar bone.

Alveolar mucosa: The mucosa which covers the alveolar bone.

Alveolar process: The thickened ridge of bone that contains the tooth sockets on bones and is also referred to as the alveolar bone.

Alveolar ridge: One of the two jaw ridges either on the roof of the mouth between the maxilarry teeth and the hard palate or on the bottom of the mouth behind the mandibular teeth.

Alveologingival fibers: The fibers collected into fiber bundles within the subepithelial connective tissue of the gingiva that extend from the crest of the alveolus and insert into the dense irregular collagenous connective tissue of the attached and free gingiva.

Alveolus: Areas in the jaws in which the roots of teeth are held in the alveolar process of maxilla with the periodontal ligament, sometimes referred to as tooth sockets.

Amalgams: A commonly used dental restorative material which is a mixture of mercury with at least one other metal, such as silver, tin, copper and zinc.

Ameloblasts: Cells which secrete the enamel proteins enamelin and amelogenin which will later mineralize to form enamel on teeth, the strongest substance in the human body.

Amelogenesis: The formation of enamel on teeth and occurs during the crown stage of tooth development after dentinogenesis, which is the formation of dentin.

Amourphous calcium phosphates: Used in dental products for the remineralization of demineralized tooth surfaces.

Amylase: An enzyme that breaks starch down into sugar and is present in saliva, where it begins the chemical process of digestion.

Anaerobic bacteria: Bacteria that survive only in the absence of oxygen.

Angled filaments: Arrangement of toothbrush bristle filaments.

Ankylosis: The fusion of the tooth to the bone which prevents the tooth from erupting.

Anorexia nervosa: An eating disorder characterized by unrealistic fear of weight gain, self-starvation, and conspicuous distortion of body image.

Anterior: Anatomical location of the front surface, such as the "front teeth."

Antimicrobial mouthwash: A mouthwash with antimicrobial properties.

Apex: Anatomically the "root tip" of the tooth.

Apexification: The process of induced root development or apical closure of the root by hard tissue deposition.

APF, acidulated phosphate fluoride: A type of fluoride used in topical fluoride agents.

Apical: Toward the root tip surface.

Apical fibers: Periodontal fibers located at the root tip surface.

Apical migration: Migration of a periodontal pocket to the root surface, which results in bone loss.

Apices: Pertaining to the area surrounding the root tip surface.

Apoptosis: A form of programmed cell death in multicellular organisms.

Approximal plaque: Plaque found on interproximal surfaces.

Arrested root caries: Carious lesions on the root surfaces that have stopped the demineralization process and have begun to remineralize.

Arthritis: A group of conditions involving damage to the joints of the body.

Articulating paper: Used to determine where cusps are occluding.

Artificially acquired active immunity: Artificially acquired passive immunity is a short-term immunization by the injection of antibodies that are not produced by the recipient's cells.

Aspartame: A dipeptide that is used as a non-nutritive, noncariogenic sweetner.

Assessment: A thorough analysis of all factors of a patient's or target population's health issues.

Assurance: Something that inspires or tries to inspire confidence.

Asthma: A chronic disease that affects the pulmonary system.

Athletic mouthguard: A thermoplastic oral appliance used to prevent dental trauma and concussions during athletic activities.

Attached gingiva: The mucous membrane extending from the mucogingival fold to the marginal gingiva on the facial side of the alveolar process.

Attachment apparatus: The tissues that invest and support the teeth for function including the cementum, periodontal ligament, and alveolar bone.

Autistic: Individuals who often have difficulty or an inability to communicate appropriately; a neurodevelopmental disability.

Automated flossers: A flossing apparatus that is automated and many patients with difficulty flossing, find automated flossers easier to use.

Autopolymerization: The ability to accomplish polymerization, scuh as during the dental sealant procedure without the use of a light source, but instead with a chemical catalyst.

Avulsion: The traumatic removal of teeth that may occur during an accident or traumatic event during sport activities.

B

Baby bottle tooth decay: Dental decay caused by the prolonged use a baby bottle or sippy cup, referred to as nursing bottle decay or more commonly early childhood caries.

Bacteremias: The usually transient presence of bacteria in the blood.

Bacterial biofilm: A biofilm is a structured community of microorganisms encapsulated within a self-developed polymeric matrix and adherent to a living or inert surface.

Bacterial endocarditis: Bacterial infection of the heart.

Bacteriostatic: Having the capability to inhibit the growth or reproduction of bacteria, which is different that bactericidal which is the capability of killing bacteria.

Bass method: A specific toothbrushing method focusing on supragingival plaque removal.

Battery-powered brushes: Toothbrushes powered by a battery, particularly useful for patients who have difficulty brushing.

B-complex vitamins: Eight water-soluble vitamins that play important roles in cell metabolism.

Behavior management: Techniques used to control behavior issues during dental services.

Behavior modification: A change in behavior due to motivation causing a shift in self-designated goals.

Beta-defensin peptides: A large family of small cationic antimicrobial peptides widely distributed in plants, mammals, and insects which display multifunctional properties with implications as potential therapeutic agents.

Bidirectional synergism: Two or more agents working together to produce a result not obtainable by any of the agents independently that can be controlled from either end and can move forward or backward with equal ease without any need to be turned around.

Bidis: A thin, often flavored, South Asian cigarette made of tobacco wrapped in a leaf, and secured with colored thread at one end.

Binding agents: Agents that are used to maintain the consistency of a toothpaste and prevent separation of the other additives.

Binge-eating disorder (BED): Individuals with this disorder eat unusually large quantities of food without control over their eating.

Biofilm: A layer of living organisms that can attach to a solid object, for instance moss or seaweed to rocks, or in a dental context, oral bacteria to the teeth.

Biopsy: The excision (removal) and microscopic examination of tissue suspected of being cancerous.

Bipolar disorder: The category of mood disorders defined by the presence of one or more episodes of abnormally elevated mood, clinically referred to as mania.

Bis-GMA: The abbreviation of the chemical name of the plastic used for sealants. (Bisphenol A-glycidyl methylacrlate).

Bitewing radiograph: a radiograph that shows the crowns of both the maxillary and mandibular teeth on the same film, and are used to detect interproximal carious lesions and when taken vertically can also detect bone loss.

Bleeding index: A record of the location of marginal bleeding following gentle probing of the free margin of the gingiva.

Body defense cells: Cells that identify the presence of antigens (foreign bodies), remove the antigens, and/or repair the damage caused by the antigens.

Body Mass Index: BMI. A medical standard for defining obesity.

Body wraps: Blanket like wraps that fully enfold a young patient to restrain body parts or patient actions during a dental procedure.

Bone marrow transplant: A procedure that transplants healthy bone marrow into a patient whose bone marrow is not working properly.

Brachytherapy: A form of radiotherapy where a radioactive source is placed inside or next to the area requiring treatment, also known as sealed source radio-therapy or endocurietherapy that is commonly used to treat localized cancers of the head and neck.

Bradycardia: A resting heart rate of under 60 beats per minute, though it is seldom symptomatic until the rate drops below 50 beat/min.

Bristles: A part of the toothbrush that is often made from synthetic fibers, although natural toothbrushes are also known in many parts of the world.

Brush test: Computer-assisted analysis of an oral brush test used to evaluate innocuous lesions.

Brushite: A mineral, formula $CaHPO_4 \cdot 2H_2O$.

Buccal: Of or pertaining to the cheek or facial area.

Buccal salivary glands: Salivary glands located within the buccal mucosa.

Buds: The tooth bud, sometimes called the tooth germ, is an aggregation of cells that eventually forms a tooth.

Buffering: The ability to neutralize acidity (of the plaque) by use of alkaline substances.

Bulimia nervosa: Binge eating. Eating a meal, and then resorting to regurgitation to eliminate the stomach contents. Often accompanied by lingual erosion of teeth from stomach acid.

Burnishing: Refers to the damaging result of not removing calculus from the tooth structure but actually allowing it to stay on the tooth surface.

C

Calcium: The fifth most abundant element by mass in the human body and a major component of teeth.

Calcium bridging: Theory that suggests that cells are held in place within biofilms by a web of polymers, but that proximity to neighboring cells is dependent on calcium bridging and that this may be manipulated to allow increased penetration of therapeutic agents.

Calcium carbonate: Calcium carbonate is a chemical compound with the chemical formula $CaCO_3$.

Calculus: Calcified deposits on the teeth, formed by the continuous presence of dental plaque, sometimes called tartar.

Caloric sugar: Sugars containing calories such as sucrose, glucose, fructose and lactose.

Canaliculi: An anatomical term used to describe a small passageway which include the small channels found in ossified bone.

Cancer: A term for diseases in which abnormal cells divide without control.

Candida albicans: A diploid fungus, which is capable of mating but not of meiosis, and a causal agent of opportunistic oral infections.

Candidiasis: A fungal infection (mycosis) of any of the *Candida* species, can be seen in the oral cavity and is referred to as thrush.

Cannula: A small diameter tip of an irrigator syringe or device that allows a deeper irrigation of a periodontal pocket.

Carbamide peroxide: A commonly used tooth bleaching agent.

Carcinogen: A substance or agent that causes cancer.

Carcinoma: Malignant neoplasm derived from epithelial tissue.

Carcinoma in situ: An early form of carcinoma defined by the absence of invasion of surrounding tissues.

Carcinomas: Malignancies that originate in the epithelial tissues.

Cardiac arrhythmias: A term for any of a large and heterogeneous group of conditions in which there is abnormal electrical activity in the heart, the heart beat may be too fast or too slow, and may be regular or irregular.

Caregiver: Members of the family, a friend, or hired personnel who assume responsibility of helping compromised persons.

Caries: A progressive destruction of any kind of bone structure, including the skull, ribs, teeth, and other bones.

Caries activity: A level of caries risk as determined by use of laboratory methods, plaque index and other evidence-based evaluations.

Caries-Activity Indictors (CAI): Evidence-based predictors of the course and outcome of the dental caries process.

Caries-free: Having no presence of carious lesions in the oral cavity.

Cariogenic: Increasing the likelihood that dental caries will develop.

Cariostatic: Acting to halt bone or tooth decay.

Carious lesion: A lesion of demineralized tooth surface.

Catheter: A tube connecting a body cavity with the exterior for purposes of irrigation or drainage.

Cavitated: An incipient lesion in which the surface zone has collapsed over the body of the lesion, thus creating an overt cavity.

Cellular immunity: Immunity resulting from a cell-mediated immune response, sometimes called cell-mediated immunity.

Cementoblasts: A biological cell that forms from the follicular cells around the root of a tooth, and whose biological function is cementogenesis, which is the creation of cementum.

Cemento-enamel junction: The junction point between the coronal enamel and the cementum.

Cementum: The surface layer of the root of the tooth.

Cerebral hemorrhage: A subtype of intracranial hemorrhage that occur within the brain tissue.

Cerebral palsy: An umbrella term encompassing a group of non-progressive, non-contagious conditions that cause physical disability in human development.

Cervical: The area of the tooth in between the crown and the root.

Cervical caries: Caries that are located on the cervical surface of the tooth.

Cetylpyridinium chloride: A cationic quaternary ammonium compound in some types of mouthwashes, toothpastes, etc.

CFUs: Colony-forming units (bacteria). The number of bacterial colonies that are found on a suitable agar after an appropriate period of incubation.

Charters technique: A toothbrushing method that focuses on circular strokes.

Chelating: Binding together.

Chemical activation: A process activated by a chemical means.

Chemical plaque control: The use of anti-microbial mouth rinses to aid in plaque control.

Chemical-cured sealants: Dental sealants that are polymerized by mixing in a chemical catalyst.

Chemotaxis: A response to a chemical signal that initiates the movement of body defense cells to an area of inflammation.

Chemotherapeutic agents: Dental agents used to prevent or maintain dental health.

Chew tobacco: A tobacco product that is placed in the mouth and "chewed" to release the tobacco product, is a risk factor in oral cancer.

Chlorhexidine gluconate: An effective antimicrobial mouth-rinse that is effective for suppressing cariogenic and periopathogenic organisms.

Chlorination: The addition of chlorine compounds to water supplies to kill pathogenic bacteria.

Chromosomes: Organized structures of DNA and proteins that are found in cells.

Chronic obstructive pulmonary disease: A disease of the lungs where the airways become narrowed.

Chronic periodontitis: The most common type of periodontal disease that is characterized by progressive loss of the bone and soft tissues that surround and support your teeth.

Clasp brush: A brush used by a patient to clean the clasps of a removable partial denture.

Classical conditioning: Suggests that individuals can become conditioned to specific stimuli to act in a specific way.

Clefting: An area of the gingival margin that becomes clefted in the middle due to aggressive brushing or other reason.

Cleft palate: An oral malformation in which there is a lack of union at the midline of the palate which may involve only a split uvula of the soft palate to a cleft of all structures of the palate and include the upper lip.

Cocci: Description of a bacterium such as a coccus, or sphere, distinguishes it from bacillus, or rod.

Cognition: Ability to concentrate and think logically.

Col: That portion of the interdental gingiva of molar teeth that is located between the oral and the vestibular papilla.

Collagen: Collagen is the protein for the framework of soft and hard tissues of the body.

Collagenase: The enzyme that attacks collagen.

Colonization: The colonizing of bacteria.

Colorado brown stain: The early designation for severe fluorosis (with brown coloration of teeth) before its etiology was known.

Community water fluoridation: The term used when adding fluoride to a community water supply for the intent to decrease the incidence of dental caries in a community.

Compliance: A willingness of a patient to follow prescribed actions.

Composites: A tooth colored dental restorative material.

Compromised individual: A person with one or more physical, medical, mental or emotional problems that limit their ability to function.

Concept: After an individual has learned a sufficient number of facts relating to a subject, by reasoning these facts begin to form an overall belief called a concept.

Concussion: The most common and least serious type of traumatic brain injury.

Congestive heart failure: A condition in which the heart cannot pump enough blood to the body's other organs.

Coronal: The area around the crown of the tooth.

Coronal caries: Caries located on the crown of the tooth.

Cost-effective analysis: A calculation of how much money is saved (or overspent) as a result of some action.

CPITN: A Community Periodontal Index of Treatment Needs: A world-wide standardized periodontal needs index based on the severity (pocket depth) exhibited by a population.

Craniofacial disorders: Refers to an abnormality of the face and/or the head.

Crevicular fluid: A tissue fluid that arises from the underlying connective tissue, flows slowly through the gingival crevice into the mouth; its two major functions are to (1) flush out catabolites, and (2) to act as a carrier for immune cells and antibodies that bathe (and protect) the four smooth surfaces on every tooth.

Cytokine: A proinflammatory blood borne agent of the body's immune system.

Cure: Occurs when a disease process terminates with a return to histologic normalcy of all tissues involved. The return to normal can be due to natural body defense mechanisms, or because of professional intercession.

D

Daily values: A new dietary reference value to help consumers use food label information to plan a healthy overall diet.

Debridement: The mechanical or chemical removal of infectious or necrotic material from an inflamed, or potentially inflamed area.

Defluoridation: The removal of naturally occurring fluoride in a community water supply, when the fluoride above the optimum level.

Dementia: The progressive decline in cognitive function.

Demineralization: The loss of mineral from the tooth because of bacterial acids, acid foods (soft drinks, acid juices, etc), or even toothbrushing abrasion.

Demographic data: Conditions relating to and having an effect on data found in a survey, such as population, socioeconomic status, race, age, unusual environmental conditions, etc.

Dentacult SM and Denticult L: Commercially available test kits that facilitate counting of mutans streptococci and lactobacilli, respectively.

Dental calculus: Mineralization of the deeper portions of plaque.

Dental caries: A carbohydrate modified transmissible localized infection caused mainly by mutans streptococci and lactobacilli.

Dental demineralization: The loss of tooth mineralization caused by dental decay.

Dental hygiene process of care: The steps or protocol used when providing comprehensive dental hygiene treatment.

Dental plaque: A combination of bacteria, saliva and complex polysaccharides on the surface of the teeth.

Dental public health: The art and science of preventing and controlling oral disease, with an emphasis on prevention, in the community.

Dental sealants: A liquid plastic that is placed on pits and/or fissures of tooth surfaces and then harden to help prevent tooth demineralization.

Dentate: With teeth. The opposite is edentulous, i.e., not to have teeth.

Dentifrice: A more scientific, but less used, term for toothpaste.

Dentinal tubules: Tubules present within the dentin.

Dentinoenamel junction: A junction of the dentin and enamel.

Dentition: The teeth, collectively

Dentogingival fiber: Gingival fibers that are inserted into the dentin.

Dentogingival junction: The junction of the dentin and gingival.

Denture adhesive: A pliable dental product used to hold a dental prosthesis in position.

Denture Liner: A resin used to coat the tissue surface of a dental prosthesis to restore or improve the conformation of the prosthesis to improve the retention of the denture.

Depressive disorders: The collective term for mental health disorders of a depressive nature.

Desquamate: To shed skin cells.

Developmental disability: A diverse group of severe chronic conditions that are due to mental and/or physical impairments.

Dextrose: Common lay designation of glucose.

Diabetes mellitus: A syndrome characterized by disordered metabolism and abnormally high blood sugar (hyperglycaemia) resulting from insufficient levels of the hormone insulin.

Diagnosis: The process of identifying a medical condition or disease by its signs, symptoms, and from the results of various assessments and diagnostic procedures.

Diastemas: Spaces between the interproximal areas of teeth.

Dietary fluoride supplement schedule: Recommended daily dosage of fluoride supplements. (applicable to fluoride drops or tablets) to bring the daily intake to the equivalent of 1 ppm.

Dietary guidance: Professional recommendations regarding an individual's nutritional habits.

Dietary Reference Intake (DRIs): To address how foods can bridge the difference between healthy individuals and those with chronic and acute disease. This also will involve a study of different vitamins, minerals as they relate to health.

Digitized radiographs: Producing images of objects by electronically detecting the arrival of x-ray photons transmitted through the object or emitted from it on various media and converting the sensed analog signals to digital signals representing the intensity of x-ray photons at each position

Disaccharide: A combination of two simple sugars. Example—Glucose + fructose = sucrose.

Disclosing agents: Agents which color dental plaque so that an individual can clearly see areas of plaque in the mouth, used during patient education.

Disclosing tablet: A tablet that is chewed to mix with saliva and then swished around the mouth to disclose (by red and purple colors) the presence and location of dental plaque on the teeth.

Distal: Away from the midline.

DNA: Deoxyribonucleic acid (DNA) is a nucleic acid that contains the genetic instructions used in the development and functioning of all known living organisms.

DNA repair: Refers to a collection of processes by which a cell identifies and corrects damage to the DNA molecules that encode its genome.

Dysgeusia: The distortion or decrease of the sense of taste.

Dysthymia: A mood disorder that falls within the depression spectrum.

E

Early and Periodic Screening, Diagnosis and Treatment (EPDST): A federal program that mandates that medical and dental services be provided to children from low income families.

Early childhood caries: Usually caused by an infant taking milk by bottle as nourishment when hungry, and then retaining the nipple and the milk in the mouth during "sleep time." Can also be caused by "demand" breastfeeding. Also called *baby bottle decay*.

Ecchymoses: Blotchy areas of hemorrhage in the skin.

Ecologic niche: The relational position of a species or population in its ecosystem.

Ectodermal dysplasias: Not a single disorder, but a group of syndromes all deriving from abnormalities of the ectodermal structures.

Edema: Swelling and inflammation.

Edentulism: Without teeth.

Efficacy: Having the ability to produce a desired effect.

Elderly: Young elderly, from 65 to 74 years of age; mid-old, 75 to 84; and 85 > oldest old.

Electrocardiogram: A measurement of the electrical activity of the heart as a diagnostic measure.

Electronic periodontal probes: Electronic probes attached to a computer that automatically triggers a measurement of pocket depth when a given pressure on the bottom of the sulcus is encountered.

Embrasure: The inter-proximal space between two adjacent teeth. Classified as class 1 embrasures that occurs when a soft tissue papilla fills the entire space, type 3 when the papilla is missing, and type 2, intermediate.

Enamaloplasty: Removing demineralized areas of tooth structure and etching and then placing dental sealant material to prevent further dental decay.

Enamel maturation: A period of one or two years after eruption during which time the enamel becomes "fully" mineralized (matured).

Enamel spindles: Short, linear defects, found at the dentinoenamel junction (DEJ) and extend into the enamel, often being more prevelant at the cusp tips.

Endodontics: The treatment of diseased root canals.

Endogenous origin: Arising from within.

Endoscope: A small probe-like videocamera for examining areas that is not readily available, for visual examination—for example, intranasal examination, colonoscopy, intraoral dental examination, etc.

Endosseous implants: Endosseous means that this type of implant is actually placed in a hole drilled in the bone and are then allowed to integrate.

Endothelial cells: The cells lining blood vessels.

End-tuft brush: Small brush head addresses special maintenance concerns including orthodontic bands, implants, and other hard-to-reach areas.

Epidemiological survey: A controlled study of the origin, presence, extent or consequences of a condition or disease.

Epilepsy: A common chronic neurological disorder that is characterized by recurrent unprovoked seizures.

Epithelial attachment: The junctional epithelial cells that attach the crevicular epithelium to the tooth.

Epithelial dysplasia: A disorder of differentiation of epithelial cells which may regress, remain stable, or progress to invasive carcinoma.

Eruptive period, pre-: Before eruption. It is a period during which teeth are developing.

Eruptive period, post-: A short, indefinite period after eruption.

Erythroplakia: Red lesions that are considered premalignant.

Erythroleukoplakia: Red and white or "speckled" lesions that are considered premalignant.

Essential oil: Any concentrated, hydrophobic liquid containing volatile aroma compounds from plants, which are called aromatic herbs or aromatic plants.

Etchant: Phosphoric acid that is used to etch the tooth surface to provide more surface area that in turn enhances retention of sealants.

Etiologic agent: Etiologic agents are those microorganisms and microbial toxins that cause disease in humans and include bacteria, bacterial toxins, viruses, fungi, rickettsiae, protozoans, and parasites.

Etiology: The cause of a disease.

Evidence-based decisions: The basing of decisions on verified research evidence that certain signs or symptoms are predictive of certain outcomes. For instance, the finding of a greater number of mutans streptococci poses a greater risk for future caries development than does a low count.

Evidence-based principles: Practice that is based on scientifically sound theories.

Exfoliate: The natural loss of primary teeth.

Exfoliative cytology: Involves the microscopic examination of cells obtained from tissues.

Excisional biopsy: A procedure for complete removal of a lump or abnormal area from the skin or other part of the body.

Exocrine glands: Opposite to endocrine glands which secrete their products (hormones) directly into the bloodstream (ductless glands) or release hormones (paracrines) affect only target cell nearby the release site.

Exodontia: Extraction is the term given to a tooth extraction.

Exodontics: The extraction of teeth.

Extra-alveolar time: The time a tooth spends outside of tooth socket such as during dental trauma and subsequent treatment.

Extracellular: Outside of the cell.

Extrinsic stain: A stain that is on the outside of the tooth surface that can be removed.

Extruded teeth: Movement of a tooth in an occlusal or incisal direction.

F

Facial: Anatomical term inferring to on or near the facial area.

Facultative aerobic and anaerobic bacteria: Bacteria that can survive in the presence, or absence of oxygen, respectively.

Filaments: The material that comprise toothbrush bristles.

Filiform: Thin, long papillae "V"-shaped cones that do not contain taste buds but are the most numerous on the tongue.

Fimbria: Small microscopic projections from a bacterial cell wall.

Fine-needle aspiration biopsy: Diagnostic procedure sometimes used to investigate superficial (just under the skin) lumps or masses.

Fissured tongue: A benign condition characterized by deep grooves (fissures) in the dorsum of the tongue.

Fistula: A tissue connection between a subsurface infected area and the surface of a mucosal membrane or skin.

Flap surgery (periodontal diseases):   The removal of a sufficient circumferential portion of the marginal gingival to lessen pocket depth and open the subgingival area to self-care preventive procedures.

Fluoridation: The addition of fluoride to public drinking water, most commonly called community water fluoridation.

Fluoride diffusion effect: Also referred to as a "halo effect." It is the caries reduction experienced by individuals not living in a water fluoridated area, but getting its benefits by eating and drinking food processed in an area with optimum water fluoride content. Also, the term applies to those who commute between fluoridated and nonfluoridated communities.

Fluoride mouthrinses: Mouthrinses that contain fluoride.

Fluoride varnish: A varnish material that contains fluoride and is used to treat hypersensitivity or to prevent decay or aid in remineralization of decay in smooth surfaces.

Fluorosis: Cosmetic deviation of enamel in development because of an excessive intake of fluoride during the development periods of the primary and the permanent teeth. Depending on amount of intake, the cosmetic effect ranges from mild veining to a severe brown coloration with a pitting of the enamel.

Fones method: A circular toothbrushing method in which the teeth are in centric occlusion, developed by the founder of dental hygiene, Dr. Alfred C. Fones.

Fossa: A depression or hollow, in general, in a bone.

Frank lesion: Same as cavitated or overt caries lesion.

Free marginal groove: The margin of the free gingival.

Fructose: A simple reducing sugar (monosaccharide) found in many foods.

Functional dentition: Dentition which functions properly.

Fungiform papilla: Mushroom shaped papillae (projections) on the tongue.

Furcation: The area of the tooth where the roots (of multirooted teeth) are joined.

Furcation areas: The space between multi-rooted posterior teeth.

G

Gag reflex: A reflex to a tendency to vomit. Often encountered when patient irritate the posterior tongue or palatal area when cleaning the teeth. Also can occur with an obnoxious taste or with some cases of pregnancy.

Gene polymorphisms: Polymorphism is a genetic variant that appears in at least 1% of a population.

Genes: A locatable region of genomic sequence, corresponding to a unit of inheritance, which is associated with regulatory regions, transcribed regions and/or other functional sequence regions.

Genome: The whole hereditary information which is encoded in the DNA (or, for some viruses, RNA).

Genomics: The study of an organism's entire genome.

Gestational diabetes: Diabetes acquired during pregancy.

Gingival crevicular fluid: Fluid that arises from the connective tissue beneath the gingival sulcus that slowly flows through the gingival crevice. Its purpose is to flush debris from the sulcus, and carry defense agents into the oral cavity.

Gingival fibers: The fibers of the gingiva.

Gingival recession: Areas of recession of the gingival which expose the root surface.

Gingival sulcus: Around each tooth there is a collar of approximately 3 millimeters on depth of soft tissue.

Gingivitis: Inflammation and infection of the gingiva caused by dental plaque.

Glass ionomer: A hard plastic with fine incorporated glass powder to resist abrasion. Used for restorations and tried as a sealant substitute.

Glaucoma: An increased intraocular pressure that, unless treated, can lead to blindness.

Glucans: A polysaccharide of D-glucose monomers linked by glycosidic bonds.

Glucosyltransferase: A type of Glycosyltransferase which enable the transfer of glucose.

Goal orientation: An objective than an individual has decided to attain; it may be only a temporary short-term goal or a long-term goal; it may be a temporary short-term goal that is powerful only until attained.

Granulocytes: A category of white blood cells characterised by the presence of granules in their cytoplasm.

Granulomas: A nodule consisting mainly of epithelioid macrophages and other inflammatory and immune cells as well as extracellular matrix.

Growth regulation: The regulation of growth.

Guideline: An established and agreed upon method for examining, treating, preventing and/or monitoring a disease.

H

Halitosis: Another term for bad breath.

Health: A state of complete physical, mental, spiritual, emotional and social well being.

Health disparities: Pertaining to populations within society that have significant rates of disease or health.

Health education: The teaching of health behaviors that bring an individual to a state of health awareness.

Health promotion: The informing and motivating of people to adopt health behaviors.

Hematopoietic cell transplantation: The intravenous infusion of autologous or allogeneic stem cells collected from bone marrow, peripheral blood, or umbilical cord blood to reestablish hematopoietic function in patients with damaged or defective bone marrow or immune systems.

Hemidesmosomes: Small stud- or rivet-like structures on the inner basal surface of keratinocytes in the epidermis of skin.

Hemophilia: A rare inherited bleeding disorder that the blood does not clot normally.

Histologic: The study of the microscopic anatomy of cells and tissues.

HIV: Human immunodeficiency virus, usually a predecessor of AIDS.

Homeostasis: Occurs when the body is in normal metabolic balance. Reference to caries: a balance between demineralization and remineralization.

Hopewood House: An orphanage in Australia that demonstrated that when children were raised on a good diet, caries was minimal. It also proved that once the children left Hopewood House and its diet, caries again became a problem, proving that the acquired low caries status of the orphanage was not permanent.

Human Genome Project: Probably the greatest health research program of the 20th century. This has been a worldwide research effort to decipher "the molecule of life"—desoxynucleic acid.

Human papillomavirus: A common sexually transmitted disease that is linked to oral cancer.

Humectants: Give toothpaste its texture as well as retain moisture so that toothpaste does not dry out.

Humeral body defenses: Genetic defense factors found in body fluids.

Hydrogen peroxide: A commonly used tooth bleaching agent.

Hydrophobicity: A repellent to water.

Hydroxyapatite: The basic building crystal in the formation of enamel rods. It is composed of mainly calcium, phosphate and hydroxyl, but also includes many other trace quantities of up to 30 or 40 elements.

Hyper-: Above normal.

Hypersensitivity: Areas of tooth sensitivity, commonly occurs when roots are exposed.

Hypertension: A medical condition in which the blood pressure is chronically elevated.

Hypo-: Below normal.

Hypoglycemic shock: A decrease in the level of blood glucose (in diabetes mellitus) that can be accompanied by a variety of symptoms from confusion to coma and death.

Hypomineralization: An area of the enamel that is not mineralized.

Hypothyroidism: A condition in which the body lacks sufficient thyroid hormone.

I

Iatrogenic disease: Disease which is caused by a health provider or health care service.

Idiopathic: An adjective used primarily in medicine meaning arising spontaneously or from an obscure or unknown cause.

Immune response: Any time a foreign substance penetrates the body's defenses, there is a cellular reaction (immune response) to seek out the antigen (foreign substance) and to neutralize or eliminate it.

Immunity: A state of having sufficient biological defenses to avoid infection or disease.

Immunization: The injection, or ingestion of an antigen into the body to cause an enhancement of the body's capability to resist disease.

Immunoglobulins: Play an essential role in the body's immune system.

Implant: A metallic "root" (the implant) that is surgically inserted into the alveolus in the space of a missing tooth. Following healing, a crown is later constructed on the "root."

Incidence: The number of newly diagnosed cases during a specific time period.

Incipient caries lesion: A pre-caries lesion that exists before cavitation. Seen on the enamel as a "white spot." It can be remineralized.

Incisional biopsy: A biopsy in which only a sample of the suspicious tissue is removed for testing.

Infection: The detrimental colonization of a host organism by a foreign species.

Informed patient consent: Before any treatment is commenced, the patient is informed verbally, or in writing of all primary and treatment options, costs and expected results.

Intense sweetener: Considered noncaloric because of their small bulk needed to deliver desired sweetness.

Interdental brushes: Toothbrushes specifically designed for removal of plaque in the interdental area.

Interdental papillae: The gingival peak between closely adjacent teeth.

Interproximal: The area between the mesial and distal surfaces of two adjacent teeth.

Intrinsic stain: A stain that was incorporated in the enamel during development or trauma and which cannot be removed without damage to the enamel.

Intrinsic stains: Tooth stains that are inside or intrinsic to the tooth.

Intruded teeth: A tooth that is "pushed" into the bone from trauma.

Iron deficiency anemia: Anemia caused by too little iron.

Irrigator: A small device containing a reservoir for water that is pumped at relatively low velocity to cleanse the interproximal spaces or loosening plaque.

Ischemia: Lack of sufficient blood to a part.

K

Kaposi's Sarcoma: An oral malignancy linked to HIV infection.

Keratin: A family of fibrous structural proteins.

Kyphosis: A curvature of the upper spine.

L

Labial: Of or pertaining to the area of the lips.

Lactobacilli: An acidogenic bacterial species that is an etiologic microorganism seen at the later stages of the incipient caries lesion.

Lamina dura: The part of the alveolar bone that lines the socket is a thin layer of dense cortical bone.

Leukoplakia: A white lesion found that is considered premalignant.

Lichen planus: A disorder of the skin and mucous membranes resulting in inflammation, itching, and distinctive skin lesions.

Life span: The maximum of life potentially possible, now considered 120 years-of-age.

Lingual: Anatomical term pertaining to the tongue.

Loss of attachment: Loss of periodontal attachment (LOA) of the tooth to the tooth socket such as in pocketing, bone loss and/or recession.

Lucency: (As applied to dental radiographs), a darker area on the x-ray indicating demineralization (caries) or the enamel, dentin or cementum.

Luxation: The dislocation or displacement of a tooth.

Lysozyme: An antibacterial enzyme found in the saliva and other fluids of the body.

M

Macroglossia: Enlarged tongue.

Malnutrition: Not receiving adequate nutrition.

Malodor, oral: A term used for halitosis or bad breath.

Manifestations: An obvious indication or specific evidence that a disease is present such as a symptom.

Marginal gingival: The margin of the gingiva.

Mastication: Occluding such as when chewing.

Materia alba: Accumulation or aggregation of microorganisms, desquamated epithelial cells, blood cells and food debris loosely adherent to surfaces of plaques, teeth, gingiva or dental appliances.

Maxillofacial surgeon: A dental specialist, specifically referred to as an oral surgeon.

Mechanical plaque control: The use of toothbrushes, dental floss, and irrigators to aid in plaque removal.

Medicament: An agent such as medicine or chemotherapeutic used to treat or prevent a disease or condition.

Menopause: The complete cessation of the female reproductive system.

Mesial: Anatomical term, toward the midline.

Methamphetamine: A street drug that when used frequently can result in "meth mouth."

Milk fluoridation: The addition of fluoride to milk to help reduce dental decay in a population.

Mineralized: The process where a substance is converted from an organic substance to an inorganic substance.

Monomer: A liquid plastic that when mixed with a catalyst, polymerizes to a hard plastic (polymer); or a liquid plastic containing a catalyst that is activated with a light (light cured).

Monosaccharide: A simple sugar, such as, fructose, and glucose.

Morbidity: A ratio of sick to a given number of persons per unit time. Example 12: 100,000/year.

Mortality: The number of deaths from a given cause in a population per unit time. Example: 1: 1000 per year.

Motivation: An inner drive of an individual to attain a self-designated goal.

Mucogingival junction: The junction of the mucosa and the attached gingiva.

Mucosal: Pertaining to the mucosa.

Mucositis: An inflammation of a mucous membrane.

Multifactorial disease process: The process whereas as several factors must coalesce in order to cause a disease.

Multiple fluoride therapy: The use of multiple forms of fluoride, such as fluoride toothpaste, fluoride mouthrinse and professional fluoride gels twice a year, to reduce dental decay.

Mutans streptococci: A causative cariogenic organism linked to the early stages of an incipient caries lesion.

MyPyramid: Used to guide an individual in healthy nutritional practices.

N

Neoplasm: Refers to a new growth and describes a cellular proliferation that has exceeded normal growth.

Nitrosamines: Cancer-causing agents found in tobacco products.

Noncarcinogenic: Not a risk factor of cancer.

Noninvasive care: Care that can be administered without damage to the body tissues.

Noninvasive caries: The beginning stages of demineralization.

O

Obturator: A specialized maxillary prosthesis constructed to facilitate speech and eating by a cleft palate individual, as well as to prevent food from entering the nasal cavity.

Occlusal surface: Each posterior tooth has five surfaces, mesial, distal, lingual, buccal and occlusal; the occlusal surface is the biting surface of the posterior teeth.

Octocalcium phosphate: The first mineral laid down for enamel formation before its conversion to hydroxyapatite.

Operant conditioning: The use of consequences to modify the occurrence and form of behavior.

Opportunistic infections: An infection caused by pathogens that usually do not cause disease in a healthy immune system.

Oral cancer: A variety of malignant neoplasms that occur in the mouth and oropharynx.

Oral hairy leukoplakia: A pathology of the associated with Epstein-Barr virus (EBV) and it occurs mostly in people with HIV.

Oral-health self-care: Any action taken by an individual to maintain optimum oral health, including carrying out daily mechanical and chemical plaque control regimens as well as complying with recommendations by the dentist or dental hygienist.

Oral lichen planus: A chronic dermatologic disease that frequently manifests in lesions of the oral mucosa.

Oropharynx: The entire are from the base of the tongue, pharyngeal wall, tonsillar fossae, and soft palate.

Oscillation movement: The movement of a powered toothbrush.

Osteoporosis: A pathology of bone marked with fragility and porosity.

OTC drugs: Drugs sold over-the-counter without a prescription.

Overt caries lesion: A cavity where the undermined enamel has broken down into a cavity, a process called cavitation. Remineralization is not a possibility (at least at this point in time, 2002).

P

Papillae: 1. The triangular soft tissue that fills the interproximal embrasures. 2. The specialized projections from the surface of the tongue that allow reception of different taste sensations.

Passive smoking: Relates to the tobacco smoke inhaled by family members or bystanders who breathe secondhand smoke.

Pasteurization: The heating of a product (usually milk) to a given temperature (often 60° C) for a given time (30 minutes) in order to kill pathogenic bacteria, and extend the time before other bacteria become pathogenic.

Peri-implantitis: Following the placement of an implant, the same meticulous self-care is necessary as with natural teeth. When this care does not materialize, the same infection and apical migration occurs to the epithelial attachment as occurs with periodontitis.

Periodontal disease indicators: Signs and symptoms that usually precede the onset of periodontal disease. Also called "markers."

Periodontal pocket: An abnormal deepening of the gingival sulcus marked by an accompanying apical migration of the epithelial attachment.

Periodontium: The four anatomical structures that support the teeth including the gingiva, periodontal ligament, cementum and alveolar bone.

Permiability (of teeth): The ability of fluids to pass from the surface to the pulp and vice versa.

Phagocytosis: The envelopment and destruction of an antigen by one of the body defense cells.

Pit-and-fissure caries: Caries located in the pit and fissure surfaces of the tooth.

Plaque index: O'Leary's index charts the location of the location of plaque on the teeth. The index of Silness and Löe is much the same with the exception that the status of the adjoining index is also recorded.

Polymerization: The reaction that occurs when the liquid resin sealant, which is a monomer, is met with a catalyst. The chemical bond repeatedly forms, increasing in number and complexity which is polymerization and results in a harded resin sealant.

Polyol (alcohol sugar): Sweeteners that have an alcohol grouping to each carbon atom of the polyol. Referred to as sugar alcohols, such as sorbitol, mannitol, and xylitol.

Polypharmacy: Excessive multiple useage of medications often seen with senior citizens.

Pontic: The artificial teeth or tooth that are (is) part of the bridge between the abutment teeth.

Potassium nitrate: A commonly used OTC desensitizing agent.

Potassium oxylate: A commonly used OTC desensitizing agent.

Prediction: A clinical decision as to the outcome of a disease process based on professional judgement and evidence-based information.

Predictive value, negative: Probability that the subject will not develop disease.

Predictive value, positive: Probability that the subject will develop disease.

Pregnancy gingivitis: Gingivitis that may occur and can be exacerbated during pregnancy.

Prevalence: The number of cases of a disease that are present in a particular population at a given time.

Primary prevention: Employs strategies and agents to forestall the onset of disease, reverse the progress of disease or arrest the disease process before secondary preventive treatment becomes necessary and can be termed dental hygiene.

Primary preventive dentistry: The preventive aspects of the dental hygiene sciences; emphasizes the use of diagnostic and therapeutic modalities to prevent disease.

Prognosis: A synonym for "prediction."

Proliferation: The multiplication of bacteria.

Prophylaxis: A cleaning, including a debridement and polishing of the hard concretions, plaque and food particles (material alba) from the tooth surfaces.

Prosthesis: An artificial replacement for a lost body part such as a bridge or dentures.

PSR (Periodontal Screening and Recording System): Similar to the CPITN, with the exception that it offers suggested treatment to match each level of severity.

Pulpal necrosis: Necrosis of the pulp that does not respond to stimulation.

Punch biopsy: A type of biopsy.

Pyrophosphates: Crystal growth inhibitors that reduce the amount of calculus formed.

R

Radiation caries: The rampant caries that often occurs because of the destruction of the oral salivary glands that have been in the x-ray beam as a part of cancer treatment.

Refractory disease: A disease that does not respond to accepted treatment therapies.

Reliability: The degree of stability exhibitied when a measurement is repeated under identical conditions.

Remineralization: The replacement of tooth mineral (hydroxyapatite) that has been lost by demineralization. The minerals needed for the remineralization are derived from the saliva (or from man-made products).

Reparative dentin: Morphologically irregular dentin formed in response to an irritant, such as caries, disease, or drilling to prepare a cavity for filling.

Risk: The probability that a harmful or unwanted event will occur.

Risk assessment: A professional judgement on an individual's susceptibility or resistance to disease, based on evidence-based information.

Risk factor: An evidence-based sign, test, or circumstance reliably associated with the onset or progression of a disease process.

Root caries: Caries located on the root (cementum) of a tooth, which frequently increases with age due to increased gingival recession, or exposure of root surfaces.

Root resorption: The resorption of root in to the alveolar bone.

Root-surface caries: Caries which occur on the root surface.

Rubber tip stimulators: Aids used to remove plaque.

S

Saccharin: A nonnutritive and noncariogenic artificial sweetener.

Saliva substitutes: Substitutes for saliva used in individuals with xerostomia.

Salt fluoridation: The addition of fluoride to salt in order to reduce dental decay in a population.

Sclerotic dentin: Dentin that has become translucent due to calcification of the dentinal tubules as a result of injury or normal aging.

Screening tests: A rapid examination to identify healthy from unhealthy individuals, and the characteristics that separate them.

Secondary caries: Caries that develop around a restoration.

Secondary prevention: Employs routine treatment methods to terminate a disease process and/or restore tissues to as near normal as possible and can be termed restorative care.

Sequelae: A pathological condition resulting from a disease, injury, or other trauma.

Sharpey's fibers: A matrix of connective tissue consisting of bundles of strong collagenous fibres connecting periosteum to bone.

Sialogogues: A medicine or substance that stimulates the flow of saliva.

Sialoliths: Calculi occurring in a salivary gland.

Sialorrhea: Drooling or excessive salivation.

Silicas: Agents used in toothpastes.

Smooth-surface caries: Carious lesions found on the smooth surfaces of the tooth.

Snyder test: A colorometric test used to estimate the relative acidogenic potential of salivary lactobacilli.

Social cognitive theory: A theory which focuses on an individual's knowledge acquisition can be directly related to observing others within the context of social interactions, experiences, and outside media influences.

Social learning theory: A theory which focuses on the learning that occurs within a social context.

Sodium citrate: A commonly used OTC desensitizing agent.

Sodium fluoride (NaF): A type of fluoride used in preventive agents.

Sodium lauryl sulfate: A detergent and surfactant found in toothpastes.

Sodium monofluorophosphate: A type of fluoride used in preventive agents.

Soft palate: An anatomical landmark directly behind the hard palate.

Soft ties: Cloth or leather straps use to immobilize uncontrollable body parts resulting from imperfect neuromuscular control.

Sorbitol: A sugar alcohol that occurs in many fruits and berries.

"Spit" tobacco: A contemptuous term for the habit associated with either chewing tobacco or use of snuff.

Staging system: A system of grading (histological subtype) and staging (clinical extent) of the tumor.

Stannous: Meaning, tin.

Stannous fluoride: A type of fluoride used in preventive agents.

Stem cells: Cells found in most multi-cellular organisms that are characterized by the ability to renew themselves through mitotic cell division and differentiating into a diverse range of specialized cell types.

Stephan curve: The relationship between acid levels (pH) at the tooth surface and time following consumption of sugar.

Stillman method: A toothbrushing method which focuses on gingival stimulation.

Stomatitis: Inflammation of the mucous lining of any of the structures in the mouth, which may involve the cheeks, gums, tongue, lips, throat, and roof or floor of the mouth.

Striae of Retzius: Incremental growth lines seen in enamel and are results of enamel's development.

Strontium chloride: A commonly used OTC desensitizing agent.

Study model: A model made of dental stone which replicates the dentition.

Subgingival: Below the gingival margin.

Subgingival and supra-gingival plaque: The plaque that is located on the tooth below, and above the gingiva, respectively.

Subluxated: Having the tooth loosened and possibly malpositioned, but retained in the jaw such as during a trauma.

Substance abuse: Abuse of a substance such as drugs or alcohol.

Substance dependence: Being dependent upon a substance such as drugs or alcohol.

Substantivity: Pertaining to the capacity of an oral antimicrobial agent to continue its therapeutic activity for a prolonged period of time.

Subsurface pellicle: Below the surface acquired pellicle.

Sucrose: A nutritive sweetener and the most commonly used tabletop sweetener, often referred to as sugar.

Sugar alcohols: Commonly used to replace sugar in food.

Sugar discipline: Restricting sugar intake as to decrease chances of decay.

Sugar substitutes: Sweetening agents that are substituted for sugar.

Sulcular epithelium: Epithelium of the sulcus.

Suppuration: Commonly referred to as a pus, a purulent discharge from an infected area.

Supragingival: Above the gingival margin.

Sweeteners: Agents used to sweeten food, gum or toothpastes.

Symbiosis (bacterial): Two or more species of bacteria that mutually support one another.

Symptom: An abnormal function or feeling which is noticed by a patient, indicating the presence of disease.

Synergistic: Systems working together.

Systemic conditions: Conditions that involve many organs or the whole body.

Systemic diseases: Diseases that involve many organs or the whole body.

Systemic fluoride: Systemic fluorides are those that are ingested into the body and become incorporated into forming tooth structures.

T

Tachycardia: Rapid beating of the heart.

Target population: A specific population that is grouped together because of one or more similarities such as age, gender, ethnicity, living situation, etc.

Taste buds: Small structures on the upper surface of the tongue, soft palate, and epiglottis that provide information about the taste of food and drink.

Tertiary prevention: Employs measures necessary to replace lost tissues and rehabilitation.

Theory of reasoned action: A theory that suggests that a person's behavioral intention depends on the person's attitude about the behavior and subjective norms.

Therapeutic: Having healing powers.

Thickening agents: Agents used to stabilize the toothpaste.

Thixotropic: A thick, viscous gel.

Tobacco cessation programs: Programs aimed at helping smokers or tobacco chewers quit.

Toothbrush abrasion: Abrasion of the tooth surface caused by brushing.

Topical fluoride: Applying fluoride to teeth already present in the mouth making them more resistant to decay.

Triclosan: A broad-spectrum antibacterial agent used in dental products.

Trismus: (As applied to dentistry). Difficulty in opening the mouth due to nerve involvement, pain and/or infection of the masticatory muscles.

V

Vaccine: The introduction of beneficial agent into the body to enhance the capability of the immune system to challenge and/or eliminate and repair the damage caused by a foreign antigen.

Validity: The reproducible accuracy of a test as a predictive measure.

Value: A strongly held belief of an individual, based on an unknown number of positive or negative concepts, that in turn are based on an unknown number of positive or negative facts.

Vasculitis: Inflammation of blood vessels resulting in the leakage of fluid and the migration of defense cells through the capillary walls.

Vasoconstriction: The narrowing of the blood vessels resulting from contracting of the muscular wall of the vessels.

Vermilion border: The border between the skin of the face and the lip.

Vipeholm: A study conducted in a mental institution in Vipeholm, Sweden. The clients were fed cariogenic snacks at different frequencies, at mealtime, between meals, etc. to see which situation was the most cariogenic.

Virulence: Refers to the degree of pathogenicity of a microbe.

W

"White spots": A white translucent area on the enamel indicating that there is localized demineralization of the enamel and possibly extending as far as the underlying dentin.

Whitlockite: A rare mineral, a form of calcium phosphate.

X

Xerostomia: Dry mouth. A lower than normal secretion of saliva (1 ml per minute). A symptom with Sjögren's disease, also following exposure of the salivary glands to cancer radiation and a common side effect to many types of medication.

Xylitol: A sugar alcohol that is used as a flavoring agent that is both non-cariogenic and anticariogenic.

Index

abrasiveness of dentifrices, 146
  damage done by, 147
  polishing agents and, 146–147
  testing, 146–147
  toothbrush, 147
abutment teeth, 106
Academy of General Dentistry, 198
Academy of Sports Dentistry, 389
acesulfame-K, 327
acid cleansers, 199
acidogenesis, 22, 30
acidogenic bacteria, 35–36
acquired pellicle, 17, 113
actinic cheilitis, 73–74
Actinobacillus, 17, 57, 59, 113
Actinomyces, 17, 54, 400
actinomycetes, 17, 18, 19, 20
Active Ageing: A Policy Framework (WHO),
  463
active immunity, 398–399
ADA Guide to Dental Therapeutics, 380
Addis, William, 122
adhesions, 18
adjunct primary treatment, 62
Administration for Children and Families
  (ACF), 411
Administration on Aging (AoA), 412
adsorption, 16n
adult dental care. *See also* women's oral health
  adolescence to young adulthood, 452, 457
  caries, 453–455
  common oral manifestations, 453
  early adulthood, 452, 457–458
  fluoride for, 459
  introduction to, 452
  mature adulthood, 452–453, 458–460
  oral and pharyngeal cancer, 455–456
  periodontal diseases, 455, 456
advantages of, 430
aerosol-generating procedures, 154
African Americans, oral cancer in, 71–72,
  73, 94, 456
Agency for Healthcare Research and Quality
  (AHRQ), 412
Agency for Toxic Substances and Disease
  Registry (ATSDR), 412
ageusia, 92
AIDS. *See* HIV/AIDS
Alaskan Natives, 412, 418
alcoholism, 72–73, 77, 485

Alcohol Use Disorders Identification Test
  (AUDIT), 77
algae, 15
alimentary tract, 15
alitame, 328
alkaline hypochlorite, 198–199
alkaline peroxide, 198
alternative restorative technique (ART), 276
Aluminum Company of America, 215
alveolar bone, 49, 51–52, 106
alveolar crest, 50, 52
alveolar crest fibers, 52
alveolar fracture, 102
alveolar mucosa, 51–52
alveolar process, 50, 100
alveologingival fibers, 51
alveolus, 100
Alzheimer's disease, 467, 468, 470, 499
amalgams, 40
ameloblasts, 16, 38
amelogenesis, 145
American Academy of Otolaryngology, 93
American Academy of Pediatric Dentistry,
  430
American Academy of Pediatrics (AAP),
  151, 390, 392
American Academy of Periodontology
  (AAP), 123, 186–187, 188, 189, 369
American Academy of Periodontology Web
  site, 59
American Association of Oral and
  Maxillofacial Surgeons, 93, 390
American Association of Orthodontists, 187,
  390
American Association of Poison Control
  (AAPC), 151
American Association of Public Health
  Dentistry (AAPHD), 413
American Cancer Association, 380
American Cancer Society (ACS), 71, 72, 73,
  78–79, 93, 415
American Dental Association (ADA), 93,
  139–140
  ADA Guide to Dental Therapeutics, 380
  alcohol-containing mouthrinses and,
    151–152
  CDT 2007–2008, 333
  chemotherapeutic agents, reviews of, 143
  Council on Dental Therapeutics, 148–149,
    282

Council on Scientific Affairs (CSA), 143,
    144, 151
  dental public health recognized by, 408
  denture cleaning recommendations, 198
  fluoridation definition, 213
  fluoride approved by, 223–224
  fluoride dentifrices accepted by, 148–149
  on fluorosis risks in infants, 227–228
  Listerine Antiseptic approved by, 153
  mouthguard use, promotion of, 388, 390
  Seal of Acceptance, 144, 149, 151, 224
American Dental Education Association, 78
American Dental Hygienists' Association,
  379–380, 390
American Dietetic Association, 321, 427
American Heart Association (AHA), 334
American Indians, 412, 418
American Lung Association, 380
American Public Health Association
  (APHA), 413
American Water Works Association
  (AWWA), 232
  Water Fluoridation Principles and
    Practices, 233
amorphous calcium phosphate (ACP), 41,
  155
amylase, 115
anaerobic glycolysis, 22
anaerobic species, gram-negative, 20
angiogenesis
ankylosis, 102
anorexia nervosa, 305
antigen I/II, 399
antimicrobials, 7
  mouthwash, 199
  toothpicks impregnated by, 180, 181
  used in irrigation, 187–188
antimicrobial therapy, 15
apex, 10
apexification, 104
aphthous-like ulcers, 482, 483
apical fibers, 53
apical migration, 10
apical tooth area, 10, 17
apices, 101
Aquafresh, 145
Aquafresh Whitening with Tartar Protection
  Toothpaste, 150
Arm & Hammer Advance White dentifrice,
  145

Arm & Hammer Dental Care, 155
Arnold, Heloise A., 463
arthritis, 477
articulating paper, 282
ascorbic acid, 299
aspartame, 327
Asperger niger, 191
Association of Local and County Dental
    Health Officers, 415
Association of State and Territorial Dental
    Directors (ASTDD), 413, 414
asthma, 484
attachment apparatus, 100
attachment loss, 48
autism, 497
autopolymerization, 275
avulsion, 100–101

Baby Boomer generation, 463, 471, 473
"baby bottle tooth decay," 305
bacteremias, 173, 189
bacteria. *See also* mutans streptococci (MS)
    acidogenic, 35–36
    adhesion, 18–19, 37
    areas of accumulation, 17
    cariogenic, 35–36
    colonization of, 15–17
    lactobacilli (LB), 37, 113, 301
    mastication of food, 17
    microbial species, 54
    mineralized, 15
    mixed-species, behavior of, 15
    in plaque, 19–20
bacterial biofilm, 7, 14–15
bacterial endocarditis, 173
bacteriocins, 17
Bacteroides, 456
baking-soda toothpaste, 148
Bandura, Albert, 354, 439–440
basal lamina, 16
Basic Screening Survey (BSS), 414
basophils, 114
bass toothbrushing method, 1131
B cells, 113
B-complex vitamins, 299
Behavioral Risk Factor Surveillance System
    (BRFSS), 414
beta-defensin peptides, 115
bidirectional synergism, 49
binge-eating disorder, 305
biochemical reaction, 15
biopsy types, 80, 82
    brush, 80–81
    fine-needle aspiration, 82, 84, 85
    punch, 84, 85
    scalpel (incisional/excisional), 81, 84–85
Biotène Mouthwash, 152–153
bipolar disorder, 480, 496
birth defects, 4
bisphenol A–glycidyl methylacrylate (Bis-
    GMA), 274, 281
bitewing radiograph, 33
Black, G. V., 30, 215
bleach, household, 199
bleeding gums, 62

blindness, 496
body mass index (BMI), 290, 292, 293
bone marrow, 113, 114
bone marrow transplant, 484
Bowen, W. H., 399
brachytherapy, 89
bradycardia, 479
BreathRx, 152
Broxadent, 133
brushite, 23
Brush Test, 81
bruxism, 497, 498
buccal gland, 116
buccal surfaces, 10
bulimia, 186, 305–307, 478
bupropion SR, 376
burning mouth syndrome, 116

CAGE, 77
calcium, 298
    bridging, 18
    carbonate, 146
    fluoride (CaF$_2$), 41
    phosphates, 459
calculus
    alkaline conditions, 23
    anti-calculus dentifrices, 150
    attachment of, 24
    in children, 23
    crystals in, 23
    formation, inhibition of, 24
    as last stage of plaque maturation, 22–24
    mineralization, 22, 23–24, 25
    removal of, 22
    on tooth surfaces of germ-free animals, 24
canaliculi, 38
cancer, 478–479
    candidiasis and, 478
    deaths in elderly, 467
    fluoride for patients, 478–479
    oral (*See* oral cancer)
    pharyngeal, 455–456
Cancer Assessment Committee of the FDA,
    328
Candida albicans, 92, 114, 115, 199–200
candidiasis, 194, 478, 482, 484
Capnocytophaga, 54
carbamide peroxide, 151
carbohydrates, 300–301
carcinogenesis, 73
carcinoma, 68
    in situ, 80
cardiac arrhythmias, 479
cardiovascular disease, 467
caries. *See also* diet and dental caries
    acidogenic bacteria, 35–36
    in adults, 453–455
    bacteria involved in formation of, 323
    cariogenic bacteria, 35–36
    cause of, 9
    in cerebral palsy patients, 498
    cervical, 89
    chewing gum and, 155–156
    as chronic childhood disease, 4
    coronal dentin, 38, 39

cost for treatments, 9
decline of, in Western countries, 300–301
development of, conditions for, 30–31, 33
in Down syndrome patients, 499
Early Childhood Caries (ECC), 305, 355,
    425, 426, 429, 430, 431, 445
in elderly, 458
in fluoride mouthrinse users, 154
genetics and, 402
immunizations for, 399–400
incidence *vs.* prevalence of, 9
incipient lesions of, 7, 10
in infants, 425–427, 429
lactobacilli and, 37
lesions (*See* carious lesions)
in mental retardation patients, 497
as multifactorial disease process, 30–31
mutans streptococci and, 36, 300
noninvasive, 10
pit-and-fissure, 10, 31, 279
plaque as cause of, 14, 40
preventing through oral self-care, 187
as public health problem, 2
rampant, 31
risk assessment form, 32
root (*See* root caries)
saturation and pH, relationship between,
    40–41
secondary/recurrent, 31, 39–40
smooth-surface, 31
S. mutans and, 300, 323, 399, 426–427
sugars and, 300, 321–323
theories of, 30
transmission, 37
cariogenic microorganisms, 30
cariogenic potential indices (CPIs), 302
carious lesions
    areas occurring in, 31
    dental sealants placed over, 282
    incipient lesion (*See* incipient lesion)
    overt/frank, 31
Carmona, Richard, 214
casein phosphopeptide (CPP), 155, 459
cavitation, 22
cellular immunity, 110, 113–114
cellular infiltrate, 58
cementoblasts, 101
cemento–enamel junction, 39
cementum, 9–10, 16, 49, 50, 51, 52, 100
cementum–dentin complex, 39
cementum resorption, 102
Centers for Disease Control and Prevention
    (CDC)
    on arthritis, 477
    Division of Oral Health, 414
    on fluoride achievements, 213
    fluoride labeling recommended by, 227
    fluoride training offered by, 234
    proficiency testing of fluoride
        concentrations, 233
    recommendations to reduce enamel
        fluorosis risk, 230
    on schoolchildren in fluoride-rinse
        programs, 235
    smoking cessation aids offered by, 380

smoking cessation strategies, 381–382
toothpick injuries documented by, 180
Centers for Medicare and Medicaid Services (CMS), 412
Cepacol, 154
cerebral palsy (CP), 497–499
cerebrovascular disease (stroke), 467
cervical tooth area, 10
cetylpyridinium chloride (CPC), 154
Chantix®, 376
Charters toothbrushing technique, 132
chelating agent, 18
chemical activation, 275
chemicoparasitic theory, 30
chemiluminescence, 80, 81
chemotactic signal, 57
chemotherapeutic agents, oral, 143–144. *See also* chewing gum; dentifrices; mouthrinses
Chesebrough-Pond, 145
chewing gum, 142, 154–155
    agents added to, 155–156
    benefits of, 142–143, 155
    safety and efficacy of, 143
    salivary flow and, 186–187
    xylitol-containing, 458–459
child development, 439. *See also* children
    adolescent, 12 to 19 years of age, 444
    culture, 445
    early, 2 to 5 years of age, 440–443
    economics, 445
    Erikson's psychosocial development, 440, 441
    gross motor skills in, 442
    parents' influence on, 444–445
    Pavlov's classical conditioning, 440
    Piaget's cognitive development theory, 439
    school-aged, 6 to 11 years of age, 443
    setting, 445
    Skinner's operant conditioning, 440
    social learning theory, 439–440
    temperament, 444
children. *See also* child development; infants
    alcohol in mouthrinses and, 151–152
    attachment loss in, 48
    calculus in, 23
    caries in, 4, 323, 425–427
    decayed, missing, and filled teeth (DMFT), 323, 327
    dental trauma in, 100, 101, 104
    flossing, 168, 169
    fluoride (*See* fluoride for children)
    gingivitis in, 48, 54, 61
    mutans streptococci in, 36, 37
    oral diseases and disorders in, 4
    packaging and labeling guidelines, 144
    school-based preventative programs, 418
    toothbrushing methods, 123, 129, 131–132, 135
    toothpick usage by, 180
    untreated dental disease results in, 5
child safety caps, 151–152
chlorhexidine, 142, 153, 186, 187, 188
chromosomes, 402

chronic obstructive pulmonary disease (COPD), 484
Church & Dwight Co., Inc., 145
Churchill, H. V., 215
Ciba-Geigy, 150
circular/circumferential fibers, 50
Citizen's Watch for Oral Health, Washington State, 417
Clark Community College, 429–430
clasp brush, 139
Clear Choice, 154
clefting, 171
cleft lip/palate, 4
clinical attachment loss, 175–176
clinical pathology, 10
clinical surveys, 414
Closing the Gap: A National Blueprint for Improving the Health of Individuals with Mental Retardation (Surgeon General), 496
cocaine use, 486
cocci, 19–20
Cochrane Collaboration, 106, 235
Cochrane Library, 107
co-discovery, 166
cold cure, 275
cold testing, 103
Colgate-Palmolive Co., 145, 150
Colgate PreviDent 5,000, 149
Colgate Pro-Health, 148
Colgate Sensitive Maximum Strength Toothpaste, 150
Colgate Tartar Control Plus Whitening Fluoride Toothpaste, 150
Colgate Total, 148, 150
Colgate Total Stripe, 145
collagen synthesis, 298–299
colonization
    disease process, colonizers responsible for, 113
    of mutans streptococci, 37
    oral flora and, 110, 113
    primary colonizers, 37
"Colorado Brown Stain," 215
Columbus Children's Hospital Dental Clinic, 428
Commission on Dental Accreditation (CODA), 496
Commit®, 375
communication, 446, 448
Community Fluorosis Index, 216, 217, 229
community water fluoridation. *See* fluoridation
complement system, 114
composites, 39
    resections, 88
comprehensive neck dissections, 88
computed tomography, 85, 88
concussions, 389, 390
condylar-displacement injuries, 390
congestive heart failure (CHF), 479
Consumer Products Safety Commission, 180
contiguous gingiva, 10
contingency management, 351

Council on Scientific Affairs (CSA), 143
counter-conditioning, 351
craniofacial disorders, 9
Crest Pro-Health, 149
Crest Pro-Health Rinse, 154
Crest Sensitivity Protection Fluoride Toothpaste, 150
Crest Tartar Control, 150
Crest Tartar Control Plus Whitening Fluoride Toothpaste, 150
Crest toothpaste, 148–149
cyclamate, 319, 328
cytokines, 58

deafness, 496
Dean, H. Trendley, 229
"Dean's 21-Cities Study," 216–217
debridement, 62
decayed, missing, and filled teeth (DMFT), 323, 327
deft/DMFT indices, 226
Delta Dental of Tennessee, 389
deltopectoral flaps, 90
dementia, 468, 499
demineralization, 10
    carious lesions, role in development of, 31, 33, 34
    defined, 41, 111
    depth of, 41
    diet and, 299
    enamel and, 111–112
    fluoridation and, 220, 222–223
    fluoride exposure, 41
    fluoride's influence on, 112
    fluoride level in saliva and, 187
    pH and, 40–41
Dental Cosmos, 215
dental floss. *See also* flossing
    agents impregnated into, 168–169
    automated flossers, 176–177
    evaluation criteria, 171
    gauze strip, 184–185
    holder, 173–174
    knitting yarn, white, 184
    pipe cleaners, 184
    threader, 174–175
    types and brand differences of, 167–169
dental hygiene care
    assessment, 333
        AHA blood pressure levels, 334
        dental/periodontal examination, 334
        diagnostic radiographs, 338
        extraoral/intraoral examination, 334
        medical/dental history, 334
        self-care examination, 338
        vital signs, 334
    creation of, 3
    diagnosis, 338–340
    evaluation, 343
    implementation, 340, 343
    introduction to, 333
    planning, 340, 341–342
    as primary preventive care, 6
    therapeutic treatment included in, 342
    treatment options, sample, 343–345

dental hygiene care assessment, 333
  AHA blood pressure levels, 334
  dental/periodontal examination, 334
  diagnostic radiographs, 338
  extraoral/intraoral examination, 334
  medical/dental history, 334
  self-care examination, 338
  vital signs, 334
dental plaque. *See* plaque
Dental Plaque Subcommittee of the Non
      Prescription Drugs Advisory
      Committee (NDAC), 144
dental prosthetics, 17
dental public health, 408
  approaches to, 408–409
    comparison of, 409
    individual rights and social protection,
      410
    population *vs.* individual, 409
    reach *vs.* intensity, 409–410
  assessment, 407, 413
    cancer registries, 413
    clinical surveys, 414
    NOHSS, 414–415
    non-clinical surveys, 414
    vital statistics, 413–414
  assurance in, 407–408, 416
  community partnerships, 415–416
  federal agencies, U.S., 411–412
  health education, 416–417
  health promotion, 417
  international agencies, 410–411
  linking people to oral health services,
      417–418
  policy development, 407
  prevention programs, support in
      implementing, 418–419
  professional organizations, 413
  state and local programs, 412–413
dental pulp. *See* pulp
dental tape, 167
dental trauma, 4. *See also* resorption
  to alveolar ridge, 100
  to anterior teeth, 100
  apexification, 104
  avulsion, 100–101
    preservation of avulsed teeth, 104–105
  categories of, 103
  in children, 100, 101, 104
  contact sports injuries, 389–390
  to dentition, 100
  displacement, 101, 106
  dry storage/dry storage time, 100
  effect of, 100
  etiology, 101
  examination, initial, 102–103
  extruded teeth, 101
  facial injuries suffered in car accidents, 9
  fractured teeth, 102, 105
  inflammatory resorption, 102
  introduction to, 100–101
  intruded teeth, 101, 104, 106
  ischemia, 101
  luxation, 101, 102, 105
  neurologic evaluation, 102, 103

pain control, 102–103
periodontal ligament damage, 101
to permanent teeth, 104–105
to primary teeth, 104
public education on, 106
pulpal necrosis, 102, 103
pulp, healing of, 105
reimplantation, 100, 104–105
replacement resorption, 101–102
research on, 106–107
soft tissue injuries, 100, 103
splinting, 105
tooth preservation, 100, 104–105
dentate patients, 9
dentifrices, 24
  abrasiveness (*See* abrasiveness of
      dentifrices)
  anti-calculus, 150
  antihypersensitivity products, 150–151
  baking soda in, 148
  chlorhexidine and, 153
  defined, 142, 144
  flavoring and sweetening agents in, 148
  fluoride in, 148–150
  humectants added to, 147
  ingredients in, 145–146
  vs. mouthrinses, 142
  packaging of, 145
  plaque control, 148
  preservatives added to, 147
  safety and efficacy of, 143
  soaps and detergents in, 147
  therapeutic agents added to, 148–150
  therapeutic *vs.* cosmetic, 145
  thickening or binding agents added to,
      147
  triclosan in, 150
  whiteners, 151
dentin, 38, 39, 471
dentinal tubules, 34, 101
  obturation of, 150
  occluding/sclerosing of, 151
dentinoenamel junction (DEJ), 31, 34, 38
dentin–pulpal interface, 150
dentition, 38
  functional, 469
  ideal, 110, 111
dentogingival unit/junction, 53
dentoperiosteal fibers, 51
denture brush, 139
dentures/removable orthodontic appliances
  adhesives, 200
  brushing, 195–198
  daily denture care, patient instructions for,
      196
  deposits formed on, 194
  disinfection of, 199–200
  for geriatric patients, 471
  immersion, 198–199
  liners, 200
  materials used in construction of, 194
  patient education, 195
  population with or in need of, 193–194
  preventive dental care, lack of, 2
  salivary flow and, 194

toothbrushes/toothbrushing, 139
xerostomia and, 200
Department of Homeland Security, 412
depression, 479–480
desensitization agents, 150–151
desquamated cells, 18
developmental disabilities, populations with
  autism, 497
  cerebral palsy, 497–499
  Down syndrome, 499
  introduction to, 496
  mental retardation, 496–497
diabetes mellitus, 480
  dental and nutritional implications, 308
  diet guidelines, 309
  periodontal diseases, 47, 49
  prevalence of, 62
  sweeteners and, 328
diagnostic modality, 6
*Diagnostic Statistical Manual of Mental
    Disorders, Fourth Edition*, 373
diastemas, 177
diet. *See also* diet and dental caries;
    nutrition
  assessment and counseling, 289
  dental demineralization and, 299
  MyPyramid, 427
  primary prevention, 289
  reference intakes, 289–290
  secondary prevention, 289
  tertiary prevention, 289
diet and dental caries
  carbohydrates and, role of, 300–301
  caries-protective foods and nutrition,
      301–302
  cariogenic potential of foods, measuring,
      302–303
  eating patterns/physical forms of food
      and, 301
  Severe Early Childhood Caries (S-ECC),
      305
dietary analysis, 7
Dietary Guidelines for Americans, 2005,
    290, 291
Dietary Reference Intakes (DRIs), 289–290
differentiation, 69
diffusion, 224
diseases and disorders, oral. *See also* caries
  categories of, 9
  in children, Surgeon General Report on,
      4
  plaque prevention, 9–11
  prevalence of, documented studies on, 9
  risk assessment form, 32
  sequelae of, 9
  systemic diseases, 3, 5–6
  tobacco-related, 366–367
disparities. *See* health disparities
dissection, 86, 88
distraction, 448
DNA, 401–402, 403
  Human Genome Project (HGP)
      401–402, 49
  repair, 69
Down syndrome, 499

dry storage/dry storage time, 100
Duval County (Florida) Health Department Dental Program, 418
dysgeusia, 89, 92
dysthymia, 480

Early and Periodic Screening, Diagnosis, and Treatment (EPSDT), 430
Early Childhood Caries (ECC), 305, 355, 425, 426, 429, 430, 431, 445
eating disorders, 305–307
ecchymoses, 485
ecologic niche, 22
edema, 58
edentulism, 30
effectiveness, defined, 410
efficacy, defined, 410
elderly. *See* geriatrics
electric vitality testing, 103
electron-beam therapy, 89
embrasures, 167
enamel
   demineralization, 22, 34
   dentin and, 38
   epithelium, 16
   extrinsic/extrinsic stains, 145
   inorganic phase of, 111
   inter-rod areas of, 38
   linear hypoplasia, 296
   matrix, 16
   remineralization of, 34
   remnants of enamel-forming organ, 16
   rods, 34
   space, 16
   spindles, 38
   yellowing of, 146
enamel fluorosis, 215, 227–231
   in children, 227–229, 230–231
   Community Fluorosis Index, 216, 217, 229
   in infants, 227–228, 230
   reducing risk for, 230–231
enamel-forming organ, 16
enameloplasty, 273
endodontic lesions, 59
endogenous origin, 16, 17
endosseous, 192
endosseous implants, 192
end rounding, 129, 130
Enfamil, 105
Environmental Protection Agency (EPA), 227, 233
eosinophils, 114
epilepsy, 480–481
epithelial atrophy, 89
epithelial dysplasia, 69–71
epithelium, 110–111
Erikson, Erik, 440
Erikson's psychosocial development, 440, 441
erythematous candidiasis, 482
erythroleukoplakia, 74, 75
erythroplakia, 74, 75
essential oil mouthrinses, 153–154
estrogen, 452–453, 456, 457

estrogen replacement therapy, 452–453
etchants, 279
ethylenediaminetetraacetic acid (EDTA), 18
etiology of disease, 9
exfoliate, 104
exfoliative cytology, 80–81
exocrine glands, 115
exodontia, 223
exogenous antimicrobial agents, 15
exogenous origin, 17
external-beam radiotherapy, 89
extra-alveolar time, 100, 101
extracellular coatings, 15
extractions, 2
Extra Strength Aim, 149
extrinsic stains, 145

facultative anaerobes, 18n
Fagerstrom Test for Nicotine Dependence (FTND), 376
Fauchard, Pierre, 30
FDI World Dental Federation, 411
Federal Bureau of Prisons, 412
Federal Food, Drug, and Cosmetic Act, 321
Federally Qualified Health Centers (FQHC), 418
Federal Trade Commission (FTC), 143
fetal alcohol syndrome, 496
filaments (nylon bristles), 122, 129
fimbriae, 18
fine-needle aspiration biopsy, 82, 84, 85
First Five Oral Health training program, 427
First Smiles Program, 429–430
floating amalgams, 457
flossing, 7. *See also* dental floss
   bacterial endocarditis, 173
   behavior, adopting, 172–173
   children and, 168, 169
   clinical attachment loss and, 175–176
   damage from, 171–172
   methods of, 169–171
   objectives of, 167
fluoridation. *See also* fluoride; fluoride for children
   action of, mechanisms of, 220, 222–223
   anti-fluoridation groups, 230
   benefits and effectiveness of, 214, 223–226
   chemicals and technical systems used, engineering aspects of, 232–233
   cost of, 234–235
   definition and background of, 213–215
   diffusion, 224
   dilution, 224
   discontinuation of, effects of, 226–227
   growth, 220
   as a health-promotion activity, 417
   history of
      clinical discovery phase of, 215–216
      demonstration phase of, 217–218
      epidemiologic phase of, 216–217
      technology transfer phase of, 218–220
   hyperfluoridation, 234
   hypofluoridation, 233–234

   introduction to, 213
   laws, 417
   levels, optimal, 231
   milk, 235
   monitoring and surveillance of, 233–234
   as population-based method of primary prevention, 214–215
   remineralization/demineralization, 220, 222–223
   risk communication (*See* risk communication in fluoridation)
   salt, 235
   state populations on fluoridated systems, percentage of, 221–222
fluoride. *See also* fluoridation
   for cancer patients, 478–479
   demineralization/remineralization, 112
   in dentifrices, 148–149, 151
   for Down syndrome patients, 499
   fluorosis (*See* enamel fluorosis)
   in gum, 155–156
   HAP, FHA, CaF$_2$, relationship between, 41
   for infants, 429
   levels, optimal, 231, 232
   Maximum Contaminant Level Goal for, 229
   in mouthrinses, 142, 154
   for older adults, 459
   remineralization and, 41
   sealants, fluoride-releasing, 276
   supplement schedule, 1994, 230
   systemic, 220, 222
   and tooth decay, research on, 216–217
   toothpicks impregnated with, 180–181
   topical, 220, 222
   varnishes, 429
fluoride for children
   benefits and effectiveness of, 223–226
   discontinuation of, effects of, 226–227
   dosage schedule for, 229–230
   enamel fluorosis, 227–229, 230–231
   ingestion for children under age of 2 years, 230
   in mouthrinses, 154
   research on benefits of, 216–219
   school-based weekly fluoride rinse programs, 235
fluorapatite, 111
fluorhydroxyapatite (FHA), 41
fluoride
   burnishing, 181
   long-term exposure to, 41
   products, 7
   releasing materials/composites, 40
   stannous, 188
   varnish, 150
Fluoride in Drinking Water: A Scientific Review of EPA's Standards, 228
fluorine, 213
fluorosis. *See* enamel fluorosis
focal alopecia (hair loss), 89, 91
focal hyperpigmentation, 89
Fones, Alfred C., 2–3, 123
Fones toothbrushing method, 132, 133

Food and Drug Administration (FDA), 142, 143
  approval, stages of, 142
  aspartame labeling and, 327
  call for rulemaking, 144
  chlorhexidine approved by, 142
  cyclamates banned by, 319
  dental radiographs during pregnancy, 428
  desensitization agents approved by, 150
  food additives approved by, 321
  label and packaging recommendations, 143–144
  Neotame approved by, 328
  OTC product reviews and regulation, 143
  plaque-control rinses approved by, 142
  role of, 412
  saccharin banned by, 327
Food and Nutrition Board (FNB), 289
Food Guide Pyramid, 293, 427
food labels, 294–295
fossa, 277
"4 city study," 216, 217
Framework for Theory Development (ADHA), 333
freebase cocaine, 486
free marginal groove, 50
fructans, 21
functional status, 467–468
fungiform papillae, 139
furcation area, 53
The Future of Public Health (Institute of Medicine), 407
The Future of Public Health in the 21st Century (Institute of Medicine), 407

gastrointestinal tract, 110
gene polymorphisms, 403
generalized ligament laxity, 499
generalized resistance resources (GRRs), 356–357
genes, 402
genetics
  caries, 402
  gene therapy, 403
  Human Genome Project (HGP), 401–402
  periodontal diseases, 402–403
  research, 49
genome, 401–402
genomics, 60–61
Georgia Department of Audits (GDOA) Report, 415
Georgia Oral Health Coalition (GOHC), 415
Georgia State Oral Health Program, 415
geriatrics
  aging issues, 307
  caries, 458
  cognitive changes, 468
  community-dwelling seniors, 466, 470
  cumulative effects of oral diseases, 470
  death, leading cause of, 467
  dental providers, 473
  dental treatment needs of, 471
  dentures and, 471
  frail elderly, 465–466
  functionally independent, 465

functional status, 467–468
  health of, 466–467
  health promotion, 471–472
  introduction to, 463
  living arrangements of, 465
  long-term care, 470
  nursing home population, 466
  nutrition, 307–308
  oral manifestations, common, 469
  osteoporosis, 467
  periodontal diseases in, 458
  physiological changes, 467
  population characteristics, 463–465
  preventative strategies, 471
  public policy, 472
  senior-friendly dental practice, 471
  Surgeon General's report on, 470–471
  systemic diseases and, 470–471
  WHO definition of "elderly" and "old," 465
gestational diabetes, 480
gingiva, 15, 49–52
  bleeding, 10
  plaque-induced/non–plaque-induced, 59
gingival bleeding, 10
gingival crevice. *See* gingival sulcus
gingival crevicular fluid (GCF), 53
gingival fibers, 50
gingival recession, 16
gingival sulcus, 10, 17, 22, 52, 53
gingivitis, 7, 10, 47, 48
  in adults, 455
  in cerebral palsy patients, 498
  in children, 48, 54, 61
  chronic stage of, 58
  defined, 47
  dentifrices used to control, 148, 149
  diagnosis of, *vs.* periodontitis diagnosis, 56
  microbial species, in children *vs.* adults, 54
  plaque and deepening pockets, 56–57, 60
  as precursor to periodontitis, 56
  prevalence of, 48
  subgingival/supragingival plaque, 56
gingivodental/dentogingival fibers, 50–51
glass ionomers, 40
  cement sealants, 276
GlaxoSmithKline, 145, 150
Glide, 169
glucans, 18, 21
glucosyltransferase, 18
glucosyl transferase (GTFs), 399–400
glycemic response, 328
glycoproteins, 17n, 18, 297
gram-negative anaerobes, 61
granular cells, 57
granulocytes, 114
granulomas, 111
growth regulation, 69

hairy leukoplakia, 76
halitosis, 139, 152
  origin of, 189
  reasons for, 189–190
  tongue and, 190
  volatile sulfur compounds (VSC), 190

Hanks balanced salt solution (HBSS), 105
Harper's Weekly, 133
health. *See* dental public health
health behavior models. *See also* health education
  Health Belief Model, 349–350
  implementing, 359
  locus of control (LOC), 356
  sense of coherence (SOC), 356–357
  social learning theory (SLT), 354–356
  summary of, 358
  theory of reasoned action, 352–354
  transtheoretical model and stages of change, 350–352
Health Belief Model, 349–350
health, defined, 6
health disparities
  in dental care for children, 4
  dental sealant use, 283
  in elderly, 465–466
  by income, 4, 5
  of racial and ethnic groups, 5
health education. *See also* health behavior models
  adult, 359–360
  history of, 348
  introduction to, 348
  motivating patients, 360
  motivational interviewing, 360–361
  oral health application, 361
  self-efficacy, 351
  vicarious learning, 352
health promotion theory, 458
Health Resources and Services Administration (HRSA), 411–412
health self-care. *See* oral self-care
Healthy People 2000, 61–62
Healthy People 2010, 93, 219, 365, 366, 417
hematopoietic cell transplantation, 484
hemidesmosomes, 16, 18
hemiglossectomy, 86
hemophilia, 481
hereditary ectodermal dysplasias, 4
hereditary fructose intolerance (HFI), 322
herpes simplex virus, 482, 483
herpetic lesion, 111
histadine, 118
histological normality, 10
HIV/AIDS, 9, 114, 308–309, 412, 481–483
homeostatis, 115
horizontal fibers, 52–53
horizontal toothbrushing technique, 133, 134
hormone replacement therapy, 452–453
host defense mechanisms in the oral cavity. *See also* demineralization; remineralization; saliva
  dentition, ideal, 110, 111
  epithelium, 110–111
  immune system and, 113–115
  introduction to, 110
  normal oral flora and, 113
  oral flora and, 110, 113
Human Genome Project (HGP), 401–402, 49
human papillomavirus (HPV) infections, 72, 74, 76

humectants, 147
humoral immunity, 110, 113–114
hydrofluosilicic acid (H2SiF6), 232
hydrogen bonding, 18
hydrogen peroxide, 151
hydrophobicity, 18
hydrophobins, 18
hydroxyapatite (HAP), 23, 41, 111, 118
hydroxyproline, 298–299
hyperfluoridation, 234
hyper-IgE syndrome, 119
hyperlipidemias, 329
hypersensitivity, 142
  antihypersensitivity products, 150–151
hypertension, 483–484
hyperthyroidism, 487
hypochlorite, 58
hypofluoridation, 233–234
hypogeusia, 92
hypomineralization, 298
hypothiocyanate, 118
hypothyroidism, 487, 488

iatrogenic disease, 458
immune evasion, 69
immune system
  beta-defensin peptides, 115
  Candida albicans, 114
  cellular and humoral components of, 110,
    113
  complement system in, 114
  leukocyte adhesion disorder (LAD), 115
  myeloid system of granulocytes, 114–115
immunity
  defined, 398
  types of, 398–399
immunizations, 398–399
  for caries, 399–400
  immunity and, 398–399
  for periodontal diseases, 400–401
immunocompromising conditions, 308–309
immunoglobulins, 110, 118–119
  A (IgA), 118–119, 398, 399–400
  D, 119
  E, 119
  G, 118
  M, 118
immunologic defense, 57
immunopathologic reaction, 57
immunosuppression, 484
immunosuppressive disease, 88
implants, 192–193
incidence, defined, 9
incipient lesion, 7, 10, 31, 33–34
  bacterial biofilm, direct connection of,
    34–35
  defined, 31
  demineralization, 31, 33, 34
  detection of, 33
  early stages of, etiologic and histologic
    standpoints, 31, 33
  features of, 31, 33
  incipient lesion (*See* incipient lesion)
  physical and microscopic features of, 31,
    33

pore spaces of different zones, 34
remineralization, 33, 34
stages of development, 31
studies of, 33
zones of, 33–34
income disparities, 4, 5
Indian Health Service (IHS), 412, 418
infants, 424
  anticipatory guidance schedule, 429
  caries in, 425–427, 429
  dental evaluations, reasons for, 429
  early dental care, 430
  enamel fluorosis in, 227–228, 230
  First Smiles Program, 429–430
  fluoride supplementation, 429, 431
  low birth weight (LBW), 424, 425
  mutans streptococci in, 37
  oral cavity, 111
  oral health education, 430
  preterm birth (PTB), 424–425
  preventative intervention, early, 430–432
    advantages of, 430
    clinical findings, 434
    concluding the appointment, 433
    counseling, 432
    examination, 432–433
    guidance, anticipatory, 433
    interview, 430–432
    recall schedule, establishing, 433
  preventive strategies, 428
  sugars in baby foods, 429
  toothbrushing of, 432, 433
infection, defined, 110
inflammatory exudate, 23
inflammatory–immune systems, 17
in situ involvement, 10
Institute of Medicine, 214, 227, 407
instrumentation, subgingival mechanical, 57
insurance coverage, 3, 4
Intensity-modulated radiotherapy, 89
interdental gingiva, 51
interdental papillae, 51
interdental toothbrushes, 177–179
interleukin-1B (IL-1B), 58, 402–403
International Association of Dental Trauma,
    104
International Federation of Dental
    Hygienists (IFDH), 411
International Liaison Committee on Dental
    Hygiene, 411
InterPlak, 123
interproximal tooth area, 10
interproximal toothbrushes, 177–179
interradicular fibers, 53
inter-rod space, 34
interstitial irradiation, 89
intertubular dentin, 38
Intraoral cone, 89
intrinsic stains, 145
investigational new drug (IND), 143
iron deficiency anemia, 298
irrigation
  antimicrobial use, 187–188
  bacteremias, irrigation-induced, 189
  devices, 187

effects of, 188
  tips and units, 188–189
irrigator, 154
ischemia, 101

Jenner, Edward, 398
Job syndrome, 119
Journal of Dental Education, 78
junctional epithelium, 47, 53

Kaposi's sarcoma, 76, 482, 483
keratin, 111
kidney disease/failure, 485
knitting yarn, white, 184
Koop, C. Everett, 214, 407
kyphosis, 467

labial salivary gland, 116
laboratory tests, 7
Lactobacillus, 113
Lactobacillus rhamnosus GG, 301
lactoperoxidase, 118
lamina dura, 102
laser Doppler flowmetry, 103
lectins, 18n
LED Dental, Inc., 81
Leonard toothbrushing technique, 132
Leptotrichia, 54
leukocyte adhesion disorder (LAD), 115
leukocytes, 18
leukoplakia, 74, 75
Lever Brothers, 145
lichenoid reactions, 471
lichen planus, 74
life expectancy, 458
Life magazine, 388
light activation, 274
light-cured dental sealants, 275
light-emitting diodes (LED), 275
linear gingival erythema, 483
lingual brackets, 176
lingual gland, 116
lingual thyroid, 488
lingual tooth surfaces, 10
lip biting, 497
Listerine Antiseptic, 153, 154, 188
LL-37, 115
locus of control (LOC), 356
long-term care, 470
loop method of flossing, 170–171
loss of attachment, 47, 48, 60
luxation, 101, 102
  crown fractures, 105
  lateral, 106
  loss of tooth, 102
lymphocytes, 114–115
lymph system, 113–114

macroglossia, 499
macrophages, 58, 114
magnetic resonance imaging, 85, 88
major depression, 479–480
malnutrition, 296–298
mannitol, 324
mantle dentin, 38

marginal gingiva, 8, 9, 13, 50, 51, 52
marginal resections, 88
marijuana use, 76, 486
Maryland Department of Health and Mental
    Hygiene, 415
Maryland Oral Cancer Prevention Coalition,
    415–416
Maryland Oral Cancer Prevention Initiative,
    416
Massachusetts Interscholastic Athletic
    Association, 389
mastication of food, 17
materia alba, 18
maxillary sinuses, 499
maxillofacial surgeon, 85
McKay, Frederick, 215–216
mechanical displacement, 17
Medicaid, 4, 408, 412, 416, 418
    Early and Periodic Screening, Diagnostic
        and Treatment benefit, 418
Medical Expenditure Panel Survey, 414
medically compromised populations
    arthritis, 477
    bulimia, 478
    cancer, 478–479
    cardiac arrhythmias, 479
    congestive heart failure (CHF), 479
    depression, 479–480
    diabetes mellitus, 480
    epilepsy, 480–481
    hemophilia, 481
    HIV/AIDS, 481–483
    hypertension, 483–484
    organ transplants, 484
    pulmonary disease, 484
    renal disease/failure, 485
    substance abuse disorders, 485–487
    synopsis of medical conditions, 488–490
    thyroid dysfunction, 487–488
Medicare, 412, 418
menopause, 452, 457
Mentadent, 149
mental retardation, 496–497
methamphetamine use, 486, 487
microbiota, 16
microcephaly, 496
microwave radiation, 199
milk
    fluoridation, 235
    as tooth preservative, 105
Miller, W. D., 30, 323
mineralization, 22, 23–24, 25
minerals, dietary, 298, 458
Misch, Carl E., 106
modified neck dissections, 88
modified toothbrushing technique, 133
Mohammed, 122–123
motile/non-motile cells, 20
motivational interviewing, 360–361
mouth disease, as public health problem, 2
mouthguards
    AAP classification of sports, 392
    activities requiring, 391
    for cerebral palsy patients, 498–499
    contact sports injuries and, 389

custom-made, 391, 392, 394
defined, 388
dental provider's role in use of, 394
as a health-promotion activity, 417
historical perspective of, 388
mouth-formed (boil-n-bite) mouthguard,
    391, 392, 393
National Facial Protection Month, 390
NCAA guidelines for, 389
protection and prevention, 390–391
stock mouthguard, 391, 393
types of, 391, 393
use of, 388–389
Mouth Hygiene (Fones), 123
mouthrinses, 142
    active ingredients in, claimed, 151
    alcohol in, 151–152, 154
        children and, 151–152
    child safety caps on, 151–152
    chlorhexidine in, 142
    vs. dentifrices, 142
    fluoride, 235
    halitosis and, 152
    safety and efficacy of, 143
    school-based weekly fluoride rinse
        programs, 235
    therapeutic, 151
        cetylpyridinium chloride (CPC), 154
        chlorhexidine gluconate, 153
        essential oil, 153–154
        fluoride rinses, 154
        xerostomia, 152–153
    zinc sulfate as anti-plaque ingredient, 151
mucogingival junction, 51
mucosal surface, 16
mucositis, 89, 91–92
multidimensional health, 6
multiple sclerosis, 496
mutans streptococci (MS)
    adherence to the tooth, 37
    caries, role in development of, 36
    in children, 36, 37
    colonization of, 37
    physiologic characteristics, 36
    sucrose and, 37
Mycostatin Pastilles, 199
MyPyramid, 293–294

National Academy of Sciences, 289
National Alliance Football Rules
    Committee, 389
*A National Call to Action to Promote Oral
    Health* (U.S. Surgeon General), 4–5
National Cancer Institute, 366–367
National Center for Health Statistics
    (NCHS), 414, 486
National Collegiate Athletic Association
    (NCAA), 389, 390
National Eating Disorders Association, 306
National Facial Protection Month, 390
National Federation of High School
    Associations' Ice Hockey Rules
    Committee, 389
National Fluoridation Report, 2002, 219
National Football League, 389

National Governors Association (NGA), 416
    Center for Best Practices, 416
National Health and Nutrition Examination
    Survey (NHANES), 228, 369, 414
National Health Interview Survey (NHIS),
    414, 471
    1983, 195
    1990, 186
National Hockey League, 389
National Institute for Dental and
    Craniofacial Research (NIDCR),
    412, 416
    "State Models for Oral Cancer Prevention
        and Early Detection," 416
National Institute of Dental and Craniofacial
    Research, 189, 216, 415
National Institute of Dental Research, 216,
    224, 366–367, 469
National Institutes of Health (NIH), 216,
    403, 412
National Labeling and Education Act of
    1990, 294
National Oral Health Information
    Clearinghouse, 93
National Oral Health Surveillance System
    (NOHSS), 414–415
National Preventive Dentistry
    Demonstration Project, 235
National Research Council (NRC), 228–229
National Sanitation Foundation (NSF)
    International, 232, 233
National Spit Tobacco Education Program
    (NSTEP), 417
National Youth Sports Foundation for the
    Prevention of Athletic Injuries, 389
neck dissections, 88
necrotizing disease, 59
necrotizing ulcerative gingivitis (NUG), 59
necrotizing ulcerative periodontitis (NUP),
    59, 483
neohesperidine dihydrochalcone, 328
neoplasm, 68
neotame, 328
Neotame approved by, 321
neurotoxicity, 92
neutrophil function, 59
neutrophils, 114
new drug application (NDA), 143
New York State Department of Health, 428
New Zealand Ministry of Health, 235
Nicoderm CQ®, Nicotrol®, 375
nicotine replacement therapies (NRT),
    374–375
    dosing of, 375–376
    gum, 375
    inhaler, 375
    lozenge, 375
    nasal spray, 375
    non-NRT medications, 376
    transdermal patch, 375
non-restorative repair, 41
nonspecific plaque hypothesis, 53–54
Notre Dame, 388
NovaMin, 459
Novello, Antonia, 214

nutrition. *See also* diet; sweeteners
  aging issues, 307–308
  deficiencies, oral symptoms of, 297
  diabetes mellitus and, 308, 309
  eating disorders, 305–307, 457
  guidelines for Americans, 290–293
    food labels, 294–295
    MyPyramid, 293–294
  immunocompromising conditions, 308–309
  introduction to, 288–289
  minerals, 298, 458
  nutrients, availability of, 17
  optimal, 295–296
  oral cavity and, factors affecting, 295–296
  oral surgery and intermaxillary fixation, 309–310
  periodontal disease and, 303, 304
  during pregnancy, 427
  protein/calorie malnutrition, 296–298
  taste perception and sensation, 317–318
  vitamins, 298–299, 458
nutritionally healthy habits
  sugar discipline, 7
Nuva-Seal, 282

Oasis Mouthwash, 152
obesity, 328
oblique fibers, 53
obturation of dentinal tubules, 150
occluding of dentinal tubules, 151
occlusal fissures, 10, 17
occlusal forces, 53
odontoblastic process, 38
odontoblasts, 38
Office of Public Health and Science in the
  Office of the Secretary, USDHHS, 412
Office of the National Fluoridation
  Engineer, 215
operant conditioning, 440
opportunistic infections, 9
Orajel Sensitive Pain Relieving Toothpaste
  for Adults, 150–151
Oral B Hummingbird, 176
oral brush test, 80–81
oral cancer, 9. *See also* oral cancer
    screening/examination; oral lesions;
    squamous cell carcinomas
  in adults, 455–456
  in African Americans, 71–72, 73, 94, 456
  alcohol-containing rinses linked to, 152
  chemopreventive agents, 74
  clinical manifestations of, 79
  defined, 68–69
  epithelial dysplasia, 69–71
  formation of, 69
  grading, 86
  immune deficiency's role in, 76
  incidence rates, 71–72
  marijuana's role in, 76
  in minority populations, 71
  mortality rate, 71, 72
  prognosis, 86
  as public health problem, 2

registries, 413
risk factors, 72
  age, 73
  alcohol, 72–73
  race and ethnicity, 72, 73
  tobacco, 72
  ultraviolet radiation, 73–74
signs and symptoms of, 76
squamous cell carcinomas, 69, 75, 86, 87
staging scale, 86
tobacco-related, 367–368
treatment options, 86 (*See also* radiation
    therapy)
  chemotherapeutic agents, 86, 90
  considerations regarding, 86, 88
  health care professionals involved in, 92
  reconstruction, 90–91
  resection/dissection, 86, 88
  side effects from, treatment of, 91–92
  surgery, 88
Oral Cancer Foundation, 93
oral cancer screening/examination. *See also*
    biopsy types
  aids for, 80–82, 83
  alcohol assessment, 76–78
  American Cancer Society
    recommendations, 78–79
  American Dental Education Association's
    competencies, 78
  consistency and thoroughness in, lack of, 79
  cultural sensitivity, 94
  in dental setting, 78
  dental team's role in, 93
  free public health screenings, 94
  imaging, 85
  medical provider's responsibility in, 78
  public education, 93
  steps involved in, 79
  tobacco assessment, 76
  visual and tactile examinations, 78
oral candidiasis, 89
oral cavity, 68–69
  nutrition affects on, 295–296
  odors originating in, 189–190
oral cleanliness, defined, 166–167
oral contraceptives (OCs), 456
oral flora, 113, 114
oral hairy leukoplakia (OHL), 482
oral health
  active aging as component of, 465
  defined, 452
Oral Health America, 417
*Oral Health Care During Pregnancy and
    Early Childhood Practice Guidelines*
    (New York State Department of
    Health), 428
Oral Health in America (Surgeon General
    report), 195, 470
*Oral Health in America: A Report of the
    Surgeon General*, 214
Oral Health Section of the APHA, 413
oral lesions
  erythroleukoplakia, 74, 75
  erythroplakia, 74, 75

hairy leukoplakia, 76
human papillomavirus (HPV), 72, 74, 76
Kaposi's sarcoma, 76
leukoplakia, 74, 75
lichen planus, 74
oral malodor. *See* halitosis
oral microflora
  antimicrobials, 187–188
  subgingival periodontopathic, irrigation
    and, 187–188
oral papillomas, 486
oral prophylaxis, 56
oral self-care, 166. *See also*
    dentures/removable orthodontic
    appliances; flossing; irrigation;
    toothbrushing; toothpicks
  comprehensive oral assessment,
    components of, 164
  dental hygiene assessment, 338
  frequency of, 166–167
  interproximal supplemental aids, 165
  interproximal supplemental aids, list of,
    165
  peri-implant, 192–193
  plan for, based on evidence-based
    principles, 165
  preventing caries, 187
  Process of Care Model, 163
  re-care (follow-up) visits, 163
  rinsing, 185–187
  supplemental self-care aids, list of, 165
oral surgery/intermaxillary fixation,
    309–310
  for oral cancer, 88
  preventive dental care, lack of, 2
oral vestibule/palate, 53
organoleptic assessment, 152
organ transplants, 484
oropharyngeal cancers. *See* oral cancer
oropharynx, 68, 69
orthodontic appliances, 132
osseointegrated implants, 90
osteoblasts, 101
Osteopathic Heritage Foundation, 428
osteoporosis, 457, 467, 487–488
osteoradionecrosis, 89, 92
otolaryngologist, 85
overt cavitation, 9–10
overt/frank lesion, 31
over-the-counter (OTC) agents, 143–144
  anti-calculus dentifrices, 150
  antihypersensitivity products, 150–151
  desensitization agents, 150
  for extrinsic/intrinsic stain removal, 145
  FDA reviews and regulation of, 143–144
  fluoride levels in, 149–150
  mouthrinses, 151
    anti-plaque/anti-gingivitis mouthrinse,
      153
  to occlude exposed dentinal tubules,
    143–144
  for tobacco cessation, 374
  triclosan in, 150
  whiteners, 151
overt lesion, 10

packaging and labeling guidelines, 144
palatal gland, 116
palate, 69
palatoglossus muscle, 68
palatopharyngeal muscle, 68–69
palisades, 20
palpation, 78
Pan American Health Organization (PAHO), 411
papillae, 51
parotid gland, 115
passive immunity, 398
pathogenic microorganisms, 14
patient autonomy, defined, 348
patient history, 7
Pavlov, Ivan, 440
Pavlov's classical conditioning, 440
pectoralis major mucocutaneous flaps, 90
pediatrics. *See also* child development; children; infants
 behavior management, 445
 communication, 446, 448
 dental treatment, implications for, 446, 447
 distraction, 448
 Early Childhood Caries (ECC), 445
 introduction to, 438
 population characteristics, 438
 positive reinforcement, 448
 preventative strategies, 445
 tell-show-do technique, 448
 voice control, 448
pellicle, 16
 acquired, 17
 glycoproteins, carbohydrate components of, 17
perfusion, 103
periapical radiograph, 33
Peridex, 154
peri-implantitis, 192, 193
peri-implant mucositis, 192
perikymata, 24
perimenopause, 452, 457
periodontal abscess, 59
periodontal debridement, 7
periodontal diseases, 2, 9, 47. *See also* gingivitis; periodontitis
 biofilm and self-care, 57, 61
 bleeding gums, 62
 cause of, 9
 cellular defense in, 57–58
 in cerebral palsy patients, 498
 classifications of, 58–59
 dental hygiene care assessment, 339–340
 diagnosis and treatment, challenges of, 49
 in elderly, 60, 458
 genomics, 60–61
 gingival lesion, 54–56
 gingival sulcus, 53
 gingivitis, 7, 10
 gram-negative anaerobes, 61
 humoral defense, 58
 immunizations for, 400–401
 immunopathologic reaction, 57
 incidence *vs.* prevalence of, 9
 leukocyte adhesion disorder (LAD), 115

loss of attachment, 47, 48, 60
 mild and severe forms of, 47
 nutrition and, 303, 304
 overt lesion, 10
 periodontal microflora, 53–54
 periodontitis, 47
 plaque as cause of, 14
 pocket depth, 56–57, 60
 prevalence of, 49
 prevention, primary, 62
 progression of, 47
 risk factors, 47, 60–62, 456
 smokeless tobacco-related, 368–369
 socioeconomic status, 60
 systemic disease and, 48–49
 therapy, 57
 tobacco-related, 368–369, 455, 459
 treatments for, 455
 volatile sulfur compounds (VSC) in, 190
periodontal ligament, 49, 52–53, 100
 preservation of, 105
 space, loss of, 102
periodontal pockets, 49, 56–57
Periodontal Risk Calculator, 62
periodontas ligament damage, 101
periodontitis, 9–10
 aggressive, 59
 categories of, 59
 chronic, 59
 defined, 47
 developmental or acquired deformities and conditions, 59
 diagnosis of, *vs.* gingivitis diagnosis, 56
 endodontic lesions, 59
 necrotizing disease, 59
 periodontal abscess, 59
 prevalence of, 48
 severe generalized, 48
 systemic, 59
periodontium, 10
 alveolar bone, 49, 51–52, 100
 attachment apparatus, 100
 cementum, 49, 50, 51, 52
 gingiva, 49–52
 gingival unit, 100
 periodontal ligament, 49, 52–53
periomylosis, 457
periosteum of alveolar bone, 50
periradicular inflammation, 102
peritubular dentin, 38
perseveration, 496
petechiae, 485
pH
 measuring, using Stephan curve, 40
 plaque and the Stephan curve, 113
 saturation, relationship of, 40–41
phagocytic cells, 114
pharyngeal arches, 68
pharyngeal cancer, 455–456
pharynx, 68
phosphate abrasives, 146
phosphorus, 298
photoactivation, 274
photocure, 274
physicochemical reaction, 15

Piaget, Jean, 439
Piaget's cognitive development theory, 439
pica, 497
pilin, 18
pilocarpine, 89
pipe cleaners, 184
pit-and-fissure caries, 10, 31, 279
pituitary gland, 452
plaque
 acquired pellicle, 17
 adherent/loosely adherent, 57
 approximal, 19
 bacterial colonization, 15–17
 bacteria in, 19–20
 bacterial adhesion, 18–19
 biofilm, 7, 14–15
 calculus (*See* calculus)
 colonizers, 19
 control of, by patient, 7
 dentifrices used to control, 148
 formation of, 17–18, 19
 interproximal removal of, benefits of, 162
 matrix, 20
 metabolism, 20–22
 mouthrinses used to control, 151, 153
 pH, measuring, 40
 prevention, 9–10
 removal of, 22, 57, 166
 subgingival, 19, 20, 23, 56–57, 62
 sucrose and, 37
 supragingival, 19, 22, 56–57, 62
 zinc sulfate as anti-plaque ingredient, 151
plaque diseases, 9
 etiology of, 9
 incipient lesions, 7, 10
 interim stages of, histological and clinical pathology, 10
 overt cavitation, 9–10
 overt lesion, 10
 periodontitis, 9–10
 preventive objective, 9–10
 in situ involvement, 10
PLUNC (palate, lung, and nasal epithelium clone), 115
poliomyelitis, 8
polishing agents, 146–147
polymerization, 274–275, 275
polymethylmethacrylate (PMMA), 273
polymorphonuclear neutrophil (PMN), 57–58
polyols, 324–326
 mannitol, 324
 sorbitol, 324
 xylitol, 324–326
polysaccharides
 coats, 20
 extracellular, glucans and, 18, 21
 intracellular, 20, 21
 as major constituent of plaque matrix, 20
polytetrafluoroethylene (PTFE) floss, 167–168
pore space, 34
Porphyromonas gingivalis, 59, 113, 400
positron emission tomography, 85
potassium nitrate, 150–151

poverty. *See* health disparities
Prader-Willi syndrome, 496
precontemplator, 351
predentin, 38
pregnancy, 423–424
  damage to teeth during, 457–458
  dental radiographs and, 428
  gestational diabetes, 480
  gingivitis, 458
  infections during, 424
  nutrition during, 427
  Oral Health Care During Pregnancy and
    Early Childhood Practice
    Guidelines, 428
  periodontal interventions on, effect of,
    424–425
  Prenatal Education and Treatment project,
    428
  preventive strategies, 427–428
  synthesis of prostaglandins, 456
  treatment necessities, modifications in, 428
pregnancy granulomas, 456
Prenatal Education and Treatment project, 428
prevalence, defined, 9
preventive dentistry. *See also* primary
    preventive care
  comprehensiveness of, 7
  constitutional causes, study of, 3
  economic benefits and enjoyment of life, 9
  facial injuries suffered in car accidents, 9
  historical aspect of, 2–5
  insurance coverage for, 3
  lack of, impact on public health, 2
  moral commitment of health providers,
    8–9
  in poor children, 4
  secondary, 6, 7, 8
  tertiary, 6, 7, 8
  tooth loss, 8, 9
Prevotella intermedia, 456, 457
primary colonizers, 19, 37
primary dental care, technological advances
    in, 398
  genetics, 401–403
  immunizations, 398–401
  preventative modalities, 398
  stem cells, 403–404
primary prevention, 289
primary preventive care
  approaches to, strategic, 7–8
  as dental hygiene, 3, 6
  practitioner and patient responsibilities in,
    8
  therapies and services, 7
Process of Care Model, 163
Procter & Gamble, 149, 150, 154
progesterone, 456, 457
prognathic mandible, 394
proliferation, 68
prophylactic odontotomy, 273
prophylaxis, 17
"Protect Your Fangs" campaign, 389
proteins, 402
proteolysis, 39
proteolytic enzymes, 199

proteome, 402
proximal surfaces, 19
ptyalism, 117
public health agencies, core functions of,
    407–408
public health, defined, 407
Public Health Service Report, 226–227
pulmonary disease, 484
pulp, 38
  chamber, 34
  death of (necrosis), 102, 103
  dentin–pulpal interface, 150
  endodontic procedures on, 102
  healing of, 105
  polyps, 111
pulpal necrosis, 102, 103
pulpal neural response, 150
punch biopsy, 84, 85
purging behavior, 457
putrefaction, 189–190

qualified health claims, 295

race and ethnicity, 72, 73
radiation therapy, 88–89
  indications for, 88
  radiotherapy, 86
  toxicity and side effects of, 89–90
  types of, 89
radiographs, 10, 33
  bitewing, 33
  for dental hygiene care assessment, 338
  diagnostic, 338
  for oral examination, 7
  periapical, 33
  pregnancy and, 428
radiotherapy, 86
rampant dental caries, 31
Recommendations for Using Fluoride to
    Prevent and Control Dental Caries
    in the United States (CDC), 230
Recommended Dietary Allowances (RDAs),
    289–290, 294
reconstruction, 6, 90–91
re-contouring, 101
Reducing Tobacco Use (Surgeon General),
    381
reimplantation, 100, 104–105
Rembrandt, 154
remineralization, 7
  arrestment phenomenon of, 112
  carious lesions, 33, 34
  conditions in the mouth, 112
  defined, 41, 111
  depth of, 41
  enamel and, 111–112
  fluoridation and, 220, 222–223
  fluoride exposure, 41
  fluoride's influence on, 112
  fluoride level in saliva and, 187
  salivary, 112
remodeling, 101
renal disease/failure, 485
reparative dentin, 38
repeated mild brain injuries, 389

replicative senescence, 69
Report on the Health Consequences of
    Smoking (Surgeon General), 365
resection, 86, 88
resorption
  inflammatory, 102
  replacement, 101–102
  root, 101, 102
  surface, 101
restorations, 2, 17
restorative care, 6
revascularization, 102
"The Rights of the Child," articles 2 and 24
    (UN), 430
rinsing of the mouth, 185–187. *See also*
    mouthrinses
risk communication in fluoridation, 236–237
  myths and actions related to, 237–238
  principles of, 238
  public's level of outrage, factors affecting,
    236–237
  Ten Deadly Sins of Communication, 238
rolling toothbrushing technique, 131–132
root
  lesions in elderly, 458
  periradicular inflammation, 102
  resorption, 100, 101
  sensitivity, 150–151
root caries
  arrested, 39
  vs. coronal caries, 39
  in men *vs.* women, prevalence of, 39
  in older adults, prevalence of, 38
  risk factors, 39
  root-surface, 31
rotated teeth, 167

saccharin, 319, 327
saccharose (common sugar), 318
Safe Drinking Water Act, 228
saliva. *See also* xerostomia
  acquired pellicle, 17
  amount secreted, 117
  artificial, 152
  bacterial colonization of the mouth, 15–17
  calcium bridging, 18
  Candida albicans and, 114
  composition of, 117
  halitosis and, 190
  homeostatis, role in, 115
  as a host mechanism, 115
  immunoglobulin A (IgA) production, 118,
    398, 399–400, 400
  oral homeostasis and, 115
  organic components of, 118–119
  pH of, 40
  protective functions of, 116
  pure, 116
  radiation treatments for cancer and, 89
  secretion of, 117
  stimulated/unstimulated saliva flow, 117
  substitutes, 92, 117
  suppression of salivary flow, 117–118
  viscosity of, 117
  whole, 116

salivary flow
    carie prevention and, 186
    chewing gum and, 186–187
    dentures and, 194
salivary glands
    defensive system functions of, 116–117
    enzymes produced by, 118
    major, 115
    minor, 115–116
    organic molecules secreted by, 118
salivary mucins, 118
salivary peroxidase, 118
salivary proteins, 118
salivary remineralization, 112
salt fluoridation, 235
salutogenesis model. *See* sense of coherence
    (SOC) model
Satcher, David, 214
saturation, 40–41
scalpel biopsy (incisional/excisional), 81,
    84–85
schizophrenia, 496
sclerosing of dentinal tubules, 151
sclerotic dentin, 38
scrub toothbrushing technique, 133, 134
scurvy, 298–299
    rebound, 299
sealants, 3, 7, 273–274
    with bonding agents, 276
    chemical-cured, 275
    colored *vs.* clear, 276–277
    dental providers, 282–283
    disparities in use of, 283
    economics, 283
    filled/unfilled, 274
    fluoride-releasing, 276
    glass ionomer cement, 276
    historical perspective, 273
    introduction to, 273
    light-cured, 275
    polymerization of, 274–275
    retention, 277
    self-cured, 275–276
    self-etching light-cured, 276
    teeth selected for, criteria for, 277–297
sealants, placement of, 279
    application of sealant, 281
    drying tooth surface, 280–281
    increasing surface area, 279
    occlusal and interproximal discrepancies,
        282
    over carious lesions, 282
    pit-and-fissure depth, 279
    preparing the tooth, 280
    retention of sealants, evaluating, 282
    surface cleanliness, 279–280
seatbelts, 9
secondary colonizers, 19
secondary prevention, 289
secondary/recurrent caries, 39–40
secretory immunoglobulin A (sIgA), 297
segmental resections, 88
selective neck dissections, 88
Selenomonas, 54
self-care, 7. *See also* oral self-care

challenge of, 62
defined, 166
plaque biofilm, removal of, 57, 61
self-cured dental sealants, 275–276
self-efficacy, 354–356
self-etching light-cured dental sealants, 276
senile dementia of the Alzheimer's type
    (SDAT), 468
sense of coherence (SOC) model, 356–357
    oral health applications, 357
Sensodyne, 152
Sensodyne Fresh Impact, 145
Sensodyne Fresh Mint Toothpaste, 150
Severe Early Childhood Caries (S-ECC), 305
Sharpey's fibers, 24
sialogogues, 92
sialoliths, 117
sialorrhea, 117
sign, defined, 76
significant scientific agreement (SSA), 295
siwak, 122
Sjögren syndrome, 117–118, 152
Skinner, B. F., 354, 440
Skinner's operant conditioning, 440
Smith toothbrushing method, 133, 134
smokeless tobacco
    chew tobacco, 370–371
    Fagerstrom Test for Nicotine Smokeless-
        Tobacco Dependence, 376
    periodontal disease related to, 368–369
    related oral lesions, 4
    snuff, 370, 371, 372
    Snuff Dipper's Pouch, 368
smoking. *See also* tobacco
    vasoconstriction caused by, 111
Smoking Cessation Leadership Center, 459
social cognitive theory (SCT), 354
social learning theory (SLT), 354–356,
    439–440
Social Security Act, Title XIX of, 418
sodium bicarbonate, 146, 155
sodium fluoride (NaF), 146, 149, 232
sodium lauryl sulfate (SLS), 147
sodium monofluorophosphate (MFP), 146,
    149
sodium silicofluoride (NaFS), 232
soft palate, 68
soft tissue necrosis, 92
solid organ/tissue transplant, 484
soluble pyrophosphates, 150
sorbitol, 155, 324
Special Supplemental Food Program for
    Women, Infants, and Children
    (WIC), 305
specific immunity, 398
specific plaque hypothesis, 54
spectrographic analysis, 215
spina bifida, 496
spirochetes, 17, 20
Splenda, 327
spool method of flossing, 169–170
squamous cell carcinomas
    grading system for, 86
    prevalence of, 69
    TNM staging system for, 87

stagnation, 17
stain removers, 151, 155
stannous fluoride (SnF₂), 149–150, 188
Staphylococcus, 199
State Children's Health Insurance Program
    (SCHIP), 4, 408, 416, 418
statherin, 118
stem cells, 403–404
Stephan curve, 40, 113
Stephan, Robert, 40
stevia/steveoside, 328
Stillman toothbrushing method, 132
stomatitis, 194
streptoccus m.
    caries and, 300
streptococci
    actinomycetes linked to, 18
    as early colonozer, 19
    hydrophobicity of, 18
    mineralization of, 23
    as non-motile cells, 20
    universally found in mouths, 19
Streptococcus gordonii, 113
Streptococcus mitis, 113
Streptococcus mutans (S. mutans), 113
    caries and, 399
    caries in infants and, 426–427
    chlorhexidine, 186
    denture adhesive, inhibited by, 200
    in normal oral flora, 113
    sorbitol and xylitol fermentation and, 155
    sucrose as energy source of, 20
    tongue cleaning and, 191
Streptococcus oralis, 113
Streptococcus sanguis, 20, 113
striae of Retzius, 34
Stripe dentifrice, 145
subgingival plaque, 19, 20, 23
sublingual gland, 115–116
subluxation, 105
submandibular gland, 115, 117
Substance Abuse and Mental Health
    Services Administration
    (SAMHSA), 412
substance abuse disorders, 485–487
    alcoholism, 485
    cocaine, 486
    marijuana, 486
    methamphetamine, 486, 487
    tobacco use, 485–486
substantivity, 153
subsurface pellicle, 16
sucralose, 327–328
sucrose
    caries and, relationship between, 300
    constituents of, 320
    consumption figures, 300
    as energy source for plaque metabolism,
        20–21
    health aspects of, evaluation of, 321
    osmotic effects of, 20
    plaque and, 37
    for synthesizing intracellular
        polysaccharides, 20
    uses of, 320

sugars. *See also* sucrose
    in baby foods, 429
    caries and, 321–323
    consumption and caries, relationship
        between, 300
    discipline, 7
Sulcabrush, 179
sulcular epithelium, 10, 52
Support for People with Oral and Head and
        Neck Cancer, 93
supragingival plaque, 19, 22
Surveillance, Epidemiology, and End
        Results Program (SEER), 71, 73,
        76
sweeteners. *See also* sucrose; sugars
    behavioral disorders, 329
    diabetes and glycemic response, 328
    history of, 318–320
    hyperlipidemias, 329
    intense, 326
        acesulfame-K, 327
        aspartame, 327
        neotame, 328
        saccharin, 327
        sucralose, 327–328
    introduction to, 317
    market areas, 319
    non-nutritive
        approved in U.S., 326
        not approved in U.S., 326, 328
    obesity, 328
    polyols as, 324–326
    sugars and caries formation, 321–323
symbiosis, 22
symptom, defined, 76
synergistic effects, 186
synthesis of prostaglandins, 456
systemic diseases, 3, 5–6, 48–49, 59

tachycardia, 479
tags, 277
Tang dynasty, 122
target populations
    infants, 424
    pregnant women, 423–424
Task Force on Community Preventive
        Services, 283
taste, loss of/altered, 92
T cells, 113
telangiectasias, 89
tell-show-do technique, 448
temperament, in child development, 444
temporomandibular joint (TMJ), 477
Ten Deadly Sins of Communication, 238
terminal sulcus, 191
Terry, Luther, 214
tertiary prevention, 289
Texas Health Steps Program, 235
thaumatin, 328
theory of reasoned action
    behavioral beliefs and normative beliefs,
        353
    oral health applications, 353–354
therapeutic modality, 6
thermal testing, 103

Third National Health and Nutrition
        Examination Survey (NHANES III),
        38, 299, 300
throat disease, 2
thyroid dysfunction, 487–488
thyrotoxicosis, 487
tissue remodeling and migration, 69
Title XIX of the Social Security Act, 418
T lymphocytes, 114
tobacco. *See also* tobacco use
    bidis ("poor man's cigarette"), 370
    cessation, 61–62
    kreteks (clove cigarettes), 370
    oral cancer and, 72, 76–77
    periodontal disease and, 47, 61
    smokeless (*See* smokeless tobacco)
    types, toxins, and carcinogens, 369–372
    water pipes, 370
tobacco cessation
    alternative methods, 377
    counseling, 459
    first-line medications, 374 (*See also*
        nicotine replacement therapies
        (NRT))
    insurance coverage for, 381
    intervention (*See* tobacco-cessation
        intervention)
    nicotine withdrawal symptoms, 373
    OTC or prescription treatments, 374
    pharmacotherapy for, 374
    second-line therapies, 376
    Smoking-Cessation Initiative, 379–380
tobacco-cessation intervention, 377
    health history of tobacco use assessment,
        378
    levels of, 379–380
    motivational interviewing, 377
    PHS guidelines' 5 A's, 377–379
    PHS's 5 R's, 379
    program, establishing, 380–381
    Stage-of-Change Model in, 378
Tobacco Settlement Funds Program,
        Maryland, 416
tobacco use. *See also* tobacco cessation
    behavioral and social addiction, 373–374
    biochemical dependence on, 372–373
    characteristics of smokers, 366
    cultural, 371–372
    dependence as a mental disorder, 373
    Diagnostic Criteria for dependence on, 373
    dose response, 368
    health consequences of, 365
    main-stream smoke, 369
    morbidity, mortality, U.S. trends, 365–366
    oral cancer and, 367–368
    oral diseases and lesions related to,
        366–367
    periodontal disease related to, 368–369,
        455
    population characteristics of, 485–486
    prevention strategies, 381–382
    reverse-smoking, 371
    second-hand smoke, 366
    side-stream smoke, 369
    as a substance abuse, 485–486

Tolerable Upper Intake Level (UL), 290
toluidine blue dye (tolonium chloride), 80
tongue
    bacteria, removal of, 17
    brushing, 139
    cleaners, 139, 190–192
    fissured, 139
    hairy, 191
    halitosis and, 190
    lesions, 86
    mucosal surface of, 16
    thrusting, 497
tonsillar fossae, 69
tonsils, 16, 114
toothbrushes
    abrasion, 147
    ADA acceptance program for evaluation
        of, 139–140
    bristles
        end rounding, 129, 130
        nylon *vs.* natural, 129
        shape and texture of, 129
    for cerebral palsy patients, 498
    for dentures and removable orthodontic
        appliances, 139
    designs of, manual, 123–129
    efficiency and safety evaluations, 138
    handle designs, 129, 131
    history of, 122–123
    interdental/interproximal, 177–179
    introduction to, 122
    laboratory testing procedures, 138
    for older adults, 459
    powered, 136–137
        battery, 123, 135
        design of, 133, 135
        first invented, 123
        InterPlak, 123
        ionic, 135
        mechanical, 135
        methods and uses of, 135–137
        movements of, 135
        power sources, 135
        sonic-powered, 123, 135
    profiles, 129
    replacement of, 139
    tongue brushing, 139
    uni-tuft, 179
toothbrushing, 7, 62, 130–131. *See also* oral
        self-care
    bacteria, removal of, 17
    bass method, 131
    Charters technique, 132
    children and, 123, 129, 131–132, 135
    clinical assessment of, 138–139
    of dental implants, 192
    of dentures, 195–198
    disclosing agents, 138–139
    Fones method, 132, 133
    horizontal technique, 133, 134
    of infants and toddlers, 432, 433
    Leonard technique, 132
    modified brushing technique, 133
    rolling technique, 131–132
    scrub toothbrushing technique, 133, 134

toothbrushing (*continued*)
  Smith method, 133, 134
  Stillman method, 132
  time and frequency of, 138
  of tongue, 191–192
  toothbrush abrasion, 139
tooth eruption, 15–17
tooth germs/buds, 104
tooth loss, 8, 9
  edentulism, 30
toothpaste. *See* dentifrices
toothpicks, 180–181
  children and, usage by, 180
  fluoride-impregnated, 180–181
  historical use of, 180
  holder, 181
  injuries, 180
  proper use of, 180, 181
  rubber or plastic tips, 183–184
  wooden or plastic triangular stick, 182–183
transseptal fibers, 50, 51
transtheoretical model and stages of change, 351–352
trauma. *See* dental trauma
traumatic brain injuries, 496
Treating Tobacco Use and Dependence (PHS), 374, 377, 380
triclosan, 148, 150
Trident Advantage gum, 155
triethylene glycol dimethacrylate (TEGDMA), 274
trismus, 478
tumor-nodemetastasis (TNM) system, 86, 87
type 1 diabetes, 480
type 2 diabetes, 480

ultrasonic cleaning, 199
U.S. Census Bureau, 463
U.S. Consumer Products Safety Commission, 152
U.S. Department of Health and Human Services (USDHHS), 411
U.S. Federal Drug Administration (FDA)
  nicotine dependence treatments, OTC, 374, 375, 376
U.S. Pharmacopoeia Convention (USP), 143
U.S. Preventive Services Task Force guidelines, 289
U.S. Public Health Service (PHS), 216, 217, 231

Commissioned Corps, 412, 418
5 A's, 377–379
5 R's, 379
Treating Tobacco Use and Dependence, 374, 377, 380
U.S. Surgeon General, 470, 496. *See also* U.S. Surgeon General oral health report of 2000
Closing the Gap: A National Blueprint for Improving the Health of Individuals with Mental Retardation, 496
geriatrics report, 470–471
Oral Health in America (Surgeon General report), 195, 470
Oral Health in America: A Report of the Surgeon General, 214
Reducing Tobacco Use (Surgeon General), 381
water fluoridation and, 214
U.S. Surgeon General oral health report of 2000
  findings from, major, 5
  framework for action, 5
  oral diseases and disorders in children, 4
  oral tissues, information derived from examining, 2
  themes included in, 4
U.S. Task Force on Community Preventive Services, 226, 227
uni-tuft brush, 179
University of Maryland Dental School, 415
urethane dimethacrylate (UDMA), 274

varenicline, 376
Veillonella, 20, 113
VELscope (Visually Enhanced Lesion Scope), 81, 82, 84, 85
vermilion (red) border, 68
Viaspan, 105
vicarious learning, 352
vinegar, 199
Vipeholm study, 322
vital signs, 334
vital statistics, 413–414
vitamins, 298–299, 458
  vitamin A deficiency, 298
  vitamin C
    deficiency (scurvy), 298–299
    excess, 299
  vitamin D, 298

ViziLite Plus, 81–82
voice control, 448
volatile sulfur compounds (VSC), 152, 190

Washington Dental Service Foundation, 306
water fluoridation. *See* fluoridation
Waterpik Power Flosser, 176
Wellbutrin®, 376
whiteners, 151
whitlockite, 23
whole saliva, 116
wide local excision, 88
Women, Infants, and Children (WIC), 408–409, 429–430
Women's Health Initiative Study, 453
women's oral health, 456–457
  hormonal changes and imbalances, 452, 453
  hormone/estrogen replacement therapy, 452–453
  menopause/perimenopause, 452, 457
  oral contraceptives (OCs), 456
  osteoporosis, 457, 467
  Women's Health Initiative Study, 453
World Health Organization (WHO), 77, 214, 220, 231, 235, 324
  Active Ageing: A Policy Framework, 463
  definition of "elderly" and "old," 465
  Department of Chronic Diseases and Health Promotion, 410
  Global Oral Health Program, 410–411
  health defined by, 6

xerostomia, 31, 89, 92, 116
  alcoholism, 485
  dental implants and, 193
  in denture wearers, 200
  in elderly, 307, 470
  halitosis, contributing to, 189
  mouthrinses, 152–153
  renal disease/failure, 485
  Sjögren syndrome, 117–118
xylitol, 37, 155, 324–326, 427, 430, 458–459

Zila Pharmaceuticals, 80, 81–82
zinc chloride, 152
zinc deficiency, 298
zinc sulfate, 151
Zyban®, 376